Introductory Maternal-Newborn Nursing

301

Cecilia L Amaro

Tri City

986 9129

marine

Introductory Maternal-Newborn Nursing

NANCY A. DiDONA, RN, MSN, CNS

Faculty, Pace University
Pleasantville, New York

Former Faculty, Iona College
Yonkers, New York

MARGARET G. MARKS, RN, BSNE

Former Instructor
Juniata-Mifflin Area Vocational Technical School
Lewistown, Pennsylvania

RHONDA KUMM, RN, MSN

Developmental Consultant
Health Care Consultant
Hunt Valley, Maryland

J. B. Lippincott Company

Acquisitions Editor: Jennifer E. Brogan
Coordinating Editorial Assistant: Danielle J. DiPalma
Project Editor: Barbara Ryalls
Indexer: Katherine Pitcoff
Design Coordinator: Kathy Kelley-Luedtke
Designer: Anne O'Donnell
Cover Designer: Jerry Cable
Production Manager: Helen Ewan
Production Coordinator: Nannette Winski
Compositor: Compset Inc.
Printer/Binder: Courier Book Company/Kendallville

6 5 4 3 2 1

Library of Congress Cataloging-in-Publication Data

Introductory maternal-newborn nursing / Nancy DiDona,
    Margaret B. Marks.
        p.   cm.
    Includes bibliographical references and index.
    ISBN 0-397-55008-1
    1. Maternity nursing.   I. DiDona, Nancy A.   II. Marks, Margaret G.
III. Kumm, Rhonda.
    [DNLM: 1. Maternal-Child Nursing.   WY 157.3 I62 1996]
RG951.I58   1996
610.73'678—dc20
DNLM/DLC
for Library of Congress
                                        94-39719
                                        CIP

The material contained in this volume was submitted as previously unpublished material, except in the instances in which credit has been given to the source from which some of the illustrative material was derived.

Any procedure or practice described in this book should be applied by the health-care practitioner under appropriate supervision in accordance with professional standards of care used with regard to the unique circumstances that apply in each practice situation. Care has been taken to confirm the accuracy of information presented and to describe generally accepted practices. However, the authors, editors, and publisher cannot accept any responsibility for errors or omissions or for any consequences from application of the information in this book and make no warranty, express or implied, with respect to the contents of the book.

The authors and publisher have exerted every effort to ensure that drug selection and dosage set forth in this text are in accordance with current recommendations and practice at the time of publication. However, in view of ongoing research, changes in government regulations, and the constant flow of information relating to drug therapy and drug reactions, the reader is urged to check the package insert for each drug for any change in indications and dosage and for added warnings and precautions. This is particularly important when the recommended agent is a new or infrequently employed drug.

Materials appearing in this book prepared by individuals as part of their official duties as U.S. Government employees are not covered by the above-mentioned copyright.

9 8 7 6 5 4 3 2 1

I lovingly dedicate this book to my husband, Bob, and my sons, Robby and Gregory. Without their support, love, and never-ending patience, this text would have remained an unfulfilled dream for me. Many thanks to the three most important men in my life, and to my family and friends who encouraged and helped me along the way.

Nancy A. DiDona

Reviewers

Debbie L. Brown, RN, MSN
LPN Instructor
Wallace Community College–Dothan
Member, Alabama Council of Practical Nurse Educators
Dothan, Alabama

Deborah Cooper Connelly, RNC, MSN, CDE
Chair, Practical Nursing Department
Bishop State Community College, Southwest Campus
Mobile, Alabama

Sherry G. Fader, BSN, MSN, RNC
Chair, Registered Nurse Program
Quincy College
Quincy, Massachusetts

Doris Falconer, RN, BSNE, MN
Consultant, Vocational Nursing Program
Formerly Director, Vocational Nursing Program
Ukiah Adult School
Ukiah, California

Meridythe Grey, RNC
Former Nursing Instructor
James Lorenzo Walker Vocational Technical Center
Surgical Assistant
Naples OBGYN
Naples, Florida

Margrit E. Hayes, BSN, RN
Instructor
Otsego Area School of Practical Nursing
Milford, New York

Dorothy Insolera, RNC, MSN
Associate Professor
College of Saint Mary
Omaha, Nebraska

Bettyann Milliron, RNC
Instructor
Juniata–Mifflin Area Vocational Technical School
Lewistown, Pennsylvania

Kathy S. Newton, RN, MSN
Nursing Faculty
Kellog Community College
Battle Creek, Michigan

Karen A. Paterno, RN, MSN
Associate Professor/Department Chairman
Odessa College–Andrews Extension
Andrews, Texas

Kathleen Simpson, MSN, RNC
Perinatal Clinical Nurse Specialist
St. John's Mercy Medical Center
St. Louis, Missouri

Bennita Vaughans, BSN, MSN
Nursing Instructor
Trenholm State Technical College
Montgomery, Alabama

Beth Donaher-Wagner, RN, MSN
Women's Center Educator
Lehigh Valley Hospital
Allentown, Pennsylvania

Contributors

Jana L. Atterbury, RNC, MSN, BSN
Lecturer, Division of Maternal-Fetal Medicine
Department of Obstetrics & Gynecology
University of South Alabama
Mobile, Alabama
Chapters 11, 13

Jeanne Grover Bidwell, RN, BSN, MSEd
Coordinator
Ostego Area School of Practical Nursing
Milford and Oneonta, New York
Chapter 16

Ardith D. Birkman, RNC, MSN
Coordinator of Women's/Children's Services
Home Technology Healthcare
St. Louis, Missouri
Chapter 8

Lynne Hutnick Conrad, RNC, MSN, BSN
Perinatal Clinical Nurse Specialist
Albert Einstein Medical Center
Philadelphia, Pennsylvania
Self-Assessments
Nursing Care Plans

Nancy A. DiDona, RN, MSN, CNS
Faculty, Pace University
Pleasantville, New York

Former Faculty, Iona College
Yonkers, New York
Chapters 1–10

Nancy Jane Donoho, RNC, MSN
Maternal/Infant Clinical Nurse Specialist
Fort Sanders Health System
Knoxville, Tennessee
Chapter 10

Teresa Amber Sanders Jennings, RNC, MSN, NNP
Nursing Instructor
Motlow State Community College
Tullahoma, Tennessee
Chapter 18

Patricia Laing-Arie, RN
Instructor, Program of Practical Nursing
Meridian Technology Center
Stillwater, Oklahoma
Chapter 19

Margaret G. Marks, RN, BSNE
Former Instructor
Juniata–Mifflin Area Vocational Technical School
Lewistown, Pennsylvania
Chapters 11–20

Linda Punch, BSN, RNC, ACCE
Nurse Manager, Women's and Children's Services
St. Francis Regional Medical Center
Wichita, Kansas
Chapter 16

Patricia A. Scott, MSN, RNC, NNP
Neonatal Clinical Specialist/Neonatal Nurse Practioner
Summit Medical Center
Nashville, Tennessee
Chapter 17

Judy E. White, RN, MA, MSN
Associate Professor
Rockland Community College
Suffern, New York
Chapter 20

Preface

The inspiration for **Introductory Maternal-Newborn Nursing** arose from the need voiced by nurse educators in practical nursing for a current textbook with essential qualities, such as easy readability, conciseness, accuracy, and positive stimulation to learn. This book was created to meet those requirements. The family-centered focus demonstrates nursing care that respects the patients as individuals yet appreciates them as part of families and society. We feel that improved nursing care for the woman, the fetus, and the family, from the moment of conception until postpartum healing occurs, is vital for the continuation of society's health and well-being.

Features

Many challenges face today's students and instructors. As information in nursing increases, there is less time available to cover it. The content, features, and design of this book were planned to assist instruction and enhance student learning. The attractive, consistent checklist format serves to highlight important information and to keep the student interested and focused.

There are numerous photographs and line art drawings with color overlay throughout. These help the learner to visualize important content, specific situations, and equipment. Various boxes appear in the text, providing additional relevant information. This material includes significant assessments, teaching strategies, and supplemental information.

Each chapter incorporates many outstanding educational tools to assist both the student and the instructor in highlighting important information.

Chapter Pedagogy

- **Objectives:** Listed with each chapter opener are behavioral Objectives. These help the learner to focus on critical topics.

- **Terminology:** An alphabetized list of vital terms appears at the beginning of each chapter. All terms are defined and highlighted in the text and aid the learner in developing pertinent vocabulary.
- **Chapter Outline:** A chapter outline offers an insightful overview of the content and organization of each chapter.
- **Review and Preview:** A synopsis of the current chapter and a brief overview of the next chapter are provided at the end of each chapter. This helps the reader to better understand the overall organization.
- **Key Points:** Summary statements that correspond with the objectives, called Key Points, follow each chapter. Recapping the most significant points contained in the chapter, they verify when the learner has met the objectives.
- **Self-Assessment:** Each chapter provides the learner with multiple-choice questions based on the chapter's content. They are designed to test knowledge and to prepare the learner for the course as well as the licensure examination.
- **Bibliography:** An extensive bibliography at the end of each chapter guides the learner toward additional information on the chapter content.

Key Features

- **Checklists:** Nursing Diagnoses Checklists, Assessment Checklists, and Family Teaching Checklists appear throughout the text. These checklists provide quick-reference information, reinforce major points and concepts, and help students to understand and retain key material.
- **Nursing Care Plans:** Care plans include information on assessment, diagnosis, planning, intervention, and evaluation of the patient and/or family in particular situations.
- **Cultural Considerations:** Cultural diversity and awareness are key issues in the administration of

health care. Each chapter discusses issues involved in the nursing care of the culturally complex family.

· **Adolescent Considerations:** Adolescent pregnancies pose many potential problems for the teenager, neonate, family, and society. Each chapter assesses and discusses the areas of concern for the adolescent relevant to the content of the chapter.

· **The Role of the Nurse:** The role of the nurse responsible for the care of the patient and/or family is summarized at the end of each chapter.

Instructor's Manual and Testbank

The combined Instructor's Manual and Testbank is the perfect complement to classroom instruction. The Instructor's Manual includes helpful teaching strategies, discussion topics, and teaching/learning activities. To assist in measuring content comprehension, 500 multiple-choice questions are provided in the Testbank portion of the manual.

Acknowledgments

I wish to extend my deepest appreciation and gratitude to the many individuals involved in the creation of this first edition of **Introductory Maternal-Newborn Nursing.** The atmosphere fostering support and encouragement from all the involved participants was invaluable to me in preparing this manuscript.

Special thanks go to the following committed people at J. B. Lippincott Company:

Jennifer E. Brogan, Editor

Danielle DiPalma, Coordinating Editorial Assistant

Eleanor Faven, Senior Developmental Editor

Donna Hilton, Publisher

Diana Intenzo, Former Publisher

For their guidance and hard work, I am indebted to the developmental editors, Rhonda Kumm and Crystal Norris, as well as the many dedicated contributors and reviewers previously listed.

I also wish to thank Peggy Marks for joining me in developing this text. Her input and writing ability has added tremendously to the quality and substance of this first edition.

Nancy A. DiDona

Contents

Introductory Maternal-Newborn Nursing

Family-Centered Maternal Care

CHAPTER 1

Directions in Family-Centered Maternal-Newborn Care

◈ OBJECTIVES

When the learning goals of this chapter are met, the reader will be able to:

◆ Describe the types of families in today's society.

◆ Discuss the philosophy and goals of family-centered maternal-newborn care.

◆ List the members of the maternal-newborn health care team, including some of the other professionals who may be called on to provide comprehensive care.

◆ Identify the trends in maternal-newborn nursing.

◆ Discuss the issues in maternal-newborn care.

◆ Explain the importance of considering the cultural practices and beliefs of the woman and her family.

◆ Describe the goals of maternal-newborn nursing care.

◆ Identify standards of maternal-newborn nursing care.

◆ Discuss the steps and activities of the nursing process, including documentation requirements for nursing care.

TERMINOLOGY

Abortion

Certified nurse midwife

Clinical nurse specialist

Culture

Family

Family-centered care

Infant mortality rate

Maternal mortality rate

Maternal-newborn care

Nurse practitioner

Nursing process

One of the most exciting events for a family is the addition of a new member. In today's society, the family is being redefined by a number of social factors, including divorce, adoption, and the blending of separate families through remarriage. Yet the miracles of conception, pregnancy, and childbirth still capture the imagination.

Although childbirth is considered a family-centered event, in the United States and Canada it is an event that is usually managed by a professional health care team. **Maternal-newborn care** is a nursing discipline that specializes in providing this care to the woman and fetus during pregnancy as well as to the neonate. The maternal-newborn health care team tries to help the family meet the challenges of pregnancy and childbirth so that they can participate more fully in the joys.

Traditionally, the importance of the family has been the basis of **family-centered care.** This type of care emphasizes building a trusting relationship between health care providers and the family that both recognizes and supports the special needs of the family, which can be difficult. It may at times seem incompatible with the health care team's primary goal, which is to promote the health and well-being of the pregnant woman and the fetus. Today's nurses are well equipped to meet this challenge (Fig. 1-1).

The goal of this text is to provide the reader with a solid foundation on the principles and practices of maternal-newborn nursing with an emphasis on the family. The antepartum, intrapartum, and postpartum periods are covered in detail. These periods are defined as follows:

> *Antepartum period:* that period of time between fertilization of the ovum (conception) and the first true uterine contraction (labor). This term is used to refer to the mother, and the period itself is often referred to as pregnancy or the prenatal period.

> *Intrapartum period:* refers to that period of time that begins with the first true uterine contraction and ends with the birth of the neonate. It is also known as labor and delivery.

> *Postpartum period:* refers to the period of time that begins with the birth of the neonate and ends 6 weeks later.

Care of the normal newborn, including the assessments and interventions practiced in normal situations, are given primary emphasis. High-risk conditions are also addressed.

This first chapter describes the types of families the nurse may come across. The goals, trends, and issues related to maternal-newborn care are also covered, as is the nurse's role in promoting healthful practices that relate to pregnancy and childbearing. Further, it

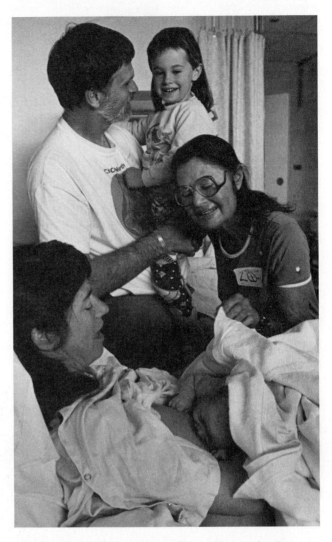

Figure 1-1. *The birth experience is considered a family-centered event. (Photo © Kathy Sloane)*

introduces for discussion the rising incidence of pregnancy among adolescents, which presents today's health care professionals with many challenges. A complex matter, it is explored in the following chapters in sections entitled *Adolescent Considerations.*

Because the multicultural makeup of the United States and Canada is becoming increasingly more complex, today's nurses must be sensitive to the ethnic and cultural practices of families in their care. This includes guarding against letting their own cultural prejudices affect the quality of the care they provide. The chapter opens the discussion on these and other cultural considerations. Culture and ethnicity are examined in further detail in sections entitled *Cultural Considerations,* which appear at the ends of chapters as appropriate.

The chapter ends with a presentation of nursing standards of care and the nursing process. These frameworks help to organize nursing care that treats the whole person and not just the physical condition.

The Contemporary Family

An individual belongs to many different groups during his or her lifetime, but none is more important than the family. The family is to society what the cell is to the body: its most basic unit. Values, traditions, ethnicity, and often religious beliefs are passed from one generation to the next through the family.

Family Function

Simply stated, a **family** is a unit of two or more persons who remain united over a period of time, share common beliefs, and support each other physically and emotionally. In its simplest form, the family is made up of two individuals who love and support each other. If the partners decide to become parents, either through sexual reproduction or adoption, the family expands to accept the addition of each new family member.

Family members may live in one household or share interests despite physical separation (as is the case when one or both partners serve in the armed forces or a child leaves home to attend college). Healthy families are all alike in that they function to meet the broad range of needs of their members.

Some of the most common needs fulfilled by the family include reproduction, the provision of basic needs (food, shelter, clothing), and the socialization of its members. Socialization is the process by which family members are educated in the beliefs, customs, cultural traditions, and ethnic and religious practices of their society.

Family Structure

Families come in all sizes and styles: there are the traditional nuclear and extended families; the single-parent, step-parent, and adoptive varieties; and several other types that range from cohabitating to communal groups. Display 1-1 explains the various family types and their distinguishing characteristics (Also see Fig. 1-2). Because it is essential that nonjudgmental health

---

DISPLAY 1-1
Family Types and Their Defining Characteristics

Adoptive:	These families include at least one child and may be headed by a single parent, married or cohabitating partners, or homosexual couples. The texture of these families is often enriched by cross-cultural adoption.
Blended:	Formed from at least two previously defined families. Subtypes include the step-parent, adoptive, and communal families.
Cohabitating:	Families headed by partners who are not legally married. They may have children from previous marriages or relationships, adopted children, or their own biologic offspring.
Communal:	Several families living together who share the responsibilities of work and childcare.
Extended:	A family unit that has been expanded to include relatives outside the nuclear family (eg, grandparents, aunts, and uncles).
Nuclear:	Made up of husband, wife, and their biologic children. In traditional nuclear families, the male is the principal wage earner. In two-career families, both parents work outside the home; in role-reversal families, the woman becomes the primary breadwinner, and the man assumes childcare responsibilities.
Same-sex:	Families headed by homosexual or lesbian partners. They may parent children from previous partnerships. They also may produce their own biologic children by taking advantage of the current reproductive technologies.
Single-parent:	Never-married or divorced parent of at least one child. Childcare is shared with relatives or hired child caretakers.
Step-parent:	Family headed by a couple who were previously married to others. They jointly parent the children from their respective marriages.

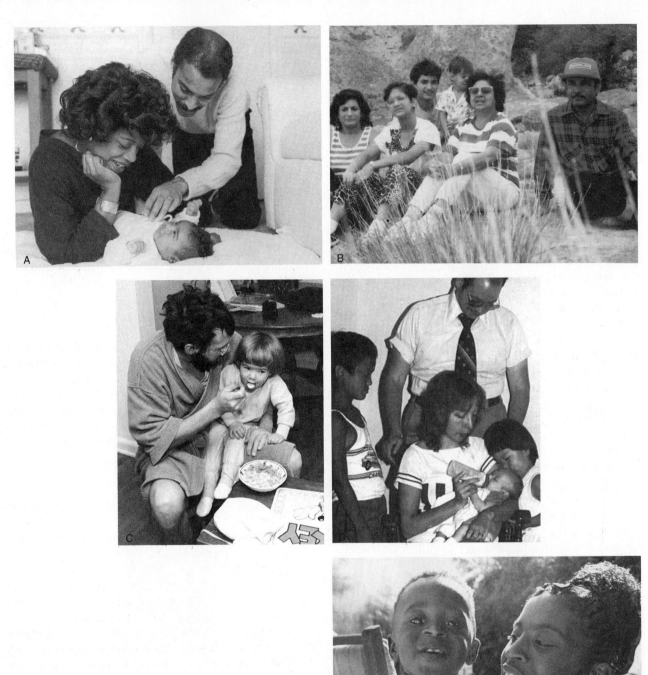

Figure 1-2. *Today there are many widely accepted types of family units.* (***A***) *Nuclear families;* (***B***) *Extended families;* (***C***) *Dual-working parents, where both parents share in child care, perhaps along with a third-party caregiver;* (***D***) *Adoptive families;* (***E***) *Single-parent families (Photos © Kathy Sloane)*

care be provided to *all* individuals, it is recommended that maternal-newborn nurses familiarize themselves with the family types they may encounter. The more comfortable nurses are with different family types, the easier it will be for them to provide competent, nonjudgmental care.

Family-Centered Maternal-Newborn Care

The word *obstetrics* is believed to be Latin in origin and can be traced back to either *obstetrix* (midwife) or *obstare* (which means to stand by or in front of). Up until the end of the 19th century, obstetrics was equated with midwifery, the tradition of women assisting other women during home-centered childbirth.

By the late 1800s, however, midwifery had become a specialty taught in male-dominated medical schools. During that period, the person *standing by* to assist in childbirth was frequently a *midman* or a *man-midwife*. This change in personnel at the mother-to-be's bedside introduced a new era in maternal-newborn care. Childbirth had, in effect, ceased to be viewed as a natural event, which midwives observed passively. It became instead an event that offered many opportunities for medical intervention.

Today's emphasis on natural childbirth is the family's attempt to return childbirth to the heart of the family, where it can be experienced as another normal life event. Natural childbirth has several advantages that define it as family-centered: it emphasizes health promotion and wellness, focuses on the prevention of illness, and allows the family to make decisions about everything from health care providers to birthing sites. Natural childbirth is also responsible for the returning popularity of nurse midwives.

Goals of Maternal-Newborn Health Care

The goals of family-centered maternal-newborn care are as follows:

To ensure the health and well-being of the mother and child during the antepartum, intrapartum, and postpartum periods. This is done by providing nursing interventions for teaching and counseling the family as appropriate

To promote family involvement in the pregnancy and throughout the birthing process

To ensure family adaptation to the new member

To provide culturally competent care that recognizes the family's social, cultural, and religious beliefs

To identify families at risk and provide interventions

To educate the family about the responsibilities of parenthood

Maternal-Newborn Health Care Professionals

Maternal-newborn health care professionals include the obstetrician/gynecologist specialist, certified nurse midwife, nurse practitioner, clinical nurse specialist, pediatrician, and neonatologist. Other significant health care professionals may interact with pregnant women and their families as needed. Examples include a geneticist, a dietitian, a social worker, and an infertility specialist.

Obstetrician/Gynecologist Specialists

The obstetrician/gynecologist is a licensed medical-surgical clinician who specializes in diseases of women, care of fetuses and pregnant women, labor and childbirth, and postpartum care. To become an obstetrician/gynecologist, the individual must first successfully complete a medical program and then apply for a 4-year residency in obstetrics and gynecology.

Certified Nurse Midwives

The **certified nurse midwife** provides normal gynecologic care for the nonpregnant woman and supports, counsels, and monitors pregnant women throughout the birthing process. In normal childbirth experiences, certified nurse midwives follow the course of labor and childbirth while encouraging family participation. The certified nurse midwife may prescribe medication and perform specified procedures (eg, episiotomy).

To receive certification as a midwife, a registered nurse must be certified by an accredited program (such the one offered by the American College of Nurse Midwifery, Washington, DC) or attend a Master's-level program to gain specialized skills. Display 1-2 provides profiles of two certified nurse midwives.

Nurse Practitioners and Clinical Nurse Specialists

Nurse practitioners and clinical nurse specialists are registered nurses with advanced education and training. The **nurse practitioner** in women's health works with the physician or nurse midwife. The nurse practitioner may see patients to obtain histories and physicals, as well as manage care from the antepartum through the postpartum periods. Preparation may be

DISPLAY 1-2
Certified Nurse Midwife Profiles

Profile #1: Kathy Horgan, Certified Nurse Midwife*

Kathy began her nursing career when she attended Bellevue School of Nursing in New York. She fell in love with maternal-newborn care at Columbia Presbyterian Hospital while working alongside a nurse midwife. The experience led her to pursue a 1-year certificate in nurse midwifery at Downstate University in Brooklyn.

Kathy motivates nursing students to consider nurse midwifery. "Certified nurse midwives have become so politically correct and consumer demanded [that they] will be delivering all normal births in the near future. Be proactive instead of passive and encourage the mother to do the same. We empower people to take control of their lives and their well-being."

Profile #2: Sylvia Blaustein, Certified Nurse Midwife†

Sylvia, who is employed by a private obstetrics group in downtown Manhattan, states, "Midwives support and celebrate the normalcy of birth and life." She has proved that by encouraging women to deliver their newborns without medications or episiotomies. She lets them know that they can eat, drink, and even walk around during labor.

"Many physicians support the certified nurse midwife for normal birth and respect us as colleagues," says Ms. Blaustein. "Being a certified nurse midwife offers incredible job and financial opportunities for nurses today."

One of the greatest cost savings for the certified nurse midwife is in malpractice insurance, which is less than one tenth that of an obstetrician. Statistics show that when care is provided by certified nurse midwives, the incidence in low-birthweight neonates decreases, breast-feeding increases, compliance with recommended practices increases, and Apgar scores (values rating the infant's physical condition immediately after birth) are higher.

To students considering midwifery Sylvia suggests, "Go for it with a passion and love. It is very fulfilling and allows the nurse to be a part of the fun of pregnancy and childbirth. I feel blessed!"

*Kathy Horgan is an assistant professor of clinical obstetrics and gynecology at New York Medical College and the director of Nurse-Midwife Services at St. Agnes Hospital in White Plains, New York.

†Sylvia Blaustein is a graduate of Columbia University with a Master's degree in nurse midwifery.

achieved in 1 year by attending a certificate program or through a Master's degree program. Nurse practitioners are not licensed to deliver the neonate, although they may be required to do so in the absence of trained personnel.

Like the nurse practitioner, the **clinical nurse specialist** manages the gynecologic and childbearing health concerns of women. The clinical nurse specialist graduates from a Master's program and may provide direct nursing care or coordinate research activities. Health promotion and parent teaching are key areas for clinical nurse specialist participation. Today, it is common for clinical nurse specialists to advance to the nurse practitioner level in the hopes of furthering their ability to address women's health issues.

Pediatricians and Neonatologists

Pediatricians are responsible for the diagnosis, treatment, health, and well-being of infants and children. To become a licensed pediatrician, one must first complete a medical degree and then a specialized 4-year residency in pediatrics. The neonatologist is a pediatrician who receives additional preparation in caring for neonates (a newborn infant up to 6 weeks of age).

Often, the neonatologist is present during the births of high-risk neonates.

Other Health Care Professionals

Several other health care professionals may be called on to assist the maternal-newborn team in meeting the health care needs of the family. Geneticists may counsel and provide testing for families at risk for genetically determined disorders. Dietitians may educate the family about nutrition and infant feeding. Social workers may be asked to assess the family's ability to meet the infant's needs within their current living situation. Each care provider participates in the well-being of the woman, the growing fetus, and the family. Together, the members of the maternal-newborn health care team provide quality coordinated care.

Trends in Maternal-Newborn Care

As health care consumers become more knowledgeable about the increasingly more sophisticated developments in medical technology, they demand a greater say in the decision making that affects their health in general. Furthermore, they expect all of this high-quality care—including skilled health care professionals, safe techniques and facilities, and comprehensive health care plans for the whole family—to be provided at a reasonable cost. Maternal-newborn care is also influenced by consumer demand.

Some of the consumer-inspired trends in maternal-newborn care include a variety of birthing options, the freedom to choose support persons, sibling involvement in the birthing process, technologic advances, managed care and case management, early discharge, and community-based care.

Birthing Options

Traditionally, home birth was the only option available for most women, many of whom lived far from hospitals or were unable to pay for the hospital stay. As the store of medical knowledge grew in the Western world, birth was moved from the home to the hospital. Childbirth was viewed as a medical secret, to be handled behind the closed doors of hospital delivery rooms. This meant that family members were prevented from participating in one of its most important events.

The natural childbirth movement has brought birthing options full circle, with a twist or two along the way. Deliveries now take place in birthing facilities that offer all the comforts of home and many of the advantages of medical technology. Home births, too, have once again become popular.

Hospital-based Childbirth

Hospitals, or acute care facilities, have modernized their attitudes and facilities to meet consumer demands for accessible, family-centered maternal-newborn care. These facilities offer a range of outpatient services for everything from antepartal care and postpartum follow-up. The typical maternal-newborn department has labor-delivery-recovery room suites (LDRs), a newborn nursery, and a postpartum unit.

In addition to providing health care services, hospitals have also changed long-standing policies to meet the needs of today's modern family. For example, the length of the hospital stay has been dramatically reduced to provide for the earliest possible discharge for the healthy woman and neonate. Some of the factors that health care providers consider in determining discharge dates include the presence of complications, the health insurance coverage of the family, and the woman's desire for an early discharge.

Hospitals have also updated their labor and delivery areas to create atmospheres that welcome the par-

ticipation of family members during all phases of the birthing experience (Fig. 1-3). Even visiting hour policies have been changed to allow siblings and members of the extended family greater flexibility in exercising their visitation rights.

Birthing Centers

Birthing centers provide a middle-of-the-road alternative for families who want the comfort of a home birth without losing the benefit of readily accessible medical care.

The calm, relaxed environment of the birthing center allows the family to experience the intimacy of childbirth without unnecessary medical distractions. But because the birthing center is located either within a hospital or fairly close to one, qualified personnel and emergency equipment are always at hand. As an added safety precaution, only women who are not considered at risk are appropriate candidates for childbirth in these centers. If there is a potential or actual problem, the pregnant woman and family are referred to the nearest hospital for treatment.

Home Birth

Women with uncomplicated pregnancies and low risk factors may choose to deliver at home with the help of nurse-midwives. Women who choose home birth are encouraged to gain a solid understanding of the birthing process. This allows them to participate more fully in all of its stages. Understanding the process and anticipating its stages also reduces the perception of pain and results in fewer complications. The home may be the preferred setting for the family who wishes to include small children and extended family members in the birthing event.

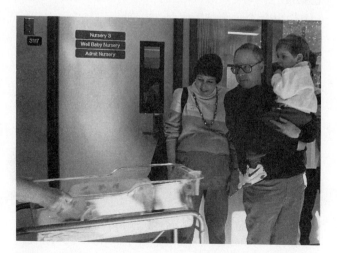

Figure 1-3. *The pregnant woman and her partner may tour the facility where their baby will be born. They are encouraged to include their families. (Photo © Kathy Sloane)*

Choice of Support Person(s)

A woman should have the right to choose as her support person for labor and childbirth the person who will provide her with the greatest encouragement and comfort. Although the husband may be considered the most logical choice in our society, individual and cultural preferences may influence a woman to select her sexual partner, sibling, mother, grandmother, aunt, friend, or any combination of these persons (Fig. 1-4) to fill the role. The support person who attends childbirth classes will have a greater understanding of the birth experience.

Technologic Advances

The rapid rate of technologic advances means that more women with high-risk pregnancies are able to deliver live neonates. The chances that these neonates will survive are greater than ever before. But this medical technology comes with a high price tag, which makes it unavailable to the poor and the homeless. Part of the nurse's responsibility is to educate the pregnant woman and her family about their potential risk factors and counsel them to adopt healthful habits. This preventive education can greatly reduce the costs of "curing" the damage caused by the preventable complications associated with pregnancies among adolescents, women older than age 35, and alcohol and drug abusers. It also ensures that high-tech medical interventions are used only as a last resort.

Managed Care and Case Management

In the United States, managed care is a system of health care delivery through the combined efforts of a team of specialists. In maternal-newborn care, nurses, nurse mid wives, obstetricians, and other health professionals provide the woman and her family with managed care. It concentrates on the physiologic, psychologic, and psychosocial needs of the family unit. Under this system of care, the nurse case manager also plans and implements timely, cost-efficient treatments. The delivery of managed care is documented on Managed Care Paths, which are similar to Nursing Care Plans (NCPs). They differ from NCPs in that they include input from all the disciplines involved in the case, and not just nursing input.

Early Discharge and Family Teaching

There are two principal reasons for early postpartum discharge: some insurance plans require it, and many women prefer to get back to the familiar atmosphere of home as soon as possible. Regardless of when the woman is discharged, the nurse will need to make arrangements for scheduling family education classes. When early discharge is planned, family education can be started during the antepartal period. More frequently, however, the nurse finds that opportunities for family teaching must fit into the new family's busy schedules in creative ways.

Classes designed to educate the family on infant care and routine postpartum guidelines can be incorporated into office or clinic appointments. The nurse is also free to show educational films and set up demonstration classes, which are very effective in representing behavioral models for the family to imitate. After the birth, the nurse can visit the home or organize local classes that address specific needs such as fatigue after childbirth, feeding at night, infant crying and its mean-

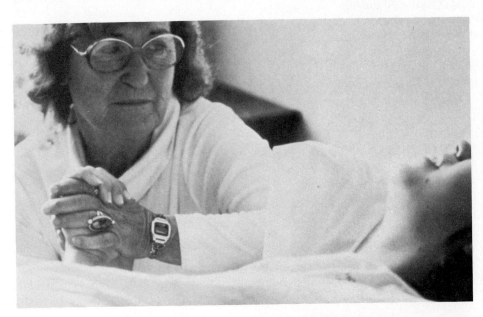

Figure 1-4. *The support person may be a friend or family member. (Photo © Kathy Sloane)*

ing, and fitting parenting into established lifestyles. The chief benefit of family education is that it provides the family with the information they need to care for their newborn with confidence.

Home Health Care

It is important to provide adequate postpartum follow-up care for families who are discharged early from the health care facility. Home health care provides this follow-up care.

These follow-up visits typically include a complete assessment of the physical condition of the woman and newborn, as well as an assessment of the family's adjustment to birth after the postpartum period. Very often, problems that the family may consider unique and complex can be easily solved by consulting with the nurse. The family is often relieved to learn that other families are dealing with similar issues.

Home health care allows families to freely express their concerns and doubts in a relaxing atmosphere. And when they are relaxed, they learn better. Home health care decreases health care costs by reducing the number of staff members needed to care for and educate the family.

Issues in Maternal-Newborn Care

Despite the advances made in women's health care and maternal-newborn care, health care providers realize there are still many issues that need to be addressed. These issues, which include mortality and morbidity, adolescent pregnancy, contraception, and "safer sex," are introduced in this section. They are discussed further in other chapters of the text as appropriate.

Morbidity and Mortality

The U.S. Office of Vital Statistics in Washington, D.C., collects data on the number of births, the incidence of diseases (morbidity), and the number of deaths (mortality rates) of fetuses, infants, and childbearing women. These statistics are important because they paint an accurate picture of the health of the nation's women and their children. This, in turn, helps government to allocate resources to those most in need. What the statistics show is not always encouraging.

For example, data show that the number of women who died in childbirth (**maternal mortality rate**) in the United States declined between 1970 and 1990. However, a similar improvement in the **infant mortality rate** has not yet been achieved. Although infant

death rates have fallen around the world, the relative ranking of the United States has worsened. This is due in large part to complications associated with low birth weight, which account for about two thirds of infant deaths in the United States. Clearly, it takes more than superior medical interventions to produce healthy babies.

According to the National Center for Health Statistics, the single most reliable predictor of infant mortality is poverty, and not race or ethnicity. It seems that the individuals least able to gain access to private health care have the highest mortality and morbidity rates.

How can health care be adequately provided to families of low income? Should money be invested in developing technology to save a few neonates, or is it wiser to invest in providing basic health care across all socioeconomic groups? These are some of the questions currently being debated as the United States tries to provide quality care to all of its citizens.

Adolescent Sexual Activity and Pregnancy

Sexual activity and pregnancy among adolescents are major health issues in the United States and Canada. The United States has the highest incidence of adolescent pregnancies among the westernized countries. In fact, it has been estimated that in the United States alone an adolescent gets pregnant every 30 seconds. Every 13 seconds, an adolescent contracts a sexually transmitted disease (STD).

The obvious costs of adolescent pregnancies include the expense of clothing, feeding, and sheltering the child. Also, if the adolescent must stay home to care for her infant, she may have to give up or at least postpone plans to finish her education. She also may feel cheated by the toll the growing fetus takes on her still-maturing physical and emotional capacities. In short, she gives up her own childhood to care for her baby. Some of the hidden costs of pregnancies among adolescents include its association with maternal poverty, which often gets "handed down" to each new generation; its link to an increased risk for alcohol and substance abuse; and its association with juvenile delinquency.

Sexually transmitted diseases can have long-term effects on the reproductive health of families. These effects can range from simple discomfort to altered self-perception. Infertility and death (in the case of acquired immunodeficiency syndrome [AIDS]) can also result. Some STDs can be transmitted to the fetus during pregnancy or during childbirth. The fetus or neonate can develop a number of serious and sometimes life-threatening conditions, depending on the infection. Because STDs are largely preventable, the nurse can teach the family to protect themselves against the most serious damage caused by these diseases.

Pregnancy After Age 35

Many women work, for a variety of reasons. Some work because they need or want to contribute financially to the household. Others live alone and work to support themselves. Still others enjoy the thrill of establishing their careers. Whatever the reason, many women find themselves making a trade-off between working and having babies during the years of peak fertility.

This has led to an increase in the number of women who are postponing childbearing until after age 35.

Some of the risks associated with childbirth after age 35 are identical to those that make childbirth risky for adolescents. These include high maternal and perinatal mortality rates. Women older than age 35 also are at greater risk of bearing children with Down syndrome. And because they frequently release more than one ovum during ovulation (even without the aid of fertility drugs), they are more likely to give birth to twins and triplets. Multifetal pregnancies are a concern because they are typically associated with low-birthweight neonates.

Health care professionals must not only find ways of providing appropriate care to the older pregnant woman, but they must also help childbearing women over age 35 maintain their reproductive health so that they can become pregnant in the future if they choose to do so.

Contraception and "Safer Sex"

Contraception is a means of preventing unwanted pregnancies and actively planning desired pregnancies. Contraceptive methods should be safe, effective, and affordable. They are also more likely to be used if they are convenient to use and produce few side effects. The types of methods available and those most commonly used are discussed in Chapter 3.

The challenge for maternal-newborn nurses is to provide families with the information they need to practice responsible sexuality without seeming to impose moral, religious, or cultural beliefs. It is particularly important to maintain this nonjudgmental attitude when discussing "safer sex."

Because sexuality is a highly charged emotional topic, the nurse's job in teaching "safer sex" has many potential pitfalls. How do nurses keep from promoting ideas that they find acceptable (such as abstinence) without seeming to disapprove of the sexual choices of the women in their care?

Nurses can make it clear that recommendations for "safer sex" are given for one reason only: to protect the reproductive health of the woman, her sexual partner, and the child (the one she may be carrying and the one she may plan to have in the future). Sexually transmitted diseases and guidelines for "safer sex" are discussed in detail in Chapter 4.

Abortion

Abortion is defined as the termination of a pregnancy before the fetus reaches the age at which it can survive outside the uterus. It may be achieved by mechanical or chemical means, or it may occur as a natural, spontaneous process.

The use of abortion to terminate unwanted pregnancies was legalized in the United States in 1973. Since that time, it has been the center of controversy.

Advocates of abortion often refer to the landmark case of Roe *v.* Wade to support the woman's right to choose abortion. Prolife supporters believe that the fetus's right to life is more important than the mother's right to abort. Many prolife advocates do not believe abortion is an alternative under any circumstance.

As long as abortions are performed, legal and ethical issues related to its practice will continue to arise. It is important that nurses avoid expressing their personal beliefs in caring for women and families who are trying to decide whether abortion is the right option for them.

Families At Risk

There are a number of physical, socioeconomic, and psychological factors that place a family at risk during pregnancy, labor, birth, and during the postpartum period. Within the family, there may be drug and alcohol abuse, physical violence or sexual abuse, and a number of psychological issues and challenges. There may be health problems such as hypertension, diabetes, poor nutrition, and STDs. Family-centered maternal-newborn care focuses on reducing these risk factors. The identification of risk factors, means of testing for them, and treatment options for reducing them are discussed in the appropriate chapters.

Legal and Ethical Considerations

Technologic advances in medicine can cure, create, and save lives, but they can also raise many ethical issues that confound our legal systems as well as our consciences.

Reproductive technologies can, for example, allow infertile couples to conceive. But who has the right to determine which ova fertilized in vitro will be implanted and thus given a chance at life? Genetic research and testing can detect a variety of features about the unborn, including gender, congenital abnormalities, and chromosomal defects. This technology can be used to help parents-to-be decide if they want to continue or discontinue the pregnancy. With this technology in hand, society may be able to design genetically "desirable" humans. However, who will decide what a desirable human being is? Tissue cultivated from aborted fetuses may be used for advancing medical practice. But if there is social intolerance of abortion, can society ever support the use of the tissue harvested from the procedure?

◆ *Cultural Considerations*

Culture is a way of perceiving and interpreting the world that is taught from birth through the processes of language acquisition and socialization. It is specific to members of a society living within a region and evolves as a pattern of complex responses to environmental factors. Most importantly, it is dynamic, changing over time.

It is vital that nurses and other health care professionals provide quality, culturally sensitive care to all. To do this, they must be aware of the practices, customs, and beliefs within the communities they serve. Every attempt should be made to understand and respect the customs of the families in their care. Although there may be times when the nurses do not understand cultural traditions, this lack of understanding should never prevent them from providing adequate health care (Fig. 1-5).

It is also essential that nurses not make assumptions about a family's beliefs and practices based solely on their physical appearance, primary language, or socioeconomic status. Although certain cultural generalizations may hold true under some circumstances, they do not necessarily apply in every instance. The individuality of the woman and her family often influence the practice of observing cultural traditions. Nurses who recognize the importance of treating every family as a unique system will be able to provide sensitive care.

◆ *Providing Maternal-Newborn Nursing Care*

Nursing practice is determined by a variety of standards and guidelines. It is based on scientific principles and procedures and implemented to promote wellness and prevent illness. Maternal-newborn nursing care incorporates nursing knowledge and skill to care and to support the woman, family, and fetus during pregnancy. It also helps the family to adjust to the physiologic, psychologic, and psychosocial changes that occur during and after pregnancy.

The **nursing process** serves as a framework for providing comprehensive family-centered nursing care

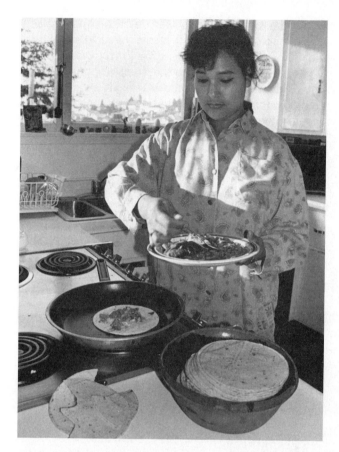

Figure 1-5. *The nurse needs to be aware of culturally significant dishes when advising the pregnant woman about nutrition. (Photo © Kathy Sloane)*

that ensures continuity as well as individualization of nursing care.

Standards of Care

Standards of care establish guidelines for providing health care. Hospitals and home care agencies are required to set these standards based on guidelines set up by an accrediting agency. The Joint Commission of Accreditation of Hospital Organizations (JCAHO), as well as federal and state governments, establish minimum standards that must be met to receive accreditation and reimbursement.

Nurses are responsible for understanding and practicing according to the established standards of their facilities. Additionally, nursing actions must meet the nurse practice acts of the state in which the nurse is practicing. The education, certification, and licensure of the individual nurse determine the types of interventions he or she may perform. For example, some states allow licensed practical nurses to give medications, whereas other states reserve this practice for registered nurses. Formed in 1949, the National Federation of Licensed Practical Nurses (NFLPN) is an organization for licensed practical nurses that describes their role in clinical practice today. All nurses need to familiarize themselves with their state's Nurse Practice Act.

Nurses must be aware that their responsibility for practicing within the boundaries of care set up by their employing facilities and state in which they work is legal and binding. Jeopardizing patient safety or providing substandard care can result in legal action against the nurse and the nurse's employing agency.

Nursing Process

Because women and their families are unique, each day brings a new set of challenges for even the most experienced nurse. Nursing care is not a routine set of tasks performed daily. Rather, it is a flexible system of responses based on a structured problem-solving approach that is used to assess the family's health care needs.

The **nursing process** is a method of providing comprehensive nursing care to women and their families. Nursing process follows five steps: assessment, nursing diagnosis, planning, implementation, and evaluation. Display 1-3 provides a checklist of the five steps of the nursing process.

Assessment

The assessment step focuses on the gathering of information that is essential in planning nursing care. Subjective (feelings, opinions, thoughts) and objective (observations, facts, measurements) data are collected through a variety of techniques. Physical examination shows normal and abnormal findings. The woman's past and present medical, gynecologic, and obstetric histories are obtained through interview. The family's strengths, weaknesses, psychosocial factors, and cultural beliefs are identified.

Diagnosis

The selection of an appropriate nursing diagnosis is based on data analysis. The identification of the problem is the first of three phases of a complete and accurate nursing diagnosis statement. Next is the related identification of factors that have contributed to the problem. The last phase consists of listing the signs and symptoms associated with the assessed data that led to the appropriate nursing diagnosis. For example: Anxiety related to unplanned pregnancy as shown by a statement of concern and worry that she was not ready to be pregnant.

A nursing diagnosis is directed at eliminating or reducing problems and risks associated with a medical diagnosis. The North American Nursing Diagnosis

---

DISPLAY 1-3
The Five Steps of the Nursing Process

Assessment

History	Observations
Physical	Laboratory findings
Interview	Data gathering

Nursing Diagnosis

Analyze data

State patient problems
    Actual
    High-risk

State nursing problems

State collaborative problems

Planning

Prioritize

State expected outcomes

Select nursing actions

Design plan of care

Collaborate with patient and family

Implementation

Perform nursing actions

Document nursing care provided

Gather activities

Promote self-care activities

Evaluation

Evaluate actual outcomes

Revise expected outcomes

Revise plan of care

Association (NANDA) has created a list of acceptable nursing diagnoses. These diagnoses allow the nurse to intervene with appropriate problem-solving strategies. These intervention strategies can change, depending on the complications associated with illness or the risk of illness. Nursing diagnoses most commonly related to family-centered maternal-newborn care are discussed in each chapter where the role of the nurse is considered.

Planning

During the planning phase of the nursing process, expected outcomes are defined for the elimination or reduction of problems identified in the nursing diagnosis. The nurse works with the family on setting goals, defining expected outcomes, determining whether the outcomes are met, and deciding what goals must be met first.

Intervention

In the intervention phase, the nurse carries out specific nursing actions to meet the expected outcome criteria. The NCP typically involves the woman and her family. It is put into effect to meet their needs by teaching, supporting, guiding, and offering them a way to actively participate in problem resolution. Nursing activities are communicated to other health care personnel through the NCP.

Evaluation

In this phase, the nurse decides whether the problem has been solved. The nurse collects information and then decides if expected outcomes were met. The factors that may have contributed to the success or failure of a plan are also pinpointed. The effectiveness of care is assessed, the NCP is redesigned as needed, and the process is repeated until the desired outcome is achieved.

Nursing Care Plans

The NCP is an individualized plan of care that includes assessment data, nursing diagnoses, goals and expected outcomes, and nursing interventions. The care plan is a formalized means of documenting nursing care to ensure that nurses and other health care team members provide continuity of care. The style and format of the NCP may vary, but all care plans typically incorporate the various steps of the nursing process. Including the woman and her family in the process is an important step toward achieving the expected outcomes.

Standardized care plans for specific conditions or patient problems may be provided in various settings. Nurses are cautioned to assess and evaluate each individual, relying on the standardized care plans only as examples or models. Several sample NCPs appear in this text. Keep in mind, however, that NCPs must be individualized to meet each patient's needs.

Documentation

Documentation of nursing care is critical, particularly because it can be used as legal proof of the activities and care provided during hospitalization and home and office visits. Observations, physical findings, nursing interventions, treatments, patient response, and compliance are examples of information included in the patient record. Forms and documentation practices may vary from one facility to the next. Narrative notes or check-off sheets may be used, but the key lies in accurately recording the various activities and findings.

The timeliness and the accuracy of the documentation are both important. Nurses should document after the actual observation or intervention is completed, taking care not to alter or falsify the records in any way.

◆ The Role of the Nurse

Nurses are important members of the health care team whose responsibilities include the promotion of healthful self-care behaviors, education, improved compliance with established standards of care, and advocating the highest level of health care possible for the family. Throughout the text, the role of the nurse is highlighted.

REVIEW AND PREVIEW

This first chapter provided an overview of family-centered maternal-newborn care, including its goals and related trends and issues. Family involvement and cultural sensitivity were also emphasized. Nursing care planning and the use of nursing process were discussed as frameworks for meeting individual and family health care needs.

The following chapter, *Reproduction and Human Sexuality*, presents a scientific foundation for understanding the male and female reproductive systems, including a discussion of how they are controlled by hormonal influences. Sexual development, the sexual response cycle, and responsible sexuality are also discussed.

◆ KEY POINTS

- Family-centered maternal-newborn care emphasizes the family as the unit of care. Family members actively partici-

pate in their own health care by working with the health care team. The goals of family-centered care include: promotion of health and well-being for the woman, neonate, and the growing family while respecting the family's unique characteristics.

- Maternal-newborn health care team members include: obstetrician/gynecologist specialists, certified nurse midwives, nurse practitioners, clinical nurse specialists, nurses, pediatricians, and neonatologists. Dietitians, social workers, and genetic counselors are just some of the additional health professionals who may provide care to the family.

- Trends in maternal-newborn health care include providing a choice of birthing options, choosing support persons, technologic advances, managed care, early discharge, family teaching, and home health care.

- Important issues in the delivery of maternal-newborn care include the incidence of morbidity and mortality, adolescent

SELF-ASSESSMENT

1. A neonatologist should be present at which of the following deliveries?

○ **A.** A patient with gestational diabetes
○ **B.** A patient with a history of heart disease
○ **C.** A cesarean delivery
○ **D.** A patient at 30 weeks' gestation

2. Goals of family-centered maternity care include all of the following EXCEPT:

○ **A.** Respect of cultural practices
○ **B.** Prevention of illness
○ **C.** Making decisions for the family during the intrapartum period
○ **D.** Health promotion

3. Which nurse's note is an example of the evaluation phase of the nursing process?

○ **A.** "Patient is requesting epidural anesthesia during labor."
○ **B.** "The patient will gain 15–20 pounds during the pregnancy."
○ **C.** "The patient states incisional pain has decreased following the administration of Demerol."
○ **D.** "Patient denies any headache or visual changes."

4. Which of the following factors plays the greatest role in predicting infant mortality?

○ **A.** Mother's age
○ **B.** Economic status
○ **C.** Race
○ **D.** Ethnic background

5. Data regarding maternal/fetal morbidity/mortality rates indicates which of the following trends?

○ **A.** Maternal mortality is increasing
○ **B.** Infant mortality has dramatically decreased
○ **C.** The rate of preterm deliveries has decreased
○ **D.** Low birth weight is a major problem in the United States.

pregnancy and "safer sex" practices, increased incidence of childbearing in women older than age 35, contraception, families at risk, and abortion. Legal and ethical issues in maternal-newborn practice continue to emerge in response to technologic advances.

◆ Individual cultural practices and beliefs directly affect the health-related beliefs and behaviors of the woman and her family.

◆ Standards for health are included in all areas of nursing practice. These standards allow nurses to implement the nursing process for the health and well-being of the woman, fetus, and family in an organized fashion. These standards also allow the nurse and family to anticipate pregnancy outcomes.

◆ The nursing process includes five steps: assessment, nursing diagnosis, planning, implementation, and evaluation. The nurse collects data, analyzes the findings, develops related nursing diagnoses, and designs a plan of care. The woman and her family participate in the care to meet the goals they set with the nurse. Evaluation looks at whether the outcomes are achieved. The process continues with all elements of care documented in the patient record. Nursing care plans, narrative notes, or flow sheets may be used to record nursing care.

BIBLIOGRAPHY

Arnold, L., & Grad, R. (1992). Low birth weight and infant mortality: A health policy perspective. *NAACOG's Clinical Issues in Perinatal and Women's Health Nursing, 3*(1), 1–12.

Boyle, J. S., & Andrews, M. M. (1990). *Transcultural concepts in nursing care.* Philadelphia: J.B. Lippincott.

Carpenito, L. J. (1993). *Nursing diagnosis: Application to clinical practice* (5th ed.). Philadelphia: J.B. Lippincott.

Carpenito, L. J. (1991). *Nursing care plans and documentation: Nursing diagnosis and collaborative problems.* Philadelphia: J.B. Lippincott.

Fiesta, J. (1991). Obstetrical liability. *Nursing Management, 22*(5), 17.

Giuliano, K., & Poirier, C. (1991). Nursing case management: Critical pathways to desirable outcomes. *Nursing Management, 22,* 52–58.

Kurzen, C. (1993). *Contemporary Practical/Vocational Nursing* (2nd ed.). Philadelphia: J.B. Lippincott.

Mathews, J., & Zadek, K. (1991). The alternative birth movement in the United States: History and current status. *Women and Health, 17*(1), 39–56.

May, K. A., & Mahlmeister, L. R. (1994). *Maternal & neonatal nursing: Family-centered care* (3rd ed.). Philadelphia: J.B. Lippincott.

North American Nursing Diagnosis Association. (1993). *Classification of nursing diagnoses: Proceedings of the Tenth Conference.* Philadelphia: J.B. Lippincott.

National Center for Health Statistics. (1992). *Health: United States—1990.* Washington, DC: US Government Printing Office.

Norbeck, J., & DeJoseph, J. (1992). *Predictors of pregnancy complications in lower socioeconomic status women.* Bethesda, MD: National Institutes of Health, National Center for Nursing Research, Grant RO 1 NR 01459.

Reeder, S. J., Martin, L. L., & Koniak, D. (1992). *Maternity nursing: Family, newborn, and women's health care* (17th ed.). Philadelphia: J.B. Lippincott.

Reinisch, J. M., with Beasley, R. (1990). *The Kinsey Institute new report on sex.* New York: St. Martin's Press.

Rosdahl, C. B. (1991). *Textbook of basic nursing* (5th ed.). Philadelphia: J.B. Lippincott.

Schlatter, B. (1991). Nurse-midwifery: The profession and the challenges it faces. *Journal of Perinatal and Neonatal Nursing, 5*(3), 25–33.

Sullivan, E. (1992). Nurse practitioners and reimbursement. *Nursing and Health Care, 1*(5), 236–239.

Thomas, C. L. (Ed.). (1993). *Taber's cyclopedic medical dictionary.* Philadelphia: F. A. Davis Company.

Yoder, M. (1993). *Nursing diagnosis vignettes in maternal-child health.* Baltimore: Williams & Wilkins.

CHAPTER 2
Reproduction and Human Sexuality

◈ OBJECTIVES

When the learning goals of this chapter are met, the reader will be able to:

◆ List and describe the internal and external male reproductive organs.
◆ Define spermatogenesis and describe the route the sperm must travel to reach the ovum.
◆ Identify and describe the internal and external female reproductive organs.
◆ Explain the structure and function of the ovaries, including the primordial follicle, graafian follicle, and corpus luteum.
◆ Discuss the structure and function of the musculature and endometrial lining of the uterus.
◆ Name the bones of the pelvis while describing the difference between the true and false pelves (plural of pelvis).
◆ Explain the phases of the ovarian and uterine cycles and the hormones involved in menstruation.
◆ Explain male and female responses during the four phases of the sexual response cycle.
◆ Describe the physical and psychological reproductive changes that take place during adolescence and puberty.
◆ Develop an awareness of individual customs and beliefs that influence human sexuality.
◆ Identify characteristics of a nurse that demonstrate an awareness of individual customs and beliefs that influence human sexuality.

TERMINOLOGY

Corpus luteum	Ovum
Epididymis	Oxytocin
Estrogen	Primordial follicles
Follicle-stimulating hormone (FSH)	Progesterone
Luteinizing hormone	Puberty
Menstruation	Sperm
Orgasm	Testosterone
	Vas deferens

The miracles of conception, pregnancy, and childbirth are made possible by sexual reproduction, which allows for the union of the male and female sex cells (**sperm** and **ovum,** respectively). Both the male and female must reach sexual maturity before they are capable of sexual reproduction. Sexual maturity is reached when the reproductive system is fully developed, an event that marks the end of **puberty.**

Puberty

Puberty is a period of rapid change during which boys and girls undergo a number of dramatic physical changes as they make the transition from childhood to adulthood. These physical changes, which produce gender traits such as breasts and facial hair, are referred to as secondary sexual characteristics.

In boys, puberty occurs between the ages of 13 and 15, a period marked by a growth spurt that leads to increases in muscle mass, height, and weight. **Testosterone,** the primary male hormone, deepens the voice and causes hair growth of the axilla (armpits) and on the face, chest, and genitalia. The penis and scrotum enlarge to adult size. Nocturnal emissions, or wet dreams, also begin to occur.

Girls, who mature a few years earlier than boys, usually go through puberty between the ages of 9 and 16. Secondary sexual characteristics become apparent with the enlargement of breasts and the growth of leg, axillary, and pubic hair. As with boys, the genitalia increase in size at this time. **Menstruation,** the monthly discharge of blood and tissue from the uterus, usually begins between 12 and 13 years of age. (Refer to Human Sexuality on page 31 for a discussion of the emotional issues that become important during puberty.)

The Male Reproductive System

The male reproductive system is made up of both internal and external organs. These organs work together to allow the male to produce healthy sperm that are capable of fertilizing the female's ovum.

The External Reproductive Organs

The external organs include the penis and the scrotum. The penis allows for copulation (sexual union with a partner) and urination. The scrotum houses several internal organs necessary for the production of sperm. In the sexually mature male, pubic hair extends from the base of the penis towards the anus. Hair growth is also present on the scrotum.

Penis

The penis is a cylindrical organ that is made up almost entirely of erectile tissue covered with skin. This erectile tissue becomes erect or stiff when filled with blood. It is arranged in three columns in the penis: the two side columns are the corpora cavernosa (or cavernous bodies); the corpus spongiosum (or spongy body), which contains the urethra, is the third column. It lies between the corpora cavernosa.

Sperm and urine exit the body through the urethral meatus, which is located in the glans penis, the cone-shaped tip of the penis (Fig. 2-1). In uncircumcised males, it may be covered by a loose fold of skin called the prepuce, or foreskin. (Some males may have had the foreskin removed during circumcision for religious, cultural, or hygienic reasons.)

When the cavernous bodies in the penis are empty, the penis is limp, or flaccid. An erection occurs when the cavernous bodies become engorged with blood as the result of physical stimulation or sexual imagery. During an erection, the penis becomes stiff and elongated, allowing the male to penetrate the female and deposit his sperm near her cervix.

Scrotum

The scrotum consists of two external pouches that hang just below the shaft on either side of the penis. Each scrotal sac contains a testis, epididymis, and part of the spermatic cord. The muscles that support the scrotum are sensitive to temperature changes. Cold external temperatures, physical exercise, and sexual stimulation can all cause the scrotal tissue to contract, thus drawing the scrotum closer to the body for warmth.

This ability to reposition the scrotum either closer to or farther away from the body is important for the control of testicular temperature. (See *Sperm and Semen* for more information.)

The Internal Reproductive Organs

The internal male organs produce, store, and deliver sperm. A sophisticated ductal system helps the sperm travel from the testes, where they are formed, to their final destiny outside the body. The internal reproductive structures include the testes, the epididymides (plural

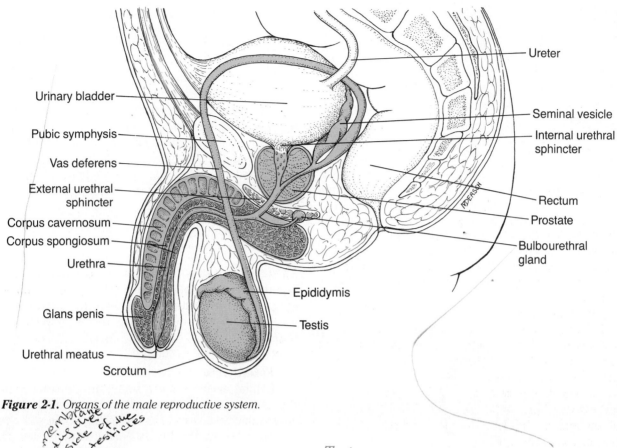

Figure 2-1. *Organs of the male reproductive system.*

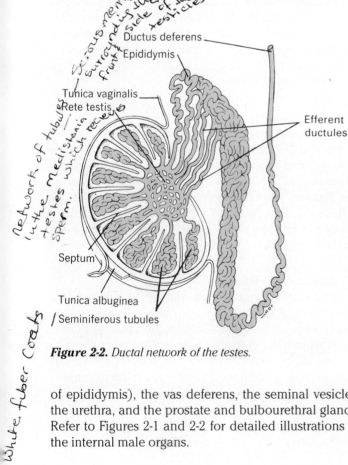

Serous membrane surrounding the front side of the testicles (handwritten)

Network of tubules in the mediastenia testes which recervs sperm. (handwritten)

White fiber coats (handwritten)

Figure 2-2. *Ductal network of the testes.*

of epididymis), the vas deferens, the seminal vesicles, the urethra, and the prostate and bulbourethral glands. Refer to Figures 2-1 and 2-2 for detailed illustrations of the internal male organs.

Testes

The testes, or <u>male gonads,</u> are solid, oval-shaped organs approximately 2.5 cm (1 inch) wide and 3.5 to 5 cm (1.5 inches) long. The testes' (plural of testis) most important contributions to male sexuality are their production of sperm and male hormones (androgens). Testosterone is the most important of the androgens.

For spermatogenesis (the production of sperm) to take place, the testes must be completely descended from the abdominal cavity. Under normal circumstances, both testes descend through the inguinal canal from the male abdomen into the scrotum at around the seventh month of fetal development.

Sperm and Semen

Spermatogenesis, which begins during puberty, is most efficient when the testes are a few degrees cooler than body temperature. The scrotum provides the ideal temperature. Significant increases or decreases in body temperature can affect the testes' ability to produce sperm. Illness, wearing clothing that is too tight, soaking in hot tubs, and exercising can all cause fluctuations in testicular temperature that can impair spermatogenesis. In males with cryptorchidism (undescended testes), the testes remain in the abdominal cavity rather than descending into the scrotum during fetal development or early childhood. The high temperature of the abdominal cavity prevents the testes from producing sperm and causes permanent sterility.

Spermatozoa, or mature sperm, are produced in the seminiferous tubules that make up the 250 to 400 lobules of each testis. A mature sperm, which has a head, neck or middle piece, and a long tail (Fig 2-3), resembles a microscopic tadpole. The head is made up of the nucleus, which contains 23 chromosomes, and the acrosome (the caplike structure containing enzymes to facilitate the penetration of the ovum). The chromosomes are the father's contribution to his offspring's genetic makeup. Connecting the tail to the head is the middle piece, or neck, where mitochondria produce energy for the swimming action of the tail.

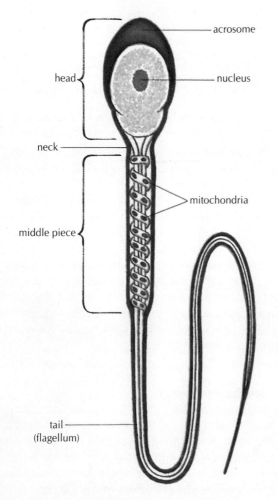

Figure 2-3. *Mature male sperm structure. (Chaffee, E. E. & Lytle, I. M. [1980]. Basic physiology and anatomy [4th ed., p. 549]. Philadelphia, Lippincott.)*

Sperm are released during reflexive expulsion of semen from the urethra called ejaculation. The average volume of ejaculate is 2 to 5 mL and contains between 60 and 150 million sperm/mL. Even though the ejaculate is rich with sperm, only one spermatozoon at a time is able to penetrate and fertilize the ovum.

The combined secretions of the epididymides, seminal vesicles, and the bulbourethral and prostate glands are known as the seminal fluid (semen). This fluid serves three important functions: it nourishes the sperm, balances the pH of sperm before they leave the body, and enhances their motility (their ability to move).

Ducts

An elaborate system of ducts is found within the testes.

The tubelike path in each testis includes the epididymis, the vas deferens, and the seminal vesicle. Figure 2-2 illustrates the complex ductal system in the testis.

Epididymis

Behind each testis is a small, firm, oblong storage site called the **epididymis.** This long, coiled canal is approximately 600 cm (20 feet) long when stretched. Although the sperm are produced in the testes, they mature and gain motility in the epididymis. A small amount of seminal fluid (semen) is added to the sperm as they leave the epididymis and continue on their journey into the vas deferens.

Vas Deferens

The **vas deferens,** also called the ductus deferens, is the tube that carries the sperm from each testis to the urethra. It is approximately 45 cm (18 inches) long. Beginning on the posterior border of each testis, each vas deferens joins the spermatic cord (from which the testes are suspended) and then weaves its way through the pelvis. The two vas deferens eventually meet at the seminal vesicles.

Seminal Vesicles

The seminal vesicles are the saclike structures located behind the bladder near the prostate. During ejaculation, sperm travel through the tubes of the vas deferens into the ejaculatory ducts (the point at which the vas deferens and the seminal vesicles meet). The seminal vesicles respond by secreting a thick, nutrient-rich fluid that combines with sperm. The sperm will exit the penis from this point via the prostate gland and the urethra. Display 2-1 provides a checklist of the male reproductive system.

Urethra

The male urethra is longer than the female urethra. This passageway begins in the bladder and passes through the prostate gland. The urethra allows semen and urine to exit the body through the urethral meatus.

Prostate Gland

The prostate gland surrounds the urethra below the neck of the urinary bladder. Prostatic secretions, which are alkaline, counteract the acidic nature of the fluid from the seminal vesicles, thereby neutralizing the pH of the sperm. The lower pH enhances the sperm's ability to survive in the acidic environment of the vagina.

Bulbourethral Glands

The bulbourethral glands (Cowper's glands) open into the urethra alongside the prostate gland. These small, pea-shaped glands secrete a thick, clear fluid that provides lubrication as the sperm leave the penile urethra. Bulbourethral secretions are also alkaline, and like the prostatic secretions, they increase sperm motility.

Hormonal Influences

Testosterone is produced in the Leydig cells within the testes. This hormone is responsible for the development of the secondary sex characteristics in the male. The mature male's voice is low because of the influence of testosterone. The presence of body hair, muscle mass development, strengthening of the bones, and the enlargement of the penis, scrotum, testes, prostate gland, and seminal vesicles are all attributable to the influence of testosterone.

The Female Reproductive System

The female reproductive system is made up of the external and internal reproductive organs (or genitalia) and several structures that play an auxiliary role in reproduction, such as the mammary glands (breasts) and the bony pelvis. The maturation and operation of the female reproductive system are controlled by several hormones.

The External Reproductive Organs

The external female genitalia include the mons pubis, perineum; and the vulva, which consists of the labia majora, labia minora, clitoris, vestibule of the vagina, and the vaginal opening. The size, shape, and color of the external genitalia vary from woman to woman.

Although the urethra is more properly classified as part of the urinary tract, it is discussed in this section because it lies so close to the external genitalia. Figure 2-4 illustrates these structures.

Mons Pubis

The mons pubis is the fatty cushion of tissue that overlays and protects the symphysis pubis (bony pelvis). Sometimes called the mons veneris, the mons pubis is covered by a thick layer of skin, which sprouts a growth of coarse hair during puberty. As with the size and shape of the external genitalia, the length and coarseness of pubic hair varies among women.

Labia Majora and Labia Minora

The labia majora are the two folds of fatty, hair-covered skin that lie protectively on either side of the vaginal vestibule. The labia minora are the smaller, more delicate folds of tissue that can be found upon separating

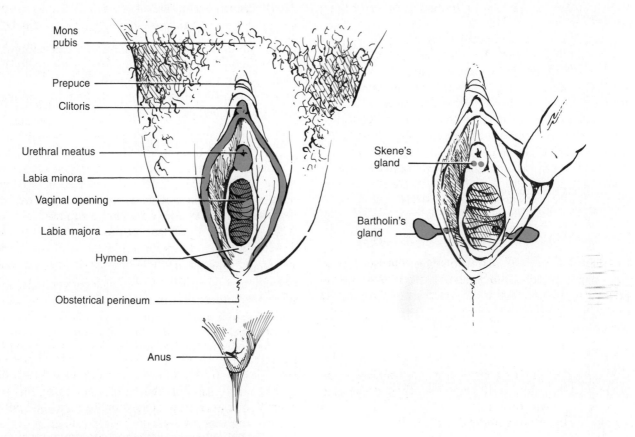

Mons pubis

Prepuce

Clitoris

Urethral meatus

Labia minora

Vaginal opening

Labia majora

Hymen

Obstetrical perineum

Anus

Skene's gland

Bartholin's gland

Figure 2-4. *Female external reproductive organs.*

the labia majora. The labia minora are supplied with an extensive network of blood vessels and nerve endings, which enhances the woman's sexual arousal.

Clitoris

The clitoris is a small bud of erectile tissue that is partially hidden by the anterior portion of the labia minora. The rich supply of blood vessels and nerve endings makes this organ extremely sensitive to stimulation.

Vestibule

An almond-shaped area called the vestibule lies between the labia minora. The openings of six structures are contained in the vestibule including: two Bartholin's glands, two Skene's ducts, the urethral meatus, and the vagina. The hymen is a thin mucous membrane that partially covers the entrance to the vagina. Using tampons, engaging in vigorous exercise, experiencing direct trauma, masturbating, and engaging in sexual intercourse are just some of the ways in which this thin membrane may be torn.

Urethra

The female urethra originates in the urinary bladder neck. It ends just below the clitoris as the urethral opening (urethral meatus), through which urine is discharged from the body. It is shorter than the male urethra, thus making the female more susceptible to urinary tract infections.

Skene's Ducts and Bartholin's Glands

Skene's ducts lie just inside of and posterior to the urethra, for which they produce a lubricating substance. Bartholin's glands, however, are located on either side of the vaginal vestibule, near the vaginal opening. During sexual arousal, these glands secrete a clear, lubricating fluid with an alkaline pH that encourages sperm motility and viability.

Perineum

The perineum is the area located between the vulva and the anus. It is composed of skin, muscle, and fasciae (fibrous membranes that support, cover, and separate muscles as well as unite skin with underlying tissue).

The muscles that support the perineum include the levator ani muscles (which form the floor of the pelvis), superficial and deep perineal muscles, and the external anal sphincter. The pudendal arteries and nerves supply the muscles, fascia, and skin of the perineum.

It is important to support the perineum during delivery of the neonate's head and shoulders, because the perineum, which stretches significantly during childbirth, is likely to tear. It may be necessary to perform an episiotomy (incision) in the perineal area to prevent tears in the underlying supporting muscles.

The Internal Reproductive Organs

The internal reproductive organs in the female include: the ovaries, fallopian tubes, uterus, cervix, and the vagina. Figure 2-5 illustrates the anatomy of the internal genitalia.

Ovaries

The ovaries, or female gonads, are two oval-shaped organs about 4 cm long and 2 cm wide. They are located in the pelvic cavity on either side of the uterus and held in place by the uterine broad ligament.

At birth, each female has in her ovaries countless thousands of immature follicles (**primordial follicles**). These follicles mature into graafian follicles, each of which contains one ovum. Throughout the reproductive years, a mature ovum is released each month during the process of ovulation.

In addition to producing ova, the ovaries secrete the hormones that regulate the female's reproductive cycle. Chief among these hormones are estrogen and progesterone. **Estrogen,** which is secreted by the graafian follicles, stimulates the development of secondary sexual characteristics, such as the breasts. **Progesterone,** the hormone secreted by the **corpus luteum** (the yellowed body formed within a ruptured ovarian follicle), is responsible for preparing and maintaining the lining of the uterus for implantation of the ovum. This hormone also enables breast cells to produce milk. (See page 28 for a more detailed discussion of the menstrual cycle.)

Ova

The female ovum (egg cell) contains 23 chromosomes within its nucleus (refer to Chapter 9; *Normal Fetal Development*). It is only through union with the sperm, which also contains 23 chromosomes, that the ovum becomes capable of transmitting its genetic gift to the offspring that results from the fertilization.

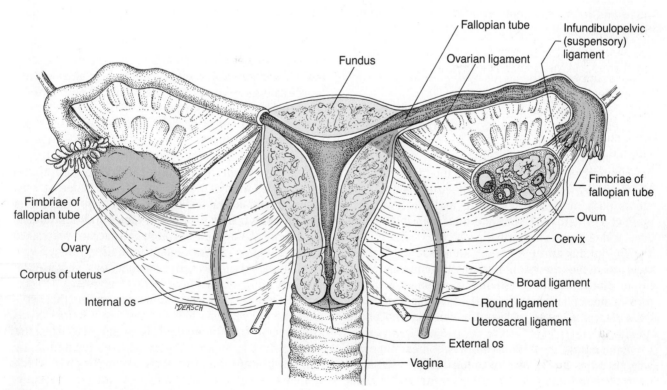

Figure 2-5. *Female internal reproductive system.*

Fallopian Tubes

The fallopian tubes connect with the lateral angles of the fundus, or base, of the uterus and end, one near each ovary. Each 8 to 12 cm (~4 inches) tube widens into a funnel-shaped opening, to which fingerlike projections are attached (see Fig. 2-5) During ovulation, these fingerlike projections (fimbriae) sweep the ovum into the fallopian tube.

The ovum is coaxed toward the uterus by tubal contractions and the wavelike action of the cilia lining the fallopian tube. Under normal circumstances, fertilization takes place in the fallopian tube, after which the ovum descends into the uterus for implantation. (Further discussion of fertilization and fetal development is found in Chapter 9.) If the ovum is not fertilized, it is expelled from the body with the female's menstrual flow.

Uterus

The uterus is a muscular, pear-shaped organ located in the center of the pelvic cavity. It is designed to nourish and protect the embryo as it develops into a fetus capable of surviving outside the mother's body. In its nonpregnant state, the uterus is roughly the size of a woman's fist. However, during pregnancy it expands to hold the developing fetus.

The uterus is stabilized within the pelvic cavity by broad and round ligaments. The lower portions of the broad ligaments are sometimes called the cardinal ligaments. They are thicker and, along with the uterosacral ligaments and pelvic muscles, provide further support. Blood is supplied to the uterus by the uterine and ovarian arteries.

Several distinct areas make up the uterus: the fundus (or main body of the uterus); the isthmus (the point at which the organ narrows), and the cervix (its lowermost, cylindrical portion). During labor contractions, uterine muscles push the fetus from the mother's body. Muscle fibers in the middle (myometrial) layer of the uterus push the fetus downward, and the lower segment of the uterus stretches and thins, causing the cervix to dilate, permitting birth through the vagina.

The fundus and the corpus are made up of three layers of tissue: the endometrium (the mucous membrane that lines the inner organ) myometrium (the middle, muscular layer of tissue), and the perimetrium (the outermost layer, which also encloses the entire uterus)

Each month, the endometrium becomes congested with blood as it prepares for the arrival of a fertilized ovum. If fertilization does not occur, the endometrial lining is shed during menstruation. However, if conception does take place, the fertilized ovum implants itself in the blood-rich uterine wall.

Cervix

The cervix, or neck of the uterus, is a cylindrical structure approximately 2.5 cm (1 inch) in length that protrudes into and is anchored in the vagina. It can be seen during a pelvic examination. It is normally pink, but during pregnancy its color deepens to purple. The cervix has an internal and external os, which constrict its upper and lower ends, respectively (See Fig. 2-5).

Vagina

The vagina is the muscular tube located in front of the rectum and behind the bladder that allows for the passage of menstrual flow, receives the penis during sexual intercourse, and is the passageway through which the fetus is delivered during uncomplicated childbirth. It is 7.5 to 10 cm (3–4 inches) long and connects the uterus to the external genitalia.

The thin walls of the vagina are covered with ridges called rugae. They allow the vagina to stretch as the fetus passes through the birth canal. Display 2-2 provides a checklist of the female reproductive system.

Pelvis

The pelvis is made up of four bones: two innominate bones (hip bones), the sacrum, and the coccyx, and the ligaments uniting them. The female pelvis is larger and wider than the male pelvis because it must support and protect the growing fetus. It also must allow for the fetus's safe passage through the vagina. (See Figure 2-6 for a diagram of the bony pelvis.)

Each hip bone is actually made up of three separate bones: the ileum, ischium, and pubis. The symphysis pubis is the point at which the hip bones join at the midline in the front of the pelvis. The mound created by the union of the two bones is also referred to as the mons pubis. The back of the pelvis is formed into a completed circle as the ileum of each hip bone meets the sacrum. The point at which the sacrum meets the ileum is called the sacroiliac joint. The coccyx is a small triangle of fused vertebrae that ends the vertebral column.

The linea terminalis is an imaginary line that separates the pelvic basin into the true (or inferior) pelvis and the false (or superior) pelvis (see Fig. 2-6). The false pelvis serves to support the growing uterus and guide the fetus toward the true pelvis. The true pelvis, which is made up of an inlet, a cavity, and an outlet, is the deeper of the two basins. It has to be, to accom-

DISPLAY 2-2
The Female Reproductive System

External Structures

Mons pubis:	protects bony pelvis
Labia majora:	protects vulva
Labia minora:	protects vulva
Clitoris:	female erectile organ
Vestibule:	location of Bartholin's glands, Skene's ducts, urethra, and vagina
Urethral meatus:	opening that allows passage of urine
Perineum:	muscular area between vulva and anus

Internal Structures

Ovaries:	seat of hormonal activity that controls ovulation
Fallopian tubes:	coax ovum into uterus
Uterus:	environment for fetal development
Cervix:	dilates to allow passage of fetus into vagina
Vagina:	permits menstrual flow, sexual intercourse, childbirth
Pelvis:	supports reproductive organs and developing fetus

Accessory Organs

Breasts:	lactation organs

modate the delivery of the fetus. Measurements of the various diameters of the pelvis are discussed in Chapter 6.

Breasts

Although the mammary glands, or breasts, are not technically part of the reproductive system, they are discussed here because of the important role they play in the production of milk for the nourishment of the newborn.

The glandular tissue of each breast contains 15 to 20 lobes, each of which in turn contains between 20 and 40 lobules. Located within the lobules are milk-secreting glands called the alveoli. The alveoli and ducts from the lobules are surrounded by myoepithelial cells.

After childbirth, the breasts produce milk in response to the release of the hormone prolactin from the anterior pituitary gland. It is prolactin that stimulates the cells in the alveoli (acini cells) to produce milk. The newborn cannot, however, get its supply of milk without the help of another hormone, oxytocin. On release from the posterior portion of the pituitary gland, **oxytocin** causes the myoepithelial cells to contract, squeezing milk toward the lactiferous ducts, where it is stored until the newborn sucks on the nipple.

The pigmented area surrounding each nipple is called the areola. Special glands, called the tubercles of Montgomery, secrete a substance that lubricates the nipples. This lubricant protects the areolae (plural of areola) from cracking when the newborn is nursing. Figure 2-7 demonstrates the glandular tissue and ducts of the mammary gland.

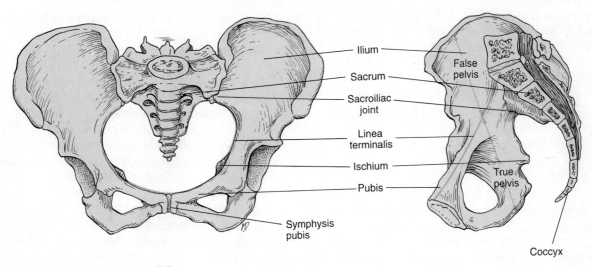

Figure 2-6. Bony female pelvis. **A.** Front view showing linea terminalis (pelvic brim). **B.** Side view showing true and false pelvis.

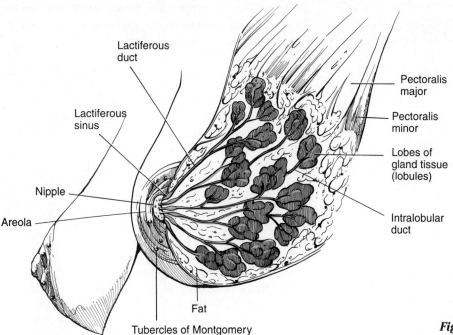

Lactiferous duct

Lactiferous sinus

Nipple

Areola

Pectoralis major

Pectoralis minor

Lobes of gland tissue (lobules)

Intralobular duct

Fat

Tubercles of Montgomery

Figure 2-7. *Glandular tissue and ducts of the mammary gland.*

Hormonal Influences

Hormones are substances that are released into the bloodstream from glandular tissue in one part of the body and carried to an area in another part of the body, where they stimulate or increase activity. The proper functioning of the female reproductive system is controlled by a series of hormones secreted by several endocrine (ductless) glands throughout the body. The entire process of hormonal release begins with the hypothalamus's secretion of gonadotropin-releasing hormone (GnRH). The anterior pituitary gland responds by secreting two gonadotropins (hormones that act on the gonads) that influence ovarian activity: **follicle-stimulating hormone** (FSH) and **luteinizing hormone** (LH). Some of the other hormones that play important roles in the female menstrual cycle are estrogen and progesterone (ovarian hormones) and prolactin. In the sections that follow, each hormone is further described within the context of its role in the female reproductive system.

The Menstrual Cycle

In the female, sexual maturity is marked by menarche (the first menstrual cycle). It signals the beginning of a series of periodically recurring changes in the hormonal status of the female. These hormones cause the buildup and shedding of the endometrium of the uterus. Shedding of the endometrium marks the end of a menstrual cycle in which conception did not take place.

The average length of the menstrual cycle is 28 days, with a normal range from 28 to 34 days. It should be noted, however, that the length of the menstrual cycle varies from woman to woman. Illness and stress may sometimes cause month-to-month variations in the same woman. The length of the cycle is determined by counting the number of days from day 1 of menstrual flow to the beginning of the next period. The flow lasts between 4 and 7 days, with a total blood loss of approximately 60 mL (2 ounces).

The menstrual cycle can be broken down into two subcycles: the ovarian cycle, during which the ova mature, and the uterine cycle, which refers to the periodic buildup of the uterus as it prepares to receive the fertilized ovum.

Ovarian Cycle

The ovarian cycle includes two phases: follicular (days 1–14) and luteal (days 15–28). During the follicular phase, FSH stimulates the primordial follicles in the ovary. The growing follicles respond by secreting estrogen, which prepares the lining of the uterus for the arrival and possible implantation of the ovum.

Increasing estrogen levels in the bloodstream signal the hypothalamus to stop producing FSH, whereupon a progesterone surge takes place. This progesterone surge stimulates the production of LH, which enhances the maturation of the follicle. The rupture of a graafian follicle on the 14th day results in ovulation, the release of a mature ovum. Variations in the length of a typical menstrual cycle are influenced by the length of this first stage.

The second phase of the ovarian cycle is the luteal phase. It begins after ovulation and ends with the start of the menstrual flow. The ruptured follicle, influenced by LH, becomes yellowish and increases in size to form the **corpus luteum** (yellow body). Progesterone levels continue to remain high.

If the ovum is not fertilized within 48 hours of its release, the corpus luteum begins to break down, thus reducing the levels of progesterone and estrogen. When levels of these hormones are low, the endometrium begins to shed, signaling menstruation.

Conversely, if conception occurs, the corpus luteum continues to secrete progesterone and estrogen. These hormones maintain the uterine endometrium until the placenta takes over.

Uterine Cycle

The uterus responds to the hormonal activities of the ovaries by either building up the endometrium in preparation for the implantation of the fertilized ovum or shedding the rich lining during menstruation. The uterine cycle is defined by four phases. These phases are the proliferative, secretory, ischemic, and menstrual. Figure 2-8 highlights the activities of each phase of the normal menstrual cycle.

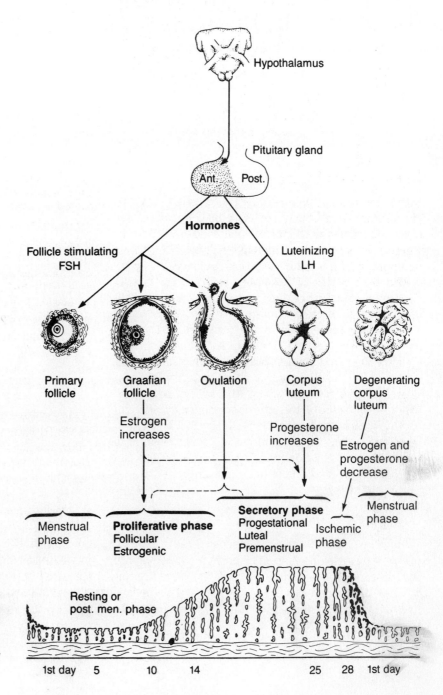

Figure 2-8. Hormonal control of the normal menstrual cycle.

Proliferative Phase

In a normal 28-day cycle, the proliferative phase immediately precedes ovulation. During this phase, the uterine endometrium is readied for the arrival of the mature ovum. As ovulation approaches, rising estrogen levels cause the cervical mucus to become clear, thin, and elastic. The elasticity of the cervical mucus (termed *spinnbarkheit*) enhances the sperm's motility, in essence increasing the female's fertility.

Secretory Phase

During this phase, which averages 10 to 14 days in length, progesterone levels increase and the developing corpus luteum further encourages the thickening of the endometrium. This blood-enriched environment awaits the ovum. If fertilization and implanta-tion occur, progesterone levels continue to increase. This inhibits the maturation and release of other ova and signals the uterus to continue to support implantation.

Ischemic Phase

If fertilization does not occur, levels of estrogen and progesterone decrease. The endometrium reacts by shrinking and shedding from the uterine walls. This stage typically lasts about 2 days.

Menstrual Phase

This period is characterized by uterine bleeding and shedding of the endometrium. It lasts between 4 and 5 days. At the end of this phase, the ovarian follicles renew their cycle of maturation. Display 2-3 pro-

---

DISPLAY 2-3
Female Reproductive Cycle Phases and Hormones

Ovarian Cycle

Follicular phase (days 1–14):	maturation of ovum
Ovulation (day 14):	expulsion of ovum
Luteal phase (days 15–28):	awaiting fertilization

Uterine Cycle

Proliferative phase (7–8 days):	build-up of endometrium
Ovulation (lasts 1 day):	expulsion of ovum from graafian follicle
Secretory phase (10–14 days):	progesterone levels rise
Ischemic phase (2 days):	when pregnancy does not occur, progesterone and estrogen levels decline
Menstrual phase (4–5 days):	shedding of endometrial lining

Female Hormones

Gonadotropin-releasing hormone (GnRH):	produced in the hypothalamus; acts on the pituitary to stimulate the release of LH and FSH
Estrogen:	produced by the ovaries; responsible for the development of secondary sexual characteristics
Progesterone:	secreted by the corpus luteum (and later the placenta); controls the changes in the endometrium as it prepares for the implantation of a fertilized ovum
Follicle-stimulating hormone (FSH):	produced by the anterior pituitary; stimulates follicle growth
Luteinizing hormone (LH):	secreted by the anterior pituitary; encourages growth of the corpus luteum
Oxytocin:	secreted by the pituitary, stimulates release of milk from mammary glands
Prolactin:	released by the pituitary; works with estrogen and progesterone to stimulate breast growth and production of milk

vides a checklist of female reproductive cycle phases and hormones.

Menstrual Cycle Variations

There are a number of factors that can lead to variations in the menstrual cycle across individuals and from month to month for the same individual. For example, taking oral contraceptives decreases the amount of menstrual flow, whereas using an intrauterine device (IUD) increases the flow.

Some women experience little or no discomfort during the menstrual cycle, and others experience full-blown premenstrual syndrome (PMS). (See Chapter 4 for a discussion of this and other menstrual conditions.) This collection of symptoms occurs several days before the onset of menses (blood flow) and lasts up to or for a few days afterwards. It is characterized by headache, bloating, heaviness of the lower abdomen and legs, tenderness and swelling of the breasts, and cravings for salty foods and sweets. Psychologic symptoms of PMS are often as distressful to the woman as physical complaints. These may include feelings of depression and irritability.

Treatment for PMS is dependent on the cause and symptoms. Mild over-the-counter analgesics, a low-sodium diet, avoidance of caffeine, stress-reducing activities such as walking, and an understanding response from family members when emotional upsets occur have all been effective.

◆ Human Sexuality

Human sexuality is necessary for the reproduction of the species. It is also a complex means of communication between individuals. The ways in which human sexuality is expressed are as varied as the individuals who engage in its practice. Although it is impossible to understand all of the cultural influences that may affect the practice of human sexuality, a basic understanding of human sexual responses will prove useful.

Sexual Intercourse

Sexual intercourse, also known as coitus, refers to the insertion of the erect penis into the vagina. During intercourse, the male makes thrusting motions. This creates friction as the penis rubs against the vaginal walls and clitoris. This friction often results in **orgasm,** the release of tension at the climax of sexual intercourse. In the male, orgasm is typically accompanied by the ejaculation of semen.

Human Sexual Response

Almost 50 years ago, Drs. William Masters and Virginia Johnson (Masters & Johnson) observed subjects during sexual activities in the interest of learning more about how men and women respond physiologically to masturbation and sexual intercourse. As a result of their scientific studies, Masters & Johnson described four phases in the human sexual response cycle: excitement, plateau, orgasm, and resolution.

Sexual Response in the Male

All of the senses: touch, taste, smell, sight (which includes giving and receiving visual cues), and sound (the production of or response to verbal advances) participate in sexual arousal. In the male, arousal in the excitement phase is marked by an erection. Erections occur in response to vasocongestion, a swelling of blood vessels. At the same time, heart rate, blood pressure, and respirations increase. The skin may become flushed.

The plateau phase is a more advanced stage of arousal that occurs before orgasm. Small amounts of semen (preejaculate) may be released from the urethral meatus at this point.

Muscle contractions (myotonia) of the genitalia mark the orgasmic phase of the sexual response cycle. In males, orgasm is usually accompanied by ejaculation and followed by a refractory (resting) period. During the refractory period, the male is resistant to further stimulation. In the final, resolution phase, the body gradually returns to its prearousal state.

Sexual Response in the Female

The phases of sexual arousal are similar for the female. During the excitement phase, the female experiences engorgement of the external genitalia (vasocongestion), vaginal lubrication, and erection of her nipples. Blood pressure, heart rate, and respirations increase. The skin may be flushed. The clitoris retracts and the vagina lengthens as the cervix and uterus are elevated during the plateau phase of sexual arousal. Orgasm is the result of multiple, strong contractions of the pelvic muscles (myotonia). The orgasmic phase is the peak of sexual arousal and is intensely pleasurable for the woman. Women may require direct stimulation of the clitoris to achieve orgasm. Although both men and women can experience multiple orgasms, women are able to go through the response cycle repeatedly without experiencing a refractory period. As resolution occurs, the internal and external genitalia return to their prearousal state.

If orgasm does not occur for either partner, vaso-congestion causes a feeling of heaviness and aching in the genitalia. Resolution is delayed because of prolonged physical arousal of the genitalia.

Responsible Sexuality

Responsible behavior is one of the results of developing socially accepted values and ethical practices. Responsible sexuality is a natural by-product of this behavior. But how does the individual arrive at his or her own definition of responsible sexuality? There is no single answer to this question, but there are a few useful generalizations that can be made of individuals who practice responsible sexuality.

Sexually responsible individuals carefully consider how the sexual choices they make can affect their sexual partners as well as any offspring that may result. They may express their respect for each other's emotional well-being by delaying sexual activity until they have determined what role it will play in their relationship. They may even decide that sex outside of marriage is inappropriate for them. Practicing "safer sex" is another way that sexually active persons can demonstrate their respect for their own physical and reproductive health as well as that of their partners. They also may insist on mutual monogamy as a means of getting the physical and emotional security they desire. The ability to make joint decisions about pregnancy and contraception are two other important indi-

cators of sexual responsibility. Above all else, sexually responsible persons openly communicate their desires and concerns to their partners. The Checklist, Responsible Sexuality, includes information the nurse may provide when teaching families to promote responsible sexuality.

Adolescent Considerations

Adolescence is a time of great transition for both sexes. The physical changes brought on by puberty often lead to feelings of self-consciousness and confusion. Young adolescents who experience delayed puberty or early-onset puberty may feel awkward even though their rate of maturation is perfectly normal for them.

Developing positive attitudes about the healthy expression of human sexuality can be difficult for adolescents, who may be facing the challenge of defining their own sexuality for the very first time. These feelings may be subtle (perhaps they have begun to fantasize about sexual activity with someone of the opposite sex) or dramatic (as may be the case for adolescents who find themselves attracted to someone of the same sex). In this case, feelings of shame, embarrassment, and denial may flood the young person's mind and increase their confusion. Because adolescents may be trying to establish a delicate balance between defining themselves as separate from their parents while enjoying the acceptance of a peer group, they may be unable to discuss their confusion with anyone. A nurse who understands the potential problems of adolescence can gently encourage the expression of troubling feelings by being open and nonjudgmental in interacting with adolescents.

Cultural Considerations

The individual's idea of human sexuality may be influenced by myths and cultural beliefs. Family planning, the importance of procreation, reproductive maturity, and sexual behaviors are all examples of areas on which an individual's cultural background may have a profound influence.

Some cultures celebrate puberty with practices such as male and female circumcision, separation of adolescent males from their mothers, and female cleansing rituals. Others may place great value on producing male offspring. Still other cultures may regard sexual activity as strictly for reproduction. The experience of sexual pleasure and satisfaction may even be forbidden.

✔ **FAMILY TEACHING CHECKLIST**

Responsible Sexuality

To promote health and well-being, the nurse includes the following information in family teaching:

Factual information can be obtained through sex education.

Monogamy has several important emotional and health-related benefits.

Sexually responsible individuals make choices based on the impact that their actions will have on self and others.

"Safer sex" activities can greatly reduce the risks of unwanted pregnancies and sexually transmitted diseases.

Partners who make joint decisions on childbearing have stronger relationships.

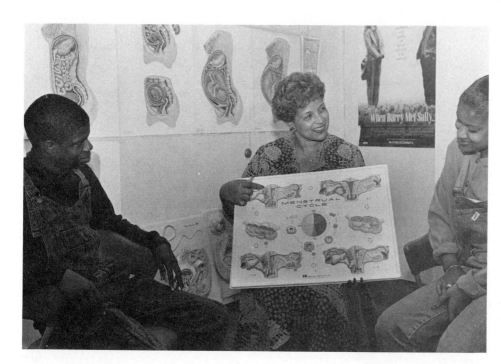

Figure 2-9. *Teaching an adolescent about human sexuality and responsible sex is a way the nurse can promote healthy sexual behaviors.*

Exploring how cultural beliefs influence values and decision making will provide the nurse with a greater understanding of and appreciation for an individual's behavior as it relates to reproduction.

The Role of the Nurse

Human reproduction requires a complex interplay between organs, glands, ducts, and hormones. Understanding these normal physiologic processes allows the nurse to provide safe, effective nursing care. By teaching individuals about these changes, nurses can relieve the family's unnecessary fear, stress, and anxiety.

Adolescents are especially vulnerable to misunderstanding the changes taking place in their bodies during puberty. Nurses can support individuals and guide them through the process of sexual maturity. By remaining open and nonjudgmental, the nurse can encourage adolescents to ask questions about human sexuality and sexually responsible practices (Fig. 2-9).

The nurse needs to be aware of personal feelings about human sexuality. Understanding a variety of sexual behaviors and practices within the context of the individual's background is necessary. The nurse who is able to provide culturally sensitive nursing care is one who carefully considers the beliefs and practices of others in an unbiased manner.

In the role of counselor, the nurse encourages, open discussions about human sexuality and reproduction. This openness can lead to freer communication of sexual desires between partners. The Nursing Diagnoses Checklist provides a list of nursing diagnoses related to reproduction and sexuality.

✓ NURSING DIAGNOSES CHECKLIST

Nursing Diagnoses Related to Reproduction and Sexuality

Anxiety, related to confusion concerning gender identity

Body Image Disturbance, related to human sexual development

Ineffective Denial, related to homosexual feelings

Altered Growth and Development, related to delayed sexual development

Knowledge Deficit, related to reproduction

Parental Role Conflict, related to unfavorable adolescent behaviors

Self Esteem Disturbance, related to physiologic changes associated with puberty

Altered Sexuality Patterns, related to impaired sexual development

SELF-ASSESSMENT

In the diagram provided, label the following male reproductive structures and organs:

Scrotum	Urethra	Vas deferens (ductus deferens)
Testis	Urinary bladder	Seminal vesicle
Prostate gland	Glans penis	
Bulbourethral gland	Epididymis	

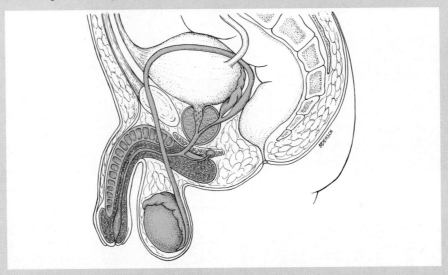

In the diagram provided, label the following female reproductive structures and organs:

Ovaries	Fallopian tubes	Implantation site
Ovarian ligament	Uterine fundus	Cervix
Ruptured ovarian follicle	Uterine corpus	Vagina
Fimbriae		

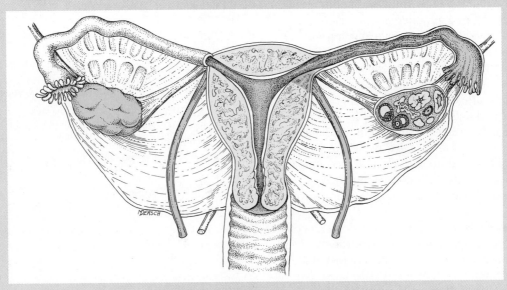

1. Decreased secretion of estrogen and progesterone results in:

○ **A.** Ovulation
○ **B.** Formation of the corpus luteum
○ **C.** Menstruation
○ **D.** Thin, elastic cervical mucus

2. What is the role of secretions from the prostate gland and bulbourethral glands?

○ **A.** Increase the concentration of sperm in the semen
○ **B.** Increase sperm motility
○ **C.** Increase acidity of semen
○ **D.** Help with the development of secondary sex characteristics

3. Which hormone is responsible for milk production?

○ **A.** Prolactin
○ **B.** Progesterone
○ **C.** Oxytocin
○ **D.** Estrogen

4. Why are women more prone than men to develop urinary tract infections?

○ **A.** The location of the urinary meatus
○ **B.** The acidic pH of urine
○ **C.** The length of the urethra
○ **D.** The abundance of ducts and glands around the urethra

5. Ovarian functioning is influenced by secretion of which two gonadotropins?

○ **A.** Prolactin and oxytocin
○ **B.** Estrogen and progesterone
○ **C.** Follice-stimulating hormone (FSH) and luteinizing hormone (LH)
○ **D.** Gonadotropin-releasing hormone and estrogen

REVIEW AND PREVIEW

This chapter opened with a discussion of the importance of puberty as the process through which boys and girls reach sexual maturity and become capable of reproduction. The basic anatomy and function of both the male and female reproductive systems was outlined. Hormones and the reproductive organs affected by their influence were also discussed. Information on the pelvis and the mammary glands was also included.

Human sexuality was discussed, with emphasis on the importance of responsible sexual activity. Adolescent and cultural considerations and their impact on nursing care concluded the chapter.

The following chapter will discuss fertility and family planning options. Discussions of alternative methods of birth control will include both their advantages and disadvantages. Infertility, including diagnosis and treatment, will also be explored.

◈ KEY POINTS

◆ The reproductive tract of the male consists of the testes, within the scrotum, epididymides, vas deferens, seminal vesicles, and urethra. In a healthy male, these structures work together to generate sperm for depositing in a receptive female. The male ejaculates spermatozoa, formed as a result of spermatogenesis. The addition of fluids secreted by the prostate and bulbourethral glands to the sperm lubricates their passage as they exit the male's body and balances their pH so that they can better survive the acidic environment of the female's vagina. Once deposited inside the vagina, the sperm then travel upward into the uterus and fallopian tubes, where they attempt to fertilize an ovum.

◆ The female external reproductive structures include the mons pubis, labia majora and minora, clitoris, vestibule, and urethral meatus. The area between the vagina and anus is referred to as the perineum. The ovaries, fallopian tubes, uterus, and cervix are found internally. The vagina connects the internal and external genitalia.

◆ At birth, the ovaries are filled with hundreds of thousands of immature follicles (primordial follicles), each of which contains an ovum. Ovulation begins when one follicle matures, thus becoming a graafian follicle, and releases a mature ovum. If the ovum is fertilized by a sperm, the ruptured follicle forms the corpus luteum. The corpus luteum then secretes hormones that support the uterine endometrium for implantation.

◆ The uterus has three layers, endometrium, myometrium, and perimetrium. Each month, the internal layer, or endometrium, prepares a nourishing bed to support the fertilized ovum. If conception does not occur, the endometrial lining sheds during menstruation. The uterus functions to nourish, support, and expel the growing fetus.

◆ The pelvis consists of two innominate bones (hips), the sacrum, and the coccyx. These four bones form a circle. The pelvis may be visually divided into the true pelvis, the lower deeper basin, and the false pelvis. The false pelvis is the upper basin. This is where the fetus grows within the uterus. The true pelvis is the lower, deeper basin. It allows for the passage of the fetus during childbirth.

◆ Under the influence of several female hormones, fertilization, fetal growth and development, and menstruation are possible. The uterine cycle prepares the endometrium for implantation through four phases: proliferative, secretory, ischemic, and menstrual. The ovaries prepare for conception during the follicular and luteal phases of the ovarian cycle.

◆ Masters and Johnson observed subjects during sexual arousal and orgasm. They described four stages of sexual excitement in both men and women. These stages are excitement, plateau, orgasm, and resolution.

◆ A variety of physical and psychological changes occur in adolescence. There is a wide range of normal variation. Both sexes experience an increased growth of genital and body hair.

◆ Nurses need to be sensitive to variations in individuals' customs and beliefs about sexuality and reproduction. A nonjudgmental approach encourages communication and expresses understanding. Educating, counseling, and promoting sexual responsibility are important roles for nursing.

BIBLIOGRAPHY

Bozett, F., & Hanson, S. (1991). *Fatherhood and families in cultural context.* New York: Springer.

D'Avanzo, C. (1992). Bridging the cultural gap with southeast Asians. *American Journal of Maternal Child Nursing, 17,* 204–207.

Kenney, J., & Tash, D. (1992). Lesbian childbearing couples' dilemmas and decision. *Health Care of Women International, 13* (2), 209–219.

Masters, J., Johnson, V., & Kolodny, R. (1992). *Human sexuality* (4th ed.). New York: Harper Collins.

Mathews, J., & Zadek, K. (1991). The alternative birth movement in the United States: History and current status. *Women and Health, 17*(1), 39–56.

May, K. M. (1992). Social networks and help-seeking experiences of pregnant teens. *Journal of Obstetric, Gyncologic, and Neonatal Nursing, 21*(6), 497–502.

May, K. A., & Mahlmeister, L. R. (1994). *Maternal & neonatal nursing: Family-centered care* (3rd ed.). Philadelphia: J. B. Lippincot.

Pilliteri, A. (1992). *Maternal and child health nursing: Care of the childbearing and childrearing family* (1st ed.). Philadelphia: J. B. Lippincott.

Reeder, S. J., Martin, L. L., & Koniak, D. (1992). *Maternity nursing: Family, newborn, and women's health care* (17th ed.). Philadelphia: J. B. Lippincott.

Reinisch, J. M., with Beasley, R. (1990). *The Kinsey Institute new report on sex.* New York: St. Martin's Press.

Rosdahl, C. B. (1991). *Textbook of basic nursing* (5th ed.). Philadelphia: J. B. Lippincott.

Stainton, M. C., McNeil, D., & Harvey, S. (1992). Maternal tasks of uncertain motherhood. *Maternal-Child Nursing Journal, 20,* 113–123.

Thomas, C. L. (Ed.). (1993). *Taber's cyclopedic medical dictionary.* Philadelphia: F. A. Davis.

Thompson, M., & Peebles-Wilkins, W. (1992). The impact of formal, informal and societal support networks on the psychological well being of black adolescent mothers. *Social Work, 37*(3), 322–328.

CHAPTER 3
Family Planning and Infertility

◈ OBJECTIVES

When the learning goals of this chapter are met, the reader will be able to:

◆ Define fertility, infertility, and family planning.

◆ Discuss the key factors that might influence an individual's preferences for various contraceptive methods.

◆ Explain why coitus interruptus and vaginal douching are not reliable methods of preventing pregnancy.

◆ Discuss natural family planning, including the activities that individuals and couples must routinely monitor.

◆ List the four barrier methods that prevent union of the sperm and ovum, including the rationale for spermicidal use with barrier methods.

◆ Explain the advantages and disadvantages of the intrauterine device (IUD), implants, and sterilization.

◆ Discuss the use of oral contraceptives, with detail on how the pill is taken, side effects, contraindications, and patient teaching implications.

◆ Identify the three most common causes of male infertility.

◆ List the location and cause of the most commonly occurring female infertility problems.

◆ Describe diagnostic and treatment options for male and female infertility.

TERMINOLOGY

Abstinence	Diaphragm
Basal body temperature	Fertility
Billing's cervical mucus method	Infertility
Calendar method	Intrauterine device
Cervical cap	Sterilization
Coitus interruptus	Symptothermal method
Condom	Vaginal sponge
Contraceptive	

Chapter 2 described the male and female reproductive systems and how they function together to support fertility. In the female, *fertility* is defined as the ability to conceive, support, sustain, and bear new life. In the male, fertility depends on the production of sufficient numbers of healthy sperm that are capable of reaching and penetrating the ovum. This chapter discusses two challenges to fertility: controlling it through the use of *contraceptives* (methods that work against conception) and *infertility* (the inability to reproduce sexually).

Fertile couples can practice contraception by using techniques and devices that interrupt or prevent fertilization from occurring. Barrier methods prevent sperm from reaching the ovum. Intrauterine devices (IUDs) irritate the uterus and thereby prevent the implantation of the fertilized ovum. Hormonal contraceptives (which can be taken orally, administered by injection, or implanted) alter the body's ability to produce viable ova. This chapter discusses these and other widely used contraceptive methods and also presents the advantages and disadvantages of each. Wherever necessary, contraindications to the use of a specific contraceptive also are given.

To provide quality care and effective counseling, nurses need to have a solid understanding of all the contraceptive options available. It is equally important that they be familiar with the problems unique to infertile couples.

Infertility in a woman is defined as the inability to conceive after 12 months of sexual intercourse without contraceptives. A man is considered infertile if he is unable to impregnate a woman after this same period of trying. Because infertility is a very stressful condition for both partners, it requires a great deal of understanding and sensitivity on the part of health care providers.

Family Planning

Family planning refers to the deliberate planning and spacing of conception. Couples who use this strategy actively avoid unwanted pregnancies with the aid of any of several effective contraceptive methods.

Choosing a Contraceptive Method

There are a number of practical factors to consider when choosing a contraceptive method, including its effectiveness, safety, expense, and availability. But choosing a contraceptive method is also a very private matter that requires that the individual address deeply held and very personal beliefs about his or her sexual-

ity. Even so, nurses can play an important role in providing accurate patient teaching that allows individuals to make contraceptive choices that are right for them. For example, women who are uncomfortable touching their genitals will not want to use diaphragms and cervical caps. Couples who value spontaneous intercourse will probably choose hormonal contraceptives over barrier methods. Nurses who can engage clients in an open discussion about their needs and preferences are better able to match clients with the contraceptive methods that best fit their needs.

Because cultural and religious factors often influence an individual's views on sexuality, nurses need to be careful to approach contraceptive counseling in a nonjudgmental way. The nurse's primary concerns are to see to it that the contraceptive method selected safely and effectively prevents pregnancy without interfering with the individual's health or ability to reproduce in future.

Abstinence

Abstinence is defined as the total avoidance of sexual activity, although it is frequently used to refer to refraining from sexual intercourse. There are several advantages to practicing absolute abstinence: there is no expense involved, and it is 100% effective in preventing pregnancy and the spread of sexually transmitted diseases and infections.

Two of the major disadvantages of sexual restraint are that it limits the natural, sexual expression of love and affection between partners and requires a great deal of self-control to practice.

Coitus Interruptus

Coitus interruptus refers to the early withdrawal of the penis from the vagina before ejaculation takes place. Coitus interruptus is frequently practiced because it is a simple, inexpensive method that does not require the purchase of any devices.

The disadvantages of coitus interruptus far outweigh its advantages. The timing of early withdrawal of the penis is critical and requires great willpower and control on the part of the man. But even if the timing is mastered, there is no guarantee that preejaculatory fluid (seminal fluid that is released into the vagina before ejaculation) has not been deposited in the vagina. Because preejaculatory fluid may contain sperm capable of fertilizing an ovum, there is a high probability that conception will occur using coitus interruptus.

Postcoital Douching

The cleansing of the vagina with a plain, medicated, or antiseptic solution is called douching. Postcoital douching (vaginal douching immediately following ejaculation) is done in an attempt to kill the sperm before they reach the ovum. Because sperm travel so quickly, it is highly unlikely that the douche solution will immobilize or kill them before they enter the cervix in search of the ovum. This practice is, therefore, not recommended as a reliable contraceptive method.

Natural Family Planning   *Test*

Natural family planning (NFP) methods work on the principle that conception can be effectively planned or prevented by accurately pinpointing ovulation and either engaging in or postponing sexual intercourse to obtain the desired results.

The effectiveness of natural family planning depends on the accurate recording and interpretation of many physiologic changes. For those couples trying to avoid pregnancy, there is the additional challenge of practicing abstinence before, during, and after ovulation to avoid periods of increased fertility. On the other hand, those using this method to enhance their chances of conception will have to time their copulations (sexual intercourse) to occur during times of peak fertility. Both strategies require that the partners agree to actively participate in natural family planning from month to month.

There are four basic strategies for predicting ovulation: the calendar method, taking basal body temperature measurements, charting changes in cervical mucus (Billing's method), and the symptothermal method.

Calendar Method

The **calendar method,** previously known as the rhythm method, enables the woman with regular menstrual cycles to determine when ovulation occurs. This method is most reliable in women who have predictable cycles with minimal variation. Cycles that occur every 24 to 28 days have their fertile phases between the 6th and 17th days of the ovarian cycle. Conception can be avoided if the woman does not engage in sexual intercourse during this period.

There are several reasons why this method of contraception appeals to couples: there is no need for medical prescriptions or assistance, there are no devices to apply or insert, and the related costs (for the calendar) are very low. Some of the disadvantages include the difficulty of tracking the menstrual cycle, which may be irregular from month to month; the difficulty of accurately recording menstrual cycles and

carefully monitoring the calendar; and the need to practice abstinence without error during the 2-week period of increased fertility. The effectiveness of the calendar method may be increased by using it in combination with other accepted methods of contraception.

Basal Body Temperature Method   *Test*

Basal body temperature (BBT) is the temperature of the body at rest. By charting the daily rise and fall of basal body temperature, a woman can determine with a fair amount of accuracy when she will ovulate. This allows her to predict times of peak fertility as well as "safe" periods, during which fertilization of the ovum is least likely to occur. This safe period corresponds to the luteal phase of the menstrual cycle. (See Chapter 2 for a review of the menstrual cycle.)

Each morning before rising and performing any activity, the woman takes her temperature and records her findings on a special chart/graph (Fig. 3-1). A decrease in BBT usually occurs just before ovulation. It then rises and remains elevated for several days (indicating ovulation). The rise in basal body temperature is caused by an elevation in progesterone levels, which prepares the endometrial lining for implantation.

A couple can avoid conception by practicing abstinence for a period that extends from a few days before the anticipated rise in basal body temperature until 3 or 4 days afterwards. If, however, this method is being used to predict times of peak fertility, the couple can plan to have intercourse on the day of the decline in the woman's temperature or on the following evening.

The advantages of the BBT method are similar to those discussed for the calendar method. There are several reasons why this method may be difficult to use. Elevations in body temperature may result from conditions that are not related to changes in hormonal levels. For example, illness, immunizations, and drug use can all cause increases in body temperature. Additionally, the woman must be able to read and record body temperatures with consistent accuracy. There are now specially designed thermometers that make reading temperatures easier, but temperature changes must still be charted on a daily basis. Omitting just a few daily temperature readings may result in a woman's missing the critical changes in her body that predict ovulation.

As with the calendar method, the BBT method can be enhanced by using other contraceptives during periods of fertility.   *Test*

Cervical Mucus Method (Billing's Method)

Changes in the consistency of cervical mucus generally follow a predictable pattern in ovulating women. Af-

How to Use the Temperature Method

Days of the month

| 5/7 | 5/8 | 5/9 | 5/10 | 5/11 | 5/12 | 5/13 | 5/14 | 5/15 | 5/16 | 5/17 | 5/18 | 5/19 | 5/20 | 5/21 | 5/22 | 5/23 | 5/24 | 5/25 | 5/26 | 5/27 | 5/28 | 5/29 | 5/30 | 5/31 | 6/1 | 6/2 | 6/3 | 6/4 | 6/5 | 6/6 | 6/7 | 6/8 |

Days of your menstrual cycle

| 1 | 2 | 3 | 4 | 5 | 6 | 7 | 8 | 9 | 10 | 11 | 12 | 13 | 14 | 15 | 16 | 17 | 18 | 19 | 20 | 21 | 22 | 23 | 24 | 25 | 26 | 27 | 28 | 1 | 2 | 3 | 4 | 5 |

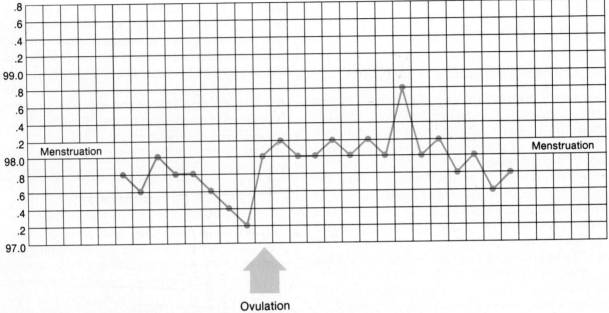

Figure 3-1. The rise and fall of the BBT over a complete menstrual cycle, including the fertile and safe periods.

ter ovulation and around the time of menstruation, there is very little cervical mucus. What cervical mucus there is is generally thick, cloudy and varies in color from white to yellowish. As ovulation approaches, the cervical mucus undergoes a number of changes that make the woman's reproductive tract more hospitable to sperm. The amount of mucus secreted increases, and it becomes thin, clear, and very stretchy.

The elasticity of the cervical mucus (or spinnbarkheit) can be tested by placing a drop of the mucus between two slides and stretching it. This stretchability is what allows the sperm to travel through the cervix more easily (Fig. 3-2). The time immediately before ovulation and the 3 days after ovulation (peak spinnbarkheit) are considered the most fertile times in a woman's cycle.

By observing the changes in her cervical mucus (Billing's method), a woman can pinpoint the times of peak and diminished fertility. Those wishing to avoid conception can abstain from sexual intercourse or use another reliable form of birth control during the fertile period.

This method of contraception has all the advantages of the other natural family planning methods. There are, however, various, nonhormonal factors and conditions that can alter the consistency of cervical mu-

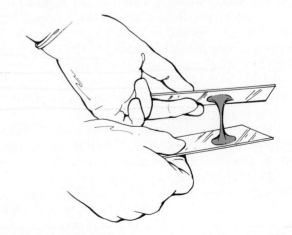

Figure 3-2. Spinnbarkeit character of cervical mucus during the ovulatory period.

cus. Douches, spermicides, lubricants, and yeast infections can all make it difficult to accurately assess cervical secretions. Refer to Chapter 2, *Hormonal Influences,* to review the normal hormonal changes that occur during the ovarian cycle.

Symptothermal Method

The **symptothermal method** allows couples to predict ovulation with greater reliability by using a combination of techniques: tracking the menstrual cycle, determining cervical mucus characteristics, noting the brief monthly abdominal pain that may signify ovulation (mittelschmerz), and monitoring BBT on a daily basis. Once the couple has targeted when ovulation will occur, they can alter their sexual behavior to decrease or increase the chances of conception. The Checklist, Natural Family Planning, lists the important components of natural family planning including the advantages and disadvantages of each method.

Barrier Methods

Contraceptives that use a physical barrier to prevent the sperm from reaching the ovum are called barrier methods. These barrier methods include: male and female

---

✓ **FAMILY TEACHING CHECKLIST**

Natural Family Planning

The nurse includes the following information in family teaching to promote health and well-being:

Calendar Method: based on regularly occurring 24- to 28-day cycles with fertile phase between the 6th and 17th days of ovarian cycle

Advantages: free; no devices, special medical management, or prescriptions needed

Disadvantages: increased risk of pregnancy with irregular cycles; lengthy period of abstinence

Basal Body Temperature Method: determination of ovulation based on decline and sudden increase in temperature

Advantages: free; works when cycle is irregular; accurate when practiced faithfully

Disadvantages: temperature variations not related to hormonal activity can result in miscalculating ovulation; accurately reading thermometer sometimes difficult; requires a day-to-day commitment; lengthy period of abstinence

Cervical Mucus Method: assessment of consistency of cervical mucus (mucus is clear and stretchable during ovulation)

Advantages: free, no devices needed

Disadvantages: period of abstinence can be extensive if cervical mucus is slow to change

Symptothermal Method: documentation of menstrual cycles, sexual activity, cervical mucus, basal body temperature, and abdominal discomfort associated with ovulation (mittelschmerz)

Advantages: increased effectiveness through a combination of all natural family planning methods

Disadvantages: lengthy periods of abstinence

condoms, diaphragm, cervical cap, and vaginal sponge. The effectiveness of these barrier contraceptives is enhanced when they are used in combination with spermicides (chemical agents that kill sperm).

Because none of the barrier methods is considered especially effective when used alone, it is generally recommended that two or more methods be used in combination.

Condom

The **condom** is a thin, flexible sheath made of rubber (usually latex) or natural membranes that is worn by either the male or female to contain ejaculated semen. In this way, sperm contained in the semen are prevented from entering the female's reproductive tract and fertilizing any ova that might be present.

Male Condom

As early as the 16th century, medicated linen sheaths were used to protect the tip of the penis from venereal infection. By the 17th century, condoms were ineffective constructions of animal guts and fish membranes that had been sewed shut at one end. They were doing double duty as a prophylactic and a contraceptive device.

Today, condoms, which are sold over-the-counter, are made of either latex or natural membranes (usually the intestinal lining of a sheep). Each condom is individually wrapped and pre-rolled for ease of application (Fig. 3-3). Condoms also come with a variety of other features. They may be coated with a lubricant, have reservoir tips for more effective collection of se-

men, or be ribbed (textured) to increase penile sensitivity.

The condom can be applied by either partner. It must be carefully rolled over the erect penis so that there is a small space left at the tip to serve as a reservoir for semen. (Some condoms have built-in reservoir tips, which make fitting the condom onto the penis easier.)

When applying the condom, care must be taken not to rip or puncture the membrane. To prevent the condom from breaking or becoming dislodged from the penis during insertion and withdrawal from the vagina, its rim must be held closed against the base of the penis.

When used properly, condoms provide a high degree of reliability in preventing pregnancy. When used in combination with spermicidal foam, their effectiveness approaches that of oral contraceptives. (See Table 3-1 for contraceptive failure rates.) Because they are inexpensive, easily obtained, and disposable, male condoms are often a preferred method of contraception. Condom use has the added benefit of providing some protection against sexually transmitted diseases (refer to Chapter 4 for further detail), especially when used with spermicides. It should be noted that although latex and natural-membrane condoms are both effective contraceptive devices, only the latex condom protects against the transmission of the human immunodeficiency virus (HIV).

Table 3-1. *Contraceptive Failure Rates* *

Method	Failure Rate (%)†
Male sterilization	0.15
Female sterilization	0.4
Oral contraceptives	3
Intrauterine device	3
Condom	12
Condom with spermicide	3
Diaphragm	18
Sponge	
Nulliparous user	18
Parous user	18
Cap	18
Coitus interruptus	18
Periodic abstinence	20
Spermicides	21
Chance	85

*Adapted from Trussell, J., Hatcher, R., Cates, W., Stewart, F., & Kost, K. (1990). Contraceptive failure in the United States: An update. *Studies in Family Planning*, *1*(1), 52.
†This failure rate is the estimated rate of accidental pregnancies when couples use the method in a "typical" fashion (ie, use is not always consistent or correct).

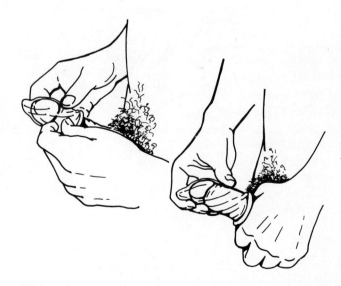

Figure 3-3. The male condom.

Condoms are sometimes viewed as inconvenient for any of several reasons. They can cause a rash in the genital area if either partner is allergic to the latex or the spermicidal lubricant with which they are coated. Some couples dislike having to interrupt sexual activity to apply the condom. Many males object to condoms because they dull sensation in the genitals. This problem can generally be relieved by using two condoms. Wearing a looser, more comfortable condom directly over the penis and covering that with a snugger condom increases friction, which enhances penile sensation.

Female Condom

The female condom is a double-ringed sheath that fits into the vagina (Fig. 3-4) so that the ring on its internal end fits snugly around the cervical os. This sheath covers the cervix, vagina, and extends from the vagina to cover the external genitalia.

As with the male condom, the female condom must be inserted and removed with care to avoid breakage or accidental spillage of the contents. For best results, it should be removed immediately after intercourse.

Some of the advantages of the female condom are that it is sold over-the-counter in a standard size and is easy to use. Because it provides some protection against sexually transmitted diseases, its availability al-lows women to take a more aggressive role in protecting themselves from HIV and other sexually transmitted diseases. Some couples do not like inserting the female condom because they believe it destroys the spontaneity of sexual expression.

Because the female condom has been on the market for such a short time, there has not been much research on its effect on either partner's sensations and experience of sexual enjoyment. It is unknown whether the female condom increases the risk of toxic shock syndrome (TSS). Refer to Chapter 4, *Women's Health Care,* for information about TSS and the signs and symptoms of this syndrome. The Checklist, Condom Use, offers family teaching tips for healthy condom use.

Diaphragm

The diaphragm is a dome-shaped device made of plastic or rubber (latex) that fits snugly over the cervix to create a physical barrier between the ovum and any sperm that might be present. Diaphragms come in sizes ranging from 7 to 10 cm in diameter. The size and fit are determined and checked by a doctor, nurse midwife, or nurse practitioner during a pelvic examination.

Properly fitted diaphragms used correctly are effective in preventing pregnancy. The success rate of this

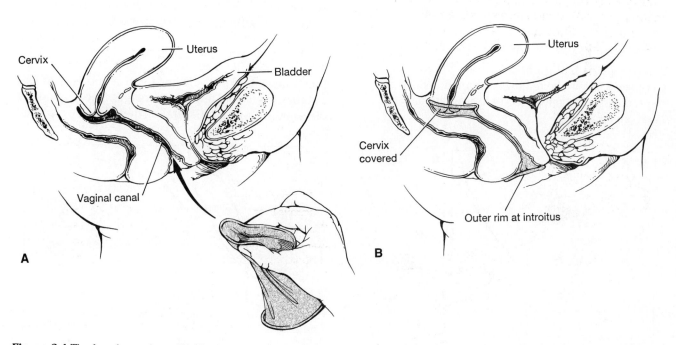

Figure 3-4. The female condom. (**A**) The flexible rim on the closed end of the condom (WPC-333) is grasped, and the condom inserted high in the vagina with the rim around the cervix. (**B**) When in place, the flexible rim at the open end of the condom is at the vaginal introitus.

✓ FAMILY TEACHING CHECKLIST

Condom Use

The nurse includes the following information in family teaching to promote health and well-being:

Male Condom:	rolled onto erect penis, while allowing room for semen; held against the base of the penis during insertion and withdrawal to prevent accidental dislodgment; care is taken to prevent accidental tearing or breaking of the condom
Advantages:	inexpensive; available over-the-counter; offers some protection against sexually transmitted diseases; disposable; when used in combination with spermicides or other barrier methods, rate of effectiveness reaches about 97%
Disadvantages:	when used singly may lead to decreased sensitivity to sexual stimulation; spontaneous intercourse may be interrupted
Female Condom:	fits into vagina, where it is anchored to the cervical os; covers vagina, cervix, and external genitalia; care must be taken to avoid breakage
Advantages:	offers some protection from sexually transmitted diseases; allows woman to control prophylaxis
Disadvantages:	spontaneous intercourse may be interrupted; unknown if sheath is associated with increased incidence of toxic shock syndrome

barrier method is enhanced by coating the inside of diaphragm and its rim with spermicidal cream or jelly before it is inserted.

The diaphragm can be inserted up to 6 hours before sexual intercourse (Fig. 3-5A). For best results, the diaphragm is left in place for 6 to 8 hours after intercourse. It should be removed, cleaned, refilled with the spermicide, and reinserted before additional acts of intercourse.

Proper care of the diaphragm includes checking it for rips and tears on a regular basis. It must also be cleaned and dried after each use to protect the rubber from deteriorating. It is important that no petroleum-based products be used on the diaphragm, because they can also lead to the breakdown of the rubber. Diaphragms are relatively inexpensive and easy to use, but they do have a few disadvantages. They cannot be obtained without a prescription, they must be replaced

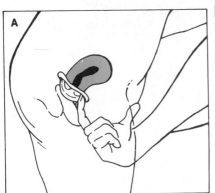 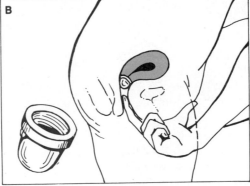 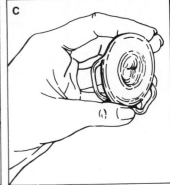

Figure 3-5. (*A*) *The diaphragm is a dome-shaped device that fits over the cervix and against the vaginal walls.* (*B*) *The cervical cap is a smaller cup-shaped version of the diaphragm, which has a stronger suction, tighter fit, and covers only the cervix.* (*C*) *The vaginal sponge provides both a physical and chemical barrier.*

every year, and a woman must be refitted for a new diaphragm after childbirth and after extreme weight changes. Some women consider inserting a diaphragm messy, and they dislike that it interferes with spontaneous sex. Other women are uncomfortable inserting the diaphragm because they do not like touching their genitals. The diaphragm is not recommended in women with a history of TSS (refer to Chapter 4).

Cervical Cap

The **cervical cap** is a rubber, cup-shaped appliance that, like the diaphragm, covers the cervix. The cap, which is held in place by natural suction (see Fig. 3-5B), is used with spermicides. It can be left in place for up to 48 hours, during which time sexual intercourse can take place repeatedly without reapplying spermicides. The cervical cap, like the diaphragm, is fitted by a health care provider. However, it may be more difficult to remove than the diaphragm because of the suction it creates. It is not recommended for use by women with a history of TSS.

Vaginal Sponge

The **vaginal sponge** is a pillow-shaped barrier contraceptive that is typically made of polyurethane. It is inserted into the vagina until it covers the cervical os. Most contraceptive sponges contain spermicides, which are activated when the sponge is moistened with water before insertion. The sponge should be left in place after intercourse for between 6 and 24 hours. It is available without prescription and designed to fit all women (see Fig. 3-5C). It is disposable after one use. Women who have a history of TSS (see Chapter 4) are discouraged from using the vaginal sponge.

Spermicides

Spermicides, chemical agents that kill sperm before they fertilize the ova, come in a variety of forms: creams, foams, jellies, films, and suppositories, all of which can be inserted in the vagina. Unfortunately, spermicides are minimally effective in preventing fertilization when used alone. Their effectiveness increases if they are used in combination with a condom or diaphragm.

To be effective, spermicides must be inserted high in the vagina, near the cervix. This can be accomplished by using the tamponlike plastic applicator that comes with the spermicide. Spermicides should be inserted no more than 30 minutes before intercourse, and they must be reapplied before each additional act of intercourse. Douching for hygienic purposes should not occur for at least 8 hours after the last intercourse.

Spermicidal agents are inexpensive and do not require a prescription. In addition, nonoxynol-9 and octoxynol have been shown to kill HIV and the human papillomavirus (HPV) under laboratory conditions. Couples may be inconvenienced by the need to apply spermicides before sexual activity begins. However, the chief disadvantages of spermicides are that they can cause allergic reactions, and they sometimes have unpleasant odors and tastes.

Intrauterine Device

The **intrauterine device** (IUD) is a flexible appliance made in a variety of shapes from a number of different materials. All of them are small enough to be inserted into the uterus through the cervix. Once inserted, the IUD creates a localized inflammation within the uterus, which prevents the fertilized ovum from implanting itself in the uterine wall. The most frequently used IUDs are the Progestasert and Copper-T 380. Figure 3-6 illustrates the placement and approximate size of an IUD.

Intrauterine devices are generally inserted in a health care facility during a pelvic examination. Before inserting the IUD, the physician, nurse midwife, or nurse practitioner determines whether the woman is an ideal candidate for the device. Women at risk for developing pelvic inflammatory disease (PID) (eg, those with multiple sexual partners) and women who have had problems previously with IUDs are not good candidates for the IUD. Because the IUD is inserted by a trained technician under sterile conditions, there is little risk of the woman's developing PID from insertion alone.

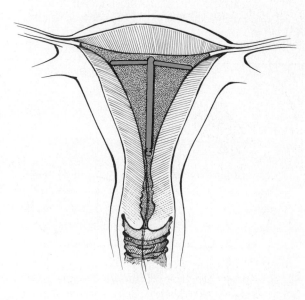

Figure 3-6. *The intrauterine device.*

During a pelvic exam, the IUD is guided through the vagina and cervix into the uterus. The woman may experience cramping and pain or pinching during insertion. This can be relieved by giving her a mild oral analgesic or muscle relaxant.

The tail (string) attached to the IUD can be used for periodically checking the placement of the device. It also is used by the health care provider for removing the device.

The IUD may become dislodged and be expelled, particularly during the first two to three menstrual cycles after insertion. The woman is encouraged to check placement of the device frequently during this time. Couples are encouraged to keep backup methods of contraception on hand in the event the IUD is expelled.

One of the the biggest advantages of the IUD is that it remains effective for up to 6 years, which allows the woman and her sexual partner to participate in spontaneous sexual activity. Some of its disadvantages include its association with the increased incidence of PID, the risk of uterine rupture, dysmenorrhea (painful menstruation), bleeding, and ectopic pregnancy (implantation of the fertilized ovum in the fallopian tube). The Checklist, Warning Signs for IUD Users, provides a family teaching list of warning signs for IUD users to report.

✔ FAMILY TEACHING CHECKLIST

Warning Signs for IUD Users

The nurse includes the following information in family teaching to promote health and well-being:

· Report any abnormal vaginal bleeding or discharge

· Keep a record of any delayed or missed periods and discuss with health care provider

· Report abdominal pain or cramps, with or without fever

· Consider any exposure to sexually transmitted diseases and discuss with health care provider

· Discuss any pain experienced during intercourse

· Report and seek health care if the tail (string) is missing

· Report any unexplained fever, shaking, chills

· Report backache not relieved by conventional measures

· See health care provider annually for monitoring of changes in the device

Hormonal Contraceptives

A variety of synthetic hormonal products are highly effective in preventing pregnancy. These hormonal contraceptives, which can be administered orally, as intramuscular injections, or implanted in the arm, work in one of several ways depending on their content.

Estrogen-based contraceptives suppress the secretion of follicle-stimulating hormone (FSH). This halts follicular development, which stops ovulation. Some hormonal contraceptives rely on progesteronelike synthetics (progestins) to suppress the secretion of luteinizing hormone (LH). Under these hormonal conditions, ovulation will not occur even if the follicle does manage to mature. Progestin also thickens cervical mucus (which makes it difficult for sperm to move through the female reproductive tract) and causes changes in the endometrial lining that make implantation of the fertilized ovum impossible. There are also oral contraceptives that combine progestins and estrogen.

Physicians, nurse midwives, or nurse practitioners usually prescribe the lowest possible blending of hormones to prevent ovulation. Table 3-2 describes the common side effects of synthetic hormones found in oral contraceptives. If indicated, higher doses can be prescribed as long as the woman does not experience harmful side effects (See *Disadvantages* below).

Hormones in oral contraceptives typically induce menstruation approximately 4 days after the last pill is taken. The monthly hormonal cycle begins again in a regular pattern under the influence of the synthetic oral hormones. All of the phases of the ovarian cycle occur as usual except for ovulation, which is inhibited.

Birth Control Pills

Oral contraceptives (commonly known as the "pill") are by far the most popular hormonal contraceptives. These pills are prepackaged in special cases for ease of dispensing. Each day's dose is labeled for easy identification. The woman is instructed to take one pill at the same time every day, beginning on day 1 of the menstrual cycle. She continues taking the oral contraceptive through day 21. On days 22 through 28, the woman is not required to take any oral contraceptive. However, some pill packages contain a round of placebo pills for days 22 through 28. Placebos are inactive substances given simply to make it easy for the woman to maintain the pattern of taking a pill every day at the same time. The level of hormones must be consistently maintained, so the woman must be sure not to miss even a single daily dose.

In the event the woman does miss a daily dose, she should take her pill as soon as she remembers the missed dose. If she misses two pills within the first 14

Table 3-2. *Common Hormonal Side Effects of Oral Contraceptives*

Estrogen		Progestin	
High Levels	Low Levels	High Levels	Low Levels
Nausea and vomiting	Amenorrhea	Acne	Menstrual flow increase
Edema	Hot flashes	Appetite increases	Spotting
Headaches	Nervousness	Depression	Delayed menses
Weight gain	Irritability	Weight gain	Weight loss
Fibroid enlargement	Lower sex drive	Hair loss	Dysmenorrhea
Hypertension	Spotting	Breast tenderness	
Lactation suppressed		Lower sex drive	
		Tiredness	

(handwritten annotation: Low Blood Flow)

days of her cycle, she should take the two pills she missed on the day she remembered and two pills the following day. If sexual intercourse is to take place within this period of reduced contraceptive effectiveness, the woman and her partner should use a backup contraceptive. The combination of spermicidal foam and condoms is recommended.

Advantages

If the pills are taken correctly, the estimated failure rate for oral contraceptives is approximately 3% to 4.5%. In addition to their high rate of effectiveness, oral contraceptives are convenient to use, and they do not interfere with spontaneous sexual expression.

Disadvantages

As with all contraceptive methods, there is a risk of pregnancy if the "pill" is not used correctly and consistently. For all its contraceptive benefits, the "pill" does not protect the woman from sexually transmitted diseases.

Because some women experience unpleasant side effects from the synthetic hormones in the pill, all women who are considering this method of contraception need to complete a thorough health history and physical examination. Side effects may include nausea and vomiting, weight loss or gain, abdominal cramping, bleeding outside the normal menstrual cycle, breast tenderness, headaches, swelling, hair loss, or mood changes.

Should a woman on the pill decide that she wishes to become pregnant, she is instructed to discontinue taking the pill. It may take 2 to 8 months for ovulation to return after the daily doses are discontinued. If ovulation does not return within this period, the clinician may prescribe hormonal therapy.

Contraindications

Not every woman is a good candidate for oral contraceptives. Those who smoke, are older than age 40, or nearing menopause are discouraged from taking birth control pills. Women with heart disease, hypertension, diabetes, and liver disease are also ineligible for hormonal contraceptives. Epilepsy, migraine headaches, and some types of cancer may be worsened by oral contraceptives.

Morning-After Pill

Morning-after pills contain high doses of one or more synthetic hormones that work by inhibiting implantation of the fertilized ovum in the uterine wall. These pills must be taken within 24 hours of coitus to be most effective.

The chief disadvantages of this method are that it is largely unavailable except in emergency situations such as rape; pregnancy may still occur even after the pill has been taken, and the drug may in fact cause fetal abnormalities if the woman is pregnant while taking the drug.

Mini Pill

The mini pill contains progestins only, which work by making implantation impossible. Some women prefer this type of oral contraceptive because the adverse effects of estrogen are eliminated. The mini pill is taken for the entire 28-day menstrual cycle and is considered very effective. (see Table 3-1 for a list of the common side effects of estrogen.) Family teaching information that draws attention to danger signs that may accompany oral contraceptive use are identified in the Family Teaching Checklist.

Norplant System

In 1991, the Food and Drug Administration approved the use of the Norplant system for use in the United States. Since then, this method of implanted hormonal contraception has become increasingly popular.

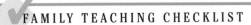

✔ FAMILY TEACHING CHECKLIST

Danger Signs That May Accompany Hormonal Contraceptive Use

The nurse includes the following information in family teaching to promote health and well-being:

· Report any unusual leg pain
· Contact health care provider for severe or recurring headaches
· Recognize and report any visual disturbances
· Notify health care provider immediately of any chest pain
· Report any signs of new weakness or loss of strength on either side of body
· Report dizziness or fainting spells
· Contact health care provider for unexplained nausea and vomiting
· Report problems and discontinue use with loss of hair and heavy vaginal bleeding outside of normal cycle

The Norplant system consists of a set of six capsules that slowly release levonorgestrel (a progestin) into the bloodstream. These "capsules" are actually thin, flexible tubes about the size of matchsticks. They are surgically inserted under the skin on the inside of the upper arm (Fig. 3-7).

Levonorgestrel prevents pregnancy by altering cervical mucus, making it inhospitable to sperm; preventing implantation; and in some cases by suppressing ovulation.

The Norplant system, which is very effective in preventing pregnancy, can be left in place for up to 5 years. Several of the benefits of using this system are that there are no estrogen side effects, the implants can be removed at any time, and there is no interference with the spontaneity of sexual expression. Despite its advantages, the Norplant system is not for everyone. Because the implants are inserted during a surgical procedure, there is the risk of infection. Since it is a hormonal therapy, there are potential side effects that make it an unacceptable contraceptive methods for some women. Some of the side effects include headaches, nausea, irregular menstrual cycles, increases or decreases in menstrual flow, and cervicitis (cervical inflammation). Norplant does not provide protection against sexually transmitted diseases.

Injectable Contraceptives

A woman can choose to receive intramuscular injections of Depo-Provera, a long-acting progestin, every 3 months. As with other hormonal contraceptives, Depo-Provera works through several mechanisms: it alters cervical mucus so that it becomes unreceptive to sperm, and it impairs ovulation and implantation.

The hormone injections are long-lasting and extremely effective in preventing pregnancy. There are, however, several important disadvantages to hormonal injection therapy. Some women may consider the injections themselves painful. Although the suppression of ovulation is reversible, it can take up to a year for normal ovulation to resume once the injections have been discontinued. The Food and Drug Administration is currently trying to determine whether the drug causes birth defects and maternal side effects.

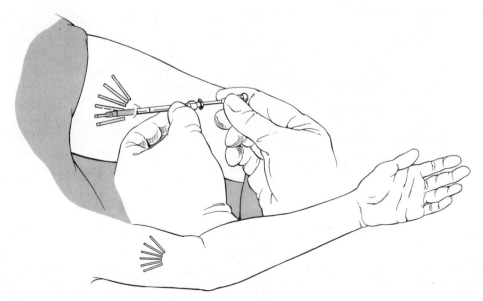

Figure 3-7. *The Norplant implant.*

This contraceptive method is not administered to women with breast cancer or abnormal vaginal bleeding.

Sterilization

Sterilization, which involves surgically altering the body so that it cannot reproduce, is a popular contraceptive choice among married couples 30 years or older who have finished with childbearing. Although some instances of male sterilization can be reversed with microsurgery, the permanent, irreversible nature of sterilization should be stressed.

Tubal ligation (tying of the tubes) is the usual method of sterilization in the woman. In the male, vasectomy (cutting and tying of the vas deferens) results in sterility.

Male Sterilization

A vasectomy is a surgical procedure in which the vas deferens, the tubes that carry sperm from the testes to the urethra, are cut and tied. The incisions are then sutured. This surgical procedure can be performed in an outpatient surgical center or office setting, under either local or general anesthesia. The nonabsorbable skin sutures used are removed in 7 to 10 days.

Typically, a small incision is made into each side of the scrotum. Each vas deferens is then located, pulled through the incision site, and cut and tied off (Fig. 3-8). A vasectomy does not alter male sexual function in any

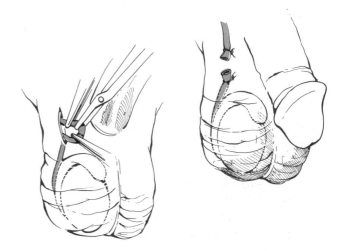

Figure 3-8. *Male sterilization. Vasectomy procedure. The vas deferens is located and cut.*

way. The man's sexual drive remains unchanged, and his testes still continue to produce sperm. But because the vas deferens have been cut, sperm are prevented from leaving the testes by traveling through the ductal system. These sperm are simply reabsorbed into the testes.

Because there are still sperm in the ductal system even after the vasectomy has been performed, additional contraception should be used until two consecutive sperm-free samples have been obtained.

Risks associated with vasectomy include pain, bleeding, and less frequently, postoperative infection.

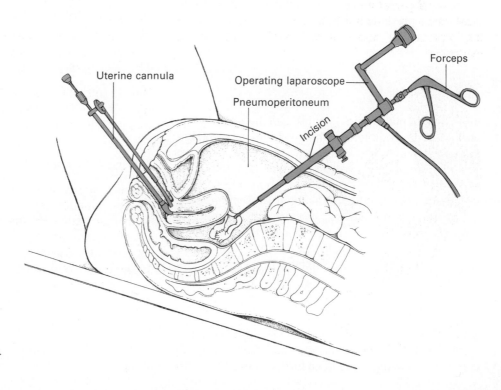

Uterine cannula

Forceps

Operating laparoscope

Pneumoperitoneum

Incision

Figure 3-9. *Female sterilization. Laparoscopic tubal ligation.*

Ice packs can be applied to the scrotum to reduce localized swelling for the first 24 hours. Scrotal support is recommended to reduce excessive tension and discomfort in the groin. Generally speaking, there are no restrictions on physical activities, with the exception of lifting heavy objects.

Female Sterilization

A tubal ligation, in which each fallopian tube is *ligated* or tied off, is the most common form of female sterilization. This procedure is most often performed with the aid of a laparoscope (an instrument that allows one to view the inside of the abdominal cavity). In Figure 3-9, the laparoscope also doubles as a surgical tool for ligating the tube.

A small incision is made through the umbilicus. The tubes are located and cut, tied, or clipped with an operating laparoscope. To increase the chances of reversing the procedure, the fallopian tubes can also be blocked with silicone plugs instead of ligated. Absorbable sutures are used to close the incision site after the procedure.

Side effects from this surgery include mild discomfort, infection, perforated bowel, and potential hemorrhage. Many pregnant women who desire tubal ligation often have the procedure performed during the postpartum period. The tubes are easily accessible during cesarean birth and may be ligated simultaneously with a planned abdominal birth.

Sterilization has the lowest failure rate of all the contraceptive methods currently available (Table 3-1). However, the irreversible nature of sterilization procedures may prevent individuals from seeking this option.

◆ Infertility

Infertility in males and females can be broadly described as the complete or limited ability to reproduce. Primary infertility is diagnosed when a pregnancy has never occurred after 1 year of unprotected intercourse. Secondary infertility is diagnosed when one successful pregnancy has occurred without subsequent pregnancy. There are a variety of causes of infertility. To pinpoint the potential causes of infertility, both partners have to provide detailed health and sexual histories and have a physical examination.

Male Infertility

Male infertility is the inability of the male partner to produce sufficient quantities of sperm that can successfully reach the ovum in the fallopian tubes. Ejaculatory problems, sperm abnormalities, or testicular causes may contribute to male infertility.

Ejaculation Problems

Premature ejaculation takes place shortly after sexual arousal. When this occurs, a large number of sperm may be lost before they are deposited within the vagina. There are a variety of techniques that can correct premature ejaculation, among them trying alternative positions for intercourse, receiving counseling, and performing various exercises such as squeezing the penis for a few seconds when near ejaculation.

Premature ejaculation may be a sign of a serious physical problem such as diabetes or prostate and urinary infections, so it is important that the man be examined.

Testicular Causes and Sperm Abnormalities

If the testes produce abnormally low levels of testosterone, it can affect spermatogenesis, resulting in a decrease in the production of sperm. If sperm production drops below 60 million per ejaculation, infertility is the result. The presence of a varicocele, or swelling of the spermatic cord, has been associated with increased vascular congestion and warmth of the scrotum, which leads to infertility.

Decreased sperm motility (the ability to move spontaneously) may prevent the sperm from reaching the ovum, and abnormally shaped sperm may contribute to infertility by failing to penetrate and fertilize the ovum. Nursing diagnoses related to family planning and infertility are provided in the Nursing Diagnoses Checklist.

Female Infertility

Female infertility may result from ovarian, tubal, uterine, cervical, and vaginal abnormalities, or any combination of these problems.

Ovarian Causes

Ovarian causes of infertility include failure of primary ovarian function, adhesions or excessive scar tissue formation, endometriosis, hypothyroidism, tumor of the pituitary, and endocrine problems. Hormone levels may be too low for the ovum to adequately mature. If progesterone production from the ovaries is limited, the endometrium of the uterus will not prepare for implantation. The woman may have anovulatory cycles (during which she does not release a mature ovum) even though the uterus prepares for implantation. Irregular ovulation can also be a factor in reduced fertility.

✓ NURSING DIAGNOSES CHECKLIST

Nursing Diagnoses Related to Family Planning and Infertility

· Anxiety, related to infertility

· Body Image Disturbance, related to varicocele

· Decisional Conflict, related to in vitro fertilization

· Altered Family Processes, related to inability to conceive

· Fear, related to invasive surgical procedure (laparoscopy)

· Hopelessness, related to infertility

· Ineffective Individual Coping, related to guilt associated with infertility

· Knowledge Deficit, related to available contraception options

· Sexual Dysfunction, related to use of barrier contraception

· Spiritual Distress, related to religious beliefs imposing on family planning

Tubal Abnormalities

Any condition that completely blocks the fallopian tubes or causes removal of the tubes (salpingectomy) makes it impossible for the mature ovum and sperm to unite. Congenital abnormalities and endometriosis associated with the buildup of scar tissue can block the passage of the tubes. Pelvic inflammatory disease, which is commonly associated with sexually transmitted diseases, often results in scarring within the fallopian tubes. It is also associated with the use of IUDs. A woman using an IUD who contracts a sexually transmitted disease is at great risk for developing PID.

Uterine Abnormalities

Uterine-related infertility can be the result of congenital abnormalities, fibroid tumors, scarring of the endometrium, and uterine infection. If progesterone levels decrease, the fertilized egg may travel to the uterus only to be unable to implant itself within the endometrium. Even if successful implantation occurs, the uterus may be unable to support and maintain the resulting pregnancy.

Cervical Causes

Cervical malformations, particularly scarring of the cervical opening (cervical os), may hinder the passage of

sperm. Likewise, if the cervical os dilates unexpectedly after fertilization has occurred, the conceptus (the products of conception) may be expelled from the uterus. Under these circumstances, the cervix is said to be incompetent to support the increasing weight of the growing fetus. Cervical mucus with a pH outside the normal range of 7.6 to 8.0 may contribute to infertility by inhibiting the sperms' passage or killing them off completely.

Vaginal Causes

Vaginal malformations may prevent sperm from entering the cervix and uterus. These abnormalities may be congenital or the result of adhesions from past surgeries and infections. Vaginal secretions that do not fall within the normal pH range endanger sperm survival by creating an environment in which they cannot survive.

Diagnosis of Infertility

In diagnosing the causes of infertility, both partners are assessed. Sexual and reproductive histories are taken, physical examinations are performed, and laboratory tests are run. Because approximately 60% of all infertility problems can be traced back to problems with the female's more complex reproductive system, women are generally tested more extensively than men in trying to determine the causes of infertility. Table 3-3 summarizes the variety of diagnostic tests used to diagnose infertility.

Treatment of Infertility

Treatment of infertility is based on the specific cause or causes. Couples need clear explanations of the options to make informed decisions about treatment.

Treatments range from noninvasive approaches to microsurgery. In the man, there is very little that can be done to treat sperm problems. There are, however, two types of artificial insemination techniques, each of which can be used to treat different types of sperm-related infertility homologous and heterologous. Concentrated specimens of the man's own sperm can be used for the homologous insemination of his female partner (see later discussion). If sperm abnormalities are genetically caused, the couple can explore the possibility of trying heterologous insemination, in which sperm is obtained from a donor. If male infertility is caused by varicoceles (enlargement of the veins of the spermatic cord), surgery can be performed to decrease venous congestion and scrotal warmth.

Complications caused by the ovaries' failure to release ova can be treated by prescribing medications that stimulate hormone release, which in turn promotes ovulation. Abnormal pH problems are usually corrected by

Table 3-3. *Male and Female Diagnostic Tests for Infertility*

Test	Purpose	Method
Hormone testing (women: prolactin, thyroid, adrenal, LH, FSH; men: LH, FSH, and testosterone)	To determine normal endocrine functioning	Blood Urine (LH, FSH)
Semen analysis	To determine normal sperm count, motility and morphology, and normal pH and viscosity of semen	Masturbated sperm sample
Menstrual cycle mapping	To determine normalcy of menstrual patterns over 6-month period; to track ovulatory and anovulatory cycles	Basal body temperature
Cervical mucus evaluation	To determine qualities of cervical mucus, which reflect normal functioning: elasticity (spinnbarkheit), presence of cells, debris, organisms	Cervical mucus
Postcoital test (women)	To test receptivity of cervical mucus to sperm penetration	Cervical mucus (1–2 days before ovulation) immediately after intercourse
Endometrial biopsy	To determine if cyclic development of endometrium is normal	Suction biopsy of uterine lining
Hysterosalpingogram	To determine if fallopian tubes are patent	Injection of radiopaque dye through cervix, with serial x-rays to track dye through cervix, uterus, and tubes
Laparoscopy	To permit direct observation of ovaries, tubes, and uterus	Insertion of lighted scope into abdomen under general anesthesia

FSH, follicle-stimulating hormone; LH, luteinizing hormone.

using douches to stabilize vaginal pH. Directly treating the causes of inflammation within the female reproductive system may allow the fertilized egg to pass through the fallopian tubes down to a welcoming uterine environment. An incompetent cervix may be surgically repaired so that the uterus can maintain the pregnancy until the fetus can survive outside the uterus.

In vitro fertilization (IVF), the process in which ova are fertilized outside of the body and redeposited in the uterus, is another option for treating infertility. Couples considering IVF may experience doubt, failure, and guilt. A complete explanation of the procedure, including its advantages and disadvantages, must be given. This should include discussing the risk of multiple and ectopic pregnancies. Couples should be warned that repeated procedures may be required because there is only a 10% to 19% chance of a viable pregnancy resulting from IVF. Additionally, the high price of IVF makes it unaffordable for many couples.

Adolescent Considerations

As sexual activity among young persons increases, so does the need for increasing their awareness and knowledge of the contraceptive methods available to them. For many adolescents, education on the availability and use of safe and effective contraception is obtained in school and local clinics and health centers. These places provide confidential counseling and testing for pregnancy, HIV, and other sexually transmitted diseases. Even so, many adolescents fail to take advantage of the information and services available to them until they have tested positive for pregnancy or a sexually transmitted disease. Nurses can have a positive impact on the long-term health of the adolescents in their care by teaching them the benefits of practicing responsible sexuality, which is designed to preserve their own as well as their partners' reproductive health. The more adolescents understand about their role in protecting the health of their reproductive systems, the more responsibility they are likely to take for maintaining it.

Cultural Considerations

There are many religious and cultural beliefs that influence the individual's preference for various methods of fertility management. For example, Roman Catholics may follow strict church teaching, which prohibits the practice of artificial contraception, promotes the use of natural family planning, and considers abortion a mortal sin. Mormons may choose not to practice contraception as a means of showing their spiritual commitment to increasing the size of the church's congregation. Women of many cultures (eg, Bahamian, Cuban, and Puerto Rican) are uncomfortable using hormonal and intrauterine contraception because they alter the monthly menstrual cycle. Native American women, however, believe that menstrual blood flow keeps the body in harmony. As a result, they may choose the IUD because it is associated with increased blood flow. The use of the IUD may, however, be rejected by women who have religious or cultural objections to the way in which it works (ie, preventing implantation by making the uterus "reject" the fertilized ovum).

Nurses need to be sensitive to these and other culturally determined beliefs about contraception. This is particularly important in dealing with minorities, who may believe that the effort to get them to adopt family planning or contraception is a racist plot to limit the growth of the nonwhite population in the United States.

Nurses who are aware of the cultural contexts in which contraceptive decisions are made are better able to address the individual's concerns about the appropriateness and effectiveness of the various contraceptive methods available to them.

The Role of the Nurse

Nurses can have a positive impact on the ways in which couples approach family planning. By providing accurate information about the benefits and risks associated with the available methods of birth control, including explaining failure rates and presenting acceptable alternatives, nurses can help couples to control their reproductive destinies.

Nurses also can help infertile couples cope with the feelings of disappointment and loss that come along with the diagnosis of infertility. The care and understanding displayed by nurses may ultimately involve helping the infertile couple to accept their inability to bear children.

REVIEW AND PREVIEW

In this chapter, two different challenges to fertility were discussed: contraception and infertility. The wide variety of contraceptive methods available today were described in terms of their effectiveness in controlling fertility, including the advantages and disadvantages of each. Wherever necessary, valuable information on contraindications were included. By gaining a solid understanding of the available methods of contraception, nurses can effectively counsel and teach individuals about their proper use.

Technologic advances in obstetric and gynecologic care have made it possible to diagnose and treat the causes of male and female infertility. Even so, infertility is a uniquely stressful situation for couples. Nurses need to provide families with opportunities for expressing their feelings of frustration and grief.

The next chapter discusses women's health care. Emphasis is placed on health promotion, including monthly self-evaluation for normal and abnormal findings in the breasts. The ever-present problem of sexually transmitted diseases is presented with information about how to reduce the risks of contracting each disease.

⊙ KEY POINTS

- ◆ Fertility is broadly defined as the ability to reproduce. In the female, fertility is the ability to conceive, support, sustain, and give birth to offspring. Fertility in the male is defined by the ability to produce sufficient quantities of healthy sperm capable of penetrating an ovum. Infertility is defined as the inability to successfully achieve desired fertilization after

12 months of regular, unprotected sexual intercourse. Family planning methods allow couples to actively prevent or enhance fertilization.

- ◆ Contraceptive methods are chosen based on a variety of factors, including cultural and religious affiliations, sexual behaviors, desire for spontaneity, cost, effectiveness, availability, side effects, and user acceptance.
- ◆ Neither coitus interruptus nor vaginal douching is a reliable method of preventing conception. Coitus interruptus is ineffective because small amounts of preejaculatory seminal fluid may be released into the vagina before ejaculation. This fluid may contain enough viable sperm to result in fertilization. Douching is ineffective because the sperms' movement toward the ovum generally outpaces the douche solution.
- ◆ Natural family planning includes closely monitoring BBT, tracking menstrual cycles to determine ovulation based on mucus characteristics, and maintaining personal records of sexual and ovulatory activities.
- ◆ Spermicides may be used with barrier devices to enhance their effectiveness. Condoms can prevent conception and reduce the risk of acquiring sexually transmitted diseases. Latex varieties also protect against the transmission of HIV.
- ◆ Implants, intrauterine devices, and sterilization are all highly effective means of contraception. Each method is easy to use, offers a high degree of protection from fertilization, and allows partners to participate in spontaneous sexual behavior. Some of the shared disadvantages of these methods include the need to consult a physician and undergo a procedure, and the potential for infection. Sterilization is often rejected because of the irreversible nature of the procedure.

◆ SELF-ASSESSMENT

1. Inadequate amounts of which hormone can prevent implantation of a fertilized ovum?

○ **A.** Estrogen
○ **B.** Progesterone
○ **C.** Prolactin
○ **D.** Follicle stimulating hormone

2. How would you advise a woman who forgot to take one birth control pill yesterday?

○ **A.** Forget that pill and continue the pack as prescribed
○ **B.** Take a "morning after" pill for the next 3 days
○ **C.** Take 2 pills that day and continue the pack as prescribed
○ **D.** Do not complete the pack and use another method of contraception

3. Which of the following factors is least likely to cause male infertility?

○ **A.** Sperm count
○ **B.** Sperm motility
○ **C.** Man's age
○ **D.** Presence of a varicocele

4. By what action does an intrauterine devices (IUD) prevent pregnancy?

○ **A.** Preventing ovulation
○ **B.** Decreasing production of estrogen and progesterone
○ **C.** Creating a physical barrier to sperm
○ **D.** Preventing implantation

5. Which contraceptive method is safest for a woman with a history of toxic shock syndrome (TSS)?

○ **A.** Female condom
○ **B.** Cervical cap
○ **C.** Diaphragm
○ **D.** Vaginal sponge

◆ Oral contraceptives are highly effective in preventing pregnancy when taken consistently for the prescribed period. A woman who complains of headaches or has an elevated blood pressure should stop taking the pill. Its use is contraindicated in women with existing medical conditions that could increase in severity.

◆ Male infertility is the result of either testicular or ejaculatory problems. Sperm abnormalities also may prevent the male from impregnating his female partner.

◆ Female infertility can be caused by ovarian, tubal, uterine, cervical, or vaginal abnormalities. Hormonal dysfunction is associated with anovulatory cycles and the prevention of implantation.

◆ Samples of semen, cervical mucus, and endometrial tissue are tested when infertility is suspected. Some of the infertility treatment options currently available include donor sperm and IVF.

BIBLIOGRAPHY

Amar, L. (1991). Male infertility. In C. Garner (Ed.), *Principles of infertility nursing.* Boca Raton, FL: CRC Press.

Blenner, J. (1991). Health care providers' treatment approaches to culturally diverse infertile patients. *Journal of Transcultural Nursing, 2*(2), 24–27.

Boyle, J. S., & Andrews, M. M. (1990). *Transcultural concepts in nursing care* (1st ed.). Philadelphia: J.B. Lippincott.

Davis, D., & Dearman, C. (1991). Coping strategies of infertile women. *Journal of Obstetric, Gynecologic, and Neonatal Nursing, 20*(3), 221–224.

Enmans, J. (1992). Teens and contraception: Encouraging compliance. *Contraception Report, 11*(6), 4–7.

Franklin, M. (1990). Recently approved and experimental methods of contraception. *Journal of Nurse Midwifery, 35*(6), 365–376.

Hahn, S. (1992). Caring for couples considering alternatives in family building. In C. Garner (Ed.), *Principles of infertility nursing.* Boca Raton, FL: CRC Press.

Kelley, K. F., Galbraith, M. A., & Vermund, S. H. (1992). Genital human papillomavirus infection in women. *Journal of Obstetric, Gynecological, and Neonatal Nursing, 21*(6), 503–516.

King, J. (1992). Helping patients choose an appropriate method of birth control. *American Journal of Maternal Child Nursing, 17*(2), 91–100.

Lommel, L., & Taylor, D. (1992). Adolescent use of contraceptives. *NAACOG Clinical Issues in Perinatal and Women's Health Nursing, 3*(2), 199–208.

Low, M. (1992). Personal values and contraceptive choices. *NAACOG Clinical Issues in Perinatal and Women's Health Nursing, 3*(2), 192–198.

May, K. A., & Mahlmeister, L. R. (1994). *Maternal & neonatal nursing: Family-centered care* (3rd ed.). Philadelphia: J.B. Lippincott.

Reeder, S. J., Martin, L. L., & Koniak, D. (1992). *Maternity nursing: Family, newborn, and women's health care* (17th ed.). Philadelphia: J.B. Lippincott.

Sharts-Engel, N. (1991). Levonorgestrel subdermal implants (NORPLANT) for long-term contraception. *American Journal of Maternal Child Nursing, 16*(4), 232–236.

Taymor, M. (1990). *Infertility: A Clinician's Guide to Diagnosis and Treatment.* New York: Plenum Publishing.

Tillman, J. (1992). An old disease: A contemporary perinatal problem. *Journal of Obstetric, Gynecologic, and Neonatal Nursing, 21*(3), 209–213.

CHAPTER 4
Women's Health Care

◈ OBJECTIVES

When the learning goals of this chapter are met, the reader will be able to:

◆ Explain the frequency, purpose, and normal findings of the pelvic examination and Papanicolaou test.

◆ Describe the importance of performing monthly breast self-examinations to detect breast changes.

◆ Discuss endometriosis, including its symptoms, possible causes, the sites where it commonly occurs, and available treatment options.

◆ Identify the most common sexually transmitted diseases, including human immunodeficiency virus (HIV), and discuss the ways in which they are transmitted, treated, and prevented.

◆ Discuss the normal physiologic changes a woman experiences during aging, with particular emphasis on menopause.

TERMINOLOGY

Acquired immunodeficiency
  syndrome

Amenorrhea

Chlamydial infection

Dysmenorrhea ⌣

Endometriosis

Fibrocystic breast disease

Gonorrhea

Human immunodeficiency virus

Menopause

Menorrhagia ⌣

Metrorrhagia ⌣

Papanicolaou smear

Premenstrual syndrome

Syphilis

Toxic shock syndrome

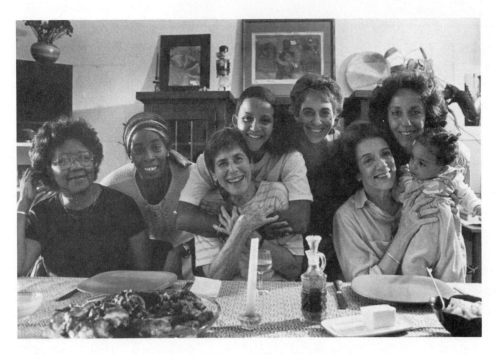

Figure 4-1. *Women's health care needs change throughout the lifespan and require special attention for disease prevention and health management. (Photo © Kathy Sloane)*

Awoman's health care needs change throughout the course of her life. Indeed, the reproductive health issues that concern a woman during adolescence and the reproductive years differ significantly from those that concern her during menopause (Fig. 4-1).

This chapter addresses a wide range of reproductive topics, including gynecologic assessment, menstrual disorders, pelvic infections, sexually transmitted diseases, and menopause. Important information on the detection, diagnosis, and treatment of breast cancer is also given.

Gynecologic Assessment

Because the female reproductive system is made up of a complex network of organs and hormones, it must be evaluated frequently to make sure that it is functioning properly. During a gynecologic examination, the health care provider takes the woman's health and reproductive histories, after which physical, breast, and pelvic examinations are performed. These examinations are important for several reasons: they allow the health care provider to determine whether there are any gynecologic problems; they can help diagnose or confirm pregnancy; and they often lead to the early detection and treatment of abnormal conditions, which reduces the risk of future problems.

Breast Examination

During a routine gynecologic examination, the health care provider typically assesses the breasts for any ab-

normalities (see the section entitled *Breast Cancer* for more information). Nurses can promote excellent self-care practices by instructing women in the proper breast self-examination techniques.

Breast Self-Examination

Breast self-examination (BSE) should become part of every woman's routine self-care. This self-assessment is easy and takes no more than 10 or 15 minutes each month. This small investment of time can actually save a life. It has been shown that the breast cancer survival rate increases to 90% if cancer is detected early and properly treated.

Instructions for how to perform BSE include pointers on visually inspecting the breasts as well as palpating them (examining them by touch), both in the shower and lying down. Display 4-1 provides teaching considerations and key points for education on BSEs. The nurse explains the appropriate techniques and observes a retuDrn demonstration by the woman.

Pelvic Examination

During a pelvic examination, the health care provider examines first the external genitalia and then the internal genitalia for growths, lesions, and other abnormalities. A special instrument called a speculum is inserted vaginally to make the visual examination of the vagina and cervix possible (Fig. 4-2). It also allows the health care provider to scrape tissue samples from the cervix (and possibly the

DISPLAY 4-1
Procedure for Performing Breast Self-Examination

· Perform once a month, about 1 week after the first day of the menstrual period. This is an ideal time to feel the actual consistency of breast tissue because there is none of the swelling associated with the hormonal changes that accompany menstruation. Women who do not menstruate (eg, postmenopausal women) can select any other, easy-to-remember date.

· Inspect the breasts while looking in a mirror with your hands at your sides. Look for any noticeable dimpling, swelling, or asymmetry in the breasts. Squeeze the nipple and note any discharge. A clear, milky discharge may be associated with the use of certain drugs (eg, antidepressants, tranquilizers, and oral contraceptives), increased levels of prolactin, or a pituitary tumor. Repeat this procedure with the arms raised over the head and a third time with the hands on the hips.

· While showering, lather the breasts so that they feel smooth and soapy. With one hand raised behind your neck, examine each breast with your free hand. Use the flat part of your free hand and gently feel the entire breast for any lumps or cysts. Start at the nipple and work outward to the outermost areas of the breast. Follow in a clockwise direction and include the axilla (underarm) area. Repeat the procedure for the other breast.

· After showering, lie down and place one hand behind the head. Place a pillow under the shoulder of the breast you are about to examine. Follow the procedure you performed in the shower to locate any abnormalities or changes in the breast.

· Report any unusual lumps, dimpling, thickening of the skin, or discharge to your health care provider.

From May, K. A., & Mahlmeister, L. R. (1994). *Maternal & neonatal nursing: Family-centered care (3rd ed)*. Philadelphia: J.B. Lippincott, p. 100.

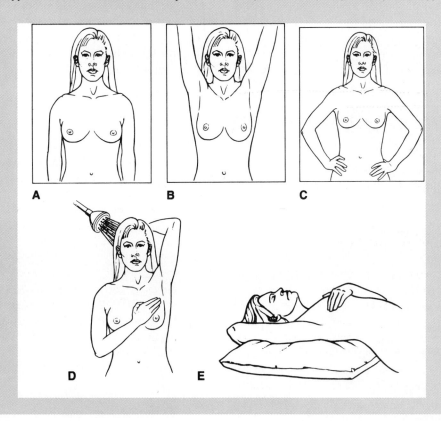

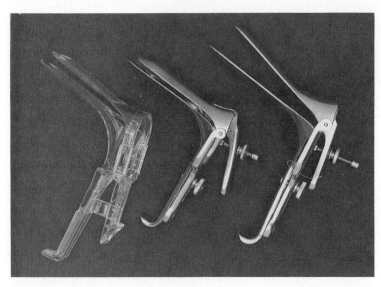

Figure 4-2. *Vaginal specula. The speculum may be made of either reusable metal or disposable plastic and is available in a variety of sizes.*

vagina) for a Papanicolaou (Pap) smear. The clinician then palpates the internal organs for abnormalities by placing several fingers of one hand within the vagina and the other hand on the abdominal wall. (See Nursing Procedure, Pelvic Examination, for a detailed description of how the examination is performed.)

The pelvic examination of a healthy, nonpregnant woman typically shows moist, pink vaginal and cervical membranes. The cervix is closed. The surfaces of the uterus and the ovaries are smooth and free of growths and abnormalities. Some of the changes in the reproductive tract that are detected during a pelvic examination can be used to confirm pregnancy. These changes include a softening and enlargement of the cervix and

uterus and a purple discoloration of the vagina. See Chapter 5, *Signs and Symptoms of Pregnancy.* Visible or palpable tumors, cysts, and other abnormalities of the vagina, cervix, uterus, and related organs require further examination and treatment. See the Assessment Checklist for a checklist of pelvic examination findings in the nonpregnant woman.

Papanicolaou Smear

A **Papanicolaou (Pap) smear** is a laboratory test used for the early detection of cancer cells in tissue samples taken from the cervix during a routine pelvic examina-

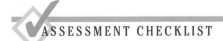

✓ ASSESSMENT CHECKLIST

Pelvic Examination Findings in Nonpregnant Women

Normal Findings

Pink, moist vaginal and cervical membranes

Closed cervical os

Smooth uterine surface

Palpable fallopian tubes and ovaries

No growths or abnormalities

Abnormal Findings

Dry, rough mucus membranes

Nonsmooth uterine surface

Difficulty palpating ovaries

Growths or abnormalities present

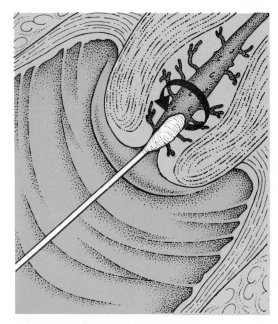

Figure 4-3. *Obtaining the Pap smear with a cotton swab.*

Pelvic Examination, Including Pap Smear and Bimanual Examination

PURPOSE: To rule out existing gynecologic problems, confirm pregnancy, reduce the risk of future complications

EQUIPMENT: Speculum, gloves, lubricant, swab or spatula, slide, fixative, adequate lighting, privacy drapes, special examination table with stirrups

Action	Rationale
Explain the purpose and steps of the procedure to the woman.	Understanding the procedure will reduce the woman's anxiety, and verbal support from the nurse will allow her to relax.
Ask her to empty her bladder.	Emptying the bladder promotes comfort and allows for the accurate manual assessment of the pelvic organs.
Give the woman privacy so that she may change into an examination gown.	Privacy and dignity are maintained.
Assist the woman into the lithotomy position (patient is on her back with the thighs flexed on the abdomen and the lower legs flexed on the thighs).	The lithotomy position allows for easier examination of the genitals and cervix.
Drape her properly when the exam begins.	Using the drape provides privacy and lessens the embarrassment felt by the patient on assuming the lithotomy position.
Stay with her throughout the procedure.	The presence of the nurse may reduce the patient's anxiety.
The examination progresses through the following stages:	
Visual inspection of external genitalia	The examiner inspects the vagina and cervix for lesions before inserting the speculum, thereby avoiding further damaging the tissue if lesions are present.
Insertion of unlubricated speculum (warm water may be used to ease insertion of speculum), visual examination of internal structures	Lubricants would interact with cells obtained for culture and cause inaccurate results.
Obtaining cell samples for a Pap smear, putting the cell specimen on a slide and spraying it with fixative	Applying fixative immediately preserves the cells for miscroscopic examination.
Performing bimanual palpation, with lubricant, if necessary	
Insertion of finger in rectum for digital-rectal examination	Digital-rectal examination sometimes necessary to better feel uterine outline.
The woman is encouraged to sit up and dress immediately after the exam.	The lithotomy position is uncomfortable, and the woman will prefer discussing the findings with the health care provider in a less vulnerable position.
A towelette is provided for the woman.	The lubricant is easily wiped off the genitalia by the woman to promote comfort.

tion. The cervical cells are collected by scraping a cotton swab or special spatula gently across the cervix (Fig. 4-3). They are then placed on a slide, sprayed with a fixative, stained, and examined by a laboratory technician for abnormalities. This test is usually accurate, but the incidence of false-negative results (when the Pap smear indicates no cellular abnormalities even though they are present) is approximately 15%.

There are a number of things that can be done to reduce the chances of obtaining a false-negative result. The woman needs to wait until her menstrual flow has stopped before having the Pap smear taken. Additionally, she refrains from douching before the pelvic exam-

ination. The health care provider ensures the accuracy of laboratory tests by not using a lubricant on the speculum (warm water may be used to ease its insertion), wiping away any vaginal discharge before the sample is taken, and spraying the slide immediately with the appropriate fixative.

The classification of Pap smear test results varies among doctors and laboratory technicians. Some commonly used terms include:

Normal: no abnormal cells found

Atypical or Inflammatory: presence of abnormal cells that are probably from a vaginal infection

Cervical Intraepithelial Neoplasia (CIN): evidence of abnormal, possibly precancerous cells (cervical dysplasia); classified according to degree of dysplasia (I, mild; II, moderate; III, severe)

Invasive Cancer: presence of actual cancer cells

Cervical cancer is considered to be highly treatable when diagnosed early. To promote the early detection of cancerous and precancerous conditions, the American College of Obstetricians and Gynecologists and the American Cancer Society recommend that all women older than age 18 have annual pelvic examinations and Pap smears, whether or not they are sexually active. There are several important exceptions to this rule: Sexually active women of *all* ages should be examined annually; women whose mothers took diethylstilbestrol (DES) during pregnancy need to be examined annually beginning at age 14; and because women who have been infected with human papillomavirus (HPV) may be at increased risk for developing cervical and vaginal cancers, they are advised to have Pap smears every 6 months. For the nursing procedure for a pelvic examination, including a Pap smear and bimanual examination, see the Nursing Procedure.

Major Gynecologic Health Concerns

Women's health care addresses a broad range of concerns, including fibrocystic disease and breast cancer, two commonly occurring conditions of the female breasts; menstrual disorders; pelvic infections, both those that cause treatable discomforts and those that can lead to irreversible infertility; preventing, diagnosing, and treating sexually transmitted diseases; and menopause.

Breast Conditions

The female's breasts change in response to the hormonal fluctuations associated with menstruation, fertilization, and lactation. In cases in which the woman is diagnosed with fibrocystic breast disease, palpable lumps in the breast increase in pain and tenderness as the menstrual cycle approaches. Although fibrocystic breast disease is often benign (not cancerous), women who have it are 2 to 5 times more likely to develop breast cancer than are those who do not have it.

Fibrocystic Breast Disease

Fibrocystic breast disease is the most common benign breast condition found in women. It typically occurs in women between the ages of 35 and 50.

Hormonal imbalances of progesterone and estrogen may be the cause of the irregularities in the breast tissue. Fibroid cysts are often felt on the surface of the breast, usually in the upper, outer quadrant. These cysts are smooth, round, fluid filled, and freely movable. It should be noted that cancerous growths do not move about freely and are generally not tender to the touch.

Just before menstruation, women with fibrocystic breast disease frequently complain of breast tenderness and pain. Mild pain relievers may help reduce the tenderness and swelling. Some women find that eliminating caffeine from their diet relieves symptoms. Some women also report a relief of symptoms after taking 400 to 600 IU vitamin E.

Treatment consists of monitoring the disease's progress by performing monthly BSEs and undergoing annual mammograms. If a cyst is unusually uncomfortable, a needle may be inserted into it to aspirate (draw off) the fluid contained in it. Because fibrocystic breast disease is associated with an increased risk for breast cancer, it is important that routine BSEs be performed regularly.

Breast Cancer

Breast cancer is the most frequently occurring form of cancer in women in the United States today. It is estimated that 1 woman in 10 will develop breast cancer in her lifetime. Although men also develop breast cancer, it is a much less common occurrence. Only about 1000 men per year are diagnosed with the disease. The difference in breast cancer rates between the sexes is thought to be related to the female hormones.

The American Cancer Society recommends that routine, monthly BSEs and annual mammograms begin sometime between the ages of 35 and 40 years of age. The mammogram is a painless, low-risk x-ray used to detect masses and tissue changes in the breasts. At the time of the mammogram, a qualified clinician also will perform a manual breast examination. If a lump or mass is identified, it is aspirated with a needle or a biopsy is performed. To perform a biopsy, a small tissue sample is cut from the breast and examined under the microscope for precancerous and cancerous cells. See the Family Teaching Checklist for a variety of risk factors for developing breast cancer.

Treatment for breast cancer generally consists of a combination of surgery, chemotherapy, and radiation therapy. Hormone therapy may also be prescribed. Surgical options may include removal of the lump (lumpectomy), removal of a portion of the breast (partial mastectomy), removal of the entire breast and surrounding lymph nodes, pectoral muscles, and involved skin (radical mastectomy).

✔ FAMILY TEACHING CHECKLIST

Risk Factors for Developing Breast Cancer

· Delaying childbirth until after the age of 35
· Onset of menarche before the age of 12
· Menopause beginning after age 59
· Previous history of breast cancer in one breast
· Mother or maternal relatives having a history of breast cancer
· Diets high in fat and protein
· Excessive weight gains
· Stress

Chemotherapy, with or without radiation therapy, is commonly prescribed. Chemotherapeutic agents are given to the patient to stop or contain the spread of cancerous growths. They also reduce the recurrence of cancer and improve the woman's overall chances of survival.

Menstrual Disorders

Menstrual disorders occur rather frequently. Many women believe that the discomforts associated with their monthly menstrual cycle are normal. They simply change their behaviors to help them cope with the physical pain and emotional upsets. Other women suffer from menstrual disorders that are severe enough to require treatment.

The common menstrual disorders include premenstrual syndrome, dysmenorrhea, amenorrhea, menorrhagia, metrorrhagia, and endometriosis.

Premenstrual Syndrome

Premenstrual syndrome (PMS) is a recurring syndrome marked by a variety of physical and emotional discomforts such as irritability, moodiness, anxiety, depression, breast tenderness, headache, fluid retention, acne, and gastrointestinal upset. Some women also crave specific foods during this period (eg, sweet or salty foods). Symptoms begin several days before menstruation starts and generally end a few days after the onset of bleeding.

The cause of premenstrual syndrome is still a mystery. It is commonly believed to be tied to the changes in estrogen and progesterone levels that occur during the luteal phase of the ovarian cycle. Alcohol, fatigue, and caffeine are sometimes known to intensify the symptoms.

Nurses can encourage women who experience premenstrual syndrome to reduce stress and avoid activities that trigger fatigue and worsen the symptoms. Reducing sodium, caffeine, and alcohol intake may help. Because water and fruits act as natural diuretics, it is recommended that the woman eat them to rid the body of excess fluid. Physical exercise often relieves tension and elevates the level of serum endorphins, the body's natural pain killers. Mild analgesics (such as aspirin, acetaminophen, and ibuprofen) can be taken to relieve the physical symptoms of premenstrual syndrome.

Dysmenorrhea

Most women experience some degree of discomfort during menstruation, but for approximately 10% of them the pain is severe enough to require treatment. **Dysmenorrhea,** or painful menstruation, may be either primary (beginning just before the onset of menstruation and disappearing once the individual experiences childbirth) or secondary (which is associated with pelvic inflammatory disease, intrauterine device [IUD] use, endometriosis, or fertility problems).

Although the cause of this disorder is not known, it is believed to be related to the elevated levels of prostaglandins. Prostaglandins are unsaturated fatty acids that influence several functions in the body, including fluid balance, blood flow, gastrointestinal activity, and the return of the corpus luteum to its pre-ovulatory state. (See Chapter 2 for a discussion of the role of the corpus luteum in the ovarian cycle.) Prostaglandins also increase the uterus's ability to contract, which gives rise to cramps.

Diagnosis of dysmenorrhea is made during the beginning of menstruation. Lower abdominal cramping (which is sometimes described as "laborlike") is assessed for intensity, frequency, and duration. If the pain is severe and accompanies most menstrual cycles, the health care provider prescribes treatment for the condition.

Dysmenorrhea is often treated with a combination of oral contraceptive therapy and nonsteroidal anti-inflammatory drugs (NSAIDs) including aspirin and ibuprofen. These pain relievers are commonly prescribed 3 to 4 times a day for the first few days of menstruation. These pain relievers should be taken with milk or food to reduce stomach upset.

Amenorrhea

Amenorrhea is the absence or suppression of menstruation that is not associated with puberty, pregnancy, lactation, or menopause. There are several factors that can cause this condition. They include congenital abnormalities of the reproductive system; metabolic disorders such as diabetes, obesity, and malnutrition; syphilis; endocrine disorders that involve the ovaries, pituitary, thyroid, and adrenal glands; and hormonal imbalances of estrogen, progesterone, and follicle-stimulating hormone. Long-term strenuous exercise, low body fat, and emotional stress are also associated with amenorrhea.

Treatment of amenorrhea varies depending on the underlying cause. Counseling and education by the nurse help the woman to adopt healthful habits that can correct some types of amenorrhea. If specific, specialized treatment of the disorder is necessary, the nurse can refer the woman to appropriate health care providers.

Menorrhagia

Menorrhagia refers to excessive menstrual bleeding, either in amount or duration. Blood loss may be great enough to reach hemorrhagic levels, which is a life-threatening condition. Menorrhagia can be caused by endocrine gland disturbances of the pituitary, thyroid, or ovaries; uterine fibroid tumors; diseases of the endometrium; cervical polyps (usually benign tumors); infection; hypertension; diabetes; and hemolytic diseases (those that cause breakdown of red blood cells).

Treatment of menorrhagia depends on the underlying cause, but its primary goal is to control the bleeding. It may be necessary to perform surgery to remove the uterus (hysterectomy) to prevent hemorrhage and shock.

Metrorrhagia

Metrorrhagia ("breakthrough bleeding") is uterine bleeding that occurs outside the usual menstrual period. It often occurs in women taking oral contraceptives. Metrorrhagia may also be caused by uterine or cervical infection, uterine cancer, or low levels of progesterone.

Treatment of metrorrhagia is begun as soon as possible. If cancer is detected, early diagnosis and treatment decrease the chances that it will spread.

Endometriosis

Endometriosis occurs when endometrial cells, which normally line the uterus, travel outside the uterus and attach themselves to other organs and tissues. The most common sites for endometriosis are the ovaries, uterine ligaments, peritoneum (the membrane that lines the abdominal cavity), and the abdominal wall. Endometrial cells still respond to the hormonal changes of the ovarian cycle by growing in preparation for the implantation of the ovum, even though they have trav-

eled outside the uterus. This results in dysmenorrhea, painful intercourse, and pelvic pain.

Endometriosis is treated with hormonal therapy, surgery, or a combination of the two. Oral contraceptives or androgens (male hormones) may be given to suppress ovarian function. Many health care providers prescribe NSAIDs to relieve the symptoms of this disorder. Surgical intervention is also an option. Women who would like to get pregnant in the future may choose to have a laparoscopy to remove adhesions and stray endometrial cells. Women who do not wish to have children may choose to have a hysterectomy. They also may decide to have a bilateral salpingo-oophorectomy (an operation in which both fallopian tubes and ovaries are removed).

Pelvic Infections

Pelvic infections range from the uncomfortable and inconvenient to those that can cause sterility or death. Vaginitis, urinary tract infections (UTIs), pelvic inflammatory disease (PID), and toxic shock syndrome (TSS) are the pelvic infections discussed in this section.

Vaginitis

Vaginitis (inflammation of the vagina) is a fairly common problem among women. Its symptoms are increased vaginal discharge (which may have a bad odor or contain blood), irritation and itching of the vulva and perineum, and frequent or painful urination. There are a number of causes of vaginitis, including use of oral antibiotics, wearing tight clothing or synthetic undergarments, overuse of bubble baths or douche products, infection with microorganisms such as those that cause sexually transmitted diseases, poor hygiene, vitamin deficiency, and yeast infections. Pregnant women and diabetics frequently suffer from yeast infections. This is because *Candida albicans*, the organism that causes yeast infections, thrives on their sugary, acidic vaginal secretions. In these women, the vaginal discharge is white and has the consistency of cottage cheese.

Treatment of vaginitis varies, depending on the underlying cause, but may involve the prescription of antifungal vaginal creams, suppositories, or oral antibiotics. The woman is instructed to avoid sexual intercourse until the infection has cleared up. If she continues to be sexually active during treatment, it is recommended that her male partner wear a condom.

Urinary Tract Infections

The symptoms, diagnosis, and treatment of UTIs is discussed in more detail in Chapter 8. Among sexually active women, UTIs are linked to use of a diaphragm and the failure to urinate immediately after intercourse.

Pelvic Inflammatory Disease

Pelvic inflammatory disease is the result of an infection that has spread untreated from the vagina up through the cervix to the uterus, fallopian tubes, and broad ligaments. It is characterized by purulent vaginal discharge, painful urination, itching, and abdominal pain. Although it can be caused by a number of microorganisms, it is frequently the result of infection with *Neisseria gonorrhoeae* or *Chlamydia trachomatis* bacteria. Practicing "safer sex" provides the woman some protection against infections with these and other organisms.

This condition is diagnosed by taking a sexual history, including recording information on infections in partners (eg, urethritis in male partners). Blood tests typically show an elevated white blood cell count, which indicates the presence of infection. Antibiotic therapy is the treatment of choice.

The early diagnosis and treatment of PID reduces the risk of further complications and infertility. But because women are often asymptomatic in the early stages of this disease, they may not seek medical treatment. It is therefore recommended that sexually active women be tested for the most common sexually transmitted diseases at least once a year. Treatment of all symptomatic sexual partners is recommended. Follow-up examination is extremely important in reducing the spread and recurrence of the infection. The Family Teaching Checklist provides family teaching tips to help prevent vaginal infections.

Toxic Shock Syndrome

Toxic shock syndrome (TSS) is the body's reaction to the toxins (poisonous substances) produced by the *Staphylococcus aureus* bacterium. Under normal circumstances, this bacterium exists within the body without causing any difficulties. However, the use of barrier contraceptives and super absorbent tampons sometimes creates an environment in which the bacterial colonies grow out of control. When this happens, the bacterial toxins reach levels high enough to cause the following reactions: sudden fever of 39°C (102°F) or higher, vomiting, diarrhea, sunburnlike rash, vertigo (dizziness), muscle aches, hypotension (low blood pressure), and a feeling of lightheadedness. Although men and nonmenstruating women sometimes present with TSS, this disorder primarily affects women who use highly absorbent tampons.

Because the symptoms of this disease mimic those of the flu and other common viral infections, they are often overlooked. Untreated TSS can rapidly become fa-

FAMILY TEACHING CHECKLIST

Prevention of Vaginal Infections

The nurse includes the following information in family teaching to promote health and well-being:

· Practice good hygiene, which includes wiping the perineal area from front to back and washing hands before and after cleaning the perineal area
· Wear undergarments that allow circulation of air (eg, cotton or those that have cotton crotches)
· Avoid tight clothing
· Avoid excessive use of vaginal douches and bubble baths
· Change sanitary pads and tampons frequently
· Remove barrier contraceptives as indicated in directions
· Observe vaginal secretions after antibiotic treatment
· Encourage male partner to use a condom
· Report abnormal vaginal discharges, itching, burning, and painful urination
· Avoid sexual contact if you have any of the symptoms of vaginal infection

tal, so it is recommended that women read the inserts in their tampon boxes to familiarize themselves with the symptoms of this disorder. Any woman who suspects that she may have TSS should remove the tampon immediately and seek medical attention. Treatment includes the administration of appropriate antibiotics and large volumes of intravenous fluids to increase decreasing blood pressure.

Sexually Transmitted Diseases

Sexually transmitted diseases (STDs) are primarily spread through sexual intercourse or other intimate contact. This includes oral-genital, anal-genital, digital-genital, as well as genital-genital contact, both with and without intercourse. STDs can also be transmitted by other means such as sharing improperly sterilized sex toys and intravenous needles; they can be passed from mother to child during pregnancy and childbirth; and they can even be spread by nonsexual means such as sharing damp towels or washcloths.

Several common STDs include gonorrhea, syphilis, and chlamydia, all of which are caused by bacteria; trichomoniasis, a parasitic infection; and the viral diseases herpes simplex (types I and II), genital warts (which are caused by the HPV), and human immunodeficiency virus (HIV), the virus that causes acquired immunodeficiency syndrome (AIDS). It should be stressed that no prophylactic is 100% effective in preventing sexually transmitted diseases under all circumstances. But if used properly and consistently, latex condoms and spermicides containing nonoxynol-9 or octoxynol (which have been shown to kill HIV and HPV under laboratory conditions) can greatly reduce the risks of contracting or spreading most sexually transmitted diseases. These preventive measures should be practiced *every time* a couple engages in sexual activity. See *Guidelines for Practicing "Safer Sex,"* Display 4-2, for guidelines on preventing the spread of sexually transmitted diseases.

Gonorrhea — Complications of Pregnancy

Gonorrhea is caused by the bacteria *Neisseria gonorrhoeae*. In women, gonorrhea may be asymptomatic, or it may present such mild symptoms that the woman fails to report them to her health care provider. When symptoms are present, they include burning on urination or vaginal discharge. As the infection progresses, the discharge may become foul smelling, purulent, and greenish yellow. Men also may be asymptomatic, but more frequently they have purulent yellow discharge from the penis and painful urination. See Chapter 18 for a discussion of infection of the neonate.

Once infected with gonorrhea, the woman who is not pregnant is at risk for developing PID. Inflammation of the reproductive system travels upward into the cervix, uterus, fallopian tubes, and the ovaries. If treatment is delayed or not given, the infection can lead to scarring and narrowing of the fallopian tubes, which results in sterility. Pregnant women infected with gonorrhea are initially protected from the spread of infection by the cervical mucus plug. This plug stops the upward spread of the bacteria. However, once the membranes rupture, the infection spreads quickly.

Treatment in both men and women consists of antibiotic therapy for gonorrhea and the infections that tend to occur with it (see following discussion). Because antibiotic therapy can mask other sexually transmitted infections, it is important that the patient be tested for all possible infections before antibiotic therapy is begun. The drug of choice is a one-time dose of ceftiaxone, 250 mg intramuscularly, followed by the administration of oral erythromycin for 7 days. Aqueous

---

<blockquote>

◆ **DISPLAY 4-2**
Guidelines for Practicing "Safer Sex"

Nurses can counsel individuals to reduce their chances of contracting a sexually transmitted disease by teaching them the basic principles of "safer sex."

· Abstinence is the most effective means of avoiding pregnancy and preventing the spread of sexually transmitted diseases. If abstinence is not desirable, latex condoms and spermicides containing nonoxynol-9 or octoxynol should be used with each and every sexual act. Those practicing cunnilingus (oral stimulation of the vulvar region) should use dental dams (rubber sheaths found in dental supply stores).

· Practice sexuality within a mutually monogamous relationship, and limit the number of sexual partners one has during the course of a lifetime.

· Exercise caution in selecting new sexual partners. This includes avoiding sexual contact until one is sure the new partner is free of STDs.

· Anal intercourse is a very high-risk activity. This is because the rectum, which does not produce any natural lubrication, tears very easily, providing an opening for the passage of disease-causing organisms.

· There are erotic activities that couples can share with a high degree of safety. Bathing and showering together is safe as long as uncontaminated semen and vaginal fluid touch only healthy skin. Rubbing bodies together and mutual masturbation are also recommended as long as semen and vaginal fluids touch only healthy skin. Individuals with herpes and genital warts are cautioned not to engage in these practices while they have infectious sores.

· It is important that individuals not share sex toys unless they have been thoroughly washed with soap, water, and disinfectant (1 part to 10 parts water)

</blockquote>

procaine penicillin G also may be given by intramuscular injection, or intravenously if the disease has progressed. The woman as well as her sexual partners must be treated to prevent the "ping-pong" process of reinfection.

A culture taken at the end of antibiotic therapy confirms the absence of *N. gonorrhoeae*. It is recommended that the infected individual abstain from sexual intercourse until antibiotic therapy has been completed. If this is not possible, condom use is encouraged until a negative culture is obtained.

Syphilis — *complications of pregnancy*

Syphilis is caused by the spirochete *Treponema pallidum*. Transmission occurs as the small spiral-shaped organisms pass from the infected partner through blood, semen, or direct contact with skin lesions. Kissing, sexual intercourse, and oral-genital contact are all possible means of transmission.

During the incubation period, which can take from 1 week to 3 months, those infected with syphilis can transmit the disease even though they have no visible signs of infection. After incubation, the disease progresses in three stages. During the primary stage, chancre sores (small painless lesions) appear at the site where the bacteria entered the body (eg, on the genitals or lips).

The secondary stage can begin as early as 6 weeks after infection or may occur until up to 6 months later. The symptoms of this stage include fever, headache, skin rash, enlargement of the lymph nodes, chronic sore throat, and possibly weight and hair loss. After a time, these symptoms disappear, even if left untreated. Syphilis is then said to have entered its latent period. In its latent stage, there are no outward signs of infection, even though the bacteria are multiplying within the body and attacking its organs. This latency period may last for up to 30 years. During the third, or tertiary, stage of syphilis, there may be severe cardiovascular disease and neurologic damage. Death is the end result.

There are several tests used to detect *T. pallidum*. Positive results from the VDRL (Venereal Disease Research Laboratories) and RPR (rapid plasma reagin) tests must be confirmed with an FTA-ABS (fluorescent treponemal antibody absorption) test.

Treatment with intramuscular or intravenous injections of benzathine penicillin G are recommended. Partners should be treated as well. If the disease has not progressed to the late stages, recovery is excellent. Although late-stage syphilis responds to treatment, any organ damage that may have occurred is usually irreversible.

Chlamydia

The microorganism *Chlamydia trachomatis* causes a variety of disorders, including genital infections of men and women. Chlamydia often occurs with other sexually transmitted diseases, particularly gonorrhea. Symptoms of a **chlamydial infection** include: purulent vaginal discharge; frequent, burning urination; and lower abdominal cramping. It should be noted that infection with *C. trachomatis* often produces no symptoms in its early stages. If left untreated, it can lead to PID, which is associated with ectopic pregnancy and infertility.

Diagnosis of chlamydial infections in women is based on positive cervical cultures. Individuals are also tested for gonorrhea because both infections tend to occur together. Treatment for chlamydia generally involves a 10-day course of tetracycline or doxycycline for pregnant and nonpregnant women.

Trichomoniasis *read complications of pregnancy*

Trichomoniasis is usually caused by the single-celled organism *Trichomonas vaginalis*. Symptoms of this infection include itching, burning, and frothy vaginal discharge that is green or gray in color. Painful urination is often reported.

Diagnosis of trichomoniasis is generally confirmed by examining vaginal and cervical cultures under a microscope for the causative organisms. Metronidazole is often prescribed to treat trichomoniasis. However, it is not used in early pregnancy because of its association with fetal abnormalities. Vinegar douches can often relieve the pain and discomfort until metronidazole can be prescribed.

Trichomonas vaginalis thrives in the folds of the glans penis, so it is recommended that sexual intercourse be avoided until both partners have been successfully treated. If sexual intercourse cannot be avoided, a condom should be used until all symptoms have disappeared.

Herpes Simplex Virus

There are two types of herpes simplex virus, type 1 and type 2. Type 1 is generally found on the lips and type 2 in the anogenital region, but either type can occur in either location.

The onset of infection is usually signaled by an itching or tingling sensation in the affected area. Some herpes sufferers also experience headache, stiff neck, or mild sensitivity to light. After this initial stage, small bumps erupt at the site of infection. These bumps develop into blisters filled with a clear, highly infectious liquid. If they occur on mucosal tissue, these blisters

German measles – causes birth defects in the 1st 2wks. It causes chronic infection in the fetus and continue in the newborn resulting to death or hearing lose.

may break, leaving open sores. If they are located on normal skin, they crust and heal. After this first outbreak, the herpes virus goes into a latency period, during which it is inactive. But the virus can be reactivated repeatedly throughout the life of the individual.

There is no known cure for herpes simplex. Acyclovir ointment can be used to relieve the discomfort and speed up the crusting of the lesions. For serious cases of herpes infection, oral acyclovir may be prescribed, although it is not recommended for pregnant women.

Infected individuals are advised to abstain from any sexual activity while they have infectious lesions. Abstinence should be practiced from the time the infected person first feels tingling until the lesions have fully healed.

Human Papillomavirus/Genital Warts

There are many strains of HPV, the infections that cause warts. As many as 20 of these strains can infect the genitalia. The genital warts that they cause come in all shapes and sizes. They may be too small to be seen with the naked eye or large enough to block vaginal delivery. They may appear as single, pointed lesions or come in clusters of soft, cauliflower-like growths. They are highly contagious and can be spread through intimate sexual contact to infect the vagina, cervix, anus, rectum, penis, scrotum, and throat. Neonates may contract HPV of the throat during delivery. Several strains of HPVs have been linked to abnormalities in cervical cells, which may in some cases lead to cervical cancer. Any woman who suspects she may have been exposed to genital HPV should see her health care provider immediately. It is recommended that women with HPV have Pap smears once every 6 months to promote early detection of potential cell abnormalities.

Genital warts may be removed by using chemicals (podophyllin or trichloracetic acid), lasers, or surgery. Difficult-to-manage warts have been successfully treated by injecting alpha-interferon directly into the warts.

Acquired Immunodeficiency Syndrome

Acquired immunodeficiency syndrome (AIDS) is a fatal disease that is caused by HIV. As HIV attacks and destroys the body's disease-fighting T4 lymphocytes, the body loses its ability to fight off common infections. Death results from the body's inability to defend itself against repeated opportunistic infections. (Fetalneonatal risks associated with HIV infection are discussed in Chapter 20.)

During the early phases of HIV infection, the individual may remain asymptomatic or show signs of viral infection. These symptoms include fever, headache, general fatigue, and enlarged lymph nodes. As the infection progresses, the patient may display generalized lymph node enlargement, chronic viral or fungal infections, and chronic opportunistic infections (some of which were mentioned previously). A person is diagnosed with full-blown AIDS when blood tests indicate that there are fewer than 200 T cells/mm³ blood. (Normally, blood contains 1000 T cells/mm³.)

There are two tests available that are widely used to test for antibodies to HIV. They are the ELISA (enzyme-linked immunoabsorbent assay) and the western blot. A positive ELISA indicates that the person has been exposed to the HIV virus and will in all likelihood develop AIDS. To protect against false-positive results, ELISA results are confirmed with the western blot. There are tests that can be used to screen for the HIV virus itself. However, these tests are extremely expensive, require highly skilled technicians to interpret, and are still considered experimental. If a person is at high risk for contracting HIV and continues to test negative to HIV antibodies while exhibiting symptoms of infection, his or her health care provider may recommend running the more detailed tests to detect the virus itself.

Those at high risk for contracting HIV and AIDS include:

· Men who have had sexual intercourse with another man, regardless of whether they consider themselves homosexual, heterosexual, or bisexual
· Intravenous drug users and their sexual partners
· Individuals with other ulcerative sexually transmitted diseases (such as genital herpes and genital warts)
· Those who practice unsafe sexual practices (such as engaging in anal intercourse, having multiple sexual partners, and not using condoms)
· The sexual partners of those who have already tested positive for or are at high risk for contracting HIV
· Infants of mothers who are HIV positive

The risk of contracting HIV from blood products has been practically eliminated by screening donors and testing blood products before they are transfused to donors. Although the HIV virus has been found in tears and saliva, these fluids are rarely implicated in the transmission of the virus.

Treatment of AIDS generally involves managing the symptoms and relieving the patient's discomfort. There have, however, been some successes with the antiviral agent zidovudine (AZT) (which has been renamed zidovudine, or ZDV) when it is given to a person suffering from full-blown AIDS. It has been shown that administering AZT to HIV+ women who are pregnant may actually protect their unborn children from infection. The women themselves will not benefit from this preventive treatment in the absence of full-blown AIDS.

There is no cure for AIDS, so prevention of HIV infection through abstinence or the practice of "safer sex" are the best methods we now have for fighting the disease. See Display 4-2 for more detailed guidelines for practicing "safer sex."

The Normal Process of Aging in Women

In the youth-oriented culture of the United States, attention is often drawn to the negative physiologic aspects for aging, such as the decrease in muscle mass and the loss of sensory acuity. The rewards of aging, such as gains in wisdom and self-confidence, are seldom regarded as the assets they are.

For women, the process of aging is represented as particularly undesirable, for it brings with it the loss of fertility. And although many women are relieved not to have to worry about contraception and pregnancy, they tend to regard menopause as an ending rather than the beginning of a new chapter in their lives. Many of the more than 30 million postmenopausal women in the United States today accept menopause for the natural function it is. With proper diet and a few adjustments in their health care regimens, these women sail through menopause with few difficulties (Fig. 4-4).

Menopause

Menopause typically occurs sometime between the ages of 45 and 50. This "change of life," as menopause

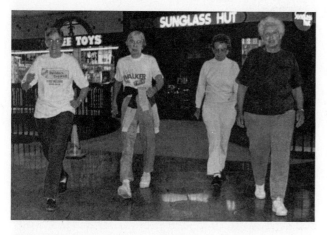

Figure 4-4. Older adults in a mall walkers club can exercise and socialize at the same time. (Photo © Kathy Sloane)

is often called, begins when the ovaries stop producing estrogen and ends when the woman's menstrual periods stop. Some women experience a gradual decrease in menstrual blood flow over time, and others may discover that their menstrual periods stop suddenly. This can take anywhere from 1 to 5 years to complete.

There are a variety of physical and psychologic changes that result from the declining levels of estrogen. (Refer to Chapter 2 for a review of the hormonal influences of estrogen.) The uterus, fallopian tubes, ovaries, and breasts gradually atrophy (shrink in size or waste away). The woman also may experience a wide range of symptoms such as irritability, insomnia, depression, weight gain, growth of facial hair, and hot flashes.

Estrogen therapy is effective in relieving the symptoms of menopause, preventing osteoporosis, and protecting against heart disease. It can also relieve vaginal dryness, thus enhancing the woman's sexual pleasure. Hormone replacement therapy is achieved by administering estrogen or a combination of estrogen and progestin in either pill or patch form.

As with any treatment, there are risks involved. Estrogen administered alone can effectively relieve many of the symptoms of menopause, but it has been associated with cancer of the endometrium. A combination of estrogen and progestin can reduce the cancer-related risks. There is, however, some worry that progestin may contribute to heart disease. Estrogen replacement therapy has also been associated with a slight increase in the incidence of breast cancer among women who have been on the hormone for 15 years or more.

Even when properly administered, hormonal therapy can produce side effects. These include vaginal bleeding (associated with progestin use), breast tenderness, fluid retention, mood changes, and pelvic cramping. Those women who are not eligible for estrogen therapy include those with breast cancer, blood-clotting disorders, and abnormal bleeding; and those who might be pregnant.

Osteoporosis

The loss of estrogen also leads to osteoporosis, a condition resulting in loss of bone mass and an increase in bone brittleness. Although this condition is associated with the normal aging process, it is more common in women who have gone through menopause. Calcium replacement and vitamin D supplements have been used to decrease the rate of bone loss. Engaging in weight-bearing exercises and adequate exposure to sunlight (which aids in the synthesis of vitamin D) also provides protection. Eliminating tobacco and alcohol consumption is also a good idea as both substances in-

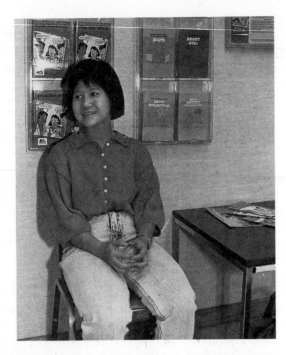

Figure 4-5. *A variety of information is available to the adolescent who may inquire about sexually transmitted diseases and contraceptive care. (Photo © Kathy Sloane)*

terfere with calcium absorption. Estrogen therapy is used to decrease the rate of bone resorption (loss of bone tissue) in menopausal women.

Adolescent Considerations

The adolescent girl should be encouraged to seek gynecologic health care as soon as she decides to become sexually active. Educating adolescents about the threats of STDs, common reproductive tract infections, and the importance of monthly BSEs can give them the knowledge they need to protect their long-term reproductive health (Fig. 4-5).

Cultural Considerations

The notion of women's health care and its importance varies from one culture to another. Even within the dominant culture, ideas of wellness change with the times. For example, today's high rates of STDs may be viewed as the result of the breakdown of the family or a failure of morality. They also can be seen as the predictable result of several related factors: improved methods of classifying and reporting diseases, our increased dependence on oral contraceptives, as opposed to the barrier methods that were popular in the 1950s; the development of antibiotic-resistant strains

of familiar diseases; and our society's preference for focusing on high-technology cures rather than on unglamorous prevention.

Nurses provide sensitive care by understanding that individuals have different ideas about reproductive health and sexuality that affect their sexual practices. Nurses who understand that not every individual is primarily concerned with maintaining perfect reproductive health can adapt their patient teaching accordingly. Carefully explaining the importance of protecting the vulnerable female reproductive system can encourage the woman to adopt sexual behaviors that ensure her long-term fertility and sexual health.

The Role of the Nurse

Nurses can teach women to have an impact on their own health and well-being simply by routinely examining their breasts and external genitalia. Effective teaching helps women identify situations that require medical intervention or follow-up.

All sexually active family members benefit from an understanding of the causes and potential sources of STDs. Because these diseases are easier to prevent than to treat, teaching the individuals how to reduce the risk of contracting these diseases can have a positive effect on their long-term reproductive health. The Nursing Diagnoses Checklist offers a list of nursing diagnoses related to women's health.

✓ NURSING DIAGNOSES CHECKLIST

Nursing Diagnoses Related to Women's Health

· Activity Intolerance, related to normal aging changes

· Body Image Disturbance, related to breast cancer

· Altered Sexuality Patterns, related to pelvic inflammatory disease

· Pain, related to dysmenorrhea

· Fear, related to positive testing for sexually transmitted disease

· Noncompliance, with gynecologic assessment related to embarrassment

· Knowledge Deficit, related to breast self-examination

· Anxiety, related to menopausal symptoms

◆ SELF-ASSESSMENT

1. To decrease the incidence of incorrect Pap smear results:

○ **A.** The patient should be instructed to douche 1 day before the test.
○ **B.** The slide should be immediately sprayed with fixative.
○ **C.** Only a water-soluble lubricant should be used on the speculum.
○ **D.** The test should not be performed during the patient's menstrual period.

2. A woman with fibrocystic breast disease should be instructed to:

○ **A.** Perform a monthly breast self-examination during her menstrual period
○ **B.** Immediately report cysts that feel smooth and are movable
○ **C.** Have a mammogram every year
○ **D.** Increase caffeine intake before her menstrual period

3. A woman with PMS should be instructed to increase her intake of which of the following before her menstrual period?

○ **A.** Oranges
○ **B.** Coffee
○ **C.** Potato chips
○ **D.** Wine

4. Dysmenorrhea is primarily due to increased production of:

○ **A.** Estrogen
○ **B.** Progesterone
○ **C.** Prostaglandins
○ **D.** Prolactin

5. Decreased estrogen production during menopause has been associated with all of the following EXCEPT?

○ **A.** Osteoporosis
○ **B.** Insomnia
○ **C.** Weight loss
○ **D.** Irritability

REVIEW AND PREVIEW

The importance of regular gynecologic assessment was discussed, with particular emphasis on monthly BSE; annual pelvic examinations; and the importance of preventing, recognizing, and treating sexually transmitted diseases.

Unit Two will focus on the issues related to the family during the antepartum period and normal fetal development.

◆ KEY POINTS

◆ Annual pelvic examinations and Pap smears are recommended for all sexually active women and all women older than age 18.

◆ Breast self-examination performed each month will familiarize the woman with her own breasts and increase the chances that she will notice and report detectable abnormalities.

◆ In endometriosis, the displaced endometrium can be found adhering to the ovaries, uterine ligaments, peritoneum, and abdominal wall. Painful menstruation is a major symptom of endometriosis. This condition can be managed with hormone therapy or surgical intervention.

◆ Premenstrual syndrome (PMS) is thought to be the result of the hormonal changes a woman experiences, particularly during the luteal phase of the ovarian cycle. Dysmenorrhea, amenorrhea, menorrhagia, and metrorrhagia are four other common menstrual disorders.

◆ Pelvic inflammatory disease is associated with a history of pelvic infections and IUD use. It typically leads to adhesions on the fallopian tubes, the buildup of scar tissue, and in some cases, infertility.

◆ Toxic shock syndrome is caused by the toxins produced by the bacterium *S. aureus*. In women, this syndrome is most often associated with tampon use and is marked by a sudden, rapid increase in temperature; rash; severe, flulike symptoms; and, if left untreated, eventual shock.

◆ Sexually transmitted diseases are most often passed between individuals through intimate sexual contact. Latex condoms and spermicides containing nonoxynol-9 or octoxynol have proven effective in stopping the transmission of HIV between individuals.

◆ Human immunodeficiency virus attacks the body's normal defense system by destroying T4 lymphocytes. Diagnosis of HIV is based on a reactive ELISA test (which is confirmed with a western blot). As the virus infects the host, the body becomes defenseless in fighting infections. Full-blown AIDS is diagnosed when there are fewer than 200 T cells/mm³ blood. Death results from opportunistic infections, which spread unchecked as the immune system collapses. There is no cure for AIDS.

◆ Menopause marks the end of a woman's reproductive life. Estrogen levels decline and the reproductive organs atrophy. Symptoms associated with menopause range from mild irritability to depression. Sleeplessness and exhaustion sometimes accompany the hot flashes for which menopause is known.

BIBLIOGRAPHY

The American College of Obstetricians and Gynecologists Patient Education Pamphlet (October 1992). *The Menopause Years.*

Corea, G. (1992). *The invisible epidemic: The story of women and AIDS.* New York: Harper Collins.

Dahl, R. (1992). Women's mental health care: Into the 1990s. *Perspectives in Psychiatric Care, 28*(4), 29–31.

Ellerhorst-Ryan, J., & Goeldner, J. (1992). Breast cancer. *Nursing Clinics of North America, 27*(4), 821–833.

Fischbach, F. (1992). *A Manual of Laboratory and Diagnostic Tests* (4th ed.). Philadelphia: J.B. Lippincott.

Fishbein, E. G. (1992). Women at midlife: The transition to menopause. *The Nursing Clinics of North America. Woman's Health.*

Ginsberg, C. (1991). Exfoliative cytologic screening: The Papanicolaou test. *Journal of Obstetric, Gynecologic, and Neonatal Nursing, 20*(1), 39–49.

Irvine, D., & Lauver, D. (1992). Addressing infrequent cancer screening among women. *Nursing Outlook, 40*(5), 207–212.

Kelley, K. F., Galbraith, M. A., & Vermund, S. H. (1992). Genital human papillomavirus infection in women. *Journal of Obstetric, Gynecological, and Neonatal Nursing, 21*(6), 503–576.

Love, C., & Seaton, H. (1991). Eating disorders: Highlights of nursing assessment and therapeutics. *Nursing Clinics of North America, 26*(3), 677–697.

Martin, L. L., & Reeder, S. J. (1990). *Essentials of maternity nursing: Family-centered care* (1st ed.). Philadelphia: J.B. Lippincott.

May, K. A. & Mahlmeister, L. R. (1994). *Maternal & neonatal nursing: Family-centered care* (3rd ed.). Philadelphia: J.B. Lippincott.

Norwood, S. (1990). Fibrocystic breast disease: An update and review. *Journal of Obstetric, Gynecologic, and Neonatal Nursing, 19*(2), 116–121.

Reeder, S. J., Martin, L. L., & Koniak, D. (1992). *Maternity Nursing: Family, Newborn, and Women's Health Care* (17th ed.). Philadelphia: J.B. Lippincott.

Rosdahl, C. B. (1991). *Textbook of Basic Nursing* (5th ed.). Philadelphia: J.B. Lippincott.

Tillman, J. (1992). Syphilis: An old disease: A contemporary perinatal problem. *Journal of Obstetric, Gynecologic, and Neonatal Nursing, 21*(3).

Tinkle, M., Amaya, M., & Tamayo, O. (1992) HIV disease and pregnancy: Part 1. Epidemiology, pathogenesis and natural history. *Journal of Gynecologic and Neonatal Nursing, 21*(2), 86–93.

The Family in the Antepartum Period

CHAPTER 5

Normal Prenatal Physical and Psychosocial Changes

◈ OBJECTIVES

When the learning goals of this chapter are met, the reader will be able to:

◆ Define and combine the terms gravida, para, primi, multi, and nulli to describe a woman's pregnancy history.

◆ List the presumptive, probable, and positive signs and symptoms of pregnancy.

◆ Determine the expected date of delivery (EDD) using Nägele's rule.

◆ Determine the desired amount of weight gain during pregnancy based on the woman's prepregnancy weight.

◆ Discuss the physical changes that occur in the maternal circulatory system to support the growing fetus.

◆ Describe the developmental tasks that indicate family adaptation to pregnancy.

TERMINOLOGY

Ballottement	Hegar's sign
Braxton Hicks contractions	Last menstrual period
Chadwick's sign	Nägele's rule
Chloasma gravidarum	Pica
Expected date of delivery	Quickening
Gestation	Radioimmunoassay
Goodell's sign	Trimester
GTPALM	

Pregnancy is defined as the period of time between conception and birth during which the fertilized ovum matures and grows in the female's uterus. This period is sometimes referred to as the antepartum, or prenatal, period. The length of pregnancy, or **gestation,** lasts approximately 280 days.

This chapter focuses on the physical and psychosocial changes the woman and her family face once pregnancy has been diagnosed. It ends by addressing several important pregnancy-related adolescent and cultural considerations.

Essential Terminology

The fetus is often described in terms of its viability, or ability to live outside the uterus. A fetus is usually considered viable if it is somewhere between 20 and 24 weeks' gestation and weighs more than 500 g (1.1 lbs). However, the legal age of viability differs from state to state.

There are many terms used to describe a woman's pregnancy history:

gravida: refers to a woman who is or has been pregnant

para: indicates the number of pregnancies that have reached the legal age of viability

primi: first

multi: indicates more than one or more than once

nulli: none or never

These terms are often combined as follows to clarify the woman's pregnancy history:

primigravida: a woman who is pregnant for the first time

multigravida: a woman who is pregnant who has also been pregnant before

nulligravida: a woman who has never been pregnant

primipara: a woman who has delivered a potentially viable fetus, whether or not it survived

nullipara: a woman who has not carried a fetus to the age of viability

GTPALM is a commonly used shorthand method for recording a woman's pregnancy history. The letters indicate the following: **G,** gravida; **T,** term pregnancies; **P,** premature births; **A,** abortions; **L,** number of living children; **M,** multiple gestations and births.

Using this system, a pregnant woman who has three living children, all of whom were single births, has had no abortions, and delivered one preterm infant who is alive and well would be defined as 4-2-1-0-3-0 (**GTPALM**).

Signs and Symptoms of Pregnancy

During pregnancy, a woman's body adapts to its role as an incubator for new life by undergoing a number of physical changes. These changes are known as the signs and symptoms of pregnancy and are classified in three groups: presumptive, probable, and positive.

Presumptive Signs

Presumptive signs are those that suggest but do not positively indicate pregnancy. These signs include amenorrhea, nausea and vomiting, breast changes, urinary frequency, fatigue, and Goodell's sign.

Amenorrhea in a healthy woman who usually experiences regular menstrual periods may suggest pregnancy. In women with irregular menstrual periods and in those who spot (bleed lightly) during early pregnancy, amenorrhea is not a reliable presumptive sign. Amenorrhea is also linked with several non–pregnancy-related conditions. These include extreme emotional upsets, fatigue, and low body fat related to anorexia or strenuous exercise. These conditions must be ruled out before pregnancy can be diagnosed.

Nausea and vomiting are associated with metabolic and hormonal changes. These symptoms occur during the first trimester in 50% of all pregnancies. This condition is often called "morning sickness" because it is present when the woman rises in the morning and goes away within hours of awakening. Nausea and vomiting can, however, persist throughout the day. Encouraging the woman to eat crackers or plain toast before rising in the morning can help relieve these symptoms.

Breast changes, such as enlargement, tingling of the nipples, and an increased sensitivity to touch are often seen in early pregnancy. The nipples and areolae may darken. By the second month, the breasts begin to increase in size.

Urinary frequency increases during early pregnancy as the enlarging uterus presses on the bladder. This symptom disappears after the first trimester, when the uterus rises in the abdominal cavity. The need to urinate frequently returns late in pregnancy as the growing fetus presses on the bladder.

Fatigue is a common complaint throughout pregnancy, although it is marked at the beginning of the first trimester. It has been associated with the increased metabolic needs of the woman and the fetus.

Goodell's sign is a softening of the normally firm cervix. It is the result of increased blood supply to the pelvic area and heightened hormone production.

Women who suspect they are pregnant may also be experiencing probable signs of pregnancy when they seek health care.

Probable Signs

Probable signs are strong indicators of pregnancy, but they do not in themselves confirm the condition. These signs can be detected by about the 12th week. Probable signs include pigmentation changes, enlarging abdomen, Chadwick's sign, Hegar's sign, ballottement, Braxton Hicks contractions, palpation of the fetal outline, quickening, and a positive pregnancy test.

Pigmentation changes occur on both the abdomen and face. The linea nigra is the darkened line that begins at the symphysis pubis and extends past the umbilicus (Fig. 5-1). **Chloasma gravidarum** refers to the uneven, brownish pigmentation of the face during preg-

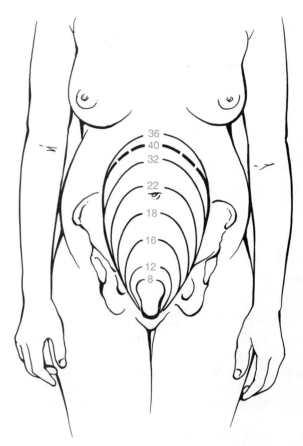

Figure 5-2. *The uterus moves upward as the fetus grows. Later in pregnancy, the fetus will descend in preparation for birth.*

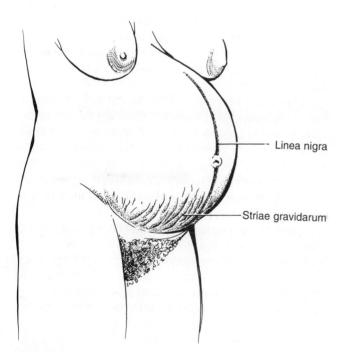

Linea nigra

Striae gravidarum

Figure 5-1. *Linea nigra appears on the abdomen as a darkened line between the symphysis pubis and the upper abdomen. This pigmentation typically fades after childbirth.*

nancy. It is often referred to as the "mask of pregnancy." The cause of this brownish pigmentation is unknown, but it is thought to be related to normal hormonal activity. Chloasma typically fades completely from the face after delivery.

Enlargement of the abdomen occurs as the uterus grows and rises out of the pelvis at about 12 weeks (Fig. 5-2). There are other medical conditions that can cause the uterus to enlarge, such as benign tumors and cancerous growths. These possible causes of uterine enlargement need to be ruled out, especially if other probable signs of pregnancy are not present.

Chadwick's sign is a purplish tinge of the vulva and vagina. It is caused by vascular congestion (an increase in blood flow) to the pelvic region. Chadwick's sign can be observed during speculum examination after the fourth week of pregnancy.

Hegar's sign is a softening of the lower uterine segment that can be felt on bimanual examination around 6 to 8 weeks' gestation. The examiner inserts several fingers of one hand in the vagina to touch the back of the cervix. At the same time, the abdominal wall is palpated above the cervix (Fig. 5-3).

Ballottement is a technique used to detect a floating object. In this case, the fetus, which is supported by the amniotic fluid, is the floating object. It can be felt rebounding against the examiner's fingers when it is given a light tap through the vagina or the abdomen. This assessment is possible during the second trimester.

Braxton Hicks contractions are irregular, painless uterine contractions that occur throughout pregnancy. The pregnant woman often describes these contractions as a tightening across the abdomen that intensifies toward the end of the pregnancy.

Braxton Hicks contractions differ from true labor contractions in that they do not lead to cervical dilatation. The examiner can detect Braxton Hick's contractions during the second half of pregnancy.

Palpation of fetal outline can be done by the examiner around 26 to 28 weeks. The examiner gently feels the abdominal area to locate the fetal body outline. Because a tumor may feel irregular, the results of palpation are not considered a positive sign of pregnancy.

Quickening describes the "fluttering sensations" felt by the woman when the fetus makes its first movements. It normally occurs around the 16th

to the 20th week of pregnancy. It may be felt as early as the 10th week, in which case it is classified as a presumptive sign. In rare cases, a woman can go through an entire pregnancy without once experiencing quickening.

Pregnancy tests can diagnose pregnancy 8 to 10 days after conception. Maternal blood or urine samples that contain human chorionic gonadotropin (hCG), a hormone produced by cells of the developing placenta, are probable pregnancy indicators.

One of the most sensitive and accurate methods of diagnosing pregnancy is the **radioimmunoassay** test. Radioimmunoassay tests can detect even trace amounts of substances such as hormones in blood plasma. With this method detectable levels of hCG can be found in maternal blood samples as early as 8 days after fertilization.

When two or more probable signs are present, pregnancy is strongly suggested. However, it is possible for some of the probable signs of pregnancy to occur in the absence of pregnancy. Women who experience uterine enlargement and amenorrhea without being pregnant are said to have false pregnancies, or pseudocyesis. This condition is usually, but not always, seen in women who are anxious to get pregnant as well as in those who wish to avoid pregnancy entirely.

Positive Signs

Positive signs must be present to confirm a diagnosis of pregnancy. These signs include the fetal heartbeat, palpation of fetal movements, and ultrasonic evidence of a fetus. A checklist of presumptive, probable, and positive signs and symptoms of pregnancy is provided in Display 5-1.

The fetal heart rate (FHR), which is rapid with a normal range of 110 to 160 beats per minute, can be detected early in pregnancy by auscultation. Auscultation is the process of listening for sounds within the body. The fetal heart tone (FHT) can be picked up with a Doppler probe from the 10th to 12th week of pregnancy. (Dopplers use a low-energy ultrasound amplifier to detect sound.)

Fetal movements also offer positive proof of pregnancy. They are typically felt by the examiner after approximately 20 weeks of gestation.

Ultrasound scanning is a useful means of confirming pregnancy and determining the gestational age of the fetus. It can be used to identify the embryo as early as the fourth week of pregnancy (see Chapter 10 for a detailed discussion of fetal assessment).

The accompanying display serves as a quick reference of the presumptive, probable, and positive signs of pregnancy.

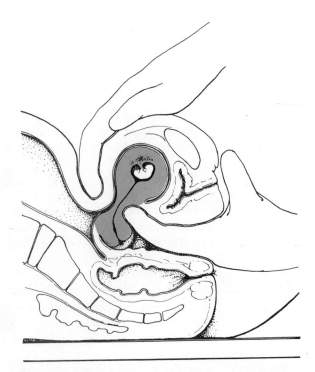

Figure 5-3. *Hegar's sign is detected at about 6 weeks' gestation. The lower uterine segment softens as a result of hormonal influences, preparing the uterus to sustain growing a conceptus.*

◆ DISPLAY 5-1
Presumptive, Probable, and Positive Signs and Symptoms of Pregnancy

Presumptive

Amenorrhea:	cessation of menses
Nausea and vomiting:	usually occurring in the morning
Breast changes:	increased tenderness and enlargement
Urinary frequency:	related to pressure of uterus on bladder
Fatigue:	increased throughout pregnancy
Goodell's sign:	softening of the cervix

Probable

Pigmentation changes:	linea nigra, chloasma gravidarum, striae gravidarum, darkening of nipples and areolae
Enlargement of the abdomen:	uterine growth and extension into abdominal cavity
Chadwick's sign:	purplish coloration of vaginal mucous membranes
Hegar's sign:	softening of lower portion of uterus
Ballottement:	rebounding of fetus in amniotic fluid
Braxton Hicks contractions:	painless uterine contractions
Palpation of fetal outline:	by trained examiner capable of identifying fetal parts
Quickening:	first perceptible fetal movements felt by the woman
Positive pregnancy test	

Positive

Fetal heartbeat heard:	typically in lower left quadrant, at 110 to 160 beats per minute
Fetal movements palpated by examiner:	palpation of abdomen for fetal limb movements
Fetal outline visualized by ultrasound:	skeletal outline seen, internal organs visualized, fetal heart beating

The Length of Pregnancy

The length of pregnancy is approximately 280 days, but there is a great deal of normal variation among women. Pregnancies may last between 240 and 300 days with perfectly fine outcomes. This is so because (1) ovulation time differs among women, and (2) there are differences in rates of fetal maturation.

After diagnosis of pregnancy is confirmed, the length of pregnancy is calculated by counting from Day 1 of the **last menstrual period (LMP).** An **expected date of delivery (EDD)** is determined by using **Nägele's rule.** To arrive at the EDD, 7 days are added to the first day of the LMP. Three months are then subtracted from this date. For example, a woman whose last menstrual period began on May 5th would have an EDD of February 12th:

May 5 + 7 days = May 12
May 12 – 3 months = February 12 (EDD).

Nägele's rule is considered a reliable means of determining EDD, even though most births occur around the EDD rather than on that date exactly.

Not all pregnancies continue to term. Some end in spontaneous abortion, which is the termination of a pregnancy before the fetus becomes viable. This may happen when an incompetent cervix dilates and the embryo is expelled from the uterus. Pregnancies that end after the fetus reaches viability but before it reaches full

Table 5-1. *Physical and Psychosocial Changes During Pregnancy by Trimester*

Trimester	Physical Events	Psychosocial Events
First	Nausea and vomiting	Happy, elated
	Breast tenderness	Doubts ability to be a mother
	Fatigue	Tolerates the discomforts of pregnancy
	Frequency of urination	Mimicry seen
	Weight gain	Accepance of pregnancy
	Estrogen and progesterone levels increase	Early mood swings
	Hegar's sign	
	Chadwick's sign	
Second	Quickening	Concern over discomforts of pregnancy
	Backaches	Fantasizes about baby
	Edema of extremities	Recognizes emotional vulnerability
	Weight gain	Desire for eating healthy foods
	Breast enlargement	Role playing
	Increased appetite	Emotional upsets
	Peaking level hCG	
	Goodell's sign	
Third	Return of urinary frequency	Desires pregnancy to end
	Fatigue	Anxious to meet newborn
	Weight gain	Physical limitations & weight gain cause sadness and concern
	Shortness of breath	
	Sleeping difficulties	Fear of labor and childbirth
	Peak prolactin level	Taking-in
		Re-forming couple relationship

term are classified as premature or preterm births. Fetuses of pregnancies that exceed the EDD by 2 or more weeks are classified as postmature (see Chapter 9).

The Three Trimesters of Pregnancy

A pregnancy lasts about 40 weeks, or 9 calendar months. These 9 months are broken down into three **trimesters** of approximately 3 months each. Each trimester is marked by specific physical changes in the woman, stages in fetal development, and psychosocial effects for the family. Periods of fetal development are discussed in Chapter 9. Physical and psychosocial effects are discussed in the following sections of this chapter. Table 5-1 compares physical and psychosocial changes during pregnancy by trimester.

◆ Physical Effects of Pregnancy

Weight gain, a decrease in energy levels, and obvious alterations in the reproductive system are just a few of the changes that the woman experiences during pregnancy. As the woman experiences pregnancy, so too does her family. Nurses who are aware of the normal physical changes that occur during pregnancy can provide anticipatory guidance and education to the childbearing family.

Weight Gain During Pregnancy

Adequate weight gain during pregnancy is necessary for the health and well-being of the woman and the fetus. A total weight gain of 10 to 14 kg (25–35 lbs) is recommended for a healthy woman of average weight. Guidelines for optimum weight gain are individualized for underweight and overweight women, but a minimum gain of 6 kg (15 lbs) is recommended.

During the first trimester, a weight gain of 1 to 2 kg (2–4 lbs) is considered average. Most weight gain occurs in the second and third trimesters. Fat deposits, products of conception, fluid retention, third-trimester fetal weight gain, and increased blood volume all contribute to the woman's total weight gain.

Changes in the Reproductive System

During pregnancy, the female reproductive system undergoes a number of changes that allow it to support the growing fetus. The uterus, cervix, fallopian tubes, ovaries, vagina, perineum, and the breasts all change significantly.

Uterus

In its nonpregnant state, the uterus is pear shaped. As the fetus grows, it expands up to 20 times its original size and becomes more egg shaped. In early pregnancy, the uterus is anteflexed, or positioned toward the front of the body. In later months, it rises from the pelvic cavity and turns slightly to the right.

The muscles of the uterus stretch and thin as it expands to support the developing fetus. Uterine blood supply increases, along with the growth of new vessels and nervous tissue. The inguinal lymphatic system, which is located in the groin area, grows to protect the reproductive system from potential infectious organisms.

In the first trimester, uterine growth exceeds embryonic growth. During this period, the uterus increases in length from approximately 7.5 cm (3 in.) to approximately 35 cm (14 in.). Its weight increases from 57 g (2 oz) to 900 g (2 lbs). In the second and third trimesters, the muscles of the uterus increase in size (hypertrophy) as the growing fetus presses on its walls.

Cervix

The cervix shortens and thins during pregnancy. It functions primarily to support the uterine contents. Cervical glands secrete a thick mucus that forms a plug in the cervical canal. This plug mixes with blood from the tiny surrounding capillaries and prevents bacteria from traveling up to the uterus (Fig. 5-4).

Fallopian Tubes and Ovaries

Blood supplied to the fallopian tubes and the ovaries increases during pregnancy. These organs become more vertical in position as the growing uterus fills the abdominal cavity. The corpus luteum enlarges, producing higher levels of estrogen and progesterone for the first 10 to 12 weeks of pregnancy. The placenta then matures and takes over hormone production for the corpus luteum, which regresses completely by midpregnancy (see Chapter 2, *Female Reproductive System*).

Vagina and Perineum

Estrogen production permits both the vagina and the perineum to stretch considerably during childbirth to allow for the passage of the fetus. There is increased

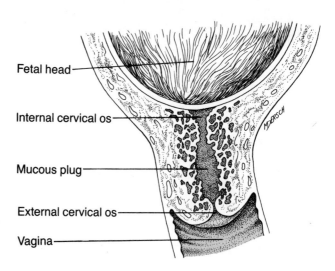

Figure 5-4. *The mucus plug serves as a protective barrier at the base of the uterus in the cervical canal.*

blood flow to the vaginal and perineal areas, along with mucosal thickening, connective tissue congestion, vaginal secretions, and hypertrophy of muscles. An acidic pH of 3.5 to 5.0 is maintained in the vagina to inhibit the growth of harmful bacteria.

Breasts

Changes in the breasts (mammary glands) begin in early pregnancy as they prepare for lactation (the production and secretion of breast milk) (Fig. 5-5). They become more sensitive to the touch. The nipples become erectile, and they, like the breasts in general, enlarge. The Montgomery glands (sebaceous glands of the areolae) also enlarge. Venous congestion and hypertrophy of breast tissue increases.

Pigmentation changes cause the areolae to get darker, and striae gravidarum (stretch marks) may develop on the outer aspects of the breasts (see *Integumentary System*, page 84, for further changes in the skin, nails, and hair).

In the latter half of pregnancy, a thick, yellowish fluid called colostrum is secreted by the breasts. Colostrum nourishes the neonate until true lactation occurs.

Changes in Other Body Systems

The reproductive system is not the only body system that changes to accommodate the growing fetus. The endocrine, circulatory, respiratory, gastrointestinal, urinary, musculoskeletal, and integumentary systems also undergo changes that enable the body to support the new life.

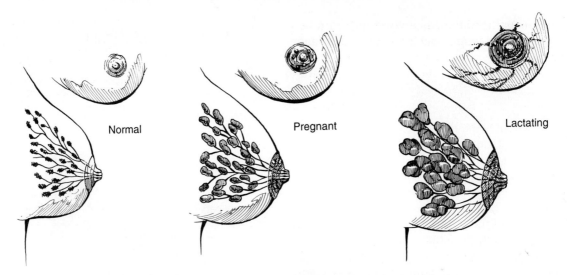

Normal   Pregnant   Lactating

Figure 5-5. *The mammary glands prepare for lactation as pregnancy progresses.*

Endocrine System

Pregnancy could not occur or be maintained without hormonal support. As we first learned in Chapter 2, estrogen and progesterone play important roles in reproductive events. Estrogen's role in pregnancy includes promoting uterine cell growth and helping prepare the breasts for lactation. It also supports increased blood flow to the developing fetus. Progesterone encourages development of the uterine endometrium. It also helps prevent spontaneous abortions by discouraging the contraction of uterine muscles during pregnancy.

In addition to estrogen and progesterone, there are several other important pregnancy-sustaining hormones. The chorionic villi are the membranes through which the developing embryo is attached to the endometrium. They secrete hCG. This hormone stimulates the corpus luteum to produce estrogen and progesterone until the placenta takes over hormone production around the end of the first trimester.

Human placental lactogen (hPL), or chorionic somatomammotropin, is also produced by the chorionic villi. It makes more protein and glucose available to meet both maternal and fetal growth needs. Because hPL increases maternal glucose levels through an anti-insulin effect, gestational diabetes may result if these levels are allowed to increase unchecked. Human placental lactogen is also important in the production of breast milk.

Secretion of aldosterone by the adrenal glands stimulates the reabsorption of water and sodium by the kidney tubules. As progesterone levels increase, sodium excretion is encouraged. The equilibrium of aldosterone and progesterone elevations is important in controlling fluid retention that may lead to hypertension.

Circulatory System

The circulatory system responds to the need to supply oxygen and nutrients to the growing fetus by increasing blood volume by up to 50%. This increase, which peaks in the third trimester, heightens blood supply for the entire body.

As blood volume increases, cardiac output increases. This is harmless in the healthy pregnant woman. However, a pregnant woman with a previous cardiac history must have her vital signs and circulatory status monitored frequently. This will allow the health care provider to manage risks to maternal and fetal well-being. Extreme elevations in blood pressure during pregnancy may indicate pregnancy-induced hypertension (see Chapter 8).

Common blood pressure changes associated with pregnancy are not usually dramatic. During the first half of pregnancy, blood pressure often decreases. It then increases to nonpregnancy levels. Heart sounds are typically regular and strong. Systolic murmurs are common. Occasionally, a diastolic or pulmonic murmur is heard. These generally regress during the postpartum period.

Supine Hypotension Syndrome

Lying in the supine position (flat on the back) can cause the enlarged uterus to press on the woman's inferior vena cava, a major vein that drains the lower portion of the body. When this happens, there is a reduction in venous return and, by association, cardiac output. Dizziness, lightheadedness, fast pulse, nausea and vomiting, and a drop in blood pressure are the important associated symptoms. Supine hypotension syndrome usually occurs in the second half of pregnancy. To decrease pressure on the inferior vena cava and promote adequate circulation, it is recommended that the woman lie on her left side and keep her head slightly elevated.

Orthostatic Hypotension

Orthostatic, or postural, hypotension, refers to the decrease in cardiac output that may occur whenever a pregnant woman rises to a standing position from a recumbent position. The sudden decrease in venous return leads to feelings of lightheadedness. This condition is dangerous because it can lead to injuries and falls. To reduce the risks of injury, pregnant women should rise slowly. They may need to sit up with support for a few minutes before actually standing. As venous blood return equalizes, the risk of injuries from falls is reduced.

Edema

Pooling of fluids (edema) in the lower extremities is common during pregnancy. As fluid gravitates toward the hands and feet, venous pressure *increases,* venous return *decreases,* and fluid seeps into surrounding tissues. This swelling is relieved by elevating and resting the affected extremity. Excessive swelling in the extremities that is not relieved by elevating the hands and feet may indicate complications such as pregnancy-induced hypertension (refer to Chapter 8).

Varicose Veins

Varicose veins are enlarged superficial veins that are engorged with blood. They are typically twisted and appear over-filled (Fig. 5-6). There are multiple causes for varicose veins, including venous congestion that remains unrelieved because of faulty valves, relaxation of the smooth muscle wall in blood vessels, increasing pressure on the inferior vena cava from the uterus, obesity, and familial patterns of varicosities. They are made worse by standing for long periods and pressure from the gravid uterus. Rest, elevation, and having the woman wear specially designed support hose can reduce the size of the enlarged vessels. Varicose veins of the rectum are known as hemorrhoids and are common in pregnancy.

An increase in blood supply, along with influence of estrogen, can also result in occasional hoarseness in the pregnant woman's voice. These vocal changes are related to swelling in the larynx caused by increased vascularization of the nasopharynx.

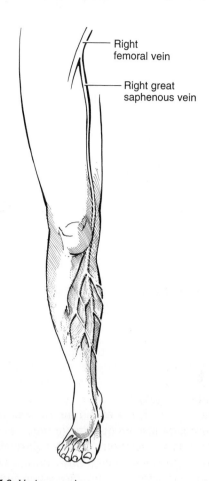

Right femoral vein

Right great saphenous vein

Figure 5-6. Varicose veins.

Respiratory System

Because both maternal and fetal blood must be adequately oxygenated, the woman's oxygenation needs increase by about 20% during pregnancy. The respiratory changes that occur result primarily from the influence of progesterone. This hormone works to relax pulmonary smooth muscle tissue, which promotes ease in ventilation. If progesterone levels are too high, hyperventilation may occur. Even though changes in the respiratory system are designed to enhance the health and well-being of the woman and fetus, they can still cause discomfort.

Nosebleeds and nasal congestion may occur, making it difficult for the woman to breathe. The pregnant woman may also find that smoking and secondary smoke also make breathing more difficult. Dust, pollen, and other pollutants in the air are particularly irritating to the respiratory systems of pregnant women.

Lying supine may cause shortness of breath because of increased diaphragmatic pressure as the uterus moves upward. The woman breathes easier when sitting in an upright position. Encouraging her to support her arms on pillows or a table will help increase lung capacity.

Shortness of breath late in pregnancy is common, but vital capacity (the amount of air that is exhaled following a full inhalation) does not diminish.

Gastrointestinal System

Changes in the gastrointestinal system are generally not serious. However, they often create some discomfort for the pregnant woman. Elevated estrogen levels and hypertrophy of gingival tissue may make gums more sensitive and prone to bleeding when brushed. Palpable lymph nodes associated with gingival hypertrophy can sometimes be felt during the first trimester. Excessive salivation, known as ptyalism, is also a common complaint; its cause is unknown. Depletion of certain vitamins can also cause drying and cracking of the lips.

In addition to "morning sickness," which is associated with elevated progesterone and hCG levels, many women experience indigestion ("heartburn"), flatulence, and constipation.

Indigestion, the result of the incomplete digestion of food, occurs most frequently during the third trimester. Associated heartburn is noticed when the acidic contents of the stomach flow upward when the woman lies down. Flatulence arises when intragastric pressure increases as the result of the heavy uterus's pressing on the stomach and bowels. A decrease in peristaltic activity and loss of muscle tone in the gastrointestinal tract frequently leads to a slowing of the passage of waste through the intestines. When this happens, water in the stools is reabsorbed, making the stools difficult to pass. The resulting constipation is another common complaint of pregnancy.

Pica

A pregnant woman may experience unusual cravings for nonfood items such as starch, clay, mothballs, wood, metal, paper and dirt. This eating disorder is called **pica.** The major danger associated with pica is the risk the woman runs for ingesting toxic substances (eg, lead, which is found in some paints) and parasites. Even when the substances ingested are not toxic, eating them sometimes prevents the woman from eating more nutritious foods. These nonfood items can also interfere with the metabolism of the proper nutrients. For example, ingesting large amounts of clay may disrupt absorption of iron and cause intestinal problems. Educating the woman and her family about the potential dangers associated with pica can reduce health risks.

Urinary System

As the uterus grows, it presses on the bladder, decreasing its capacity for storing urine. This phenomenon lasts briefly during the first trimester. It ends once the uterus lifts out of the pelvic cavity. In the last trimester, the fetus descends back into the pelvic cavity as the time for childbirth approaches. This is called lightening. Again, bladder capacity is reduced and frequency of urination returns.

Progesterone production causes the ureters to dilate. This increases the risk of urinary stasis (or stagnation of normal fluid flow), which can promote the development of infections. The nurse encourages the woman to drink plenty of fluids to decrease this risk. The kidneys respond to the increased blood volume by becoming more efficient in removing fetal and maternal waste products. There is also a slight increase in their size, which reverts shortly after childbirth.

Musculoskeletal System

As the uterus continues to grow, the pregnant woman will strive to maintain her center of gravity by adjusting her posture (Fig. 5-7). Her spine typically curves inward, and she may alter the way she walks as she tries to maintain her balance. These changes may result in complaints such as backache and leg cramps.

A hormone called relaxin, which is secreted by the corpus luteum, is thought to be responsible for increasing the mobility and softening of the pelvic joints. The relaxation and widening of joints in labor permits the fetus to pass through the bony structures of the pelvis.

There is a large abdominal muscle called the rectus abdominis. It may separate in late pregnancy or during labor from the strain of supporting the uterus. This is a fairly common occurrence, especially in obese woman or in multifetal pregnancies. The woman does not feel any pain and the separation corrects itself after childbirth.

Integumentary System

The integumentary system is made up of the skin and its attachments, including the hair and nails. It, too, responds to pregnancy by changing in several ways. Striae gravidarum, "stretch marks," may occur on the skin of a pregnant woman as it stretches to cover her expanding breasts, abdomen, thighs, and buttocks. These marks do not disappear after childbirth, but they typically lighten in color.

Other changes in the integumentary system include darkening of the nipples and areolae, the appearance of the *linea nigra,* and chloasma gravidarum (see

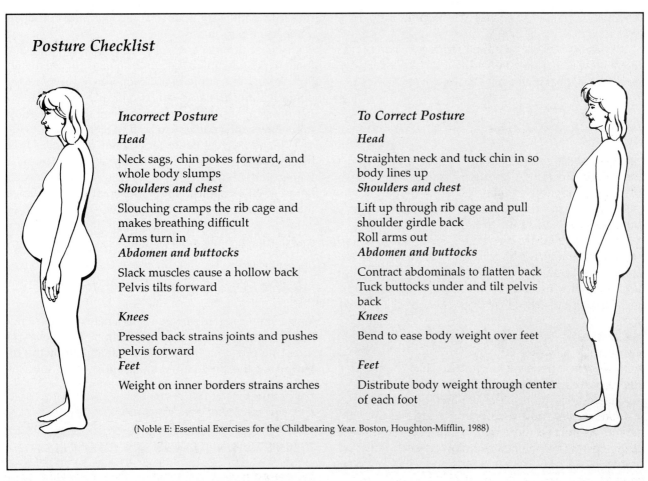

Posture Checklist

Incorrect Posture	To Correct Posture
Head	*Head*
Neck sags, chin pokes forward, and whole body slumps	Straighten neck and tuck chin in so body lines up
Shoulders and chest	*Shoulders and chest*
Slouching cramps the rib cage and makes breathing difficult	Lift up through rib cage and pull shoulder girdle back
Arms turn in	Roll arms out
Abdomen and buttocks	*Abdomen and buttocks*
Slack muscles cause a hollow back	Contract abdominals to flatten back
Pelvis tilts forward	Tuck buttocks under and tilt pelvis back
Knees	*Knees*
Pressed back strains joints and pushes pelvis forward	Bend to ease body weight over feet
Feet	*Feet*
Weight on inner borders strains arches	Distribute body weight through center of each foot

(Noble E: Essential Exercises for the Childbearing Year. Boston, Houghton-Mifflin, 1988)

Figure 5-7. *The woman's posture will change to provide adequate support and avoid discomforts from backaches and muscle strain.*

Fig. 5-1). The intensity of pigmentation changes varies normally in women according to the pigments in their skin.

Psychosocial Effects of Pregnancy

The psychosocial effects of pregnancy on the woman and her family are determined by a number of factors. These include the woman's general physical health, age, emotional maturity and stability, educational background, and work status. Financial considerations, housing issues, and marital status can also influence the reaction of the childbearing family. The timing (planned versus unplanned), both partners' feelings about pregnancy and children, and the number and ages of children already in the family affect the degree to which the family accepts the pregnancy.

Even if the pregnant woman accepts all of these changes with grace, she may experience the anxiety of a change in how she perceives herself as a sexual being.

Developmental Tasks of Pregnancy

The developmental tasks of pregnancy (mimicry, role playing, fantasy, and taking-in) were identified by R. Rubin in 1984. The accomplishment of these phases indicates that the woman is adapting positively to the reality of pregnancy and future motherhood.

In mimicry, the pregnant woman begins to associate with other pregnant women or young mothers, and possibly with her own mother. She asks questions about pregnancy and newborns to learn as much as she can about the whole experience.

During role playing, the pregnant woman may offer to babysit for a friend to practice her parenting skills. This is an important time for the nurse to encourage participation in education classes because the woman's desire to learn is heightened. This exposes her to other positive role models. It is also important that the pregnant woman learn to care for herself and her newborn through demonstrations provided at these classes.

During fantasy task accomplishment, the woman fantasizes about the sex of her newborn and delights in accepting the eventuality of her baby's gender. The last

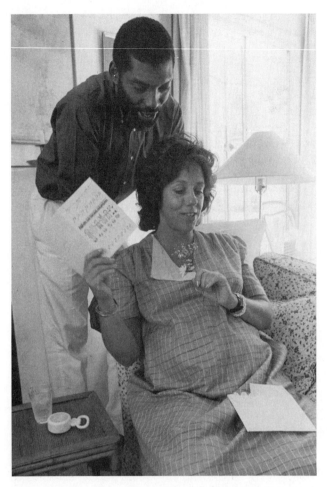

Figure 5-8. *To take an active role in the pregnancy and preparations for the baby, the father may participate in a number of activities from prenatal visits to baby showers. (Photo © Kathy Sloane)*

phase, taking-in, is marked by the pregnant woman's close watch of the behaviors of other mothers around her. Taking-in is successfully accomplished when the mother-to-be modifies the observed behaviors and makes them her own.

The partner can participate in these experiences by staying involved and learning as much as possible about pregnancy, labor, and childbirth. The couple's relationship needs to change to accommodate the growing fetus and the eventual reality of parenthood. It is particularly important that the father or partner's role not be downplayed or overshadowed by focusing all of the attention on the expectant mother (Fig. 5-8).

Adolescent Considerations

The pregnant adolescent is very often too emotionally immature to accept the realities and responsibilities of pregnancy and parenthood. She is very vulnerable, both physically and psychosocially, and is in need of supportive nursing guidance and counseling during the antepartum period.

Fear of the reactions of parents or guardians may force her to attempt to hide or terminate her pregnancy. Some pregnant adolescents even run away to avoid confrontation. Because she is typically very aware of her physical appearance, the pregnant teen may adopt unhealthy eating patterns to limit weight gain.

The adolescent father faces many challenges from his pregnant partner and her family as well as from his family and friends. He may seesaw between acceptance of his responsibility and denial of his involvement. By offering support and guidance to the adolescent father, the nurse can help him adjust to his new role during the antepartal period.

Cultural Considerations

Most cultures regard pregnancy as a natural occurrence that requires no medical intervention. For these cultures, the pregnancy outcome is influenced by the behaviors of the pregnant woman and not by those of medical personnel.

NURSING DIAGNOSES CHECKLIST

Nursing Diagnoses Related to Physical and Psychosocial Changes During Pregnancy

· Risk for Activity Intolerance, related to shortness of breath

· Body Image Disturbance, related to pigmentation changes

· Constipation, related to overcrowding of intestines by uterus

· Family Coping: Potential for Growth, related to first-time pregnancy

· Fatigue, related to pregnancy

· Risk for Injury, related to altered gait

· Knowledge Deficit, related to anticipated physical and psychosocial changes

· Altered Nutrition: Potential for more than body requirements, related to increased appetite in pregnancy

· Sleep Pattern Disturbance, related to physical discomforts

· Social Isolation, related to peer rejection of the pregnant adolescent

· Altered Urinary Elimination, related to first trimester frequency of urination

A Mexican American woman may believe that she must sleep on her back during pregnancy to prevent injury to the fetus. In the Philippines, the woman must bathe her body and cleanse her hair daily to deliver a clean neonate. Some Hispanic and Asian American cultures believe that if the pregnant woman reaches for an object above her head, the cord may wrap around the fetus's head and strangulate it.

The Role of the Nurse

The diagnosis of pregnancy is a highly charged event for the woman and her family. Lack of knowledge or understanding can produce fear and apprehension. Nurses are in a key position to calm these fears. This is done by providing the family with accurate information about the normal physical and psychosocial changes that accompany pregnancy. When the family knows what to expect during the antepartum period, they adapt more easily.

Nursing diagnoses related to normal prenatal physical and psychosocial adaptations are identified in the accompanying display. These sample diagnoses are helpful in formulating individualized nursing diagnoses as nursing care related to physical and psychosocial changes during pregnancy is planned (see Nursing Diagnoses Checklist).

REVIEW AND PREVIEW

This chapter discussed the positive diagnosis of pregnancy, including explaining its early signs and symptoms. The expected physical changes that normally accompany pregnancy were addressed. The emotional and psychosocial needs of the pregnant woman and her family were also examined.

The following chapter describes the importance of adequate antepartal care to promote maternal and fetal health. The comprehensive antepartal assessment provides vital information about the health status of the woman, the fetus, and the childbearing family, which helps nurses to identify women and families at risk.

◈ KEY POINTS

◆ The early, or presumptive, signs and symptoms of pregnancy that may cause a woman to believe that she is pregnant include amenorrhea, nausea and vomiting, breast changes, urinary frequency, and Goodell's sign.

◆ Probable signs of pregnancy include pigmentation changes, enlargement of the abdomen, Chadwick's sign, Hegar's sign, ballottement, Braxton Hicks contractions, quickening, palpation of fetal outline, and a positive pregnancy test. Two or more of these signs typically signify conception.

◆ The positive signs of pregnancy confirm diagnosis with certainty. Presence of fetal heart tones (FHT), palpable fetal movements by the examiner, and visualization of the fetal outline using ultrasound are diagnostic indicators of pregnancy.

◆ Total weight gain in pregnancy varies, but the suggested weight gain in a healthy woman is between 11 and 13 kg (25–30 lbs).

◆ The maternal circulatory volume expands by about 50% to meet the needs of the growing fetus. The blood pressure typically stays stable throughout pregnancy under normal circumstances.

BIBLIOGRAPHY

Bauxite, F., & Hanson, S. (1991). *Fatherhood and Families in Cultural Context.* New York: Springer

Boyle, J. S., & Andrews, M. M. (1990). *Transcultural concepts in nursing care.* Philadelphia: J.B. Lippincott.

Castiglia, P. T. (1990). Adolescent mothers. *Journal of Pediatric Health Care, 4*(5), 262–264.

Castiglia, P. T. (1990). Adolescent fathers. *Journal of Pediatric Health Care, 4*(6), 311–313.

Chapman, L. (1992). Expectant fathers' roles during labor and birth. *Journal of Obstetric, Gynecologic, and Neonatal Nursing, 21*(2), 114–120.

Colman, L., & Colman, A. (1991). *Pregnancy: The psychological experience.* New York: Noonday Press.

Conley, L. (1990). Childbearing and childrearing practices in mormonism. *Neonatal Network, 9*(3), 41–48.

D'Avanzo, C. (1992). Bridging the cultural gap with southeast Asians. *American Journal of Maternal Child Nursing, 17,* 204–207.

Fischbach, F. (1992). *A manual of laboratory and diagnostic tests* (4th ed.). Philadelphia: J.B. Lippincott.

Fishbein, E. (1990). Predicting paternal involvement with a newborn by attitude toward women's roles. *Health Care for Women International, 11,* 109.

Frager, B. (1991). Teenage childbearing: Part I. The problem has not gone away. *Journal of Pediatric Nursing, 6*(2), 131–133.

Hofmeyr, G., Marcos, E., & Buchart, A. (1991). Pregnant women's perceptions of themselves: A survey. *Birth, 17,* 205–206.

Love, C., & Seaton, H. (1991). Eating disorders: Highlights of nursing assessment and therapeutics. *Nursing Clinics of North America, 26*(3), 677–697.

Martin, L. L., & Reeder, S. J. (1990). *Essentials of maternity nursing: Family centered care* (1st ed.). Philadelphia: J.B. Lippincott.

May, K. A., & Mahlmeister, L. R. (1994). *Maternal & neonatal nursing: Family-centered care* (3rd ed.). Philadelphia: J.B. Lippincott.

Reeder, S. J., Martin, L. L., & Koniak, D. (1992). *Maternity nursing: family, newborn, and women's health care* (17th ed.). Philadelphia: J.B. Lippincott.

Rubin, R. (1984). *Maternal identity and the maternal experience.* New York: Springer Publishing.

Thomas, C. L. (Ed.). (1993). *Taber's cyclopedic medical dictionary* (17th ed.). Philadelphia: F. A. Davis.

SELF-ASSESSMENT

1. A pregnant woman who has had one full-term infant, 2 preterm infants (one of whom died), and 1 miscarriage would be classified as:

○ **A.** G4 P1213
○ **B.** G4 P1212
○ **C.** G5 P2114
○ **D.** G5 P1212

2. A woman complains of urinary frequency when she is 10 weeks' pregnant. Which of the following actions would be most appropriate for the nurse?

○ **A.** Notify the physician at once
○ **B.** Inform her that this is common at this point of pregnancy
○ **C.** Obtain a specimen for urinalysis
○ **D.** Ask how much fluid she normally drinks

3. Using Nägele's rule, what would be a woman's due date if the first day of her last menstrual period was April 13th?

○ **A.** December 30
○ **B.** January 7
○ **C.** January 14
○ **D.** January 20

4. A pregnant patient should be encouraged to assume which of the following positions whenever possible?

○ **A.** Supine
○ **B.** High semi-Fowlers
○ **C.** Left lateral
○ **D.** Trendelenberg

5. Potential complications from pica include all of the following EXCEPT:

○ **A.** Altered metabolism of proper nutrients
○ **B.** Excessive weight gain
○ **C.** Ingestion of toxic substances
○ **D.** Decreased appetite for nutritious food

CHAPTER 6

Prenatal Visits and Assessments

◘ OBJECTIVES

When the learning goals of this chapter are met, the reader will be able to:

- ◆ Discuss the importance of prenatal care.
- ◆ Describe the essential components of a comprehensive prenatal assessment.
- ◆ State the routine schedule for follow-up prenatal visits.
- ◆ State the recommended weight gain during pregnancy for women of normal weight, including the amount of gain for each trimester.
- ◆ Identify normal and abnormal changes in the cardiovascular system during pregnancy.
- ◆ Describe the normal findings during the pelvic examination that help the examiner diagnose pregnancy.
- ◆ List the typical laboratory and screening tests that are routinely ordered during the initial visit.
- ◆ Describe identification of women and families at risk during prenatal assessment.

TERMINOLOGY

Antigens	Indirect Coombs' test
Antibodies	McDonald's rule
Diagonal conjugate	Rh factor
Fundal height	Rubella
Hepatitis B	True conjugate
High risk	

Prenatal care is health care a woman receives during the antepartum, or *prenatal,* period. The primary goal of prenatal care is to promote the well-being of the pregnant woman and the fetus. Although this text has used the words *antepartum period* and *antepartal* to refer to this period, the term *prenatal* is used here and in the following chapters to reflect its common usage in everyday experience.

The nurse's responsibilities usually include providing treatments and assessments ordered by the care provider. The nurse also teaches positive health practices in a way that is consistent with and respectful of the family's cultural practices.

Advanced technology and increased understanding of reproduction, conception, fetal growth, and maternal adaptation to pregnancy have improved prenatal care over the last 100 years. Despite these advances, many women still do not receive adequate prenatal care. They may not seek care because of inadequate funds or a lack of health care insurance. Other reasons for poor prenatal care include ineligibility for Medicaid, inaccessibility of health care facility, substance abuse, and difficulty finding reliable transportation and child care. A pregnant woman may fail to seek appropriate prenatal care also if she is a victim of physical abuse, or if she is herself a substance abuser.

The poor and uneducated often do not have access to information concerning the importance and availability of prenatal care. And when they do, it is not always guaranteed that they will take advantage of it.

This chapter begins with a discussion of the importance of prenatal care for all pregnant women. Prenatal assessment, scheduling of routine prenatal visits, and identification of women and families at risk builds on the understanding of the normal changes that occur during pregnancy (discussed in Chapter 5).

Importance of Prenatal Care

Prenatal care is most often provided by nurses, nurse midwives, and physicians. Professionals from other disciplines, such as nutritionists, childbirth educators, and social workers, also may be involved in the care of the childbearing family.

Studies show that when pregnancy is diagnosed early and the woman and family receive consistent care, the associated risks are reduced. When pregnancy diagnosis is delayed, the woman may continue to practice behaviors that are potentially harmful to the unborn child (eg, smoking or taking certain medications). This, in turn, results in low-birthweight neonates or other negative pregnancy outcomes.

Prenatal Visits

The emphasis of prenatal care is on the reduction of maternal and fetal complication and death rates. Regular contact with pregnant women and their families allows nurses to see firsthand how the childbearing family is adapting to the physical and psychosocial changes associated with pregnancy. During these routine prenatal visits, nurses check on the progress of the woman and growing fetus and teach the family about positive self-care behaviors.

Initial Visit

The initial visit should take place as soon as pregnancy is suspected. During the initial visit, the nurse takes detailed health, gynecologic, obstetric, and psychosocial histories. These provide important information about the woman's general and reproductive health, both past and present. The identification of risk factors is an essential function of taking detailed histories.

The woman is provided privacy in a relaxing environment free of distractions before assessment is begun (Fig. 6-1). She will feel less inhibited about answering such personal questions in this type of setting. Once the psychosocial assessment has been done and the oral histories have been taken, a complete physical examination, with extensive laboratory testing, is performed. These tests include, but are not limited to, a urinalysis, complete blood count (CBC), serum electrolytes and glucose, blood typing, Papanicolaou (Pap) smear, Venereal Disease Research Laboratory (VDRL) and other cultures for sexually transmitted diseases (STDs), indirect Coombs' test, and antibody

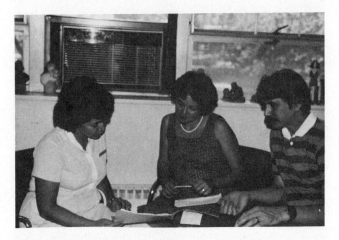

Figure 6-1. *During the initial visit and assessment of the health history, the nurse strives to provide privacy and comfort for the pregnant woman and her partner. (Courtesy of the former Booth Maternity Center, Philadelphia.)*

> **DISPLAY 6-1**
> *Prenatal Visit Schedule*
>
> | | |
> |---|---|
> | Initial visit: | Usually takes place between 6 and 8 weeks |
> | Health, gynecologic, and obstetric histories: | detailed personal and family histories taken |
> | Psychosocial assessment: | woman's and partner's attitudes toward pregnancy discussed |
> | Physical examination: | weight, vital signs, and all body systems assessed |
> | Laboratory tests: | urinalysis; complete blood count (CBC); serum electrolytes; blood typing; Pap smear; VDRL; smears and cultures for other sexually transmitted diseases (STDs); indirect Coombs' test; antibody titers for rubella and hepatitis B; screening for HIV (with consent) |
>
> Follow-up visits are scheduled as follows:
>
> Every 4 weeks until the 28th week of pregnancy
>
> Every 2 weeks from the 28th to the 36th week of pregnancy
>
> Every week until labor begins
>
> Every 3 days if pregnancy progresses past 41 weeks
>
> The health care provider performs several ongoing assessments as necessary during the initial and follow-up visits:
>
> | | |
> |---|---|
> | Pregnancy status: | normal and abnormal changes recorded and monitored |
> | Physical examination: | vital signs; fundal height; fetal heart tones; date and record first fetal movements; after 38 weeks' pregnancy, signs of impending labor |
> | Psychosocial assessment: | plans for obtaining childbirth education and neonatal care information discussed with woman and partner |
> | Laboratory tests (ongoing): | routine urine dipstick tests; CBC; Rh antibody screen at 24 to 28 weeks if necessary; repeat tests for STDs as needed; blood glucose screen at 24 to 28 weeks |
>
> Adapted from May, K. A., & Mahlmeister, L. R. (1994). *Maternal and neonatal nursing: Family-centered care* (3rd ed.). Philadelphia: J. B. Lippincott.

titers. Screening for human immunodeficiency virus (HIV) is stressed for women with significant risk factors (see Chapter 4).

Follow-up Visits

The woman is more likely to keep her scheduled prenatal visits if they fit conveniently into her schedule. Concerns about taking time off from work and finding adequate child care are examples of the types of situations that may negatively affect a woman's ability or desire to keep prenatal appointments. Follow-up visits are scheduled by considering any risk factors identified during the first visit. If there are few or no risk factors, more flexibility can be used when planning follow-up visits. If risk factors have been identified, they are clearly explained to the woman and her family. Appointments are scheduled accordingly. See Display 6-1, *Prenatal Visit Schedule,* for a recommended timetable of prenatal visits.

Prenatal Assessment

In addition to assessing the health of the woman and fetus as just described, the nurse also collects valuable information on the ethnic and cultural background of the family. This and all health-related information are recorded on prenatal forms. Appendix A presents just one example of a detailed prenatal assessment form. These forms are used to gather information during the initial visit. This information is then updated during later visits. The following sections of the chapter present essential components of a comprehensive prenatal assessment.

Health History

A thorough health history includes information specific to the woman, such as age, education level, and current occupation. Discussion about relatives' general health is helpful for evaluating the presence of or potential for heart disease, hypertension, diabetes, or obstetric complications.

A woman whose health history findings are routine is classified as low risk. Significant findings (such as a history of sickle cell anemia) may indicate that the woman or the fetus is at risk for developing complications during pregnancy. These women are classified as **high-risk** patients.

Gynecologic and Obstetric Histories

A gynecologic history includes the age of menarche (first menstruation) and the woman's description of an average menstrual cycle. The frequency of her previous gynecologic examinations as well as the results of previous Pap smears are also discussed. Any abnormal findings from earlier health checkups are explored.

The obstetric history provides information about the woman's previous pregnancies, labor, and birth experiences. The GTPALM method is used to summarize her reproductive information (see Chapter 5 for a discussion of how to record and interpret GTPALM readings). The nurse documents the number of pregnancies, gestational ages at the time of birth, birth weights of all newborns, pregnancy outcomes such as live births and stillbirths, the length of labor with each pregnancy, and significant changes that occurred with each pregnancy. All medications that were taken before this pregnancy and during previous labor experiences are discussed, as are pregnancy-related conditions and complications.

The woman is asked to recall the first day of her last menstrual period (LMP). Using Nägele's rule, the estimated date of delivery (EDD) is then calculated (see Chapter 5).

Psychosocial Assessment

Assessing lifestyles, backgrounds, and coping strategies of family members provides insight into the family's ability to adapt to the current pregnancy. Psychosocial assessment of the woman includes determining her perception of her health status, chronological age and developmental level, and whether her partner and family support the pregnancy.

The family's financial status, housing situation, number of children already in the family, future goals, and feelings about how the pregnancy will change their lives are all assessed. Psychosocial risk factors, such as alcoholism and substance abuse, are also assessed. If the family is determined to be at risk for any damaging factors, the maternal-newborn nurse may work with other health care team members to provide a multidisciplinary approach to treatment.

Weight Gain Assessment

Advances in maternal-newborn care have established that weight gain during pregnancy has a direct impact on neonatal outcomes, including birth weight. For example, pregnancy-induced hypertension and other prenatal complications are more prevalent among underweight women. Neonates of malnourished women have greater risks of neurologic damage and mental retardation, as well as low birth weight. Low birth weight is dangerous because of its association with an increase in the incidence of neonatal death.

An assessment of the woman's weight is made during the initial visit. Thereafter, weight is monitored at every prenatal visit. As described in Chapter 5, a total weight gain of 11 to 13 kg (25–30 lbs)* is recommended during pregnancy for the normal weight woman; 13 to 18 kg (28–40 lbs) for an underweight woman; and 7 to 11 kg (15–25 lbs) for the overweight or obese woman.

Younger adolescents are encouraged to gain the uppermost recommendations, and small or short women are counseled to gain weight in the lower range just described. See Display 6-2 for a more detailed prenatal weight-gain assessment.

Keep in mind that these are suggested gains. Individuals may vary in terms of their actual needs. For example, it is recommended that a woman who is pregnant with twins gain a total of 16 to 20 kg (35–45 lbs) to ensure adequate birth weights of 2500 g or greater for each of her full-term offspring.

Much of the weight a pregnant woman gains is related to the uterus, fetus, placenta, fluid retention, and increased blood volume. This weight is typically lost within approximately 6 weeks of childbirth. Weight gained as fat deposits is more difficult to lose.

---

*Using body mass index (BMI), the revised weight gain range associated with normal birth weights in singleton pregnancy is 11 to 16 kg (25–35 lbs). Source: Chez, R. A. (1993). What are the present guidelines related to weight gain in pregnancy? *AWHONN Voice,* *1*(6), 11.

DISPLAY 6-2
Prenatal Weight Gain Assessment for Women by Weight

Weight gain for 1st trimester:	1–2 kg (2–4 lbs)
Weight gain for 2nd trimester:	5–6 kg (12–14 lbs)
Weight gain for 3rd trimester:	5–6 kg (12–14 lbs)
Total weight gain for woman of average weight:	11–13 kg (25–30 lbs)
Total weight gain for underweight woman:	13–18 kg (28–40 lbs)
Total weight gain for overweight woman:	7–11 kg (15–25 lbs)
Weight gain 1st trimester:	0.5 kg (1 lb) per month
Weight gain 2nd and 3rd trimester for the normal-weight woman:	0.5 kg (1 lb) per week
Weight gain 2nd and 3rd trimester for the underweight woman:	0.5–1 kg (1–2 lbs)
Weight gain 2nd and 3rd trimester for the overweight woman:	0.25 kg (0.5 lb.)

Vital Sign Assessment

A complete set of vital signs is accurately recorded in the woman's chart during the initial visit. These baseline indicators of maternal health will be referred to later in pregnancy to identify variations around the norm. Special attention is given to the blood pressure reading. An increase of 30 mm Hg in the systolic baseline or an increase of 15 mm Hg in the diastolic baseline is a significant finding (see Display 6-3). Abnormal

DISPLAY 6-3
Report Significant Blood Pressure Findings

Notify the woman's physician or nurse midwife when:

- The systolic baseline blood pressure increases 30 mm Hg or more.
- The diastolic baseline blood pressure increases 15 mm Hg or more.
- The woman complains of headaches, blurred vision, or dizziness.
- The woman experiences pain in the upper abdomen, stomach, or liver region.
- The woman experiences unexplained nosebleeds.
- The woman experiences abnormal fatigue, insomnia, and nervousness.
- Anginal pain and shortness of breath are noted in the absence of activity.
- Confusion or seizures are present.

findings are reported to the nurse-midwife or physician. An example would be:

A woman presents with a baseline blood pressure of 108/68. If, at a future assessment, her blood pressure is 140/70, or 120/86, the woman's health care provider is notified.

Blood pressure decreases slightly in the second trimester and returns to first trimester values as pregnancy approaches 40 weeks.

Physical Examination

A thorough physical examination assesses all body systems. The skilled examiner is able to recognize and distinguish normal changes from abnormal changes, which require follow-up and treatment.

Normal and Abnormal Changes

Careful assessment of the pregnant woman gives the examiner a chance to identify 1) the normal changes associated with pregnancy as well as 2) abnormal developments and threats to maternal–fetal health. Abnormal findings may warrant special consideration and treatment during pregnancy. See Chapter 5, *Changes in Other Body Systems,* for a detailed account of normal physiologic changes and indications of abnormalities.

Pelvic Examination

During a pelvic examination, the reproductive organs are assessed for any abnormalities that may interfere with pregnancy or childbirth. Pelvic examinations are typically not repeated until the woman nears the end of pregnancy, unless she is at risk for preterm labor and birth. A description of the routine pelvic examination is found in Chapter 4 (Nursing Procedure), including detailed explanations of nursing actions and rationales.

During pelvic examination of a pregnant woman, the health care provider may put a pillow at the small of the woman's back to reduce back strain. The woman's support person also may be present.

A Pap smear is obtained during the initial visit after the vagina and cervix are visually inspected. The examiner concludes the pelvic examination with bimanual palpation of the uterus and cervix through the vagina and the rectum. Both Goodell's sign (cervical softening) and Hegar's sign (softening of the lower uterine segment) are evident in early pregnancy and detectable on bimanual palpation. The size, texture, and position of internal reproductive organs are assessed. Rectal polyps (small, usually benign growths) and hemorrhoids may be found during this part of the examination. Chapter 5 provides a detailed discussion of the expected reproductive system changes that occur during pregnancy.

Pelvic Measurements

The **true conjugate** (conjugate vera), the area between the sacral promontory and the symphysis pubis, is measured (see Chapter 2, Fig. 2-6). The true conjugate must be large enough to allow the fetus to pass through the inlet of the pelvis during vaginal birth.

The examiner obtains the measure of the true conjugate by measuring the distance between the sacral promontory and the lower border of the symphysis pubis (**diagonal conjugate**) (Fig. 6-2). If the diagonal conjugate is greater than 11.5 cm (4.6 in), the pelvic inlet is considered adequate for vaginal birth. The true conjugate is estimated by subtracting 1.5 to 2 cm from the length of the diagonal conjugate.

Fundal Height

Fundal height is the measurement used to estimate the gestational age of the fetus. Using McDonald's technique, the length from the symphysis pubis to the top of the fundus is determined in centimeters. A measuring tape that has centimeter markings is all that is needed. The zero end of the tape is gently placed at the top of the symphysis pubis and rounded over the abdomen until the uterine fundus is felt, or it can be held straight between the fingers with the hand at a right angle to the top of the fundus. The measurement of the top of the fundus is recorded as the fundal height (Fig. 6-3). Between 20 and 31 weeks' gestation, the number of weeks' gestation and the accurate fundal height measurement should be equal. For example, at 24 weeks, the fundal height should be 24 cm.

McDonald's rule determines gestational length in weeks and lunar months. To establish gestational length in weeks, the height of the fundus in centimeters is multiplied by 8 and divided by 7. To establish gestational length in months, the height of the fundus in centimeters is multiplied by 2 and divided by 7. For example, a woman with a fundal height of 20 cm multiplied by 8 and divided by 7 would be 22.8 weeks pregnant. The same woman with a fundal height of 20 cm multiplied by 2 and divided by 7 would be 5.7 months pregnant.

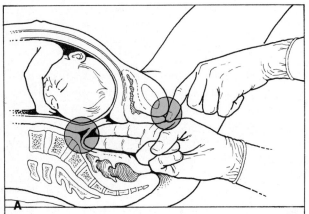 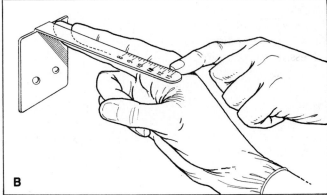

Figure 6-2. *Measurement of the diagonal conjugate. (**A**) A vaginal examination is performed to measure the diagonal conjugate. The examiner touches the sacral promontory P, then marks the hand where it touches the symphysis pubis P. (**B**) The distance between the two points is measured by subtracing 1.5 to 2 cm from this measurement. The true conjugate is measured. The size of the conjugate helps determine the woman's ability to accommodate vaginal childbirth.*

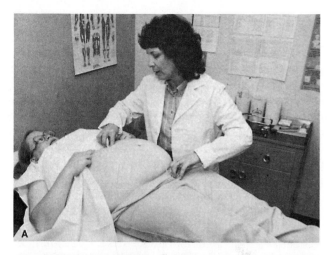

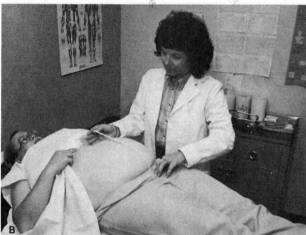

Figure 6-3. *Measurement of fundal height: McDonald's technique. (**A**) The tape measure is curved over the mother's abdomen. (**B**) The tape measure is held straight between the fingers with the hand at a right angle to the top of the fundus. (Courtesy of Media Services, Sonoma State University, Rohnert Park, CA)*

Examples of factors that create inaccurate fundal height measurement include obesity, hydramnios (excess amniotic fluid), multifetal pregnancies, a full bladder, malnourished fetuses, and fetuses that are too large or too small for their gestational ages. Ultrasound may be used to confirm gestational age if the fundal height differs significantly from the actual weeks of gestation (see Chapter 9). Display 6-4 provides a checklist for pelvic examination findings during early pregnancy.

Laboratory Tests

Laboratory tests obtained during the initial prenatal assessment include a urinalysis, CBC, serum glucose and electrolytes, VDRL, blood typing, indirect Coombs' test, screening for HIV, and antibody titers for rubella and

hepatitis B. Laboratory testing of serum and urine is very helpful in determining factors that place many women and their fetuses at risk. Often the woman may appear asymptomatic initially, but results of routine laboratory tests uncover existing abnormalities. These are typically easily treated when detected early. Normal laboratory test values and ranges are included in Appendix B.

Urinalysis

A urinalysis is performed to detect the presence of infection, glucose, or protein. The presence of any of these substances in the urine may indicate a serious condition. For example, glucose found in the urine of a pregnant woman may indicate diabetes. The detection of protein is often the first evidence of pregnancy-induced hypertension (PIH). Infection is confirmed by culture and sensitivity testing of bacteria in urine. A specimen is placed in containers with a culture medium that promotes bacterial growth. Urine testing is repeated at each prenatal visit by dipstick analysis. Results are immediate.

DISPLAY 6-4
Pelvic Examination During Early Pregnancy

Normal findings:

Pink, moist vaginal and cervical membranes

Closed cervical os

Smooth uterine surface

Easily palpable fallopian tubes and ovaries

No growths or abnormalities

Increased vascularity of vagina and cervix

Purplish discoloration

Increase in uterine size

Rising of uterus out of pelvis

Nonpurulent vaginal discharge

Abnormal findings:

Dry, rough mucous membranes

Nonsmooth uterine surface

Difficulty palpating fallopian tubes and ovaries

Growths or abnormalities

No change in vascularity

No increase in uterine size

No change in uterine position

Purulent vaginal discharge

Complete Blood Count

A CBC includes hemoglobin (Hgb) and hematocrit (Hct) levels. Sufficient levels of hemoglobin and hematocrit are necessary for oxygenating maternal and fetal blood. A decrease in the hemoglobin and hematocrit can indicate folic acid deficiency or anemia (see Chapter 8 for a discussion of anemia during pregnancy). Hematocrit and hemoglobin levels may decrease during pregnancy when total blood volume increases but the portion of red blood cells stays the same. This is called hemodilution. Levels that indicate true anemia unrelated to temporary hemodilution include a Hgb count of less than 12% and a Hct reading of less than 35%.

The CBC also identifies the white blood cell count (WBC). Elevations in WBCs may indicate an infection. A WBC count above 11,000 is cause for further investigation. The platelet count assesses blood-clotting ability. Insufficient platelets may result in abnormal bleeding or hemorrhage.

Serum Electrolytes

Electrolytes are loosely defined as the substances in a solution that conduct electrical impulses. Common electrolytes in the human body are: sodium (Na), potassium (K), and chloride (Cl). Serum electrolytes are drawn initially to assess the woman's electrolyte balance, which gives an indication of an individual's cellular and overall health. These values serve as baseline data against which future serum electrolyte values are compared. Disturbances in serum electrolyte levels can pose serious threats to the pregnant woman and her fetus (see Appendix B).

VDRL

The VDRL test or rapid plasma reagin test are used to detect the presence of syphilis, which can be transmitted by an infected woman to her fetus for many years. Untreated syphilis in the pregnant woman may result in deformities or death of the fetus; therefore, early detection is essential.

Blood Type

There are four major blood types: A, B, AB, and O. Whenever patients require a blood transfusion, they must receive blood that is compatible with their own. If they do not, they may develop an immune response, during which their body produces antibodies to the transfused blood. **Antibodies** are complex glycoproteins that destroy foreign antigens from other blood types introduced into the body to protect against infection. **Antigens** identify cells as "self" or "other." Because type O blood has no antigens, it can be transfused into persons in any blood group, as long as Rh compatibility has been as-

sured. In emergency situations, it may be necessary to transfuse a premature neonate. The mother's blood type may be used because the neonate's antibodies typically do not attack the mother's blood type.

Incompatibility in maternal–fetal ABO blood types is common and generally poses no threat to either the mother or fetus. However, Rh factor incompatibility between the woman and her fetus can be problematic. Rh factor is an antigen found in the red blood cells of approximately 90% of the population. When this factor is present, the blood is said to be Rh positive (Rh+).

Hemolytic anemia is caused when fetal red blood cells cross the placenta and enter the mother's bloodstream. Because her body recognizes these cells as "other," it produces antibodies. These antibodies, in turn, cross the placenta, enter the fetus's bloodstream, and destroy its red blood cells. Rh incompatibility, including corrective interventions, is described in Chapter 8. Appendix C illustrates the blood groups and antibody–antigen relationship.

Indirect Coombs' Test

An **indirect Coombs' test** is necessary to verify the presence of antibodies to the Rh factor in a pregnant woman who is Rh negative. If the woman's antibody titers are not sufficiently elevated, RhIgG (Rh immunoglobulin; RhoGAM) is given at 28 weeks' gestation to sensitize the pregnant woman.

Screening for HIV

A simple blood test identifies individuals with antibodies to the human immunodeficiency virus (HIV), the virus that causes acquired immunodeficiency syndrome (AIDS). After explaining the procedure for testing the blood, the nurse obtains permission from the woman to perform the analysis. See Chapter 4 for a more detailed explanation of HIV testing. If a risk for contracting HIV is identified during the health history or if the testing for HIV is positive, counseling is established for the woman and her partner.

Antibody Titers for Rubella and Hepatitis B

Antibody titers measure the amount of an antibody produced to a specific antigen. Titers for **rubella** (German measles) and hepatitis B are determined early in pregnancy to assess whether the pregnant woman is immune to acquiring these diseases. These diseases place the fetus at risk for congenital abnormalities and grave complications. If the woman's rubella titer is less than 1:10, she is not considered immune to German measles. A vaccine to provide active immunity cannot be given during pregnancy. However, the woman is vaccinated during the postpartum period. A variety of infections that may adversely affect pregnancy, including rubella and hepatitis B, are covered in Chapter 8.

Identifying Women and Families at Risk

Women from households in which substance abuse, battering, and low socioeconomic factors are present are often at risk for poor health, lack of prenatal care, psychological problems, and the development of special needs during pregnancy. Anemia, pregnancy-induced hypertension, gestational diabetes, and infections are seen frequently in these women. Health care providers depend on early prenatal assessment to counteract the effects of these risk factors and to promote a positive pregnancy outcome.

Adolescent Considerations

When added to the normal stress of adolescent growth and development, pregnancy increases the potential for poor coping skills. Take, for example, the adolescent's concern about her body image. During pregnancy there may be a desire to hide weight gain and to actually restrict intake to disguise the growing uterus. This can lead to low-birthweight neonates whose chances for survival are less than optimum.

Often, the young teenager does not understand the importance of prenatal assessments and routine health care during pregnancy. The nurse can offer help and

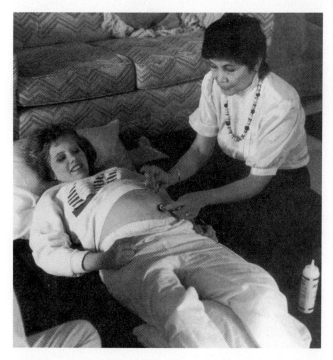

Figure 6-4. The nurse can play a vital role in helping the pregnant teen recognize that prenatal care is extremely important. (Photo courtesy of St. Anne's Maternity Home)

support in getting the adolescent to recognize that good prenatal care is essential (Fig. 6-4). Classes and support groups with other pregnant teenagers are excellent ways to provide positive peer pressure in a situation the nurse can control.

Cultural Considerations

Childbearing in the United States and Canada is often treated as a condition that requires intervention and management by health care professionals. Other cultures view pregnancy and childbirth as normal conditions that do not require any special treatment. This low-key attitude may result in a woman's failing to seek prenatal treatment or comply with prenatal treatment that has already been initiated.

Learning more about various cultural and ethnic groups will allow nurses to respect and understand the wide range of behaviors they may encounter. As long as these practices do not harm the woman or the fetus, every attempt should be made to incorporate them into the pregnant woman's daily routine.

The Role of the Nurse

Appropriate prenatal assessment requires that nurses use their expert abilities to recognize actual and potential problems. These problems may interfere with the health and well-being of the pregnant woman, the fetus, and the childbearing family. It is the nurse who collects the vital prenatal data that will be used to determine the

NURSING DIAGNOSES CHECKLIST

Nursing Diagnoses Related to Early Pregnancy

· Activity Intolerance, related to fatigue

· Anxiety, related to physical and gynecologic examination

· Altered Nutrition: Potential for more than body requirements, related to increased dietary intake in early pregnancy

· Parental Role Conflict, related to diagnosis of new pregnancy

· Altered Role Performance, related to anticipated birth

· Situational Low Self Esteem, related to decreased ability to care for self during pregnancy

SELF-ASSESSMENT

1. Decreased hemoglobin and hematocrit levels during pregnancy are due to:

○ **A.** Vasoconstriction
○ **B.** Hemodilution
○ **C.** Use by the developing fetus
○ **D.** Pregnancy-induced hypertension

2. During her first prenatal visit at 8 weeks, an overweight patient expresses concern over gaining more weight. She should be encouraged to:

○ **A.** Not worry, because the fetus needs the nutrients
○ **B.** Gain no more than 10 pounds
○ **C.** Gain between 15–25 pounds
○ **D.** Limit her daily intake to 1500 calories

3. Which lab test would you expect ordered for a woman at 27 weeks' gestation?

○ **A.** Complete blood count (CBC)
○ **B.** Rapid plasma reagin (RPR)
○ **C.** Glucose
○ **D.** Blood type and Rh factor

4. A patient's fundal height measurement is greater than expected. The physician is likely to order which of the following tests for further evaluation?

○ **A.** Ultrasound
○ **B.** Amniocentesis
○ **C.** Contraction stress test
○ **D.** Nonstress test

5. A woman's baseline BP is 104/70. Which of the following blood pressures would be of the greatest concern at 25 week's gestation?

○ **A.** 98/62
○ **B.** 130/83
○ **C.** 132/80
○ **D.** 124/88

learning needs of the family. Once these have been established, the nurse can teach health promotion based on nursing diagnoses gathered from the assessment data. The nursing care plan reflects the nursing actions that are needed to achieve positive prenatal outcomes for the woman and her growing family. Nursing diagnoses related to early pregnancy are located in the Nursing Diagnoses Checklist.

REVIEW AND PREVIEW

Early care followed by routine visits throughout pregnancy ensures better maternal and fetal outcomes. All of the components of a prenatal assessment were discussed. They included detailed physical, obstetric, and gynecologic histories; psychosocial assessment; pelvic examination; and laboratory tests. Early identification of women at risk during pregnancy was also discussed. Cultural considerations for the pregnant woman and her family and special needs of the adolescent were explored.

The following chapter discusses the nursing care provided to childbearing families during pregnancy, including preparation for childbirth. Regular visits provide excellent opportunities for pregnant women to discuss their concerns and questions with their health care providers.

◈ KEY POINTS

◆ Prenatal care is health care that is provided to the childbearing family during pregnancy. Routine assessment and screening combined with early detection of any potential problems or complications during pregnancy improve health outcomes for the woman and the fetus.

◆ Detailed health and gynecologic histories are obtained during the initial prenatal visit. Comprehensive assessment also includes psychosocial evaluation, recording of weight and vital signs, pelvic examination and Pap smear, and routine laboratory testing.

◆ Routine prenatal visits occur monthly until the 28th week of pregnancy, biweekly up to the 36th week of pregnancy, and every week after 36 weeks of pregnancy. Visits are increased to every 3 days if the pregnancy continues past 41 weeks.

◆ A variety of factors influence the woman's decision to obtain prenatal care, including age, financial status, transportation, family or partner support for the pregnancy, other child care responsibilities, work situation, educational level, and location of an available health care facility.

◆ The recommended total weight gain during pregnancy for women of normal weight is 11 to 13 kg (25–30 lbs). During the first trimester, the pregnant woman gains 1 to 2 kg (2–4 lbs). The total weight increase comes from the 5 to 6 kg (12–14 lbs) gained during each of the last two trimesters.

◆ During early pregnancy, the pelvic examination discloses the probable signs of pregnancy, including Chadwick's sign, Goodell's sign, and Hegar's sign.

◆ The fundal height estimates the gestational age of the fetus most accurately between 20 and 21 weeks' gestation. Accurate measurement uses McDonald's technique. Fundal height equals the distance in centimeters between the top of the symphysis pubis to the rounded crest of the fundus.

◆ Routine laboratory tests obtained during the initial prenatal assessment typically include: a urinalysis, a CBC, serum electrolytes, VDRL, blood typing, indirect Coombs' test, and antibody titers for rubella and hepatitis B. If the woman is determined to be at risk for HIV, she is also screened for antibodies to this virus.

BIBLIOGRAPHY

Bates, B. (1991). *A guide to physical examination and history taking* (5th ed.). Philadelphia: J. B. Lippincott.

Boyle, J., & Andrews, M. (1990). *Transcultural concepts in nursing care.* Boston: Scott Foresman.

Barnes, L. (1991). Pregnancy over 35: Special needs. *American Journal of Maternal Child Nursing, 16*(5), 272.

Carpenito, L. J. (1993). *Nursing diagnosis: Application to clinical practice* (5th ed.). Philadelphia: J. B. Lippincott.

Colman, L., & Colman, A. (1991). *Pregnancy: The psychological experience.* New York: Noonday Press.

Dineen, K., Rossi, M., Lia-Hoagberg, B., & Keller, L. (1992). Antepartum home-care services for high-risk women. *Journal of Obstetric, Gynecologic, and Neonatal Nursing, 21*(2), 121–125.

Engstrom, J., & Sittler, C. (1993). Fundal height measurement: Part 1. Techniques for measuring fundal height. *Journal of Nurse-Midwifery, 38*(1), 5–16.

Eschleman, M. M. (1991). *Introductory nutrition and diet therapy* (2nd ed.). Philadelphia: J. B. Lippincott.

Fischbach, F. (1992). *A manual of laboratory and diagnostic tests* (4th ed.). Philadelphia: J. B. Lippincott.

Kelley, S. J., Walsh, J. H., & Thompson, K. (1991). Birth outcomes, health problems, and neglect with prenatal exposure to cocaine. *Pediatric Nursing, 17*(2), 130–135.

Martin, L. L., & Reeder, S. J. (1990). *Essentials of maternity nursing: Family centered care* (1st ed.). Philadelphia: J. B. Lippincott.

May, K. A., & Mahlmeister, L. R. (1994). *Maternal & neonatal nursing: Family-centered care* (3rd ed.). Philadelphia: J. B. Lippincott.

Pillitteri, A. (1992). *Maternal and child health nursing: Care of the childbearing and childrearing family* (1st ed.). Philadelphia: J. B. Lippincott.

Reeder, S. J., Martin, L. L., & Koniak, D. (1992). *Maternity nursing: Family, newborn, and women's health care* (17th ed.). Philadelphia: J. B. Lippincott.

Roller, C. (1992). Drawing out young mothers. *The American Journal of Maternal/Child Nursing, 17*(5), 254–255.

Scherer, J. C. (1992). *Introductory clinical pharmacology* (4th ed.). Philadelphia: J. B. Lippincott.

Rose, A. (1992). Effects of childhood sexual abuse on childbirth. *Birth, Issues in Perinatal Care, 19*(4), 214–218.

Starn, J., Patterson, K., Bemis, G., Castro, O., & Bemis, P. (1993). Can we encourage pregnant substance abusers to seek prenatal care? *The American Journal of Maternal/Child Nursing, 18*(3), 148–152.

CHAPTER 7

Prenatal Health Promotion

◈ OBJECTIVES

When the learning goals of this chapter are met, the reader will be able to:

◆ Discuss the significance of meeting the nutritional needs for pregnant women.
◆ Describe how health teaching and dietary choices are modified to take special diets into consideration.
◆ State at least six areas the nurse includes in general health teaching.
◆ Identify three common discomforts associated with pregnancy and describe sample health-promoting behaviors.
◆ List the danger signs that the pregnant woman or her family needs to report.
◆ State the major threats to healthy pregnancy.
◆ Explain the goals of childbirth preparation.
◆ Describe the Dick-Read, Bradley, and Lamaze methods of childbirth.
◆ Describe situational factors that have a significant impact on pregnancy.

TERMINOLOGY

Bradley method	Minerals
Dick-Read method	Nutrients
Dyspnea	Protein
Lamaze method	Vitamins

Chapter 6 focused on the importance of performing comprehensive physical and psychosocial assessments of the woman and her family during the antepartum period. This chapter describes maternal-newborn nursing care as it relates to health promotion. Health promotion in normal pregnancy includes: nutrition counseling, teaching positive self-care behaviors, preparation for childbirth, relief of common discomforts, understanding threats to healthy pregnancy, and recognizing of danger signs.

Nutritional Counseling

One of the best ways to ensure maternal and fetal well-being is to teach the family the importance of proper nutrition during pregnancy. The nurse may work alone or with a dietitian to provide nutrition counseling to the expectant family. A sharing of pertinent nutritional information with the pregnant woman and her support person is essential.

Importance of Nutrition During Pregnancy

Pregnant women who consume a nutritionally adequate diet reduce the risks associated with poor nutrition, such as pregnancy-induced hypertension and anemia for the woman and compromised fetal brain cell development and low birth weight in the neonate.

Display 7-1 lists the risk factors that may endanger the health of the woman or fetus. Many of these risk factors are directly related to maternal nutrition.

Nutritional Requirements During Pregnancy

A woman who normally eats a balanced diet needs to make only a few changes in her diet to maintain proper nutrition during pregnancy. These changes consist of increasing daily intake of protein, vitamins, and minerals. An additional 300 calories a day is recommended by the end of the first trimester. Some woman may need to increase their caloric intake by as many as 500 calories. Dietary needs for essential **nutrients** (foods or other substances that nourish the body) and supplementation are described below.

Protein

The body's demand for "fuel" to support the growth of fetal and maternal tissues is supplied by **proteins,** which are rich in essential amino acids. The Recom-

mended Dietary Allowances (RDA) for protein during pregnancy is 60 g per day. Protein is supplied by animal and vegetable sources. These include meat, fish, poultry, eggs, beans, legumes, seeds, nuts, and low-fat milk and cheese.

Vitamins

Vitamins are organic substances needed by the body to regulate metabolism. During pregnancy, the body needs more than the usual RDAs of vitamins and minerals. The fat-soluble vitamins (A, D, E, and K) are stored in the tissue and excreted in minimal amounts. They are needed for growth, development, and the proper functioning of the body. Water-soluble vitamins (C, B-complex, and folic acid) are readily excreted once the body meets its demands for them.

Vitamin A is essential for body growth and cell reproduction. Adequate intake of vitamin A also improves the body's ability to fight off infection. Sources of vitamin A include dark green vegetables, yellow vegetables, animal liver, and egg yolks.

Vitamin D aids in the absorption of calcium and phosphorus for the formation of bones and teeth.

Sources include fish liver oil, egg yolk, butter, fortified milk and green vegetables. Vitamin D is also synthesized in the skin after exposure to sunlight.

Vitamin E creams and lotions have long been used on the skin to slow down drying and aging. However, the most important role played by vitamin E is as an antioxidant. Antioxidants are substances that help protect the body from infections and many degenerative diseases (such as cancer). Sources of vitamin E include vegetable fats and oils, grains, and eggs.

Vitamin K is essential for the formation of prothrombin, a necessary factor in normal blood clotting. It is synthesized in the large intestine. (Newborns have no vitamin K in their digestive tracts until food is ingested and the intestines produce bacteria, from which the vitamin is synthesized.) Sources of vitamin K include spinach and other dark green leafy vegetables and liver. Table 7-1 includes the recommended intake of fat-soluble vitamins.

Vitamin C (ascorbic acid) prevents scurvy and is necessary for the healing of wounds and fractures. Vitamin C deficiency in a pregnant woman can lead to imperfect formation of the fetal skeleton. Sources of vitamin C include citrus fruits and juices, most fresh vegetables, and tomatoes.

B-complex vitamins act as coenzyme factors in cell respiration, energy metabolism, and glucose oxidation. Sources of B-complex vitamins include whole grains, fortified cereals and breads, lean meats, and dairy products.

Folic acid, a B-complex vitamin, is important in the formation of red and white blood cells in bone marrow. It also helps in the synthesis of DNA, promoting healthy cell division and replication. Adequate intake of folic acid is particularly important to the pregnant woman because it regulates embryonic and fetal development of nerve cells. Sources of folic acid include kidney, liver, and green leafy vegetables. The rec-

ommended intake of water-soluble vitamins is summarized in Table 7-2.

Minerals

Minerals are inorganic materials that allow the body to perform its many functions efficiently. The primary minerals are iron, calcium, and phosphorus. As with vitamins, the body's demand for minerals increases during pregnancy.

The body requires greater supplies of iron to transport oxygen via hemoglobin between the fetus and the woman. Stores of iron in the fetal liver, which are built up during the third trimester of pregnancy, last for approximately 3 months after birth. After this period, the newborn receives sufficient amounts of iron daily from breast milk or formula. Recommended daily intake for iron is between 15 and 20 mg throughout the antepartum period. Dark green leafy vegetables, red meat, liver, eggs, legumes, and enriched or whole grain breads, and cereals are good sources of iron.

Calcium and phosphorus are essential for the formation of teeth and bones. The RDA for calcium in pregnancy is 1200 mg/day. Insufficient intake of calcium by the woman results in inadequate calcium reserves. Fetal needs for bone growth and tooth formation are met by using the woman's calcium reserves, especially during the last trimester. It is essential that the woman have enough calcium stored in her long bones to satisfy fetal needs; otherwise, this mineral will be depleted by the fetus. Today, most nutritionists recommend that the pregnant woman get her calcium by drinking four 8-ounce glasses of milk, or its equivalent, per day.

Phosphorus is found in many foods rich in calcium. These foods include milk, organ meats, grains, and legumes (beans, peas, and lentils). This mineral is needed for bone and cell growth and tooth formation.

Table 7-1. *Recommended Intake of Fat-Soluble Vitamins*

| Age in Years | Nonpregnant Intake | | | | Pregnant Intake | | | |
	Vitamin A (µg RE)*	Vitamin D (µg)	Vitamin E (mg TE)†	Vitamin K (µg)	Vitamin A (µg RE)	Vitamin D (µg)	Vitamin E (mg TE)	Vitamin K (µg)
11–14	800	10	8	45	800	10	10	65
15–18	800	10	8	45	800	10	10	65
19–24	800	10	8	45	800	10	10	65
25–50	800	5	8	45	800	10	10	65

*RE = retinol equivalents.
800 = 4,000 IU (International units)
1000 = 5,000 IU (International units)
†TE = tocopherol equivalents
From May, K. A., & Mahlmeister, L. R. (1994). *Maternal and neonatal nursing: Family-centered care* (3rd ed.). Philadelphia: J.B. Lippincott, p. 392.

Table 7-2. *Recommended Intake of Water-Soluble Vitamins*

	Age in Years			
Vitamin	11–14	15–18	19–24	25–50
Nonpregnant Intake				
Vitamin C (mg)	50	60	60	60
Thiamin (mg)	1.1	1.1	1.1	1.1
Riboflavin (mg)	1.3	1.3	1.3	1.3
Niacin (mg)	15	15	15	15
Vitamin B_6 (mg)	1.4	1.5	1.6	1.6
Folacin (μg)	150	180	180	180
Vitamin B_{12} (μg)	2	2	2	2
Pregnant Intake				
Vitamin C (mg)	70	70	70	70
Thiamin (mg)	1.5	1.5	1.5	1.5
Riboflavin (mg)	1.6	1.6	1.6	1.6
Niacin (mg)	17	17	17	17
Vitamin B_6 (mg)	2.2	2.2	2.2	2.2
Folacin (μg)	400	400	400	400
Vitamin B_{12} (μg)	2.2	2.2	2.2	2.2

From May, K. A., & Mahlmeister, L. R. (1994). *Maternal and neonatal nursing: Family-centered care* (3rd ed.). Philadelphia: J.B. Lippincott, p. 393.

Phosphorus deficiency is rare because the mineral is found in so many foods. The RDA for phosphorus is 1200 mg/day. Table 7-3 summarizes the recommended intake of minerals for pregnant and nonpregnant women.

Carbohydrate and Fat

The body's energy and metabolism needs are met with sufficient carbohydrate and fat intake. Excess carbohydrates are stored by the body as fat and increase maternal weight gain. Carbohydrate sources include starches, legumes, and grains. Although fat is necessary for the absorption of fat-soluble vitamins, the diet should supply only moderate amounts. Sources of fat include oils, nuts, meat, and butter.

Supplementation

To ensure adequate amounts of vitamins and minerals in the pregnant woman's diet, many health care providers prescribe prenatal vitamin and mineral tablets. Supplements are typically prescribed once a day. Other providers believe that if the woman's diet is adequate, supplementation is unnecessary. The pregnant woman whose diet is lacking in essential nutrients needs to be encouraged to take supplements. Some women report

prenatal vitamins taken during the first trimester result in nausea and vomiting. The woman may experience fewer gastrointestinal symptoms if she takes the supplement at the same time each day, preferably with food.

Food Pyramid

The United States Department of Agriculture (USDA) Food Guide Pyramid is an effective tool in simplifying appropriate food choices. Foods are divided into five groups and arranged hierarchically according to the frequency with which they should be consumed. The base of the pyramid reflects that carbohydrates are the largest portion of dietary intake (Fig. 7-1). Fats, oils, and sweets are at the top of the pyramid. These items should be eaten in the smallest portions. The **food pyramid** is designed to make healthy food choices easier.

Bread, Cereal, Rice, and Pasta Group

Bread, cereal, rice, and pasta serve as the foundation of the pyramid. Foods in this group make up the largest source of daily calories. Individuals are counseled to eat six to seven servings from these carbohydrate sources every day during pregnancy and lactation. An average serving is one slice of bread, three to four small crackers, or ½ cup pasta. To obtain the most

Table 7-3. *Recommended Intake of Minerals*

| | Age in Years | | | |
Mineral	11–14	15–18	19–24	25–50
Nonpregnant Intake				
Calcium (mg)	1200	1200	1200	800
Phosphorus (mg)	1200	1200	1200	800
Magnesium (mg)	280	300	280	280
Iron (mg)	15	15	15	15
Zinc (mg)	12	12	12	12
Iodine (mg)	150	150	150	150
Pregnant Intake				
Calcium (mg)	1200	1200	1200	1200
Phosphorus (mg)	1200	1200	1200	1200
Magnesium (mg)	320	320	320	320
Iron (mg)*	30	30	30	30
Zinc (mg)	15	15	15	15
Iodine (mg)	175	175	175	175

*Supplemental iron is needed daily in addition to dietary sources.
From May, K. A., & Mahlmeister, L. R. (1994). *Maternal and neonatal nursing: Family-centered care* (3rd ed.). Philadelphia: J.B. Lippincott, p. 393.

benefit from this food group, it is best to choose cereals and breads with enriched flour or whole grains. Bread, cereal, rice, and pasta provide excellent sources of energy.

Fruit Group

Fruits are good sources of vitamins C and A and fiber (in the form of carbohydrates). Fruits, which have a high flavor content, are typically eaten raw. During pregnancy and lactation, two to four servings of fruit each day are recommended. A serving is one medium apple or banana, or ½ cup cooked or canned fruit.

Vegetable Group

Vegetables are another ideal source of vitamins C and A as well as carbohydrates. To preserve the nutritional value in the vegetables, they are best eaten raw or steamed. Using the cooking liquids in soups and gravies reduces waste of valuable vitamins and minerals. Like fruits, vegetables vary by season and geographic region and can be purchased fresh, frozen, or canned. One cup raw or ½ cup cooked vegetables is a serving. Pregnant women are encouraged to include a minimum of two servings of dark green, or yellow leafy vegetables in their daily diet.

Meat, Poultry, Fish, Dry Bean, Egg, and Nut Group

Meat, poultry, fish, dry beans, eggs, and nuts are the principal sources of protein and minerals. However, milk, yogurt, and cheese are also good, less expensive sources of these nutrients. To meet the needs of the developing fetus, a daily total of three or more servings from this group are recommended. Each serving should be 5 to 7 ounces. One egg equals 1 ounces. Two tablespoons of peanut butter or ½ cup beans also equals a serving.

Milk, Yogurt, and Cheese Group

Milk, yogurt, and cheese provide essential protein, calcium, phosphorous, and zinc. Pregnant women should eat three or more servings a day from this group. One cup of milk, 8 ounces of yogurt, and 2 ounces of cheese are average servings. During lactation, servings from this food group increase to six to seven per day.

Because lactose-intolerant women cannot digest milk sugars, they should be encouraged to get their calcium from other sources. The lactose in yogurt and aged cheese has already been broken down into lactic acid, so they make two good alternatives. Other foods such as beans, greens (cabbage, kale, and collards), cauliflower, rhubarb, molasses, and egg yolks are also good sources of this mineral.

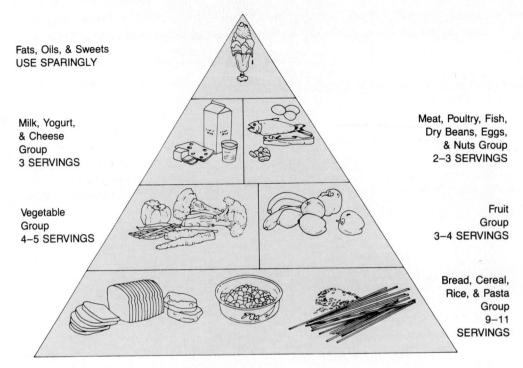

Figure 7-1. *USDA Food Guide Pyramid.*

Fats, Oils, and Sweets Group

Fats, oils, and sweets are at the top of the pyramid, indicating that they should be eaten sparingly. Chips, candy, cakes, cookies, and mayonnaise are examples of foods in this group.

Dietary Considerations

Taking a thorough dietary history for every pregnant woman helps the nurse to determine customary eating habits. With this information, the nurse suggests appropriate dietary modifications to the woman. Nutrition counseling must be individualized to incorporate the special needs and dietary preferences of the pregnant woman and her family. Examples of factors that effect dietary patterns include vegetarianism, adolescence, cultural and ethnic influences, and unsafe eating habits.

Vegetarian Diets

The vegetarian diet can vary from one individual to the next. Pure vegetarians get all of their calories from plant material. Revising diets for these women takes careful planning to include complete protein sources. Other vegetarians supplement their intake with milk and milk products (lacto-vegetarians); some of these vegetarians even add eggs to the list (lactovo-vegetari-

ans). Devising diets for these women is typically easier because they already consume animal sources of proteins.

All pregnant women, whether they are meat eaters or vegetarians, must consume adequate amounts of essential amino acids to maintain and promote maternal and fetal health. The nurse encourages the pregnant vegetarian to meet her daily protein requirements by suggesting that she include some of the following protein sources in her diet: lean meat, fish, poultry, or one egg a day. For those who avoid animal products altogether, a careful mix of legumes, nuts, and grains is recommended.

Preparation for Lactation

Preparation for lactation includes eating a well-balanced diet that is based on the food pyramid guidelines. The requirements for calcium, protein, and milk during lactation are met by drinking four 8-ounce glasses of milk a day or its equivalent. It is important that daily fluid intake during lactation remains the same as during pregnancy.

◆ Health Promotion

Teaching the pregnant woman to eliminate or reduce the minor discomforts associated with pregnancy provides her with a sense of control. It also actively involves her in promoting her own and the fetus's well-being.

Health Teaching During Pregnancy

All aspects of the woman's activities of daily living (ADL) are taken into consideration before providing health teaching. The woman appreciates understanding ways to modify her behavior to ensure a positive pregnancy experience. General health promotion guidelines are discussed in the following sections.

Elimination

The pregnant woman is encouraged to drink six to eight glasses of fluids every day, increase dietary fiber, and engage in regular exercise to improve elimination patterns. Taking over-the-counter medications (OTCs) to treat constipation is discouraged during pregnancy unless approved by the woman's health care provider.

Hygiene

Daily bathing is suggested during pregnancy because of increased vaginal discharge, sweat, and oil gland activity. Certain safety precautions are important during pregnancy. If the woman prefers to tub bathe, nonslip bath mats or safety strips should be applied to the tub surface. As pregnancy progresses, the woman may need assistance getting into and out of the bath. (See Chapter 5 for a discussion of orthostatic, or postural, hypotension and its association with falls during pregnancy.)

Many care providers discourage the use of routine vaginal douches. Because douche solutions tend to change the normal pH of the vagina, the body's natural ability to fight vaginal and uterine infections can be compromised. This poses a serious health threat to the fetus. Additionally, the increased vaginal pressure caused by forceful douching may rupture the membranes.

Breast and Nipple Care

The oily secretions produced by Montgomery's glands act as natural lubricants that protect the nipples during the postpartum period. Daily cleansing of the breasts and nipple area with plain water is recommended. Harsh or perfumed soaps may remove essential lubricants and cause dryness and cracking.

Some health care providers instruct the pregnant woman to "toughen" nipples in preparation for breast-feeding by wiping them daily with a dry washcloth, beginning at the seventh month. They may also instruct her to pull each nipple out slightly and roll it back and forth several times a day between thumb and forefinger. This practice is discouraged among women who are prone to preterm birth because it may cause uterine contractions.

Clothing

Clothing worn during pregnancy should be comfortable and loose-fitting to allow for continued abdominal growth. As the breasts enlarge, the woman needs to change her bra size to one that provides added support. Anything that constricts circulation in the lower extremities may cause edema or result in the formation of varicose veins. For this reason, knee-high stockings need to be avoided. Shoes with low or medium heels are recommended. High-heeled shoes, which cause back strain and increase the incidence of falls, are to be avoided.

Sleep and Rest

The pregnant woman requires between 6 and 8 hours of sleep each night. Ideally, a brief nap during the day would benefit the woman. Resting several times a day or every few hours will also help her to "recharge her battery" so that she can carry on with her daily life. Pregnant women who can find time to rest and relax often have trouble assuming a comfortable position. The nurse can recommend that she lie down on her back with her legs elevated, or on her side with the abdomen gently supported (Fig. 7-2). Teaching the pregnant woman to sit with her feet slightly elevated is also sure to improve her energy level and promote circulation to her legs (Fig. 7-3).

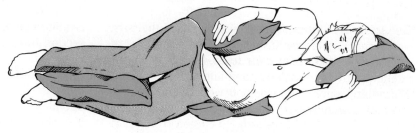

Figure 7-2. The pregnant woman may rest in a comfortable position by lying down with her body aligned and pillows supporting her legs, abdomen, and head.

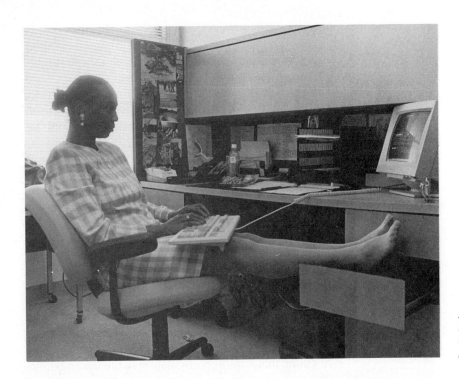

Figure 7-3. *Employed pregnant women need to elevate their feet periodically throughout the workday. (Photo © Kathy Sloane)*

Activity and Exercise

The American College of Obstetricians and Gynecologists (ACOG) published *Guidelines for Exercise During Pregnancy and the Postpartum Period* in 1985. These guidelines suggest variations for standard exercises and sports during pregnancy. The goal of any exercise program should be the safety of the woman and the fetus. Promoting adequate oxygenation, placental perfusion, venous return, and a positive emotional state are important elements of a well-rounded exercise program. Walking, swimming, and bicycling are acceptable activities to meet the needs of most pregnant women. However, a modified program of aerobics, weight training, and muscle-developing techniques can be continued into pregnancy. Adaptations in the routines are designed to minimize maternal and fetal injury. Examples of other exercises for muscle strengthening and relaxation are shown in a later display.

Employment

Many women are employed outside the home and continue to work during pregnancy. Most occupations do not present hazards to the woman or the fetus. However, jobs that require heavy lifting or place the pregnant woman in a position where balance may be altered need to be evaluated for safety. Because falls and accidents during pregnancy contribute to maternal and fetal complications, the woman's work responsibilities need to be adjusted to reduce these risks. Figure 7-4 provides an example of proper body alignment and posture for lifting objects from the floor.

Some work environments may expose the pregnant woman and her unborn child to chemicals and noxious fumes. Common household chemicals such as ammonia and lye are also dangerous to the fetus. Exposure to radiation, particularly during the first trimester, is extremely dangerous for the developing fetus.

Travel

Traveling during pregnancy is generally not restricted. Occasionally, however, women in high-risk situations and those in the last trimester of pregnancy are advised to cut down on travel. Women with previous histories of premature labor or other complications need to discuss travel plans with their health care providers.

Any travel should allow the woman to assume a comfortable position and present her with plenty of opportunities to walk around every few hours. This activity stimulates circulation and decreases fatigue. All pregnant women traveling by car need to wear seat belts, preferably a harness-type model. Today, airlines allow travel up to the seventh month of pregnancy. Overseas travel is typically not recommended after the second trimester. During the third trimester, the childbearing family is advised to familiarize themselves with the location of nearby health care facilities before traveling. In the event of an emergency, the family can seek adequate care.

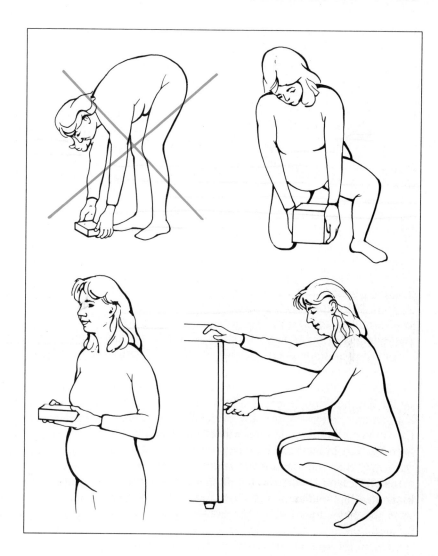

Figure 7-4. *Proper bending and lifting techniques help the pregnant woman avoid back strain.*

Sexual Activity

Sexual activity may continue during pregnancy as long as it is comfortable and desirable for both partners. The woman's sexual response may actually be heightened because of increased vasocongestion in the perineal and vulvar regions. As pregnancy progresses, the woman and her sexual partner may need to experiment with positions that provide comfort and enjoyment for both.

Occasionally, sexual stimulation may be contraindicated by a complication, such as a history of premature labor or placenta previa (see Chapter 13). The couple is encouraged to ask their health care providers questions and to explore concerns about sexual activity.

Use of Medications

Because most medications pass the placental barrier, pregnant women need to get the approval of their primary health care providers before taking any prescription or OTC medications. All medications should be given in the lowest effective doses to minimize any potential adverse effects to the fetus. They also should be discontinued as soon as possible.

Particular care should be taken during the first trimester, when drugs have the greatest teratogenic effect. Teratogenic agents are drugs and other like substances that, when ingested by the pregnant woman, cause fetal abnormalities (see Chapter 9). It is vital that these agents be avoided during pregnancy.

Health Teaching for Relief of Common Discomforts During Pregnancy

Some of the most commonly reported discomforts of pregnancy include nausea, vomiting, indigestion ("heartburn"), and constipation and flatulence; urinary frequency; shortness of breath; edema and varicose veins; and orthostatic hypotension. The causes of these symptoms are described in Chapter 5 under *Changes in Other Body Systems*. They are discussed here in terms of symptom relief.

Gastrointestinal Disturbances

Nausea and vomiting are often controlled by eating smaller, more frequent meals. Crackers or whole wheat toast can also be kept near the bed so that the woman can eat them before rising.

Having the woman avoid foods that are highly seasoned, spicy, or fried relieves indigestion. Encouraging her to remain upright for at least 30 minutes after each meal also prevents indigestion by cutting down on acid reflux. The use of antacids for indigestion is usually permissible but should be discussed with the health care provider. It is important that the pregnant woman report long-lasting gastrointestinal disturbances. They may indicate ulcers or other gastrointestinal problems, which may remain undiagnosed if they are controlled through the use of antacids.

Both constipation and flatulence can be relieved by having the woman follow a few simple guidelines. For example, engaging in daily exercise such as walking or swimming can increase gastrointestinal motility. Increasing fluid intake to at least 8 to 10 glasses of liquid each day reduces constipation by keeping the stools sufficiently hydrated. Eating more fruits, vegetables, and high-bulk items such as whole grains and fiber also helps to soften stools and ease bowel movements.

Many foods that are high in gas-producing sulfur compounds are highly nutritious and should not be avoided during pregnancy. This is especially true of beans. To reduce their gas-causing effects, beans should be boiled for 1 minute, drained, and then brought to a second boil with fresh water. Encouraging the woman to eat small, frequent meals also reduces flatulence.

Frequency of Urination

The pregnant woman is taught to attend to any and all urges to urinate, no matter how frequent. Failure to empty the bladder regularly may result in urinary stasis, a preventable cause of bladder infections. Reducing total fluid volume intake is not recommended.

Backache

It is important that the health care provider assess complaints of backache carefully to rule out urinary tract infections and premature labor. Once these causes of discomfort have been ruled out, the nurse can concentrate on teaching the pregnant woman how to avoid back strain by practicing a few simple techniques.

Because pregnancy changes the woman's center of gravity (and her posture along with it), she will need to be trained to alter her lifting and reaching techniques. Teaching her correct lifting technique and encouraging her to rest frequently and avoid strenuous activities are all part of the nurse's patient teaching efforts (see Fig. 7-4). She should also be discouraged from bending from the waist to reach for something on a low shelf, because it may place undue stress on the back.

Shortness of Breath

The pregnant woman may experience **dyspnea** (shortness of breath) as the growing uterus rises upward and presses against the diaphragm. This crowding of the lungs causes dyspnea, which is common during the latter part of pregnancy. Dyspnea is typically more pronounced when the woman is lying down. Shortness of breath that occurs early in pregnancy or while the woman is in an erect position needs to be reported to the health care provider for evaluation.

Nurses can reassure women that shortness of breath in the third trimester does not usually indicate a complication. The fetus receives adequate oxygen despite the woman's temporary discomfort. Once the fetus drops into the birth canal in late pregnancy the woman will be able to expand her lungs more fully. Dyspnea can be distressing to the woman, particularly when she is trying to sleep. The nurse can suggest that she use pillows to prop up her upper body and head. The arms need to be adequately supported.

Edema

The nurse encourages the woman to rest and elevate her lower extremities to relieve swelling. A full night's sleep is often helpful because reclining promotes venous return and reduces dependent edema. Swelling of the hands, face, or lower extremities after rest and elevation needs to be reported. These symptoms may indicate pregnancy-induced hypertension (see Chapter 8). Because edema is also affected by sodium retention, having the pregnant woman eliminate heavily salted foods from her diet is also a good idea.

Varicose Veins

It is easier to prevent varicose veins than to treat them. The woman is encouraged to avoid wearing constricting clothing, especially garments that impair circulation in the legs. Frequent changes of body position are also recommended. Women who stand for long periods are particularly encouraged to alternate their standing with sitting. Stretching and simple body movements promote circulation and reduce stasis of blood flow. Regular rest periods throughout the day and elevation of the legs for 5 to 10 minutes at a time helps to prevent varicose vein formation. Maternity support hose may even be prescribed. These are usually worn during the waking hours. Hemorrhoids can be avoided by relieving constipation and reducing the need to strain during bowel movements.

Round Ligament Pain

Lower abdominal pain in pregnancy can be associated with ectopic pregnancy, premature labor, or round ligament pain. The round ligament is attached to the uterus and extends to the broad ligament (see Chapter 2, Fig. 2-5). Sudden movements that cause strain to the body can cause round ligament pain. Although all pain in pregnancy is assessed, the woman can eliminate this discomfort by avoiding lifting and twisting in late pregnancy.

Leg Cramps

Leg cramps may be caused by decreased circulation, pressure from the growing uterus, muscle strain, excess chloride excretion, and disruption in the calcium-phosphorous ratio. Relief is typically obtained by teaching the woman to stand erect while bearing her full weight on the affected limb. Dorsiflexion of the foot may reduce the discomfort of lower extremity cramping (Fig. 7-5). Planning frequent rest periods during the day may decrease the frequency of leg cramps. Adequate intake of protein and dairy products ensures the appropriate calcium-phosphorous ratio.

Vaginal Discharge

An increase in odorless and colorless vaginal discharge is common during pregnancy. This is caused by increased estrogen levels and hypervascularity of the cervix. Vaginal secretions that are foul smelling or have a distinctive color require further evaluation.

Nurses provide reassurance that increased vaginal discharge is normal during pregnancy. In a private setting, the nurse can share practical tips with the pregnant woman to improve her personal comfort. These tips include wearing 100% cotton underwear, cleansing the vulva and perineal areas with soap and water, drying the perineal area frequently, avoiding constrictive clothing, and wearing undergarments that permit circulation of air. Douching is to avoided because it disturbs vaginal pH, thus altering the body's ability to fight bacterial infection. It may also lead to premature rupture of membranes (PROM).

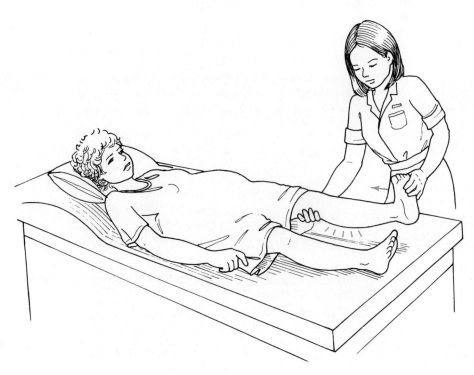

Figure 7-5. Dorsiflexion of the foot often relieves leg cramps.

Orthostatic Hypotension

The major risk associated with orthostatic hypotension is fainting, which can lead to falls and related injuries. The pregnant woman is taught to rise slowly after reclining. She needs to sit with her legs dangling and head erect for a brief period before attempting to get up and walk.

Fatigue

Fatigue during pregnancy seems to be universal and almost unavoidable. This lack of energy can begin at the onset of pregnancy and last well into the postpartum period. There are many causes for fatigue during pregnancy. Hormonal disturbances, increased circulatory workload, changes in the woman's metabolic rate, and dietary intake all affect energy levels. Most women find that they must rest throughout the day, even if it is just for brief periods.

Danger Signs to Report

An important aspect of prenatal education is teaching the family to recognize the danger signs that need to be reported to the health care provider immediately. The woman is assured that prompt medical treatment is usually sufficient to minimize the related complications and relieve their negative effects. Danger signs are listed in the Family Teaching Checklist.

Threats to Healthy Pregnancy

Smoking, alcohol consumption, substance abuse, and family violence pose serious hazards to the pregnant woman and the fetus. During prenatal visits, nurses and health care providers need to identify women and families at risk to intervene and promote healthy behaviors. Family counseling and education help convey the importance of healthy behaviors during pregnancy. Frank discussions about the adverse effects of harmful behaviors are presented in a nonjudgmental manner. Lifestyle changes are difficult to make, but pregnancy is an important life cycle event that may make behavior modification a little easier.

Smoking

Smoking during pregnancy is associated with fetuses who are small for gestational age (SGA), premature birth and low-birthweight neonates, abruptio placentae (detachment of the placenta), and spontaneous abortion. Perinatal and neonatal mortality rates are higher when the pregnant woman smokes. Although the to-

---

✔ **FAMILY TEACHING CHECKLIST**

Danger Signs to Report Promptly During Pregnancy

The nurse includes the following information in family teaching to promote health and well-being:

- Report any signs of vaginal bleeding or fluid leakage, noting color and time
- Monitor urine output for blood or reduction in output
- Recognize and immediately report symptoms of pregnancy-induced hypertension, including: weight gain of more than 5 pounds from last prenatal visit; swelling of face and fingers; persistent headache; lightheadedness or dizziness; double or blurred vision; epigastric pain
- Check body temperature if feeling hot and flushed and notify health care provider of fever greater than 38.3°C (101°F)
- Notify health care provider if vomiting persists for more than 1 day or there is difficulty keeping solids or fluids down
- Monitor fetal movement and report sudden decreases in activity level or lack of movement for more than 6–8 hours
- Consider preterm labor if experiencing low backache and uterine tightening or cramping before 36 weeks of gestation, and contact health care provider promptly

bacco industry continues to deny any connection between secondhand smoke and health threats to the nonsmoker, pregnant women are advised to seek out smoke-free environments.

Smoking endangers the fetus in two major ways: it interferes with adequate maternal nutritional intake, and the nicotine causes blood vessels to constrict. This vasoconstriction reduces oxygen supply to the placenta and, by association, the fetus. Nicotine also depletes vitamin C levels and impairs the metabolism of calcium.

The woman is encouraged to eliminate or reduce her smoking activities during pregnancy. The childbearing family can be referred to appropriate resources to stop smoking. Nicotine patches are not usually recommended during pregnancy.

Alcohol Consumption

The consumption of alcohol during pregnancy has been associated with fetal alcohol syndrome (FAS), fetal growth retardation (FGR), learning disabilities, and congenital abnormalities (see Chapter 20). Because no one knows what constitutes a safe level of alcohol intake during pregnancy, all pregnant women are advised to refrain from any alcohol consumption.

As the woman drinks, the alcohol passes through the placenta to the fetus. Damage to the fetus occurs as late as the third trimester. Newborns with FAS are born with abnormalities such as flattening of facial features, decreased head circumference, low birth weight, and hyperactivity. The nurse screens the woman carefully on her alcohol intake, paying close attention to the frequency of intake, the type of liquor, and any signs of discomfort or embarrassment demonstrated in discussing these issues. Immediate education is initiated on the devastating effects of alcohol. Eliminating drinking at any time during pregnancy can limit its ill effects on the fetus.

Substance Abuse

The use and abuse of drugs in pregnancy has crushing effects on the fetus and the neonate. These neonates are themselves born addicted to the mother's drug of choice. The crack-addicted neonate exhibits all of the signs of withdrawal within hours of birth: listlessness, poor muscle reflexes and sucking abilities, and high-pitched cries. Nursing care of newborns of drug-addicted women is discussed in Chapter 20.

Early identification and treatment of the woman who abuses substances is essential. Nurses need to be able to identify subtle and obvious signs of dependency. Subtle signs include constricted pupils, multiple dental caries, moods swings, rhinitis, and frequent falls or "accidents." Obvious signs include anorexia and weight loss, poor hygiene, infrequent or no prenatal care, irregular fast heart rate, and recurrence of sexually transmitted diseases. These women need immediate intervention and support to stop their drug use and improve their general health. After referral is made for rehabilitation and possible hospitalization, follow-up by the prenatal nurse is essential for promotion of a positive pregnancy outcome and a drug-free life for the woman.

Family Violence

Family violence cuts across race, ethnicity, and socioeconomic status. The pregnant woman who is battered and beaten, usually by her sexual partner, is at risk for injury to herself and the fetus. The nurse who suspects a woman has been beaten must be gentle but direct in asking about suspicious bruising and abrasions. This is done in a private setting and in a supportive, nonjudgmental manner. If the woman does not immediately respond to the offer of help, she may at a later time. If she does admit to family violence, assessment of injuries to her and the fetus is done first. Referral to a domestic violence agency for assistance and protection is then made to ensure her safety.

◆ Preparation for Childbirth

Through childbirth preparation classes given during the antepartum period, nurses have an opportunity to implement teaching strategies that prepare the childbearing family for labor, childbirth, and parenting responsibilities. Family teaching includes the normal physical and psychosocial changes associated with pregnancy, labor and childbirth preparation, and care of the newborn. Prenatal classes encourage women and family members to express their ideas, interests, and feelings with support and guidance provided by the childbirth educator. Group settings facilitate discussions and participants benefit from the exchange of information.

Methods of Childbirth

Family-centered maternal-newborn nursing care promotes active participation of family members during pregnancy, labor, and childbirth. The three most popular choices among the many methods of natural childbirth in this country are the Dick-Read, Bradley, and Lamaze methods. These methods have many similarities. They all focus on instructing the family in safe labor and childbirth. They each emphasize childbirth as a meaningful, shared experience.

Dick-Read Method

In the 1930's, Dr. Grantly Dick-Read, a physician from England, actively supported natural childbirth. He discovered that women who feared labor exhibited a high degree of tension. As labor progressed and tension increased, these women experienced an increase in muscular tension, which produced pain. This phenomenon became known as the fear-tension-pain syndrome.

The **Dick-Read method** promotes relaxation by eliminating the unknown. It offers factual and realistic information for the woman and her family on what to expect during labor and childbirth. Through the use of specific exercises, which include breathing and relaxation techniques, the couple feels a sense of control during labor. The woman is encouraged to concentrate on relaxing each part of her body with every contraction. Dick-Read's book, *Childbirth Without Fear*, stressed that a woman in labor should never be left alone because being alone induces fear.

Classes in the Dick-Read method are directed toward helping the childbearing family actively participate in the birth process. Teaching the woman exercises that strengthen abdominal and perineal muscles and breathing techniques for relaxation helps the couple take charge during labor. This knowledge and sense of control decreases fear and breaks the fear-tension-pain cycle.

Dick-Read supporters approve of the use of analgesics during labor as needed. However, the labor process should be as natural as possible.

Bradley Method

Named after Dr. Robert A. Bradley, the **Bradley method** supports labor as a natural process. The room is free of extraneous noises, and lighting is dim. The woman and her partner both participate in diversionary activities such as walking, listening to music, playing games, and having discussions. Most women use **tailor sitting** as a comfortable alternative when they tire of walking (Fig. 7-6A). During active labor, the woman may prefer Sim's position with pillows supporting her head and chest, and another under the forward leg (Fig. 7-6B). The woman closes her eyes during contractions, breathes slowly and deeply, and concentrates on relaxing. The Bradley method encourages breast-feeding immediately after birth to form early maternal-neonatal attachments.

Lamaze Method

The **Lamaze method** of childbirth originated in Paris after Dr. Ferdinand Lamaze attended a conference in Russia. The conference advocated the use of a technique known as psychoprophylaxis during labor and childbirth. In other words, the couple prepares for childbirth by learning techniques for mentally preventing pain. Lamaze classes are typically small. The labor coach, spouse, friend, or partner is encouraged to attend all of the classes with the woman.

The couple is taught a variety of positive behaviors that can be substituted for fear, pain, and uncontrolled responses during labor. Support pillows and position changes increase comfort for the woman. Relaxation and breathing techniques are stressed in Lamaze classes. A deep, cleansing breath is taken at the beginning of each contraction. The woman focuses on a predetermined focal point such as a picture or her partner's eyes. In early labor, breathing is slow and deep. As la-

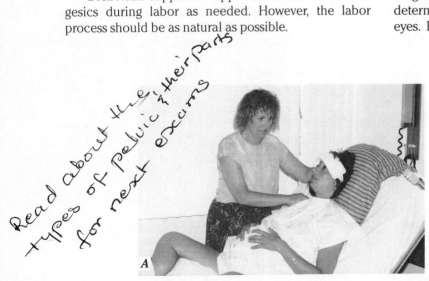
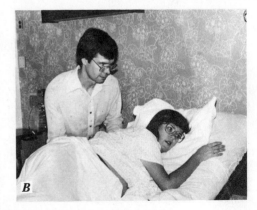

Figure 7-6. (**A**) *Tailor sitting may be a comfortable position during labor.* (**B**) *The Sims's position may be preferred during active labor to encourage rest and relaxation.*

bor progresses, breathing becomes shallow and quicker when contractions become stronger. Pant-blow breathing, quick shallow breaths alternating with forceful blowing of air out the mouth, is used in transition labor (see Chapter 11). The pattern of pant-blow breathing is quickened when the woman pushes during contractions. This is effective in promoting adequate oxygenation.

The labor coach encourages relaxation of muscles, while informing the woman when each contraction begins, reaches its peak, and comes to an end. This technique helps the woman feel each contraction has a beginning and an end in sight. During the contraction, the woman is encouraged to relax her muscles. After each contraction, she is instructed to take several deep, cleansing breaths. Praise and moral support for the woman and her partner build confidence and encourage the couple to continue.

Techniques Used During Childbirth

Breathing during contractions is paced in rhythmic patterns. Ideally, the woman stays calm and breathes in a manner that adequately oxygenates both her and the fetus. Usually the woman needs to concentrate on breathing in through her nose and out through her mouth at a comfortable rate. Two to four *deep* and effortless cleansing breaths are taken at the beginning and end of each contraction. Breathing techniques allow the woman to vary her breathing rate with the intensity of each contraction.

Prenatal Exercises

Prenatal exercises promote relaxation and strengthen targeted muscle groups. The pregnant woman needs to learn the proper way to relax all groups of muscles from her head to her toes. Strengthening pelvic, back, and abdominal muscles helps prevent back strain during pregnancy. The woman is able to push more effectively during the second stage of labor if muscle tone is maintained. See the Family Teaching Checklist, which provides family teaching exercises for strength and relaxation.

Prenatal Education Programs

Prenatal education programs provide the childbearing family with specific guidance and details concerning the physical and psychosocial changes that occur during pregnancy. Group discussions teach families the specific needs of the pregnant woman, as well as how to care for the new family member. A typical prenatal education program might meet once a week during early pregnancy and resume again in late pregnancy to reinforce health teaching.

Prenatal education programs are sponsored by local health care facilities, physicians, and birthing cen-

---

✔ FAMILY TEACHING CHECKLIST

Exercises for Strengthening Muscles and Promoting Relaxation

- Tailor sitting: Sit on floor with legs crossed and back straight. Purpose: Strengthens thigh and pelvic muscles.

- Kegel exercise: Tighten perineal muscles of anus and vagina and relax as if trying to stop and start the flow of urine. Purpose: Strengthens muscles of pelvis. This exercise can be done every few hours throughout the day.

- Pelvic tilt: Sit on floor with knees flexed and arms stretched behind the back for upper body support. Inhale and arch back inward, and exhale and arch back outward. Repetitions of 8 tilts can be done 2 to 3 times a day. Purpose: Strengthens back and abdominal muscles.

- Relaxation exercise: Sit on floor, in chair, or lie down in comfortable position and concentrate on relaxing muscle groups from head and face to fingers and toes. Purpose: Promotes relaxation and enhances ability to focus inward and concentrate

- Straight-leg lift: Sit on the floor, flex the left leg, and straighten the right leg with the right foot flexed. Lift the extended leg off the floor 4 to 6 inches while inhaling, slowly lower while exhaling. Cycles of 8 lifts 2 to 3 times a day are suggested. Repeat the exercise with the left leg. Purpose: Promotes venous blood return.

ters. Prenatal classes are most commonly taught by maternal-newborn nurses.

Choice of Birthing Experience

The woman and her partner are encouraged to discuss birthing options and individualize the birthing experience so that it is mutually satisfying. Examples of birthing options include: labor-delivery-recovery (LDR) rooms in acute care facilities, alternative birthing centers (ABC) in off-site facilities, and home birth. These options promote a family-centered approach to childbirth. Chapter 1 discusses the consumer movement and how it influenced available birthing options.

Situational Factors Affecting Pregnancy

Certain situational factors affect pregnancy in both positive and negative ways. Prenatal nutrition, healthy self-care behaviors, psychosocial stability, compliance with prenatal visit schedules, and preparation for childbirth and parenting are key areas that require close attention from the nurse. Women who may need additional guidance and support during pregnancy are single women, those older than 35 years of age experiencing their first pregnancy, and adolescents. The pregnant adolescent is discussed in the section entitled *Adolescent Considerations*.

Single Parenthood

The stress of impending single parenthood often makes pregnancy very difficult for the woman. Two of the most profound effects of that stress are experienced as financial strain and emotional distress.

Nurses can help needy single women obtain financial aid for food and adequate shelter. Referrals to social workers put pregnant women in touch with community and state resources that support pregnancy and parenthood. Pregnant single women who may be experiencing rejection, anger, or depression sometimes require immediate referral by nurses to appropriate mental health care professionals.

A single woman may be understandably fearful of being alone during labor and childbirth. Increasing her awareness of the different birthing alternatives available to her is often reassuring. Referrals to community agencies such as Parents Without Partners may provide additional support and help the single woman to maintain her dignity.

Pregnancy After Age 35

Statistically speaking, women who become pregnant after age 35 run an increased risk for delivering premature neonates who may or may not have congenital abnormalities, such as Down syndrome. These women are also at increased risk for developing pregnancy-induced hypertension.

Nurses need to stress the importance of prenatal visits for careful monitoring of maternal-fetal health and well-being. Additional testing, such as amniotic fluid sampling and genetic counseling, may be recommended by the health care provider.

Adolescent Considerations

Busy schedules, the low price and availability of fast food, and party activities are examples of some of the factors that may result in poor food choices and irregular eating habits among adolescents (Fig 7-7). Skipping meals is also fairly common among adolescent females, many of whom worry about how weight gain affects their body image. These adolescents need gentle guidance and counseling about the need for adequate nutrition to ensure the delivery of healthy neonates (See the Nursing Care Plan for the Pregnant Adolescent).

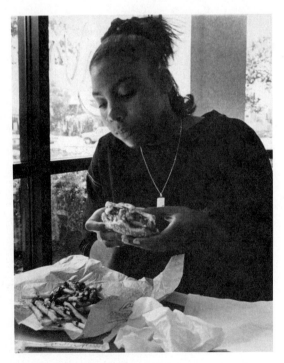

Figure 7-7. *Pregnant adolescents often make poor food choices and may require special counseling on the importance of adequate nutrition. (Photo © Kathy Sloane)*

NURSING CARE PLAN
for the Pregnant Adolescent

ASSESSMENT: Carolyn is a 16-year-old primigravida who comes for her first prenatal visit today. While waiting to be seen, you notice she is eating a bag of potato chips and drinking soda. Carolyn weighs 186 pounds and is 5'3" tall.

NURSING DIAGNOSIS #1: Alterated Nutrition: More than body requirements, related to poor eating habits

EXPECTED OUTCOMES:

1. Carolyn will gain a total of 15–20 pounds during her pregnancy.
2. Carolyn will eat three balanced meals and two nutritious snacks daily.
3. Carolyn will understand the role proper nutrition plays in fetal development.

Nursing Interventions	*Rationale*
1. Obtain a 24-hour dietary recall from the patient; refer to dietitian as needed.	1. Provides baseline from which specific learning needs can be established.
2. Provide sample menu that includes necessary nutrients and lists sources of vitamins/minerals.	2. Patient will have written information on refrigerator at home and to take food shopping for easy referral and reinforcement.
3. Describe the role vitamins and minerals play in fetal development.	3. Poor nutritional intake during pregnancy has been associated with low birth weight and poor fetal development.

EVALUATION:

1. During subsequent clinic visits, Carolyn reports dietary intake that reflects appropriate caloric and vitamin/mineral intake.
2. Carolyn gains 18 pounds during her pregnancy.
3. Carolyn takes her prenatal vitamin and iron pills as prescribed.

NURSING DIAGNOSIS #2: Knowledge Deficit, related to pregnancy, fetal development, and birth

EXPECTED OUTCOMES:

1. Carolyn will comply with instructions and recommendations made by health team.
2. Carolyn will attend prenatal classes specifically designed for adolescents.

Nursing Interventions	*Rationale*
1. Evaluate patient's level of understanding regarding pregnancy, fetal development, and birth.	1. Provides basis from which the nurse can plan future teaching. Recognizing the patient's level of knowledge and individual learning needs helps establish a feeling of trust and respect.
2. Using age-appropriate teaching strategies, provide oral and written instructions regarding pregnancy; fetal development; labor and delivery.	2. Adolescents may be reluctant to ask questions or may feel overwhelmed by extent of information provided during prenatal visit. Providing written information that can be reviewed at home reinforces instruction and may raise questions for the next visit. Prenatal classes for adolescents provide peer group discussion and support.

EVALUATION:

1. Carolyn asks questions regarding her baby's development.
2. Carolyn attends prenatal classes with her boyfriend.
3. Carolyn complies with instructions regarding self-care during pregnancy.

Deliberate and innovative nutrition planning is used to support the pregnant adolescent in choosing appropriate foods. Special classes that focus on healthful nutrition during pregnancy can be scheduled during convenient hours for teenagers. These group activities provide peer support and encourage discussion of ways to modify the diet to ensure proper nutrition. The nurse offers healthful snack ideas, including reducing between-meal snacking on empty-calorie foods and cutting down on excessive soda consumption.

Nurses can also increase the adolescent's compliance with healthful behaviors by offering easy-to-understand explanations and gearing teaching to her level of understanding. Discussing the importance of prenatal visits, practicing appropriate self-care behaviors, and preparing for childbirth are just a few of the topics that the nurse and the pregnant adolescent can work on together.

Cultural Considerations

Dietary recommendations made by nurses are generally based on Western, middle-class preferences. But nurses need to be aware that there are many cultural, ethnic, religious, and even monetary factors that may influence the pregnant woman's dietary choices and preferences. For instance, suggesting that pregnant women increase their calcium intake by ingesting greater amounts of whole-milk products is an unacceptable alternative for lactose-intolerant women. Encouraging pregnant women to get their protein from animal sources such as beef may also be inappropriate for practicing Hindus, just as encouraging pork consumption would be offensive to Muslims. There are also a whole host of other culturally determined reasons that affect eating patterns during pregnancy.

For example, some women believe that unsatisfied food cravings may produce birthmarks. If a woman subscribes to this belief, her longing for strawberries during pregnancy may be the reason her infant has its red birthmark. Although there is no harm in eating vast quantities of strawberries, the woman may incur serious health risks by ingesting nonfood substances. This practice, known as pica (geophagia), is described in Chapter 5.

Women of various cultures believe that the "hot" and "cold" properties of foods and conditions affect them and the fetus. (It is important to note that the "hotness" or "coldness" of a substance or condition is often unrelated to temperature.) These women may alter their eating patterns during pregnancy to maintain a desirable balance between hot and cold. For instance, a pregnant Puerto Rican woman may avoid "hot" foods and medications (such as iron and vitamins) because

she does not want to intensify the already hot condition of pregnancy. It is also common among Latinas and Asian women to avoid "cold" foods, such as fruits and juices, during the postpartum period. It is believed that these foods adversely effect health by delaying the emptying of the uterus.

The Role of the Nurse

The role of the nurse in providing prenatal health care is to promote positive outcomes of pregnancy for the woman, neonate, and the childbearing family. Specific nursing diagnoses for prenatal health care promotion are identified in the Nursing Diagnoses Checklist.

The nurse teaches the family about the normal changes associated with pregnancy and ways to relieve anticipated discomforts. It is important that education be presented at a level the family understands. An interpreter may be needed if a language barrier exists between the nurse and the family. Self-care guidelines regarding ADLs are discussed with the woman and her family. Childbirth education classes and prenatal education programs help prepare the family for pregnancy, labor, childbirth, and parenting. These educational groups are typically directed by nurses.

NURSING DIAGNOSES CHECKLIST

Nursing Diagnoses Related to Prenatal Health Care

· Knowledge Deficit, related to appropriate prenatal health

· Activity Intolerance, related to fatigue

· Body Image Disturbance, related to weight gain in pregnancy

· Diversional Activity Deficit, related to labor pain

· Family Coping: Potential for Growth, related to role changes as birth nears

· Fatigue, related to normal physical changes associated with pregnancy

· Risk for Fluid Volume Deficit, related to nausea and vomiting in the first trimester

· Altered Growth and Development: physical and psychosocial changes associated with pregnancy, particularly in adolescents

· Altered Nutrition: Less than body requirements, related to poor food choices

· Health Seeking Behaviors, related to need for keeping all scheduled appointments

SELF-ASSESSMENT

1. A patient complains of shortness of breath (SOB) at 35 weeks' gestation. The nurse's initial action should be which of the following?

○ **A.** Check the woman's blood pressure
○ **B.** Arrange for oxygen therapy
○ **C.** Contact the physician immediately
○ **D.** Explain this is a common finding at this point in pregnancy

2. Adequate intake of vitamin K during pregnancy helps with which of the following?

○ **A.** Blood clotting
○ **B.** Prevention of infection
○ **C.** Vitamin C absorption
○ **D.** Cell reproduction

3. To limit common discomforts of pregnancy, the woman should be instructed to:

○ **A.** Lie down after eating
○ **B.** Limit her fluid intake
○ **C.** Increase her fruit intake
○ **D.** Wear knee-high stockings

4. Management of lower leg cramping includes:

○ **A.** Dorsi-extension of the affected leg
○ **B.** Decreased milk and cheese intake
○ **C.** Avoidance of weight-bearing activity until the cramp has subsided
○ **D.** Frequent rest periods

5. Limiting sodium intake during pregnancy can help minimize:

○ **A.** Constipation
○ **B.** Edema
○ **C.** Indigestion
○ **D.** Dyspnea

REVIEW AND PREVIEW

This chapter gave an overview of nursing care during the antepartum period. Prenatal health promotion through nutrition counseling as presented. Relief of common discomforts, danger signs to report in pregnancy, and potential threats to pregnancy are important teaching opportunities for nurses. Family preparation for childbirth and prenatal education programs were described. Situational factors that affect pregnancy, including single parenthood, first pregnancies in women older than age 35, and adolescent pregnancy, were given special consideration.

The following chapter deals with families who are at risk during the antepartum period. Medical conditions such as heart disease and diabetes mellitus are described. Pregnancy-induced complications such as bleeding, *Rh* incompatibility, and pregnancy-induced hypertension follow. Information related to assessment and appropriate medical management and nursing care is also presented.

◉ KEY POINTS

◆ Proper nutrition during pregnancy promotes maternal and fetal health. The pregnant woman must balance her intake of proteins, carbohydrates, fats, vitamins, and minerals. Vegetarian diets, food preferences of pregnant adolescents, and cultural beliefs are examples of factors that must be considered in diet planning.

◆ Most women hope to continue functioning routinely in their ADLs while pregnant. However, changes in normal day-to-day activities such as bathing, elimination, eating, resting habits, employment, and travel plans may need to be made to promote the comfort and well-being of the fetus and woman.

◆ It is important that complications such as vaginal bleeding, preterm labor or rupture of membranes, absence of fetal movement, persistent vomiting, fever, and symptoms of pregnancy-induced hypertension be reported promptly. Measures need to be taken to reduce the risk of danger for the woman and fetus as soon as possible.

◆ Four areas of concern regarding major threats to the health and well-being of the woman and fetus include cigarette smoking, associated with SGA neonates; alcohol consumption, associated with FAS; substance abuse, associated with embryonic and fetal abnormalities, and withdrawal symptoms in the neonate; and family violence, associated with spontaneous abortion of the fetus and maternal physical impairments.

◆ Different methods of childbirth, such as Dick-Read, Bradley, and Lamaze, encourage pregnant women and their families to reduce the tension, fear, and pain associated with labor. Self-confidence, comfort, relaxation and control guide the couple as they master the childbirth experience.

BIBLIOGRAPHY

Boyle, J. S., & Andrews, M. M. (1990). *Transcultural concepts in nursing care.* Philadelphia: J.B. Lippincott.

Dudek, S. G. (1993). *Nutrition handbook for nursing practice* (2nd ed.). Philadelphia: J.B. Lippincott.

Eschleman, M. M. (1991). *Introductory nutrition and diet therapy* (2nd ed.). Philadelphia: J.B. Lippincott.

Falvo, D. R. (1994). *Effective patient education: A guide to increased compliance* (2nd ed.). Rockville, MD: Aspen Publishers.

Fleming, B. W., Munton, M. T., Clarke, B. A., & Strauss, S. S. (1993). Assessing and promoting positive parenting in adolescent mothers. *Maternal-Child Nursing Journal, 18,* 32–37.

Institute of Medicine, National Academy of Sciences. (1992). *Nutrition during pregnancy and lactation: An implementation guide.* Washington, DC: National Academy Press.

Kemp, V. H., & Hatmaker, D. D. (1993). Health practices and anxiety in low-income, high- and low-risk pregnant women. *Journal of Obstetric, Gynecologic, and Neonatal Nursing, 22,* 266–277.

Mattson, S., & Lew, L. (1992). Culturally sensitive prenatal care for southeast Asians. *Journal of Obstetric, Gynecologic, and Neonatal Nursing, 21,* 48–54.

May, K. A., & Mahlmeister, L. R. (1994). *Maternal and neonatal nursing, family-centered care* (3rd ed.). Philadelphia: J.B. Lippincott.

May, K. A. (1992). Social networks and help-seeking experiences of pregnant teens. *Journal of Obstetric, Gynecologic, and Neonatal Nursing, 21,* 497–502.

McClanahan, P. (1992). Improving access to and use of prenatal care. *Journal of Obstetric, Gynecologic, and Neonatal Nursing, 21,* 280–286.

Newman, V., Fullerton, J. T., & Anderson, P. O. (1993). Clinical advances in the management of severe nausea and vomiting during pregnancy. *Journal of Obstetric, Gynecologic, and Neonatal Nursing, 22,* 483–490.

Noel, N., & Yam, M. (1992). Domestic violence: The pregnant battered woman. *Nursing Clinics of North America, 27*(4), 871–884.

Omar, M. A., & Schiffman, R. F. (1993). Prenatal vitamins: A rite of passage. *Maternal-Child Nursing Journal, 18,* 322–324.

Pillitteri, A. (1992). *Maternal and child health nursing: Care of the childbearing and childrearing family* (1st ed.). Philadelphia: J.B. Lippincott.

Roller, C. G. (1992). Drawing out young mothers. *Maternal-Child Nursing Journal, 17,* 254–255.

Sampselle, C., Petersen, B., Murtland, T., & Oakley, D. (1992). Prevalence of abuse among pregnant women choosing certified nurse-midwife or physician providers. *Journal of Nurse Midwifery, 37*(4), 269–273.

Scherer, J. C. (1992). *Introductory clinical pharmacology* (4th ed.). Philadelphia: J.B. Lippincott.

Starn, J., Patterson, K., Bemis, G., Castro, O., & Bemis, P. (1993). Can we encourage pregnant substance abusers to seek prenatal care? *Maternal-Child Nursing Journal, 18,* 148–152.

USDA's food guide pyramid, Human Nutrition Service. U.S. Department of Agriculture, April 1992.

van Lier, D., Manteuffel, B., DiIorio, C., & Stalcup, M. (1993). Nausea and fatigue in women during early pregnancy. *Birth, Issues in Perinatal Care, 20,* 193–197.

Weiss, J., & Hansell, M. (1992). Substance abuse during pregnancy: Legal and health policy issues. *Nursing and Health Care, 13*(9), 472–479.

Zeanah, M., & Schlosser, S. P. (1993). Adherence to ACOG guidelines on exercise during pregnancy: Effect on pregnancy outcome. *Journal of Obstetric, Gynecologic, and Neonatal Nursing, 22,* 329–337.

CHAPTER 8

The Family at Risk During the Antepartum Period

◆ OBJECTIVES

When the learning goals of this chapter are met, the reader will be able to:

◆ Discuss factors that place expectant families at risk.
◆ Describe assessment and nursing interventions for women diagnosed with hyperemesis gravidarum.
◆ Identify implications of anemia in pregnancy.
◆ Describe the effects of the physiologic changes in pregnancy associated with thromboembolic disease.
◆ Summarize assessment and nursing interventions for women diagnosed with pregnancy-induced hypertension.
◆ Discuss implications of blood incompatibilities.
◆ Explain causes of bleeding in pregnancy.
◆ Identify implications of diabetes in pregnancy.
◆ Discuss assessment and nursing interventions for the pregnant woman diagnosed with heart disease.
◆ Identify teratogenic infections and related consequences associated with pregnancy.

TERMINOLOGY

Abruptio placentae

Disseminated intravascular coagulation

Ectopic pregnancy

Gestational diabetes

Gestational trophoblastic neoplasm

Hyperemesis gravidarum

Placenta previa

Pregnancy-induced hypertension

Prostaglandins

Sickle cell anemia

TORCH

Most women have uneventful pregnancies, but those who are at risk for complications have special needs. Nurses can help identify these women and their families for referral to appropriate resources.

Problems that can occur during pregnancy are discussed in this chapter, along with nursing assessment and management processes. The problems discussed include: hyperemesis gravidarum, anemias, pregnancy-induced hypertension (PIH), Rh incompatibility, bleeding during pregnancy, diabetes, heart disease, infections, and multifetal pregnancies.

Families at Risk

There are many factors that affect pregnancy and create special needs for the family during the antepartum period. The major factors relating to high-risk pregnancy are highlighted in Display 8-1. Medical complications are discussed in detail in the following sections.

Hyperemesis Gravidarum

Mild nausea and vomiting, known as "morning sickness," is common in early pregnancy, and usually disappears after the third month of gestation. **Hyperemesis gravidarum,** or pernicious vomiting, occurs when these symptoms become persistent and severe. Approxi-

mately 3.5 in 1000 pregnant women are affected by this condition, which can last for 4 to 8 weeks or longer. The cause is unknown. However, endocrine imbalance, the metabolic changes associated with pregnancy, and slow motility of the stomach during pregnancy are thought to produce symptoms. The highest incidence of hyperemesis gravidarum occurs in primigravidas, multifetal pregnancies, women diagnosed with hydatidiform mole, and women with a history of psychiatric disorders.

Assessment

Vomiting that persists over a prolonged period may cause symptoms of dehydration, such as decreased urinary output, electrolyte imbalance, dry skin, rapid pulse, and low-grade fever. It should be noted that severe cases of hyperemesis gravidarum are rare. The woman also may suffer from acidosis and, in severe cases, liver damage. There may be associated weight loss.

Accurate records are kept to assess the amount and character of emesis, intake and output, and daily weight. Laboratory results are observed for hematocrit, hemoglobin, electrolytes, and urine protein and acetone.

Management

Hospitalization is recommended for women whose symptoms cannot be managed at home. Goals for treatment include control of vomiting, correction of fluid and electrolyte imbalance, and adequate nutrition. The woman is given nothing by mouth (NPO) and receives liberal amounts of intravenous fluids with electrolyte and vitamin supplements for 24 to 48 hours. Sedatives and antiemetics are used to treat vomiting and nausea. A quiet environment and an understanding attitude from caregivers is necessary to decrease the woman's emotional distress. Visitors may need to be restricted.

Intravenous therapy continues until the vomiting stops. Small feedings of dry food such as toast or crackers are given every 2 to 3 hours, alternated with small amounts of water, hot tea, or ginger ale. Intake is increased as tolerated by the woman. If oral feedings are not tolerated, it may be necessary to administer high-calorie, high-vitamin fluids via nasogastric tube or intravenously. Nasogastric feedings are rarely used.

Anemias

Anemias are characterized by hemoglobin levels below 11 g/dL and hematocrit levels below 35%. Women with

122

anemia tire easily, are susceptible to infection, are at increased risk for postpartum hemorrhage, and tend to deliver small for gestational age (SGA) babies.

Iron Deficiency Anemia

Iron deficiency anemia is common in pregnancy.

As the fetus grows, it meets its needs for iron by tapping into the woman's stores of the mineral. Maternal iron stores are soon depleted unless she receives adequate amounts of iron, either through proper diet or from supplements.

Assessment

The primary symptoms of anemia are fatigue and pallor of the skin and conjunctiva. A nutritional history indicates a diet low in iron-rich foods. Laboratory tests to assess for hematocrit and hemoglobin levels are done early and are repeated throughout pregnancy.

Management

Iron supplements are essential during pregnancy. The usual daily dosage is 320 mg ferrous gluconate or 200 mg ferrous sulfate taken orally. Supplements should be taken with food to prevent gastrointestinal side effects, and with vitamin C (orange juice) to increase absorption. Women are warned that iron intake will produce black stools and may cause constipation, abdominal cramping, diarrhea, nausea, and vomiting. Reducing supplement dosage usually relieves symptoms.

Sickle Cell Anemia

Sickle cell anemia is an inherited disorder caused by abnormal hemoglobin (*hemoglobin S.*) This abnormal hemoglobin is what causes the sickling of red blood cells. Sickle cell anemia affects women of both African and Mediterranean descent, although it is primarily seen in blacks. Approximately 8% of black women are carriers only; they are usually asymptomatic. They can, however, pass the sickle cell trait on to their offspring.

During sickle cell crisis, cells clump together and cause blockage of vessels and decreased oxygen flow to maternal and fetal tissue (Fig. 8-1). The vital organs primarily affected are the kidneys, spleen, and the placenta. The crisis causes sudden, severe, generalized pain. Women with this condition are susceptible to repeated infections, particularly of the genitourinary tract; spontaneous abortion; intrauterine growth retardation; still birth; and neonatal death. The maternal

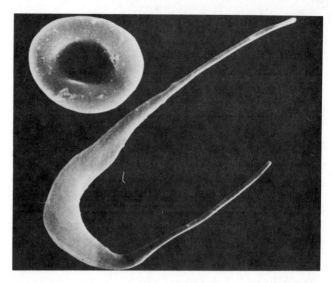

Figure 8-1. *The U-shape of the sickle cells, in comparison with the normal circular shape, often causes the cells to clump together, blocking vessels and decreasing oxygen flow to maternal and fetal tissue. (Photo by Dr. Bruce R. Cameron)*

mortality rate is significant, at approximately 2% to 7% (see Fig. 8-1).

Assessment

Women with sickle cell disease frequently have severe anemia, with hemoglobin levels of less than 9 mg/dL. They relate histories of frequent illness and recurring abdominal and joint pain, and they may appear undernourished. Pooling of blood in the lower extremities is common and typically causes ulcers on the legs and ankles.

Management

Pregnant women with sickle cell anemia should be taught good hygienic practices to prevent infection. They are also encouraged to adopt an appropriate diet, with increased oral intake of fluids and folic acid supplements. Folic acid aids red blood cell production and leads to increased levels of hemoglobin. Sickle cell crisis may be treated with partial blood exchange transfusions after 28 weeks of gestation. Sickle cell components are separated out from normal hemoglobin, and the woman's plasma and other blood components are reinfused. The woman may be on bed rest, and fetal status is monitored closely.

◆ Thromboembolic Disease

Superficial thrombosis and deep vein thrombosis (DVT) of the lower extremities is fairly common in pregnancy. Women who used oral contraception before becoming pregnant and those who have jobs where they sit for long periods are at risk. Others at risk are obese women, women on bed rest while pregnant, those older than 30, and women who have had previous pregnancies. Increased fibrinogen (a clotting factor) levels in pregnancy also contribute to the possibility of DVT.

As pregnancy advances, the uterus grows heavy and exerts pressure on vessels of the pelvis and lower extremities. Circulation becomes poor, slowing of blood flow occurs (stasis), and a clot may form and attach to the vessel wall. If the clot breaks free, it becomes an embolus, which may travel to the lungs. This condition is known as pulmonary embolus. It can be life threatening if not diagnosed and treated promptly.

Assessment

Symptoms of superficial thrombosis and DVT vary greatly, but usually the woman complains of sudden onset of pain with swelling of the extremity. There may be redness and heat at the site. The presence of Homans' sign is an early indication of DVT. To test for it, the woman is instructed to lie in a supine position while the health care provider supports the knee with one hand, using the other hand to apply pressure to the sole of the foot of the same leg. The leg is then pushed back toward the knee (flexion). If calf pain is noted, Homans' sign is present.

Management

Superficial thrombosis is treated with moist heat and elevation of the extremity. Early ambulation is encouraged. DVT is treated with intravenous heparin until the woman is pain free. Blood samples are drawn daily to test for partial thromboplastin time (PTT), a clotting factor, to aid in calculating heparin dosage. If continued treatment is required, heparin is given subcutaneously. Injections are given in the abdomen. (Injection sites are rotated to prevent tissue damage.) Heparin levels are monitored carefully because there is an increased danger of hemorrhage during birth. Epidural or spinal anesthesia is not recommended with heparin use.

Pain medication, moist heat, and elevation of the extremity help hasten recovery. Elastic support stockings should be worn when ambulation begins. Women with a history of thrombosis should be instructed to avoid sitting with their legs crossed at the knee. They are also instructed to elevate the feet when sitting and to wear elastic support stockings if they have jobs where they must stand for long periods.

Pregnancy-induced Hypertension

Pregnancy-induced hypertension (PIH) occurs in 6% of all pregnancies. This condition was previously known as toxemia, because it was believed to be caused by a toxin.

This has been proven not to be the case, although the actual cause is still unknown. Risk factors associated with PIH include a family history of hypertension, weight extremes (both too little and too much), diabetes, multiple pregnancy, hydatidiform mole, hydramnios, inadequate prenatal care, and previous history of PIH.

The occurrence of PIH is higher in young primiparas, women with chronic hypertension, and those from lower socioeconomic groups. PIH is a major cause of maternal and fetal deaths. Premature birth accounts for a large number of neonatal deaths during the first 4 weeks of life. Fetal complications include intrauterine growth retardation (IUGR) and distress caused by hypoxia. Maternal complications include hemorrhage, cardiac problems, and disseminated intravascular coagulation (DIC). PIH is classified as preeclampsia or eclampsia, depending on the severity of the signs and symptoms.

Preeclampsia/Eclampsia

Preeclampsia is a less severe disorder than eclampsia, although it may develop into eclampsia if not properly treated. The primary symptoms of preeclampsia are hypertension, edema, and albuminuria.

Under normal conditions, blood pressure does not rise significantly in pregnancy. However, if there is an increase of 30 mm Hg or more in the systolic pressure or 15 mm Hg or more in the diastolic pressure, then blood pressure is considered to be abnormally elevated. A woman with a systolic blood pressure of 140 mm Hg or a diastolic pressure of 90 mm Hg is considered hypertensive. Blood pressure should be assessed on two separate occasions at least 6 hours apart before it is diagnosed as abnormally high.

Body tissues retain fluids more readily during pregnancy. Hypertensive women have an increased tendency to retain fluids. The first sign of fluid retention may be sudden, excessive weight gain. A weight gain of 5 pounds or more during the first week is generally a sign of preeclampsia. Other signs are edema of the feet, hands, and face. Women become aware of fluid retention in the hands when they can no longer wear their rings. Most women have some edema of the hands and feet late in the pregnancy, but this usually recedes during the night. In PIH, edema of the hands and feet remains during the night. Preeclampsia can be confirmed by the presence of proteinuria and albuminuria of 1+ or 2+, or greater than 300 mg/L in a 24-hour urine sample.

In severe preeclampsia, the following symptoms may be present: 3+ or 4+ albuminuria, blood pressure of 160/110 or higher, or diastolic pressure greater than or equal to 30 mm Hg while the woman is on bed rest; extensive edema, including pulmonary; decreased urine output; weight gain of more than 2 pounds per week; nausea and vomiting; headache; epigastric pain; and increased hematocrit.

The woman with severe preeclampsia may develop hematologic complications called **HELLP Syndrome.** This acronym stands for **H**emolytic anemia, **E**levated **L**iver enzymes, and **L**ow **P**latelet count. The presenting symptoms include malaise, nausea and vomiting, and right upper quadrant abdominal pain. Later symptoms include edema, hematuria, jaundice, and generalized abdominal discomfort. These symptoms, along with potential hypertension, are seen at approximately the 17th week of pregnancy and may persist until after birth. Women with this condition are usually delivered without delay. The condition resolves soon after delivery. Blood and blood product replacements are often necessary.

Eclampsia is defined as convulsions or coma occurring in preeclampsia. Eclampsia is commonly preceded by an increase in blood pressure in the preeclamptic woman, accompanied by headache, blurred vision, epigastric pain, and nausea and vomiting.

Eclampsia occurs in approximately 1 of every 200 women with preeclampsia. The maternal death rate is 10% to 15% of all cases. Common causes of death include pulmonary edema, failure of vital organs, cardiac failure, and cerebral hemorrhage.

Assessment

Hospitalization of the preeclamptic patient is vital to control the symptoms of hypertension. Vital signs are assessed frequently. Ideally, the woman is placed in a quiet room on her left side. Blood pressure is taken from the right arm. Edema is evaluated, and daily weight is recorded every morning before breakfast. Urine is evaluated every 8 hours for proteinuria and specific gravity. An accurate record of intake and output is kept. Urine output of 30 mL/hour is considered adequate. A Foley catheter is generally inserted to drain the bladder. Seizure precautions are taken.

Deep tendon reflexes are evaluated every 8 hours by eliciting the patellar knee jerk. Response is graded from 0, no response observed, to +5, brisk response

with sustained clonus (rapid alternating involuntary contraction and relaxation of the muscle). A +5 response indicates extreme neuromuscular irritation and danger of impending convulsions.

The nurse must assess for symptoms of epigastric pain (upper abdomen), nausea or vomiting, blurred vision, and headache. These are all signs of impending eclampsia. Maternal vital signs are recorded every 4 hours. An oral airway, suction equipment, and oxygen supply are kept at the bedside in anticipation of convulsions. The bed is cushioned with seizure pads or pillows for the protection of the woman. If the nurse is at the bedside when a convulsion begins, he or she quickly inserts the oral airway. If the seizure is well under way, there is no attempt to insert an airway. During the seizure, the nurse attempts to protect the woman from injury without using force. Length of seizure, how and where it started, a description of seizure movements, aftereffects, and vital signs are recorded.

The fetus is evaluated for activity pattern and heart rate. The woman is taught to assess for fetal activity patterns by counting the number of times the fetus moves for 1 hour each day, preferably at the same time each day. Four or more fetal movements should be recorded for positive results.

Management

Home management may be possible if the woman's blood pressure is only slightly elevated. Activity is restricted, and bed rest is commonly prescribed. The woman will be seen for office visits at least once weekly. If signs and symptoms of preeclampsia persist, she will be hospitalized for closer observation and treatment. The Nursing Care Plan for the woman experiencing PIH offers further insight. Magnesium sulfate (MgSO$_4$) is commonly used to control seizures. It decreases muscle irritability and relaxes smooth muscle. Initially, a bolus of 4 to 6 g MgSO$_4$ in 150 to 500 mL 5% dextrose in water (D$_5$W) is given over 20 minutes. This is followed by a slower, continuous infusion with 20 g MgSO$_4$ in 1000 mL D$_5$W at the rate of 100 mL/hour (2.0 g/h). The nurse remains with the woman during its administration, assessing blood pressure at regular intervals. Antihypertensives such as Apresoline (Ciba Pharmaceutical Co., Summit, NJ) may be given in repeated intravenous boluses to control high blood pressure. The usual dosage is 5- to 10-mg intravenous push given every 10 to 20 minutes until blood pressure responds favorably.

Fetal nonstress tests (NSTs) are performed frequently to assess the condition of the fetus. The woman

NURSING CARE PLAN
For the Woman Experiencing Pregnancy-Induced Hypertension (PIH)

ASSESSMENT: Katrina is a 17-year-old G1 P0 at 32 weeks' gestation whose pregnancy has been uneventful up to this point. Today, her B/P is 190/98 and proteinuria +3. She complains her rings feel tight and she has a headache. Katrina is admitted to the hospital with a diagnosis of PIH

NURSING DIAGNOSIS #1: Risk for Injury, related to potential eclamptic seizure.

EXPECTED OUTCOMES:
1. Katrina will verbalize an understanding regarding the need for immediate hospitalization and treatment
2. Katrina will not experience an eclamptic seizure
3. Maternal and fetal well-being will be maximized

Nursing Interventions	*Rationale*
1. Explain pathophysiology of PIH; need for continuous monitoring and left lateral positioning.	1. Increases patient understanding to help enhance compliance with treatment. Left lateral positioning increases utero-placental and renal circulation.
2. Maintain seizure precautions: • Provide darkened, quiet environment, limit visitors • Have emergency equipment readily available • Pad side rails	2. Reduced stimuli decreases risk of seizure occurring. Prompt availability of emergency equipment speeds intervention, helping to minimize adverse maternal/fetal effects. Padded side rails decreases maternal injury during seizure.
3. Observe for signs of worsening condition: • Headache, blurred vision • Excessive weight gain • Increasing blood pressure, proteinuria and/or edema • Epigastric pain • Nausea and vomiting • Hyperreflexia	3. Prompt recognition and management of worsening medical condition helps improve maternal/fetal outcome.

EVALUATION
1. Katrina's blood pressure ranges from 126/84 to 134/88; proteinuria +1.
2. Katrina's condition does not worsen.
3. Katrina complies with the prescribed managment regimen.

NURSING DIAGNOSIS #2: Knowledge Deficit, related to cause and management of PIH

EXPECTED OUTCOMES
1. Katrina will verbalize an understanding regarding the etiology and management regimen associated with PIH.
2. Katrina will comply with treatment regimen.

Nursing Interventions	*Rationale*
1. Evaluate patient's understanding regarding PIH and provide required instruction.	1. Initial evaluation provides basis on which the nurse can plan future teaching.
2. Explain rationale for all procedures or tests before taking any action.	2. Helps maintain atmosphere of trust, decreases anxiety, and enhances patient compliance.

EVALUATION
1. Katrina verbalized good understanding of PIH and treatment regimen.
2. With a stabilized medical condition and anticipated patient compliance, Katrina is discharged home.

is monitored for contractions and fetal heart rate. An NST is reactive and is considered successful if two or more fetal heart rate accelerations are detected during a 20-minute period. Each acceleration contains 15 or more beats and lasts for 15 seconds or more. These accelerations can occur spontaneously or with fetal movement. Amniocentesis (analysis of amniotic fluid) is performed to evaluate fetal lung maturity. Fetal lung maturity is a criterion used to determine if delivery is an option. If gestation is equal to or greater than 36 weeks, or PIH is worsening, labor may be induced with Pitocin (oxytocin). Under 36 weeks, if the woman's condition permits, an attempt may be made to control symptoms while allowing the fetus time to mature.

Betamethasone may be given intramuscularly in two doses of 12 mg each, 24 hours apart, to boost surfactant production. It assists the fetus's lungs to mature if a premature birth is anticipated.

If the woman's condition is critical, immediate delivery of the fetus is necessary. This is usually accomplished by cesarean birth. The special care nursery or neonatal intensive care unit (NICU) is always notified well before the birth, so they can be present to care for the neonate. PIH resolves very quickly after delivery, but the danger of convulsions remains for up to 48 hours after delivery.

◆ Rh and ABO Incompatibilities

A small number of fetal-blood cells typically pass into the woman's bloodstream at the time of delivery. When the fetus's Rh+ cells mix with the mother's Rh– cells, the woman's autoimmune system forms antibodies in a process called maternal autoimmunization. The maternal autoimmune response is very low during the first pregnancy. As a result, problems usually do not occur. In subsequent pregnancies, however, the woman's antibodies are extremely sensitive to the presence of fetal cells in the maternal bloodstream. They react by crossing the placenta and destroying the fetal red cells. The fetus suffers severe anemia (hemolytic anemia or erythroblastosis fetalis). This condition is characterized by jaundice, enlargement of the liver and spleen, and edema. It can lead to heart failure and death as the result of kernicterus. In kernicterus, the fetal bloodstream, carrying large amounts of bilirubin from the affected liver, deposits bilirubin in the brain, which causes permanent, irreversible damage.

ABO incompatibility may occur when a woman with type O blood carries a fetus whose blood type is A or B. This incompatibility is not nearly as serious as Rh incompatibility. It typically affects the first-born infant, who develops jaundice within 24 hours of birth.

Assessment

The pregnant woman's blood type and Rh factor are determined early in pregnancy and noted on her record. If the woman and father are both Rh–, no treatment is necessary because the fetus will be Rh–. An Rh+ will be able to accommodate a fetus of either Rh status. However, if the woman is Rh– and the father is Rh+, there is a large probability (50% to 100%) that the fetus will be Rh+. In this instance, the woman is screened frequently for antibodies during pregnancy. If no antibodies are detected by 28 weeks' gestation, 1 mL (300 mg) RhoGAM (Ortho Diagnostic, Raritan, NJ) may be given intramuscularly, and no further screening is necessary until delivery. RhoGAM should also be given after each amniocentesis, abortion, or ectopic pregnancy. There is no comparable treatment for ABO incompatibility.

Management

During pregnancy, if the life of the fetus is in danger, intrauterine fetal transfusions of O– blood are frequently successful. After delivery of an Rh+ neonate, the Rh– woman and newborn have blood samples crossmatched to assess for fetal–maternal exchange during delivery. The woman is given 1 mL (300 mg) RhoGAM intramuscularly within 72 hours of delivery, before she can produce antibodies to the fetal blood cells that entered her bloodstream. The neonate is closely watched for signs of jaundice, in which case phototherapy is initiated (Fig. 8-2).

◆ Bleeding in Early Pregnancy

Approximately 20% of pregnant women experience bleeding during the first trimester. Because bleeding in pregnancy is never normal, the cause must be investigated. The cause may be spontaneous abortion, lesions or cervical polyps, ectopic pregnancy, carcinoma of the cervix, hydatidiform mole, or abnormal implantation of the placenta.

[handwritten: Pregnancy terminated 20wks: Viability]

Abortion

Pregnancy that ends before the fetus can survive outside of the uterus is termed abortion. For a fetus to survive, or to be considered viable, its gestational age must

[handwritten: Explosion of Products of Conception before the Period of Viability 20wks]

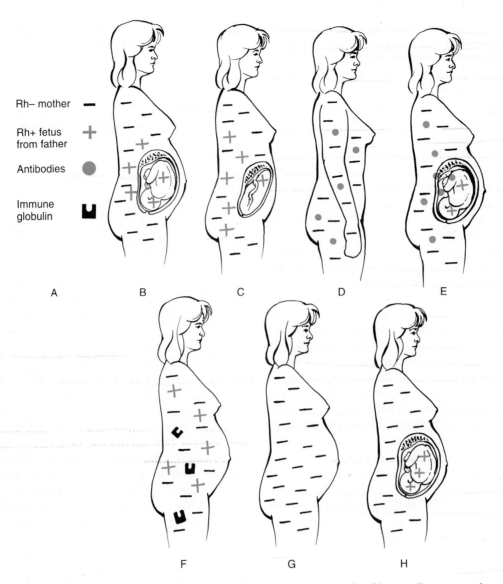

Rh− mother

Rh+ fetus from father

Antibodies

Immune globulin

A   B   C   D   E

F   G   H

Figure 8-2. (**A**) Rh− mother and Rh+ father. (**B**) When the fetus is also Rh+, small amounts of the fetus' Rh+ blood may mix with the mother's Rh−. (**C**) During delivery, more Rh+ blood escapes into the mother's system. (**D**) Untreated, the Rh+ cells remain, causing the mother to develop Rh+ antibodies to destroy foreign cells. The mother becomes **permanently** sensitized. (**E**) During a subsequent pregnancy with an Rh+ fetus, the mother contains antibodies against her fetus. Erythroblastosis fetalis may result. (**F**) To avoid sensitization, the mother should be administered immune globulin whenever Rh+ cells escape into the bloodstream and after each pregnancy. (**G**) The immune globulin attacks and eliminates Rh+ cells. (**H**) In a subsequent pregnancy with an Rh+ fetus, the mother is free from Rh+ antibodies.

be approximately 23 weeks and it must weigh at least 500 g. Abortions are either spontaneous or induced.

Spontaneous Abortion

A spontaneous abortion, called miscarriage by many, occurs without outside intervention. Approximately 10% of all pregnancies end in spontaneous abortion, most of which occur before 12 weeks' gestation. A woman who has experienced three or more consecutive abortions is diagnosed with habitual abortion. The chances that she will carry a pregnancy to term decrease with each abortion.

Spontaneous abortions may be caused by defects in the ovum or the sperm. Problems with the intrauterine environment also may be responsible for spontaneous abortion. Maternal diseases that may predispose toward spontaneous abortion include infection, diabetes, hormonal deficiencies such as low levels of thyroid or ovarian hormones, or an incompetent cervix. In many cases, the cause of abortion is unknown.

A spontaneous abortion is classified as threatened, inevitable, incomplete, complete, missed, or delayed. Signs of abortion include bleeding, abdominal cramping, and lower backache. In inevitable abortion, bleeding and abdominal cramping are accompanied by rupture of the membranes and dilation of the cervix. An incomplete abortion occurs when part of the products of conception are not expelled. The fetus is expelled, but the placenta is retained. A missed abortion occurs when the fetus dies but is not passed vaginally. If the fetus is retained for a long period, the breakdown of fetal tissues results in the release of thromboplastin, and DIC develops. Usually, labor will start spontaneously after approximately 2 weeks, and uterine contents are passed.

Incomplete Abortions

Hemorrhage may be profuse because of partial separation of the placenta from the uterine wall. Bleeding occurs because the uterus is unable to contract and place pressure on vessels located on the underside of the separated portion of the placenta. Surgical dilatation and curettage (D&C) is done to remove the retained placenta, which allows the uterus to contract and stop the bleeding.

Abortion Due to Incompetent Cervix

An incompetent cervix is one that dilates before labor occurs. This condition can be prevented by performing a McDonald or Shirodkar procedure. A pursestring suture, known as a cerclage or ligature, is placed in the cervix and holds it closed until the suture is removed when the pregnancy reaches term, or when the woman goes into labor.

Induced Elective Abortion

In 1973 the United States Supreme Court ruled that women have a right to terminate pregnancy during the first trimester. After 12 weeks' gestation, individual states have the power to regulate elective abortion and, after the age of viability, to prohibit such procedures except when the woman's life or health is endangered.

Before an elective abortion is performed, the woman receives counseling regarding the risks involved. Risks include those related to any surgical procedure and the possibility of difficulty becoming pregnant in the future. Alternatives such as continuing the pregnancy and adoption are discussed.

Assessment

Assessment of the pregnant woman who is bleeding includes taking a health history, documenting onset, duration, amount, and character of discharge. Vital signs are assessed and recorded as ordered.

Management

The methods used for elective termination of pregnancy depend on the gestational age of the fetus. First-trimester pregnancies are often terminated with D&C or suction curettage. These procedures can be performed with local anesthesia or light general anesthesia. Suction curettage involves the insertion of a curette into the uterus after the cervix has been dilated with instruments called dilators. The curette is attached to an electric pump and suctions out the contents of the uterus. D&C is also used for a spontaneous abortion when indicated.

An alternate method of dilating the cervix involves the use of *Laminaria digitata*. Dried stems of this seaweed are inserted in the cervix. Fluid from cervical tissue is absorbed by the *Laminaria* and it swells, causing the cervix to dilate and pass the developing embryo.

Second-trimester elective abortion may be performed by injection of hypertonic saline solution into the uterus under local anesthesia. After several hours, the woman goes into labor, and uterine contents are expelled. The fetus is usually dead when delivered. This procedure is contraindicated in women with hypertension, cardiac or renal disease, or severe anemia.

Prostaglandins are chemical substances that occur naturally in the body and are capable of producing powerful contraction of smooth muscle such as the uterus. They can be used to induce labor and may be given as vaginal suppositories or intramuscular injection. Side effects of prostaglandin use include nausea, vomiting, diarrhea, fever, hemorrhage, cervical laceration, and fistula (an abnormal tubelike passage) formation.

Written informed consent is obtained before elective abortions are performed. The nurse instructs the woman and her support person regarding the process and any side effects. Time is given for questions and verbalization of feelings about outcome. The woman should refrain from eating or drinking fluids for 12 hours before the procedure to lessen the danger of nausea and vomiting and subsequent aspiration of fluids.

After elective procedures, the nurse assesses for discomfort, vital signs, and vaginal bleeding for 2 to 3 hours. Analgesics are given for pain from cramping and uterine contractions. When the woman is stable, she is discharged after instruction regarding self-care and return visits. If discomfort, unstable vital signs, or excessive bleeding occur, the woman is kept overnight for observation.

Ectopic Pregnancy

Ectopic pregnancy results when the fertilized ovum implants somewhere other than in the uterus. Implanta-

Missed Abortion When the Fetus dies and does not Abort

Septic Abortion Where there are Galthogens the Woman has to go on Antibiotics. Infections

tion sites include the fallopian tube, ovary, cervix, or abdominal cavity (Fig. 8-3). Most ectopic pregnancies occur in the right fallopian tube.

Causes of ectopic pregnancy include developmental abnormalities of the fallopian tube, a previous tubal infection that narrowed the passage, previous tubal ectopic pregnancy, low levels of hormones affecting tubal motility, use of intrauterine contraceptive devices (IUDs), and tumors that distort the tube.

Rupture of the fallopian tube occurs as the fertilized egg grows in size. Rupture can be sudden or gradual. With sudden rupture, signs and symptoms include abrupt, sharp abdominal pain, hemorrhage, shock caused by falling blood pressure, and rapid pulse. Prompt diagnosis and treatment is essential. Gradual rupture results in milder symptoms. There is abdominal discomfort, and there may or may not be vaginal bleeding.

The incidence of ectopic pregnancy is 1 of every 100 pregnancies and appears to be increasing. They are common in nonwhite women, women older than 35, and those with a history of infertility. Ectopic pregnancy is responsible for 10% of all maternal deaths.

Assessment

Hormonal levels of beta-human chorionic gonadotropin (BhCG), which increase during pregnancy, are assessed to diagnose ectopic pregnancy. Vaginal probe ultrasound shows an empty uterus and may show the site of the ectopic pregnancy.

Culdocentesis shows whether there is fluid from tubal rupture in the cul-de-sac between the uterus and rectum. A needle attached to a syringe is inserted through the vagina into the cul-de-sac to aspirate any fluid accumulated there. Aspiration of more than 3 mL unclotted blood is considered a positive sign of ectopic pregnancy. A positive pregnancy test and visualization of an empty uterus by ultrasound offer confirmation.

The nurse takes a health history to assess for the possibility of ectopic pregnancy. The date of the last menstrual period, treatment for pelvic infection, use of

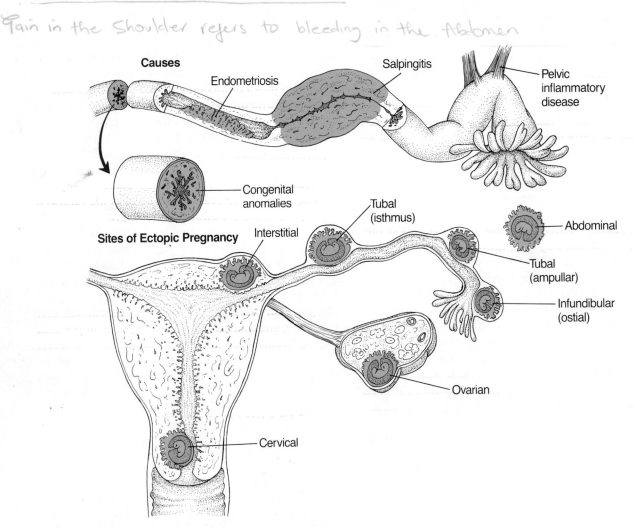

Figure 8-3. Causes and sites of ectopic pregnancy.

birth control devices, and history of previous ectopic pregnancy are all recorded.

Management

Management of ectopic pregnancy consists of surgical removal of the ruptured tube (salpingectomy), usually through laparascopy. The Rh– woman will receive RhoGAM after the ectopic pregnancy is resolved.

If there are no signs of bleeding, 1 mg methotrexate can be given intramuscularly every other day for 4 days. Methotrexate, a drug used to treat cancer, causes the products of conception to stop growing and eventually to dissolve. Levels of BhCG are assessed and found to decrease gradually.

Gestational Trophoblastic Neoplasm

Gestational trophoblastic neoplasm (hydatidiform mole) is a fast-growing, benign growth of the trophoblastic cells. These cells develop into cystic, transparent vesicles that resemble clusters of grapes. There are two categories of hydatidiform mole: complete and partial. Complete moles lack an embryo or amniotic sac. Partial moles contain an embryo and amniotic sac, usually with multiple abnormalities.

Hydatidiform mole occurs in approximately 1 in 1500 to 1 in 2000 pregnancies. Those at increased risk for developing this disorder are women from Southeast Asia or the Far East, and women older than 40 or younger than 18. The cause is unknown, but researchers speculate that poor maternal nutrition or defective ova are responsible.

Assessment

Early pregnancy appears normal, but as gestation progresses, the uterus begins to grow rapidly. The woman may experience hyperemesis gravidarum, signs of preeclampsia, and brownish vaginal discharge. The vaginal discharge may contain vesicles from the mole. Symptoms of partial mole may resemble those of incomplete abortion. Hemorrhage is an associated potential complication.

Levels of hCG are assessed. In normal pregnancy, these levels increase through the first trimester and level off. When hydatidiform mole is present, hCG levels continue to increase. Ultrasound usually confirms the diagnosis.

Management

The pregnancy is terminated, and uterine contents are emptied by suction curettage. The woman is at risk for hemorrhage, infection, and uterine perforation. If the cervix is unreceptive to dilation with dilator instruments, one of the chemical dilators, such as prostaglandin, may be used.

Follow-up care is very important for these women. There is a great risk of neoplasia (cancerous growth). Continued assessment includes ongoing study of levels of hCG and ultrasound scans of the abdomen. Assessment of hCG is done weekly until levels remain normal for 3 consecutive weeks. Levels are again assessed monthly for 6 months, then every 2 months for 6 months, and then every 6 months for a year. Regular pelvic examinations are important in detecting changes indicating abnormal tissue growth. Chest x-rays are done at regular intervals to assess for pulmonary tumors. The woman is instructed to report the presence of dyspnea, cough, or chest pain. The nurse must educate the woman and her family about the importance of follow-up assessments. Pregnancy is avoided until hCG levels are normal, which usually occurs after about a year. IUDs are contraindicated because bleeding irregularities may occur. Some health care providers prescribe chemotherapy. However, this form of treatment is controversial and needs further study.

Bleeding in Late Pregnancy

Frequent causes of bleeding in late pregnancy include placenta previa and abruptio placentae. DIC occurs as the result of other complications.

Placenta Previa

Placenta previa occurs when the placenta implants near or over the cervical os instead of in the fundus of the uterus. There are three classes of previa: marginal, where the placenta is near the os; partial, with the placenta covering part of the os; and total, with the placenta completely covering the os.

Placenta previa occurs in approximately 1 in 200 pregnancies. Uterine scarring, multiple gestation, previous placenta previa, closely spaced pregnancies, uterine tumor, and increased maternal age are all potential causes. Women are routinely hospitalized for observation and evaluation after the first bleeding episode (Fig. 8-4).

Types of Placenta Previa

Assessment

Painless bleeding is the most common symptom in placenta previa. It can occur late in the second trimester, but it occurs more commonly in the third. As the cervix begins to change in preparation for birth, the marginal or overlying placenta separates, and bleeding results.

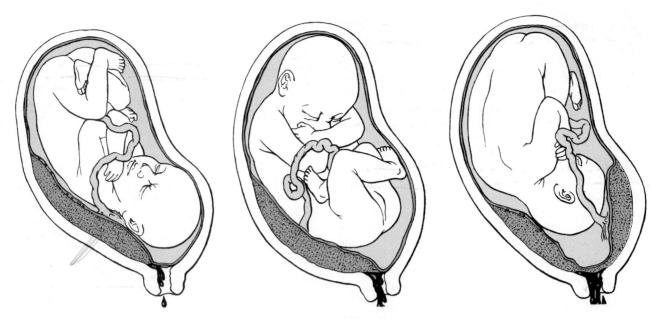

Figure 8-4. *Placenta previa.* **(A)** *Marginal implantation.* **(B)** *Partial implantation.* **(C)** *Total implantation.*

The first episode is usually not severe and stops shortly after onset. As the expected date of delivery draws near, bleeding episodes continue and grow progressively more severe.

Women diagnosed with this condition must be closely assessed for the amount and character of blood loss. Vital signs are routinely documented as well as fetal heart rate and fetal activity. Diagnosis is confirmed with abdominal ultrasound. Until the cause is determined, digital vaginal examination is strictly prohibited anytime a pregnant woman is bleeding because severe hemorrhage may result from the examination.

Management

Management depends on the gestational age of the fetus and the severity of hemorrhaging. If gestational age is less than 36 weeks, bleeding is mild, and labor has not begun, the woman may be placed on strict bed rest to give the fetus time to mature. The woman is closely observed for signs of continued bleeding and onset of uterine contractions.

Intravenous fluids are given unless blood loss is minimal. Blood transfusions may be given if loss is severe. The fetus is closely assessed for movement and heart rate. An NST (see Chapter 10) is performed daily, and betamethasone therapy is initiated. Home management is allowed if the bleeding stabilizes and fetal status remains good. The nurse teaches the woman to monitor fetal activity and limit her own activities. Enemas, douching, and sexual intercourse are to be avoided.

If bleeding becomes severe, or gestation has progressed to 36 weeks, the fetus will be delivered. Cesarean section is done unless the previa is minimally marginal.

Abruptio Placentae

Abruptio placentae occurs with premature separation of the placenta. Separation can be total or partial. Abruptio placentae occurs in approximately 1% of all deliveries and greatly compromises the well-being of the fetus. Fetal demise occurs frequently when placental separation is greater than 50%.

Causes of abruptio placentae can be external trauma to the uterus; social drug use in pregnancy, particularly of cocaine; PIH; previous abruption; folic acid deficiency; cigarette smoking; and premature rupture of the membranes. Abruptio placentae is the most common cause of DIC (Fig. 8-5).

Assessment

Classic symptoms of an abrupted placenta are heavy dark red vaginal bleeding, uterine rigidity, severe abdominal pain, and fetal distress. The nurse assesses for the character and amount of bleeding, abdominal discomfort or contractions, and fetal activity and heart tones.

If separation is central to the placenta, bleeding may be trapped and concealed. With no outlet, blood builds and causes abdominal pain and rigidity. If concealed bleeding is suggested, the abdomen should be

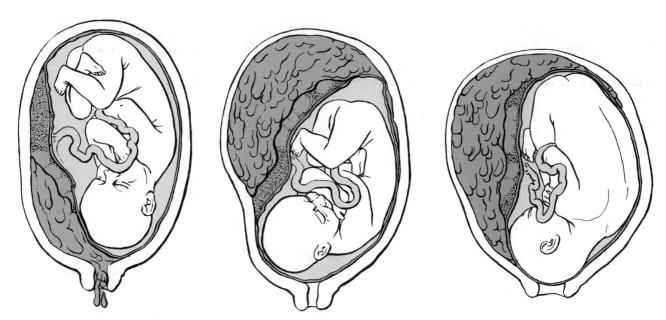

Figure 8-5. _Abruptio placentae at various separation sites._ (**A**) _External hemorrhage._ (**B**) _Internal or concealed hemorrhage._ (**C**) _Complete separation._

measured at the height of the fundus. Height of the fundus is noted by marking it with a skin marker; assessment for change in fundal height is done frequently thereafter. The woman is monitored for shock caused by hemorrhage. Because the normal physiologic changes of pregnancy result in increased maternal blood volume, the classic signs of abruptio placentae are not always noticeable.

Management

Management depends on the severity of the abruption, condition of the woman and fetus, and the size of the fetus. If either the woman or fetus is badly compromised, cesarean birth is performed. NICU is notified so that they can be present at delivery to care for the neonate. Blood transfusions are given if blood loss is severe or symptoms of DIC are present. Ringer's lactate solution is infused at the same time to aid in fluid volume replacement.

Disseminated Intravascular Coagulation

It's secondary to something else

Disseminated intravascular coagulation (DIC) is a condition in which a coagulation defect prevents blood from clotting. This results from overstimulation of the normal coagulation process. As a result, severe anemia develops and massive internal and external hemorrhage occur.

Disseminated intravascular coagulation is not a primary disorder, but a complication arising from a number of conditions. Not much is known about DIC, but events activating the coagulation process are known to precede onset. These events include infusion into the bloodstream of injured tissue; various chemical and physical agents; thrombocytopenia; severe injury to endothelial cells; immune reactions; bacterial debris or endotoxins; and red cell or platelet injury.

Assessment _Little hematomas_

Early signs of DIC include bruising of the skin, hematuria, and oozing of blood from IV or other invasive sites. As the condition progresses, symptoms include petechiae; peripheral cyanosis; and bleeding from the gums, nose, and vagina. Blood laboratory values are evaluated for coagulation factor values such as fibrinogen, platelets, prothrombin time (PT), and PTT.

Management

If coagulation factors are critically depleted before delivery of the fetus, they should be replaced, especially platelets and fibrinogen. The fetus is delivered as soon as the primary cause is corrected or stabilized. NICU personnel are present to assess neonatal status. Blood and volume replacement is accomplished by transfusion with packed cells, fresh frozen plasma, and crystalloids such as lactated Ringer's solution. The nurse assesses for vital signs, character and amount of bleeding, output of urine, and type and amount of fluids infused. Although there is a high mortality rate associated with DIC, it resolves quickly after delivery

NURSING CARE PLAN
for the Woman With Diabetes

ASSESSMENT: Diane is a 22-year-old G1 P0 whose 1-hour glucose screen at 28 weeks' gestation was 162. Gestational diabetes mellitus (GDM) was diagnosed after a 3-hour glucose tolerance test. She is extremely upset and asking what this means for her baby.

NURSING DIAGNOSIS #1: Anxiety, related to effects of hyperglycemia on fetal well-being

EXPECTED OUTCOMES
1. Diane will verbalize an understanding of steps that can enhance fetal well-being.
2. Diane's anxiety level will be decreased.

Nursing Interventions	*Rationale*
1. Encourage patient to verbalize fears and anxiety.	1. Patient may have unrealistic fears, which can be dispelled in an environment that promotes trust and understanding.
2. Explain usual management of GDM and anticipated patient's role in that regimen.	2. Increasing patient participation can help lessen anxiety as she feels in greater control of situation.

EVALUATION
1. Diane's verbal and nonverbal behaviors demonstrate decreased level of anxiety.
2. Diane plays an active role in the management of her diabetes.

NURSING DIAGNOSIS #2: Knowledge Deficit, related to treatment of gestational diabetes

EXPECTED OUTCOMES
1. Diane's fasting blood glucose levels will be less than 100 mg and 2-hour postprandials less than 120 mg.
2. Diane will understand how to follow a 2200-calorie ADA diet.
3. The fetus will not demonstrate any adverse effects of hyperglycemia.

Nursing Interventions	*Rationale*
1. Demonstrate how to perform self-glucose monitoring at home. Instruct patient to perform test 4 times/day; fasting and 2 hours after each meal.	1. Careful monitoring of glucose levels during pregnancy helps minimize maternal and fetal side effects.
2. Arrange consult with dietitian for 2200-calorie American Diabetic Association (ADA) diet.	2. Regulation of dietary intake helps control glucose levels and may prevent the need for insulin therapy
3. Arrange and explain need for prenatal tests such as nonstress tests and biophysical profiles. Teach patient how to maintain daily fetal movement chart.	3. Prenatal testing may identify early effects of GDM such as macrosomia and polyhydramnios. Decreased fetal movement may indicate fetal hypoxia, requiring prompt evaluation.

EVALUATIONS
1. The fetal weight remains within normal limits for gestational age.
2. Diane's dietary recall from the last 3 days indicates a good understanding of the American Diabetic Association (ADA) diet.
3. Diane's fasting blood sugar levels do not surpass 95; postprandial levels remain lower than 112.

Diabetes in Pregnancy

Women diagnosed with diabetes mellitus before becoming pregnant and those with unknown diabetic tendencies will experience abnormal carbohydrate metabolism. Resistance to insulin occurs as pregnancy with adequate preservation of blood volume and replacement.

progresses. Elevations of normal blood glucose levels result.

Diabetes Mellitus

Diabetes mellitus is a metabolic disorder in which the pancreas produces insufficient insulin. This condition is found in approximately 2% of pregnant women. They are at risk for PIH, infection, increased incidence of stillbirth, spontaneous abortion, preterm or early labor, IUGR, and heavier than normal fetal birth weight (macrosomia). Diabetic women often develop greater amounts of amniotic fluid (hydramnios) related to fetal hyperglycemia. Hyperglycemia in the fetus results in increased fetal urine production. Fetal use of glucose causes maternal hypoglycemia. Ketoacidosis occurs when the woman uses stored fat for her caloric needs and saves glucose for fetal needs. Effects of diabetes on the fetus include congenital abnormalities such as cardiac or central nervous system disorders, hypoglycemia, macrosomia, hyaline membrane disease of the lungs, hypocalcemia, possible traumatic delivery because of large size, and intrauterine fetal demise. *The*

Gestational Diabetes

Gestational diabetes occurs as a result of altered carbohydrate metabolism triggered by the changes in estrogen and progesterone levels associated with pregnancy. The woman typically knows little or nothing about the disorder because she has no previous history of carbohydrate metabolism problems. These women require instruction from the nurse concerning diet, self-care and hygiene, and blood glucose monitoring. Many gestational diabetics do not require treatment for abnormal carbohydrate metabolism after delivery. Between 40% and 60% of gestational diabetics develop diabetes requiring treatment in later years.

1st Initial Visit test GTT

Assessment

Control of diabetes and blood glucose levels is vital to a positive pregnancy outcome for the woman and fetus. A fasting blood glucose level of less than 100 to 120 mg/dL in pregnancy is acceptable. All pregnant women, except for known diabetics, are screened for gestational diabetes, usually between 24 and 28 weeks' gestation. A glucose challenge test is given in which 50 g glucose are ingested and glucose levels are assessed 1 hour later. If results are above 140 mg/dL, a 3-hour glucose tolerance test is necessary. It should be stressed that a pregnant woman's blood volume increases by 40% to 50% over her prepregnancy levels, peaking at 28 to 30 weeks' gestation. This increase has an impact on blood glucose results. Once diagnosed as diabetic, the woman is usually referred to a perinatologist.

Management

The prepregnant diabetic woman continues with diet, blood glucose monitoring, and insulin therapy as prescribed by her physician and nutritionist. The gesta-

tional diabetic woman receives counseling and instructions from her health care provider, nutritionist, and nurse. Often, blood glucose levels of gestational diabetics can be controlled by diet alone. Generally, a 2000- to 2400-calorie diet is prescribed. The nurse teaches the woman how to monitor her blood glucose levels, to test her urine for ketones, and how to administer insulin if required.

The fetus is assessed and evaluated frequently throughout the pregnancy. The NST is performed weekly after 34 weeks' gestation. The well-controlled diabetic may be allowed to deliver at term. Early delivery may be planned if glucose levels are not controlled, if there is a history of previous stillbirth, or if other complications have developed such as very large infant or fetal compromise. Induction of labor or cesarean birth may then be scheduled. For further information, see the Nursing Care Plan for the woman with diabetes.

140 / 90 Beginning of ↑ BP

Heart Disease

Mitral valve prolapse is the most common cardiac disease assessed in pregnancy. It affects approximately 6% to 8% of women of reproductive age and is probably genetic in origin. Other cardiac conditions that may have risk potential for pregnancy are complications from rheumatic heart disease and congenital heart disease (CHD). *Heparin is OK NO Coumadine*

Assessment

The pregnant woman with heart disease is assessed early in pregnancy, when baseline evaluations are made to decide if the pregnancy should continue. If the pregnancy is not life-threatening, the woman is monitored closely to ensure an optimal outcome for herself and the fetus.

Management

The nurse instructs the pregnant woman with heart disease regarding levels of activity, diet, and signs of impending complications. It is important that she not expose herself to children or adults with infectious diseases. The woman should report any difficulty with breathing, cough, chest pain, rapid weight gain, or edema. Edema associated with increased fluid volume levels can be very serious for the pregnant woman with heart disease. The workload of the heart is greatly compromised when blood volume levels are excessive. The fetus is assessed frequently throughout the pregnancy, with NST done weekly after the fetus is viable.

Infections

Infections in pregnancy place the woman and fetus in jeopardy for many other associated complications. Early detection and treatment are essential to avoid complications. Specific infections, their assessment, and management are discussed in the following sections.

Urinary Tract Infection

Urinary tract infections (UTIs) are common during pregnancy because the heavy uterus places excess pressure on the ureters and bladder. This results in relaxation of the urethra and urinary stasis. Both conditions place the urinary tract at risk for bacterial invasion. Bladder (cystitis) and kidney (pyelonephritis) infections are frequently diagnosed in pregnancy. Infections may be diagnosed as asymptomatic or symptomatic bacteriuria.

Assessment

Signs of bladder infection include frequency of urination, pain or burning during urination, a feeling of urgency to void, and low abdominal or back pain. Symptoms of kidney infection are fever and chills, nausea, vomiting, and flank pain. — Right over kidney is flank pain

The nurse collects a clean-catch urine specimen after instructing the woman on how to obtain the specimen. (The perineal area is cleaned and dried, after which the woman is instructed to hold her labia apart. The best urine specimen is collected midstream without having touched the skin.) The specimen is evaluated for bacteria count, after which a diagnosis is made.

Management

Oral or intravenous antibiotics are generally prescribed for bladder or kidney infection, depending on urine culture and sensitivity results. Ampicillin is the antibiotic of choice. Acetaminophen may be given orally if the woman complains of pain or discomfort from the infection. Urine culture is repeated after the course of antibiotics is finished.

Teratogenic Infections

A teratogen is any agent that interferes with fetal development. Teratogenic infections, formerly known by the acronym TORCH, can be transmitted to the fetus during pregnancy. **TORCH** was the abbreviation for the infectious conditions of *T*oxoplasmosis, *O*ther infections, *R*ubella, *C*ytomegalovirus, and *H*erpes. Other teratogenic infections that are dangerous to the fetus are syphilis, hepatitis B, and HIV.

Risk to the fetus from these infections include congenital heart defects, physical anomalies, IUGR, mental retardation, and encephalitis. The woman is routinely screened and appropriately treated early in pregnancy if infection is present. The woman is counseled regarding the effects the infection may have on the fetus, and it is her right to choose if she wants to continue the pregnancy. Universal precautions are used by health care workers when caring for women with infectious disease.

Sexually Transmitted Teratogenic Infections

The symptoms, treatments, and means of preventing gonorrhea, syphilis, chlamydia, herpes, and HIV are described in detail in Chapter 4. These teratogenic infections are described here briefly in terms of how they affect the neonate.

Gonorrhea

Pregnancy complications associated with gonorrhea include increased risk for spontaneous abortion, preterm delivery, and premature rupture of the membranes (PROM). Because the infection is transmitted to the neonate during vaginal delivery, cesarean birth is performed if infection is present at time of delivery. The greatest gonorrhea-related risk to the neonate is an eye infection called gonococcal ophthalmia, which can cause blindness. In the United States, federal law requires that every newborn's eyes be treated with an antibiotic ointment or silver nitrate drops to prevent this complication.

Syphilis

If untreated, there is increased risk of spontaneous abortion, fetal deformity, neonatal infection, or fetal death.

Chlamydia

Implications for pregnancy include PROM, preterm labor (PTL), early delivery, and low birth weight. The infection is transmitted to the fetus during passage through the birth canal. The newborn is at risk for conjunctivitis (which is treatable with erythromycin ointment) and chronic otitis media.

Herpes

Herpes can cause local infection of the neonate's skin, eyes, and nose. Systemic infection of the liver, central nervous systems, and other organs is also possible.

Trichomonas- Thick frothy discharge foul smelling treated ̄c Sulfur cream
ABC cream
Flagyl use for 7 days can't use 1st half of pregnancy *Multifetal Pregnancy* ◆ *137*
or Use warm weak vinegar douche

Although acyclovir is prescribed to treat herpes in non-pregnant women, use of this and other drugs in pregnancy is not recommended. This is because the effects on the fetus are not known. If the mother is suffering from an outbreak of herpes at the time of delivery, a cesarean birth is performed.

HIV/AIDS

There is no cure for this disease, which acts by destroying the body's immune system. It is known that 35% to 50% of all newborns test positive for human immunodeficiency virus (HIV) when the woman is HIV+. (See Chapter 4 for a discussion of recent findings related to the maternal use of AZT and its effect on the infant's prognosis.) HIV can be transmitted to the fetus at the time of birth, transplacentally while the fetus is in utero, or through breast milk.

Hepatitis B

Fluid that carries the sperm

Hepatitis B (HBV) is a virus spread through blood, saliva, semen, and vaginal secretions. Symptoms of the disorder include fever, jaundice, and an enlarged liver. The danger from this virus to the pregnancy is that it may cause preterm labor in the third trimester. The fetus will probably be a carrier if not treated. If the woman has HBV, the neonate should be injected with hepatitis B immune globulin within 12 hours of delivery, followed by HB vaccine (Recombivax). Booster injections are given within the first 2 years of life.

Cytomegalovirus   Kissing disease

Cytomegalovirus (CMV) is a common infection and cause of mental retardation and congenital deafness. It is caused by a virus from the herpes family. CMV is spread through body fluids, including breast milk, and may be contracted through sexual contact or through the respiratory tract. Those at high risk for contracting CMV include children attending day-care centers, those younger than 25, Caucasians, persons of lower socioeconomic status, and anyone engaging in unprotected sexual contact. Fifty percent of neonates with severe congenital infection die shortly after birth. There is no approved vaccine available at this time.

Toxoplasmosis

Toxoplasmosis is caused by the protozoan parasite *Toxoplasma gondii*, which is carried by cats and mice. The parasite is commonly found in cat feces. It is for this reason that pregnant women should avoid contact with kitty litter. Contamination with this parasite causes

Streptococc

malaise, lymphadenopathy, muscle pain, and a slight fever in the woman. The fetus is at risk for developing lesions of the central nervous system, anemia, and lymphadenopathy.

Rubella

Inter Uterine Growth retardation
IUGR

Rubella, also called German Measles, is caused by a virus that produces a rash after an incubation period of 14 to 21 days. It is transmitted through the upper respiratory tract via nasopharyngeal secretions. The virus is most dangerous to the developing fetus if the woman contracts the disease during the first trimester of pregnancy. The fetus may develop anomalies, particularly deafness and cataracts. Threat of spontaneous abortion is greatly increased.

Women are screened early in pregnancy for presence of rubella antibodies. A titer of more than 1:16 indicates immunity. If the woman has low or no immunity, she is given rubella vaccine after delivery. The nurse instructs her not to become pregnant for 3 months after immunization because the rubella vaccine is a live virus and can affect a developing fetus.

Tuberculosis

Tuberculosis (TB) is an infection caused by the tubercle bacillus *Mycobacterium tuberculosis*, an airborne organism. This disease primarily affects the lungs but can spread to other organs. Risk factors include lower socioeconomic status and poor nutrition. Symptoms include fatigue, weight loss, low-grade fever, and a productive cough. A positive skin test for the disease indicates the need for x-ray of the chest. A chest x-ray showing involvement of the lungs confirms the diagnosis. Sputum is tested for the presence of the tubercle.

The drug isoniazid is the treatment of choice. The drug is taken orally for at least 12 months or longer if needed and can be started in pregnancy. The fetus is not at risk for contracting tuberculosis in utero. After delivery, the mother must take precautions not to infect the newborn. This may include isolation from the infant. Breast-feeding is not recommended.

Multifetal Pregnancy

Multifetal pregnancies are considered complications of pregnancy because of the associated risks for the mother and the neonate. Maternal risks include increased incidence of PIH, PROM, PTL, and early delivery. Fetal complications include higher risk for fetal growth retardation, congenital abnormalities, umbilical cord problems, and malpresentation such as transverse lie or breech presentation.

Assessment

A multifetal pregnancy is generally suggested when the fundal height is unusually long. These pregnancies are confirmed by ultrasound in which more than one fetus is visualized or more than one fetal heart rate is heard.

Management

Management goals are to evaluate fetal growth and prevent preterm labor and delivery. If preterm labor does occur, the woman will be placed on bed rest. Fetal evaluation includes abdominal ultrasound every 3 to 4 weeks after 16 weeks' gestation to assess growth patterns.

The health care provider and expectant family discuss the appropriate route for delivery before labor begins. Route of delivery depends on presentation, gestational age, and condition of the fetuses.

If preterm labor further complicates the pregnancy, the woman is hospitalized and given medication (tocolytics) to stop contractions. The nurse must assess for maternal vital signs, uterine contractions, presence of abnormal vaginal discharge such as amniotic fluid or bleeding, fetal heart tones, and fetal activity. Women hospitalized for long periods in pregnancy need responsive support from caregivers as well as from their families. Resources such as social services, spiritual care, and occupational and physical therapy should be used.

Adolescent Considerations

With any prenatal problem, the adolescent is classified as having a higher risk for a negative pregnancy outcome than a woman who begins pregnancy with low risk.

With continual vomiting, low hemoglobin levels, abortions with associated maternal Rh− factors, history of sexually transmitted infections, and carbohydrate metabolism discrepancies, the pregnant adolescent needs very close monitoring and intense counseling.

Cultural Considerations

Culture plays an important role on the impact complications have on the family with special needs. Nutritional deficits that affect carbohydrate metabolism may be grounded in cultural roots that place the pregnant woman and family at risk. The use of herbs and homemade remedies to combat excessive nausea and vomiting may hinder a woman from seeking professional care for hyperemesis gravidarum.

Bleeding at any stage in pregnancy may be viewed as a "sign" that the woman has taken part in a forbidden cultural rite. For instance, a Vietnamese woman who does not ritually avoid weddings and funerals during pregnancy may view vaginal bleeding as a punishment for disobeying social laws. Among many Mexican American women, congenital abnormalities in the neonate may be mistakenly attributed to lunar eclipses and moonlight, and not to the actual causative infections.

Nurses caring for women at risk and their families must use discretion and facts to assist them in resolving their special needs and attaining a positive pregnancy outcome.

The Role of the Nurse

The role of the nurse in caring for the family with special needs during the antepartal period addresses the significant threats to maternal and fetal health. When complications arise that jeopardize a positive pregnancy outcome, appropriate nursing diagnoses and interventions must be taken. See the Nursing Diagnoses Checklist, which highlights some of the nursing diagnoses that assist the nurse in providing care.

✔ NURSING DIAGNOSES CHECKLIST

Nursing Diagnoses for the Family With Special Needs During the Antepartum Period

- Activity Intolerance, related to bedrest in hyperemesis gravidarum
- Ineffective Denial, related to carbohydrate metabolic disturbance in pregnancy
- Ineffective Family Coping: Compromised, related to bleeding in pregnancy
- Anticipatory Grieving, related to impending spontaneous abortion
- Knowledge Deficit, related to risk factors in pregnancy
- Powerlessness, related to blood incompatibility of woman and fetus
- Fear, related to cardiac disease in pregnancy
- Pain, related to ectopic pregnancy
- Ineffective Airway Clearance, related to active tuberculosis in pregnancy
- Risk for Infection, related to exposure to infected person(s)

SELF-ASSESSMENT

1. An anemic pregnant woman must be watched carefully for signs of:

○ **A.** Diabetes
○ **B.** Preeclampsia
○ **C.** Hepatitis B
⊘ **D.** Infection

2. Which of the following pregnant women is at highest risk of developing a deep vein thrombosis (DVT)?

○ **A.** A 16-year-old
⊘ **B.** A patient with restricted activity
○ **C.** A primigravida
○ **D.** An underweight patient

3. Methotrexate may be used in the management of:

○ **A.** Hydatidiform mole
⊠ **B.** Ectopic pregnancy
○ **C.** Hyperemesis
○ **D.** Incomplete abortion

4. What is the most common symptom of placenta previa?

⊘ **A.** Painless vaginal bleeding
○ **B.** Mild uterine contractions every 1 to 2 minutes
○ **C.** Severe abdominal pain
○ **D.** Premature labor

5. A pregnant woman with a history of cardiac disease is considered high risk due to which physiological change of pregnancy?

⊘ **A.** Decreased pulse
○ **B.** Increased respiratory rate
○ **C.** Decreaesd blood pressure
○ **D.** Increased blood volume

REVIEW AND PREVIEW

In this chapter, we discussed in detail the special needs of families at risk during the antepartum period. Many of the physiologic conditions that threaten maternal and fetal well-being were outlined. Appropriate assessment and management of the problems were explained.

In the following chapter, a detailed outline of normal fetal development throughout the trimesters is presented.

◈ KEY POINTS

◆ Hyperemesis gravidarum occurs when the normal nausea and vomiting in pregnancy threatens the well-being of the woman and fetus because nutritional consumption and stores are diminished. It has negative implications for fluid and electrolyte imbalance when not diagnosed and treated early.

◆ Anemia in pregnancy, which causes lowered levels of iron and oxygen in the maternal circulation, affects the fetus in much the same way. Hemodilution of serum levels is ruled out and appropriate interventions are initiated, such as prescribing iron supplements, to stabilize these levels.

◆ Thromboembolic disease in pregnancy can be a life-threatening situation. It causes pain in the affected lower extremity and often greatly hinders the mobility of the woman. Bed rest and anticoagulation therapy are begun and continue until symptoms subside.

◆ Pregnancy-induced hypertension, formerly known as toxemia, is an elevation of the diastolic or systolic blood pressure. Preeclampsia may result when there is a sudden increase in edema, particularly of the hands and face, a significant increase in blood pressure, and proteinuria in the woman.

◆ A woman who is Rh– may build up antibodies after her first pregnancy that will attack and destroy the blood cells of subsequent fetuses that are Rh+. These women are given RhoGAM intramuscularly at 28 weeks gestation or within 72 hours postpartum.

◆ The cause of any bleeding in pregnancy must be diagnosed and treated as soon as possible to avert potentially serious threats to the woman and fetus. Abortion, ectopic pregnancies, placental anomalies, and hydatidiform mole are the most common factors associated with bleeding in pregnancy.

◆ A woman with no previous metabolic disturbance can develop impaired metabolism of carbohydrates in pregnancy. These women are classified as gestational diabetics. They are mostly controlled with diet but are closely monitored. There are associated risks even when close evaluation measures are taken, such as increased incidence of abortion and large-for-gestational-age (LGA) fetuses.

◆ A woman with heart disease is susceptible to fluid retention, hypertension, and infections. When this same woman becomes pregnant, the heart is more compromised. These women are assessed bimonthly in pregnancy and often referred to a cardiologist to ensure a safe pregnancy and positive outcome.

BIBLIOGRAPHY

Bansen, S. S., & Stevens, H. A. (1992). Women's experience if miscarriage in early pregnancy. *Journal of Nurse-Midwifery, 37*(2), 84–90.

Boyle, J. S., & Andrews, M. M. (1990). *Transcultural concepts in nursing care.* Philadelphia: J.B. Lippincott.

Carpenito, L. J. (1993). *Nursing diagnosis: Application to clinical practice* (5th ed.). Philadelphia: J.B. Lippincott.

Corinne, L., Bailey, V., Valentin, M., Morantus, E., & Shirley, L. (1992). The unheard voices of women: Spiritual interventions in maternal-child health care, *The American Journal of Maternal/Child Nursing, 17*(3), 141–145.

Cosico, J. N., & Rothlauf, E. B. (1992). Indications, management, and patient education: Anticoagulation therapy during pregnancy. *The American Journal of Maternal/Child Nursing, 17*(3), 130–135.

Crawford, N. G., & Pruss, A. M. (1993). Preventing neonatal hepatitis b infection during the perinatal period. *Journal of Obstetric, Gynecologic, and Neonatal Nursing, 22*(6), 480–482.

Day, S., Dancy, R., Kelly, K., & Wang, W. (1993). Iron overload? In sickle cell disease?. *The American Journal of Maternal/Child Nursing, 18*(6), 330–340.

Eisele, C. J. (1993). Rubella susceptibility in women of childbearing age. *Journal of Obstetric, Gynecologic, and Neonatal Nursing, 22*(3), 260–265.

Handler, A., & Rosenberg, D. (1992). Improving pregnancy outcomes: Public versus private care for urban, low-income women. *Birth, 19*(3), 123–130.

Hodnett, E. (1993). Social support during pregnancy: Does it help? *Birth, 20*(4), 218–219.

Karch, A. M. (1992). *Handbook of drugs and the nursing process* (2nd ed.). Philadelphia: J.B. Lippincott.

May, K. A., & Mahlmeister, L. R. (1994). *Maternal & neonatal nursing: Family-centered care* (3rd ed.). Philadelphia: J.B. Lippincott.

Mays, M. (1993). Tuberculosis: A comprehensive review for the certified nurse-midwife. *Journal of Nurse-Midwifery, 38*(3), 132–139.

Reeder, S. J., Martin, L. L., & Koniak, D. (1992). *Maternity nursing, family, newborn, and women's health care* (17th ed.). Philadelphia: J.B. Lippincott.

Scherer, J. C. (1992). *Introductory clinical pharmacology* (4th ed.). Philadelphia: J.B. Lippincott.

Surratt, N. (1993). Severe preeclampsia: Implications for critical-care obstetric nursing. *Journal of Obstetric, Gynecologic, and Neonatal Nursing, 22*(6), 500–509.

Tillman, J. (1992). Syphilis: An old disease, a contemporary perinatal problem. *Journal of Obstetric, Gynecologic, and Neonatal Nursing, 21*(3), 209–213.

CHAPTER 9

Normal Fetal Development

◈ OBJECTIVES

When the learning goals of this chapter are met, the reader will be able to:

◆ Describe the structure and function of chromosomes.
◆ Explain sex determination of male and female traits.
◆ Discuss the course of development of the ovum from fertilization through implantation.
◆ Explain embryonic cell differentiation including the three primary germ cell layers.
◆ List the primary functions of the amniotic fluid and the placenta.
◆ Summarize embryonic and fetal development.
◆ State the significance of a diagnosis of postmaturity during pregnancy.
◆ Explain the two basic types of twin pregnancies.
◆ Identify six risk factors that may interfere with normal fetal growth and development.
◆ Explore the implications for nursing care related to fetal growth and development.

TERMINOLOGY

Blastocyst	Gene
Chorion	Meiosis
Chromosome	Mitosis
Deoxyribonucleic acid	Morula
Ductus arteriosus	Soma cells
Ductus venosus	Teratogen
Embryo	Trophoblast
Foramen ovale	Zygote
Gamete	

Once fertilization of a mature ovum takes place, the unique genetic code of the fetus-to-be influences its own growth and development through sequential stages. This genetic code is programmed into the fetus's **deoxyribonucleic acid (DNA),** a spiral-shaped, double helix that is often referred to as the "thread of life." This chapter explores normal fetal development from fertilization to the birth of a healthy neonate.

The Genetic Code

What we inherit from our parents comes to us through the genetic code. This complex code is determined by the sequence of genes on each chromosome and translates into the individual characteristics that make each of us unique. Figure 9-1 takes a close look at the nucleus of a human cell, where the genetic codes are contained. Each division will be discussed in the following pages.

Chromosomes

Cells are the building blocks of all organ systems. There are two major types of cells: **soma cells,** which are found throughout the human body, and **gametes** (sex cells), which are found in the reproductive glands only. The ovum and the sperm are, respectively, the female and male gametes.

The nucleus of each soma cell contains 46 **chromosomes,** arranged in 23 pairs. One chromosome in every pair is donated by each parent. Each chromosome is composed of **genes,** which are defined as segments of DNA that control hereditary traits. Twenty-two of the 23 pairs of chromosomes are known as autosomes; the remaining pair determines an individual's sex.

There are two types of cell division involved in the creation of human life: mitosis and meiosis. **Mitosis** is the process by which somatic cells "give birth" to daughter cells. Each daughter cell contains the same number of chromosomes as the parent cell. It is the process by which the body grows and somatic cells are replaced.

Meiosis, however, is the process by which the sex cells undergo two sequential cellular divisions of the nucleus. It is in this way that the number of chromosomes of these sex cells is halved. Remember, each sex cell has only 23 chromosomes. The ovum undergoes meiosis just before ovulation, and the male germ cell divides in the seminiferous tubules of the testes. When the ovum and the spermatozoon unite, a **zygote** results.

This zygote has the full complement of 46 chromosomes, arranged in 23 pairs (Fig. 9-2).

Genes

The nucleotides that make up DNA are: adenine (A), cytosine (C), guanine (G), and thymine (T). These molecules are grouped in trios (eg, CAG) to form the genetic building blocks of life.

The long chainlike DNA molecules are contained in the genes. The coded information they carry results in individual variations in eye and hair color, facial features, and body details.

Some genes are dominant, and others are recessive. Dominant genes "overpower" recessive genes. That is to say, traits associated with dominant genes occur more frequently because only one dominant gene is needed for the expression of that trait. Conversely, each parent must contribute a recessive gene to express a recessive trait. For example, the gene for brown eyes (B) is dominant over the gene for blue eyes (b). An individual will have brown eyes under two circumstances: if both parents contribute one dominant gene each (BB) and if only one parent contributes a dominant gene (Bb). Blue eyes can occur only if both parents have recessive (b) genes to pass on to their offspring.

Sex Determination

Sex determination occurs at the time of fertilization. Because the spermatozoon can have either an X or a Y chromosome, it is the male that is responsible for fetal sex determination. The Y chromosome is smaller and contains mainly genes for maleness. The female ovum always contains an X chromosome, which carries several genes for other traits besides femaleness.

A female fetus (XX) will develop when the ovum unites with a spermatozoon with an X factor. Conversely, fertilization with a spermatozoon that contains a Y factor will produce a male fetus (XY). Research states that there is an approximately 50-50 chance of either occurrence (Fig. 9-3).

Many couples mistakenly believe that they can influence sex determination by using certain sexual positions, ingesting particular foods before intercourse, or timing sex to occur at specific times during the menstrual cycle. These beliefs are often rooted in folklore. Nurses need to express in a nonthreatening manner that cultural or family practices designed to control sex determination are not grounded in scientific principles.

Amniocentesis (the analysis of amniotic fluid) after 14 weeks' gestation is the only definitive means

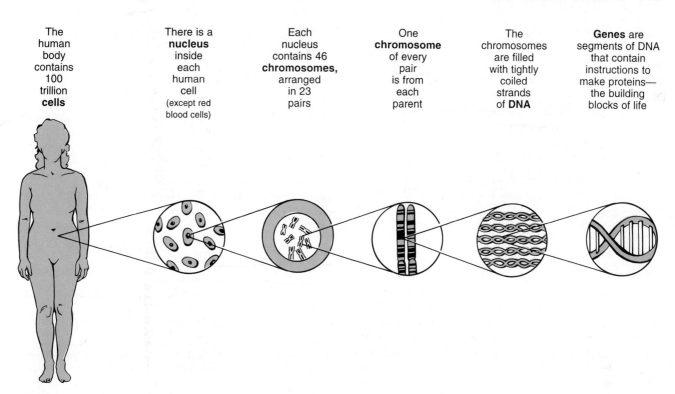

Figure 9-1. *Cellular components. (Adapted from* Time, *January 17, 1994 p. 50.)*

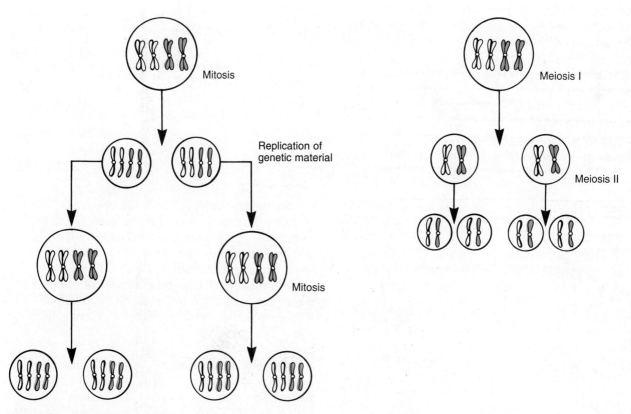

Figure 9-2. (**A**) *Mitosis of the soma cell.* (**B**) *Meiosis of the gamete.*

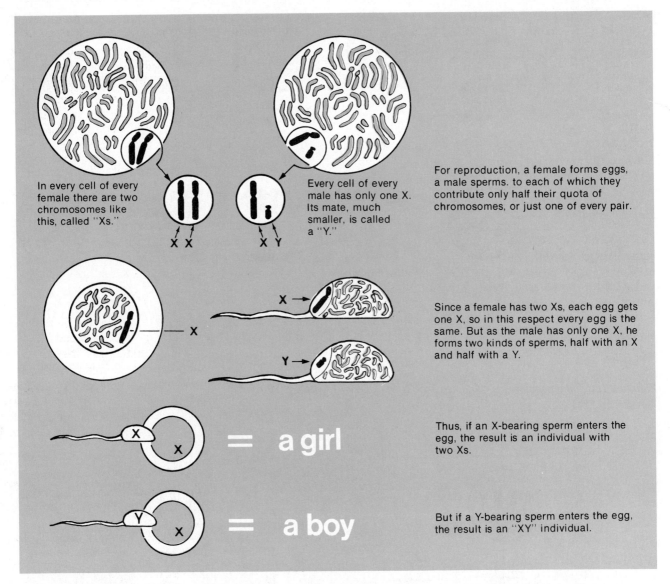

In every cell of every female there are two chromosomes like this, called "Xs."

X X

Every cell of every male has only one X. Its mate, much smaller, is called a "Y."

X Y

For reproduction, a female forms eggs, a male sperms. to each of which they contribute only half their quota of chromosomes, or just one of every pair.

X

X →

Y →

Since a female has two Xs, each egg gets one X, so in this respect every egg is the same. But as the male has only one X, he forms two kinds of sperms, half with an X and half with a Y.

X
X
= a girl

Thus, if an X-bearing sperm enters the egg, the result is an individual with two Xs.

Y
X
= a boy

But if a Y-bearing sperm enters the egg, the result is an "XY" individual.

Figure 9-3. The sex of the offspring is determined at the time of fertilization by the combination of the sex chromosomes of the spermatozoon (either X or Y) and the ovum (X).

of *diagnosing* the sex of the fetus before birth. Ultrasonography may strongly indicate the sex of the fetus, depending on fetal presentation and the examiner's ability to identify sex organs. Chapter 10 describes the procedures for ultrasonography and amniocentesis.

Fertilization

The ovum is receptive to fertilization for approximately 24 to 48 hours after release from the ovary. Fertilization normally takes place in the outermost half of the fallopian tube.

Sperm are viable for 24 to 72 hours after ejaculation into the female reproductive system. The high estrogen content of sperm enhances their motility and ability to penetrate the ovum. Prostaglandins in the semen increase smooth muscle contractions of the uterus, thus facilitating the transport of the sperm. It takes only one sperm to penetrate the ovum for fertilization to occur. Immediate cellular changes occur within the ovum, making it impossible for other sperm to enter.

After fertilization occurs, the zygote begins its rapid mitotic division in a process called cleavage. The zygote does not increase in size during cleavage because individual cells become smaller as they divide. Within 3 days, division results in a solid mass of 16 cells called a **morula.**

Peristalsis of the fallopian tubes and the wavelike motion of the cilia carry the morula toward the uterus.

Division of the morula continues until a blastocyst is formed. This **blastocyst** has several components: a fluid-filled cavity; the **trophoblast** (outer wall), which will later become the placenta; and an inner cell mass from which the **embryo** is formed. By 4½ days, the blastocyst has divided into more than 100 cells. Within approximately 6 days, the blastocyst reaches the endometrium of the uterus, where implantation normally occurs. Figure 9-4 highlights the process of fertilization.

Implantation

Sites vary, but most often the trophoblast implants itself in the upper segment of the uterus. This typically occurs within a week of fertilization. Some women may experience slight vaginal bleeding that coincides with implantation.

The trophoblast has enzyme properties that assist in implantation in three ways. First, the enzymes allow the trophoblast to embed in the uterine endometrium. Second, the trophoblast enzymes oxidize the endometrial vascular walls. Finally, the trophoblast provides the growing embryo with a link to the maternal circulatory system. (The products of conception are referred to as an embryo through the eighth week of gestation.) This link is used for the transportation of nutrients and oxygen.

The **chorion** is an extraembryonic membrane that is formed from the trophoblast. It forms the outer wall of the blastocyst. Rootlike projections called chorionic villi extend from the chorion into the endometrium. The chorionic villi are blood vessels that transport oxygen and essential nutrients from the woman's circulatory system to the developing fetus.

After the second week of pregnancy, the vascularized endometrium is called the decidua. The decidua encircles the entire interior wall of the uterus. The chorionic villi and decidua combine as pregnancy continues, eventually forming the placenta.

Embryonic Cell Differentiation

Approximately 16 days after fertilization, the blastocyst mass differentiates into three primary germ cell layers: the ectoderm, mesoderm, and endoderm. These three layers are the basis for all embryonic organ and tissue development. Each germ cell layer has specific characteristics, as shown in Table 9-1.

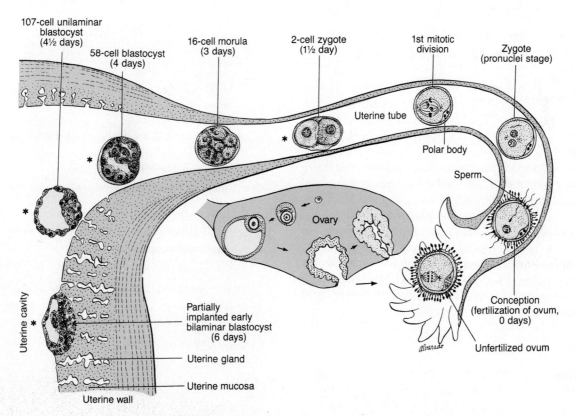

Figure 9-4. *Ovum transport and fertilization. From ovulation to fertilization to implantation, the ovum travels through the fallopian tube, experiencing a rapid miotic division. During this division the ovum evolves through several stages, including zygote, morula, and blastocyst.*

Table 9-1. *Body Structures Developing From the Primary Germ Cells*

Germ Layer	Structure Formation
Ectoderm	Skin
	Nervous system
	Nasal passages
	Crystalline lens of the eye
	Pharynx
	Mammary glands
	Salivary glands
Mesoderm	Muscles
	Circulatory system
	Bones
	Reproductive system
	Connective tissue
	Kidneys
	Ureters
Endoderm	Alimentary tract
	Respiratory tract
	Bladder
	Pancreas
	Liver

Development of the Embryo and Supportive Structures

During the first 8 weeks of pregnancy, embryonic tissues and the surrounding supportive structures are formed simultaneously. It is during this time that the embryo is at greatest risk for malformation. From the 8th week through the end of pregnancy, the embryo is known as the fetus.

The supportive structures that nourish and maintain the growing fetus are called the fetal membranes. These include the yolk sac, amnion, chorion, decidua, and the placenta. Of these, the **placenta** is singled out for its essential role in fetal nourishment and waste removal. The umbilical cord is equally important for its role in providing blood and oxygen to the fetus. Display 9-1 offers a checklist of the functions of the fetal membranes (with the placenta given special attention) and umbilical cord.

Fetal Membranes

The chorion and the amnion are formed shortly after implantation. The amnion grows and expands to accommodate the enlarging fetus. A cavity is formed, in which the fetus floats, suspended in amniotic fluid. By the end of the first trimester, the amnion (inner membrane) and chorion (outer membrane) fuse together to become the amniotic sac (Fig. 9-5).

Amniotic Fluid

Amniotic fluid is 98% water. The fluid also contains other substances, such as fetal waste products, epithelial cells, vernix, albumin, uric acid, creatinine, lecithin, sphingomyelin, and bilirubin. The fluid typically has a pH of 7.0 to 7.25 and is absorbed and replaced throughout pregnancy. The approximate volume of amniotic fluid in a full-term pregnancy is 1 liter. A volume of 2 or more liters is known as polyhydramnios, and a volume under 300 mL is termed oligohydramnios. Fetal abnormalities may be associated with oligohydramnios.

The primary function of the amniotic fluid is to protect the fetus from injury while maintaining it in a temperature-controlled environment. Its other specific functions are summarized in Display 9-2, "Functions of the Amniotic Fluid." Amniotic fluid can be analyzed in high-risk pregnancies (see Chapter 10).

Placenta

The placenta is formed from the chorionic villi and decidua. It is fully functional by the 12th week of preg-

---

DISPLAY 9-1
Key Functions of Supportive Structures

Fetal Membranes

- Contains amniotic fluid and prevents leakage
- Acts as a barrier in preventing the entrance of baceria, infection, and other substances that cause fetal harm
- Prevents prolapse of umbilical cord
- Inhibits fetal parts from adhering to uterine wall

Placenta

- Supplies oxygen and nourishment to the fetus
- Produces hormones for maintaining pregnancy
- Removes waste products from fetal circulation
- Protects fetus from harmful materials with placental barrier
- Provides passive immunity to fetus

Umbilical Cord

- Transports oxygen and nutrients to fetus
- Transports waste products away from fetus
- Anchors fetus to placenta
- Provides blood for fetal blood sampling

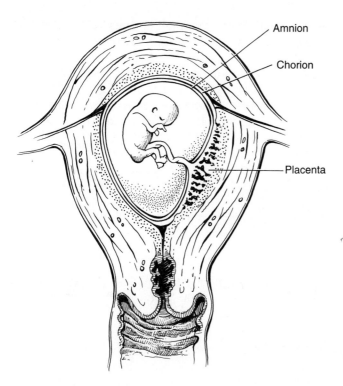

Amnion

Chorion

Placenta

Figure 9-5. *Membranes, with embryo lying within amniotic sac.*

nancy. Through the process of diffusion, the placenta transports oxygen and nourishment to the fetus. It also removes fetal waste products such as carbon dioxide.

The maternal and fetal circulatory systems are completely separate. Only an occasional break in one of the chorionic villi allows mixing of fetal and maternal blood products. Essential nutrients and oxygen in maternal circulation are collected in the chorionic villi. They are then transported to the fetus by villi capillaries. Fetal circulation accepts these nutrients and elimi-

nates waste through the placenta. Substances of high molecular weight or complex structures cannot cross the placental barrier.

Temporary immunity to a number of diseases (such as diphtheria, whooping cough [pertussis], German measles [rubella], and smallpox) may be passed from the woman to the fetus via the placenta. The placenta also produces hormones that help maintain pregnancy. These hormones include human chorionic gonadotropin (hCG), estrogen, human placental lactogen (hPL), and progesterone. For a detailed discussion of placental hormones, the reader is referred to Chapter 2.

Near the end of pregnancy, the placenta is normally 15 to 20 cm (6–8 inches) in diameter. The maternal side of the placenta is secured to the uterine wall. It has a rough and irregular texture. There are many subdivisions on this side of the placenta, called cotyledons. The fetal side of the placenta is smooth and covered with the amniotic membrane.

Umbilical Cord

The umbilical cord extends from the placenta to the umbilicus (navel) of the fetus. It forms between the fourth and eighth week of pregnancy as chorionic villi merge together. The cord normally contains two arteries and one vein. It is approximately 50 cm (20 inches) in length and is surrounded by a substance called Wharton's jelly. This gelatinous material helps protect the cord from injury.

Oxygenated blood that is rich in nutrients is transported from the placenta through the umbilical cord vein to the fetus. The enriched blood is exchanged for waste products that return to the placenta through the umbilical arteries. Arteries typically carry oxygen-rich blood to the tissues in the body. To accommodate the unique needs of the growing fetus, the two umbilical arteries and the vein function in reverse!

Harmful substances that pass the placental barrier are transported to the fetus by way of the umbilical vein. These substances may include street drugs such as crack cocaine and heroin, over-the-counter and prescription medications, nicotine, alcohol, and caffeine. Disease-producing microorganisms may also cross the placental barrier and jeopardize the fetus. The fetus is especially vulnerable to harmful substances throughout the first trimester of pregnancy.

Fetal Circulation

Fetal hemoglobin carries 20% to 30% more oxygen than adult hemoglobin. The fetus obtains this oxygen indirectly from the maternal circulatory system through the

DISPLAY 9-2
Functions of the Amniotic Fluid

· Equalizes pressure
· Prevents amnion from adhering to the fetus
· Permits floating movement of fetus
· Maintains a constant temperature surrounding the fetus
· Protects the fetus from external injury
· Provides fluid and nourishment for the fetus
· Aids in fetal lung development (surfactant)
· Prevents umbilical cord compression
· Helps mechanically dilate the cervix during early labor

umbilical vein that extends from the placenta. Oxygenated blood from chorionic villi in the placenta enters the umbilical vein. Carbon dioxide is removed by the umbilical arteries. The fetus relies on three shuntlike structures to supply oxygen and nutrients and exchange waste products. These structures are called the ductus venosus, foramen ovale, and ductus arteriosus.

The umbilical vein is joined by a vein called the ductus venosus. The **ductus venosus** transports the blood to the portal vein of the liver and the inferior vena cava. From the inferior vena cava, the oxygenated blood enters the right atrium of the heart. The blood is shunted through the **foramen ovale** to the left atrium heading toward the left ventricle and the aorta.

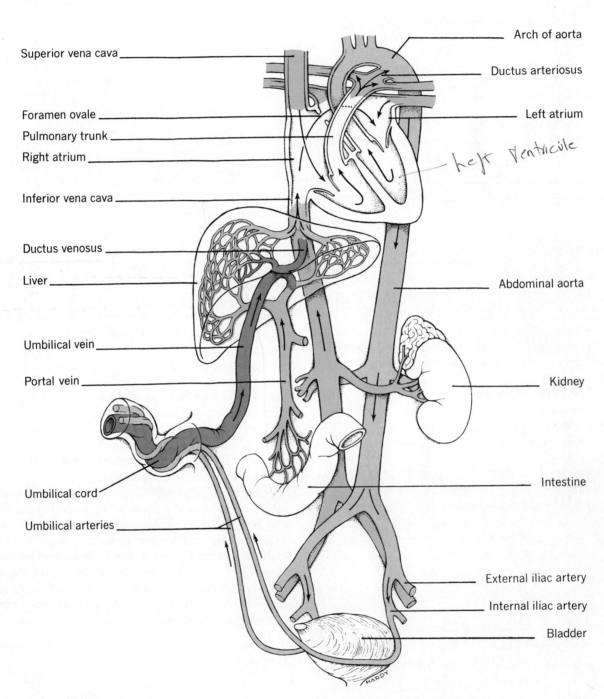

Figure 9-6. *Diagram of the fetal circulation shortly before birth. The course of blood is indicated by arrows. The umbilical vein carries oxygen-rich blood to the ductus venosus. From there it is carried to the liver and inferior vena cava to enter the right atrium of the heart. As blood shunts through the foramen ovale to the left atrium and ventricle, it enters the aorta to supply the body.*

The fetus relies on the aorta to supply oxygenated blood to the entire body. The right atrium supplies the right ventricle with oxygenated blood. Once fetal lung tissue is adequately oxygenated, the remainder of the oxygen-saturated blood exits the right ventricle through the pulmonary artery. The **ductus arteriosus** adds this blood to that in the aorta for distribution to the body tissues (Fig. 9-6).

Deoxygenated blood from the descending aorta is returned to the umbilical cord arteries. At the placental site, oxygen and nutrient exchange take place within the chorionic villi. Shortly after delivery, the circulatory system undergoes a number of dramatic changes as the neonate adjusts to extrauterine life.

The umbilical cord is clamped shortly after birth. The ductus venosus normally closes as soon as the cord is clamped. The first few respirations taken by the neonate expand lung tissue and successfully oxygenate the blood.

The foramen ovale closes soon after birth in response to increased pressure in the left side of the heart. Closure occurs when the lungs are fully oxygenated and pulmonary tension decreases. Delayed closure of the foramen ovale may result in benign heart murmurs in some neonates. The ductus arteriosus constricts as oxygen levels rise in the newborn and thereafter becomes known as the ligamentum arteriosus. Complete closure occurs approximately 3 months after birth.

Summary of Embryonic and Fetal Development

The fertilized ovum follows a fairly predictable course of growth and development on its way to becoming a viable fetus. Three periods are used to describe the developmental changes that it undergoes: the pre-embryonic, embryonic, and fetal periods. The following discussion summarizes embryonic and fetal development. Figure 9-7 depicts the development of the embryo and fetus at the end of each period.

Pre-embryonic Period: Weeks 1 to 3

The pre-embryonic period is a time of rapid development. The zygote, morula, blastocyst, and trophoblast are formed during this period. The beginnings of utero-placental circulation and chorionic villi formation also take place. Head and tail folds are visible on endoscopic examination.

The first 3 weeks of organ development are critical. During this time, the developing embryo is extremely susceptible to damage from drugs, radiation, viruses, and other factors that might disrupt the normal growth sequence. The woman, who often does not realize she is pregnant during this time, can place the embryo at increased risk by practicing unhealthy self-care behaviors.

Embryonic Period: Weeks 4 to 8

During the embryonic period, the embryo more than doubles in size, from 0.5 cm up to 3 cm (¼ to 1 in.) in length. The head enlarges, and brain development is rapid. The head encompasses 50% of the total size of the embryo. Fundamental organ development is evident. The beginnings of the circulatory system are present, and the heart is capable of pumping minute amounts of blood. There is early formation of the ears, eyes, and nose. The arms and legs are distinguishable. The umbilical cord, which contains one vein and two arteries, is fully functional. The embryonic period ends at the completion of the eighth week of gestation, marking the beginning of the fetal period.

Fetal Period: Weeks 9 to 40

The fetal period of development begins at week 9 and ends with birth. Keep in mind that normal fetal development may vary from one individual to another. However, several developmental events occur during the 9th through the 40th weeks of pregnancy.

Weeks 9 to 12

The fetus grows approximately 6 to 8 cm (2–3½ in.) in length and can weigh up to 30 g. Bone and tooth formation is evident, and fingers and toes are distinguishable. Male and female genitalia are apparent but not well defined. (It should be noted that the basic blueprint for the human creature is female. In other words, without the prompting of the Y chromosome, every fetus would develop internal and external female genitalia.)

The spleen is capable of producing red blood cells by the end of the 12th week. Small amounts of amniotic fluid swallowed by the fetus aid in fetal digestion, and the kidneys begin to produce scant amounts of urine from the amniotic fluid intake. The face has human characteristics, and the eyelids are fused together.

Weeks 13 to 16

Rapid fetal growth occurs during this time. The fetus reaches 10 to 16 cm (4–6 in.) in length and weighs approximately 120 g. Movement of fetal arms and legs may be detected by the woman. This "fluttering" sensation is called quickening. Genitourinary development at this

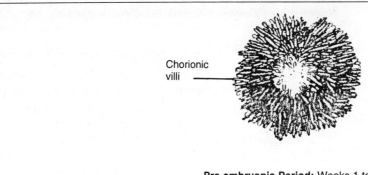

Chorionic
villi

Pre-embryonic Period: Weeks 1 to 3

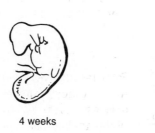

4 weeks   8 weeks

Embryonic Period: Weeks 4 to 8

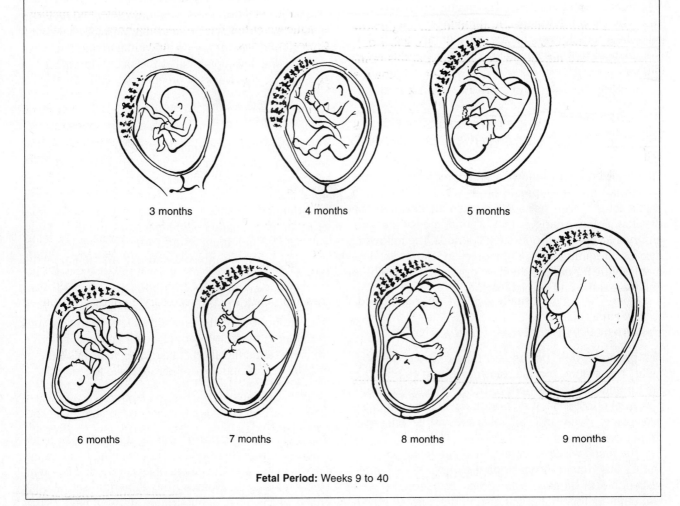

3 months   4 months   5 months

6 months   7 months   8 months   9 months

Fetal Period: Weeks 9 to 40

Figure 9-7. Embryonic and fetal development.

stage allows for the secretion of increased amounts of urine into the amniotic fluid. Black, tarry stools known as meconium form in the bowels. The fetal gastrointestinal system is sterile and will remain so until food is ingested. Sucking and swallowing reflexes function but are immature at this time.

The circulatory system develops very early during pregnancy. It is fully functional by the 20th week, although fetal heart tones can be heard for the first time at around 14 to 16 weeks' gestation. Heart tones may also be heard as early as 11 weeks.

Weeks 17 to 23

Fetal length increases dramatically to between 25 and 35 cm (10–12 in.), and fetal weight increases to between 200 and 700 g (7 oz to 1 lb 8 oz). Fine, downy hair, called lanugo covers the fetal body. Vernix, a cheeselike substance, encases and protects the delicate, wrinkled skin of the fetus. Fetal movement is more perceptible, and the heartbeat is heard on auscultation.

Weeks 24 to 27

The fetus is approximately 40 cm (16 in.) in length now and weighs from 1000 to 1200 g (2 lb 3 oz to 2 lb 7 oz). Major organs are functional. A fetus born at this point will be premature. It will, however, have a fair chance of surviving, provided there are no surfactant abnormalities. Surfactant is a phospholipid that serves two important functions: it prevents lung collapse during exhalation and reduces lung surface tension, which makes breathing easier. Production of surfactant and the development of pulmonary alveoli are both evidence of fetal respiratory maturity. The premature neonate is discussed in Chapter 19.

Weeks 28 to 31

Fetal length can increase up to 43 cm (17 in.), and weight is typically between 2.0 and 3.0 kg (4 lb 6 oz and 5 lb 7 oz). The fetus is usually viable if labor and childbirth occur at this time. Lung maturity is typically sufficient to sustain life by 28 weeks' gestation. The closer the lecithin sphingomyelin ratio (L/S ratio) is to 2:1, the greater the lung development (see Chapter 19). Strong fetal movements are felt by the woman. At this stage, the fetus can respond to external noises by moving. Scalp hair is present as lanugo diminishes, and the fetus's eyes have opened. Subcutaneous fat begins to appear as the size of the fetus increases. The testes descend into the inguinal canal in the male fetus. Fingernails cover the entire nail bed, and there is a heavy vernix coating.

Weeks 32 to 36

Fetal length approaches 46 cm (18 in.), and weight reaches 2000 to 2700 g (4 lbs 6 oz to 6 lbs). Extrauterine survival rates increase dramatically at this point. The lungs have reached maturity, and neonatal survival is likely with minimal respiratory difficulty. Surfactant levels, which are detectable in the amniotic fluid, are increasing. The fetus has more subcutaneous fat, and wrinkling of its skin diminishes. There are decreases in lanugo, vernix, and amniotic fluid. The fetus takes on more "babylike" characteristics during the eighth month of pregnancy.

Weeks 37 to 40

Fetal length averages 48 to 50 cm (20 in.), and fetal weight is approximately 3000 to 3500 g (6 lbs 8 oz to 7 lbs 8 oz). As the placenta begins to age toward the end of pregnancy, its functioning naturally decreases in preparation for childbirth. All organs and body systems are mature at this time. The eyes and limbs are fully functional, and the fetus's skin is smooth and supple. The testes normally fully descend into the scrotum before birth. Fetal development is complete, and maturity is achieved at this time. A neonate born any time after 42 weeks is considered postmature.

Postmaturity

Postmaturity refers to gestation that lasts beyond 42 weeks. Confusion about the woman's last menstrual period (LMP) or incorrect estimation of the expected date of delivery (EDD) may make it difficult to accurately predict the number of weeks of gestation. Therefore, it is important to note that not every fetus so labeled is actually postmature.

The risk of dystocia (difficult labor) increases when the postmature fetus continues to gain weight. The large size of the fetus's presenting part may make it impossible for the pelvis to accommodate vaginal childbirth. The likelihood that labor will have to be induced or a caesarean birth will be necessary increases the longer the pregnancy lasts.

A major concern in postmaturity is the decreasing efficiency of the aging placenta. As the placenta ages, the fetus may be deprived of essential nutrients, including adequate oxygenation. Fetal weight loss may result. Amniotic fluid amounts decrease (oligohydramnios) and may be meconium stained, indicating fetal distress. The fetus may aspirate meconium *in utero* and have difficulty ventilating adequately at birth. Neonates born after 42 weeks' gestation have excessive growth of fingernails and toenails. Their skin is wrinkled as the result of diminished vernix, and lanugo is not typically evident. There is also an increased risk of umbilical cord compression. Cesarean birth may have to be done if placental insufficiency is suggested or confirmed by nonstress test.

Multifetal Pregnancy

When a woman presents with an unusually high fundal height measurement, a multifetal pregnancy is suspected. Diagnosis of a multifetal pregnancy is confirmed when more than one fetal heart tone is heard on auscultation and the fetuses or amniotic sacs are visualized with ultrasonography. These pregnancies are often associated with the use of fertility treatments. Twins, which account for 1% of all births in the United States, are the most commonly occurring multifetal pregnancy (Fig. 9-8). The rate of all other multifetal pregnancies is less than 1%.

A variety of potential complications and additional risks accompany multifetal pregnancies. These include maternal hypertension, anemia, abruptio placentae, dystocia, preterm labor, prolapsed cord, postpartum hemorrhage and abnormal fetal presentations (eg, breech birth).

Twin Pregnancy

Twins can be classified as monozygotic (identical twins) or dizygotic (fraternal twins) (Fig 9-9).

Monozygotic twins are produced from fertilization of a single ovum by one sperm. The ovum splits into two identical monozygotes sometime before the 15th day of

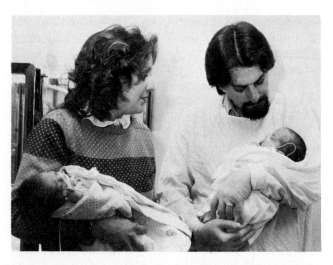

Figure 9-8. *Parents of twins need support from the nursing staff, even when twins were expected. (Courtesy of The Children's Hospital of Philadelphia)*

gestation. (When this division is incomplete, Siamese [conjoined] twins result.) The amniotic sacs and placentas may be either shared or separate. Monozygotic twins are always of the same sex. They are exact mirror-images of one another, hence the name, identical twins. Monozygotic twins tend to weigh less at birth than do dizygotic twins. They also have a higher incidence of congenital malformations and greater neonatal mortality rates.

Dizygotic twins result from fertilization of two ova by two different sperm. Each fetus has its own amniotic

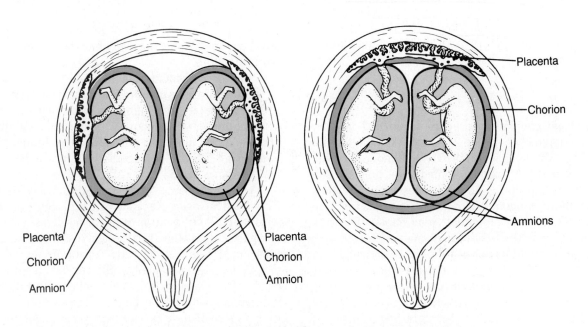

Figure 9-9. *Twin pregnancy. (A) Fraternal twins with two placentas, two amnions, and two chorions. (B) Identical twins with one placenta, one chorion, and two amnions.*

sac and placenta. Dizygotic twins can be of either the same sex or opposite sexes, and they share no more resemblance to each other than do normal siblings. Dizygotic twins are more common than monozygotic twins. They are born more frequently to women who are older, have a higher parity, or to those who take fertility drugs.

Risk Factors in Fetal Development

During the first trimester, the fetus is especially vulnerable because development of the body systems is accelerated. Many factors place the developing fetus at risk for delayed or abnormal growth. Examples include poor maternal nutrition, substance use and abuse, ingestion of harmful agents that cross the placental barrier, and inadequate prenatal care. See the Family Teaching Checklist for information regarding avoidable risk factors during pregnancy.

Chromosomal alterations and teratogens disrupt normal intrauterine fetal development. A **teratogen** is any substance or condition that causes abnormal development of the fetus. The childbearing family is able to control some of the harmful factors that may interfere with normal fetal growth and development. Understanding the damaging effects of teratogenic agents assists nurses in counseling families about known risk factors during pregnancy.

Teratogenic Factors

Teratogens range from childhood infections, such as German measles (rubella), to poisonous substances. Obvious examples of teratogens include alcohol, cocaine (including crack), heroin, nicotine, and caffeine. Maternal conditions can also threaten fetal development. Examples of maternal conditions include diabetes, heart disease, pregnancy-induced hypertension, malnutrition, and exposure to sexually transmitted infections.

Teratogenic factors can have disastrous results for the fetus. Preterm birth, mental retardation, intrauterine growth retardation, and low birth weight are just some of the risks faced by the fetus exposed to teratogens. Multiple neurologic deficits, cardiac abnormalities, and renal complications are some of the more serious results of exposure to teratogens. Table 9-2 provides information about leading teratogenic factors and their potential harmful effects to the growing fetus.

FAMILY TEACHING CHECKLIST

Healthy Prenatal Self-Care Behaviors That Promote Normal Fetal Development

The nurse includes the following information in family teaching to promote health and well-being:

- Abstain from illegal drug and substance use
- Avoid alcohol consumption
- Eliminate smoking and avoid secondhand smoke
- Check with health care provider before taking any over-the-counter or prescription medications
- Identify occupational hazards that may make the workplace unsafe
- Consult family members for any known history of genetic disorders or familial diseases
- Maintain daily healthy dietary intake
- Avoid exposure to hazardous chemicals and household cleaning agents such as ammonia and lye
- Follow instructions for daily vitamin and mineral supplementation
- Maintain a daily exercise program such as walking and spending time in the fresh air
- Avoid unnecessary activities that cause back strain, falls, and other injuries
- Seek health care immediately if a danger sign occurs
- Keep all prenatal health care appointments

Table 9-2. *Known and Potential Teratogens*

Known Teratogenic Chemicals		Potential Teratogenic Maternal Conditions and Infectious Agents	
Agent	*Related Effects*	*Agent*	*Related Effects*
Alcohol	Intrauterine growth retardation; mental retardation; maxillary hypoplasia; reduction in width of palpebral fissures; microcephaly	Cytomegalovirus	Central nervous system damage; intrauterine growth retardation
Anticancer drugs	Drug-specific effects, with wide variation from drug to drug	Diabetes mellitus	Affects various systems; caudal dysplasia or caudal regression syndrome; insulin therapy protects fetus
Anticonvulsants, hydantoins, diones	Orofacial clefts; cardiac and skeletal defects; hydantoin syndrome; trimethadione syndrome; central nervous system anomalies; developmental delay	Herpes simpex	Central nervous system anomalies; microcephaly; intracranial calcification; eye defects
Androgenic hormones, progestogenic hormones	Genital malformations, masculinization of female fetus with high doses	Phenylketonuria	Fetal death; mental retardation; microcephaly; intrauterine growth retardation
Aspirin	Heavy use related to low birth weight and bleeding after birth	Rubella virus	Cardiovascular malformations; deafness; mental retardation; cataracts; glaucoma; microphthalmia
Radiation	Microcephaly; mental retardation; intrauterine growth retardation	Syphilis	Maculopapular rash; hepatosplenomegaly; deformed nails; osteochondritis at joints of extremities; congenital neurosyphilis; abnormal epiphyses; chorioretinitis
Thyroid and antithyroid drugs	Hypothyroidism or goiter	Toxoplasmois	Hydrocephaly; microphthalmia; chorioretinitis
Smoking/nicotine	Intrauterine growth retardation; placental lesions	Varicella-zoster (chickenpox)	Skin and muscle defects; intrauterine growth retardation; limb and eye defects
Tetracycline	Hypoplastic tooth enamel; bone and tooth anomalies	Venezuelan equine encephalitis	Hydroanencephaly; microphthalmia; luxation of hip

Adapted from Beckman, & Brent. (1986). Mechanism of known environmental teratogens: Drugs and chemicals. Clin Perinatol, 13(3):649–687. Used with permission.

Chromosomal Abnormalities

Chromosomal abnormalities can cause a wide range of diseases and conditions in the fetus and the growing child. At times, the genetic alterations result in such serious congenital abnormalities that spontaneous abortion is inevitable. Abnormalities in the essential number of chromosomes or in the genetic structure of chromosomes can result in fetal death or retardation. Sex chromosome abnormalities occur infrequently. In this case, there is an extra X or Y chromosome, or an absent sex chromosome. Genetic counseling and family education regarding specific risk factors are essential. Early testing and detailed genetic histories help identify families at risk. Table 9-3 provides a sampling of some of the more common chromosomal abnormalities, the disease or condition they cause, and fetal and neonatal outcomes.

Trisomy 21: Down Syndrome

One of the most commonly known chromosomal abnormalities is trisomy 21, commonly referred to as Down syndrome. It occurs in 1 of every 800 births. The fetus with trisomy 21 has an extra chromosome on the 21st that is structurally correct. In other words, there are three copies of chromosome number 21 instead of two. The newborn characteristically has a broad flat nose, protruding tongue, and a single transverse palm crease. The mental retardation associated with Down syn-

Table 9-3. *Summary of Numeric Chromosomal Abnormalities*

Type	Synonym	Incidence	Diagnostic Features at Birth	Prognosis	Detection
Sex Chromosome Monosomy					
XO	Turner syndrome*	1/10,000 live female births Most common chromosomal abnormality in spontaneous abortions (18%)	Edema of hands and feet Increased incidence of coarctation of the aorta Somatic abnormalities may be few, and condition often is not recognized at birth	Normal intelligence Sterile	Buccal smear for X chromatin bodies may be negative. Endocrine levels are abnormal. Abnormality usually revealed in adolescence by presence of short stature, ovarian streaks, and amenorrhea. Estrogen at puberty may aid development of secondary sex characteristics.
Autosomal Trisomy					
Trisomy 21	Down syndrome	1/800 live births Most common chromosome disorder	Typical round face with flat profile Protruding tongue Epicanthal folds Brushfields' spots (speckling of irises) Simian palm creases	Mild to severe retardation Increased incidence of leukemia Congenital heart defects (40% to 60% of cases) may require surgical correction	Karyotype analysis confirms diagnosis; "older" mother is at higher risk for offspring with this syndrome.
Sex Chromosome Trisomy					
XXX	Triple X syndrome	1/1,000 female births	None	Usually normal intelligence, but slightly increased incidence of mental retardation Fertile, with normal offspring	"Older" mother is at higher risk for offspring with this syndrome. Buccal smears may reveal triple-X karyotype.
XXY	Klinefelter syndrome	1/1,000 live male births	None—signs usually appear after adolescence	Usually normal intelligence Mild mental retardation does occur Sterile	Feminine characteristics appear in puberty, including gynecomastia. Typically, sufferer is tall and gangly with small testes and underdeveloped facial and body hair. Breast reduction may be advised for psychological and cosmetic reasons.
XYY		1/1,000 live births	None	Rarely, may be associated with some intellectual impairment Fertile	Abnormality may remain undetected until revealed on karyotyping. In persons with XYY syndrome, sperm count may be reduced, and plasma testosterone levels may be high.

*Turner syndrome also can be the result of other chromosomal abnormalities, but these are extremely rare.

drome ranges from mild to severe. Amniotic fluid testing is routinely used to rule out Down syndrome in the fetuses of women older than 35. See Chapter 10 for a description of amniocentesis.

Adolescent Considerations

Fetal abnormalities are seen more often in woman younger than 21, placing the adolescent's offspring at greater risk. Nurses need to educate the adolescent about the importance of positive self-care behaviors during pregnancy. It is particularly important that the pregnant adolescent be counseled to avoid teratogens, which can lead to preventable complications. Because substance abuse during pregnancy is a significant problem among adolescents, nurses are advised to pay attention to this issue.

Cultural Considerations

There are documented genetic traits that are seen more often in specific cultures and regions. Some examples include cleft lip and palate among the Japanese, ear anomalies for Navajo Indians, phenylketonuria among the Irish, and malignant osteoporosis in Costa Ricans. Nurses need to familiarize themselves with predispositions for genetic abnormalities among various racial and ethnic groups. Encouraging families to seek prenatal counseling and genetic testing may help reduce fetal risks, allay family concerns, and ensure normal fetal development.

The Role of the Nurse

Nurses are responsible for providing supportive prenatal care, adequate prenatal screening, and assisting with data collection to obtain a thorough health history. Their work is necessary for the early identification of risk factors that could interfere with normal fetal devel-

✓ NURSING DIAGNOSES CHECKLIST

Nursing Diagnoses Related to Fetal Development

- Altered Family Processes, related to multifetal pregnancy
- Knowledge Deficit, related to normal fetal development
- Fear, related to outcome of fetal development
- Anxiety, related to postmaturity of pregnancy
- Altered Tissue Perfusion, (placenta), related to postmature neonate
- Risk for Altered Parenting, related to chromosomal abnormalities of developing fetus
- Altered Health Maintenance, related to exposure to teratogenic factors
- Risk for, Injury, related to exposure to known teratogens
- Altered Growth and Development (intrauterine), related to multifetal pregnancy
- Anticipatory Grieving, related to possible chromosomal abnormality of fetus

opment. Nurses may be involved in genetic counseling and family teaching regarding hereditary predisposition for various diseases.

Nursing care follows the organization of the nursing process during the antepartum period. Once assessment is completed, data is analyzed for the formulation of nursing diagnoses. Examples of nursing diagnoses related to fetal development are found in the Nursing Diagnoses Checklist. Keep in mind, each family and woman will have unique needs. These sample nursing diagnoses serve as examples for developing individualized nursing care plans.

REVIEW AND PREVIEW

The mechanisms of fertilization, implantation, and embryonic cell differentiation were presented. The supportive role of the fetal membranes and the umbilical cord was also discussed. Fetal circulation was described to point out how quickly the neonate adapts to extrauterine life with minimal effort.

Postmaturity beyond 42 weeks can create serious problems for the woman and the fetus. These complications were presented. The discussion of multifetal pregnancies focused on twin gestations. The discussion of teratogens was designed to increase nurses' awareness of the wide range of substances that can negatively affect fetal

outcomes. Knowledge about harmful practices enables nurses to teach childbearing families appropriate self-care behaviors.

In the following chapter, fetal assessment during the antepartum period will be presented. Diagnostic tests such as ultrasonography, amniocentesis, chorionic villus sampling, and electronic fetal monitoring will be discussed.

◈ KEY POINTS

◆ Chromosomes are cellular structures that contain segments of deoxyribonucleic acid (DNA) called genes. Each gene is

1. Which term describes the products of conception during the first eight weeks of gestation?

⊙ **A.** Zygote
○ **B.** Morula
⊘ **C.** Embryo
○ **D.** Blastocyst

2. The placenta is able to sustain a pregnancy by ___ weeks' gestation.

○ **A.** 4
○ **B.** 6
○ **C.** 8
⊗ **D.** 12

3. Which statement best describes an infant born at 28 weeks' gestation?

○ **A.** 2000 grams; fused eyelids
○ **B.** Minimal lanugo and vernix
⊘ **C.** Testes in the inguinal canal; abundant vernix
○ **D.** Dry, cracked skin; abundant subcutaneous fat

4. Monozygotic twins occur when:

○ **A.** One ovum is fertilized by two sperms
○ **B.** Two ova are fertilized by one sperm
⊗ **C.** One ovum is fertilized by one sperm
○ **D.** Two ova are fertilized by two sperms

5. Where does fertilization most frequently occur?

⊗ **A.** Fallopian tube
○ **B.** Uterus
○ **C.** Vagina
○ **D.** Endometrium

composed of nucleotides including adenine (A), cytosine (C), guanine (G), and thymine (T). Genes are responsible for determining our inherited traits. Every soma cell in the body has 46 chromosomes arranged in 23 pairs within the nucleus. Each parent contributes one gamete (sex cell) with 23 chromosomes.

◆ The determination of fetal sex occurs when the gametes from both parents unite. At that point, the female X chromosome will pair off with either an X or Y chromosome from the male. An XX match will produce a female, and an XY pairing will result in a male.

◆ Fertilization of the ovum by a spermatozoon usually takes place in the fallopian tube. As the resulting zygote travels through the fallopian tube, it begins a series of cellular divisions known as mitosis. The morula evolves and further divides to become the blastocyst upon descent into the uterine cavity. The blastocyst implants in the rich, highly vascular endometrial lining of the uterus.

◆ Approximately 2 weeks after fertilization, embryonic cell differentiation takes place when blastocyst cells develop into three primary germ layers: the ectoderm, mesoderm, and endoderm.

◆ Pre-embryonic development begins at conception and ends at 3 weeks' gestation. Embryonic development lasts through the eighth week, until the fetal period begins. The fetal period lasts until the 40th week of pregnancy. During the pre-embryonic period, early organ development and rudimentary uteroplacental circulation are established. The embryonic period is marked by continued development of organs and structures with minimal body system function. Throughout the fetal period, advanced growth and maturation occurs in preparation for extrauterine life.

◆ Any pregnancy that lasts 42 weeks or longer is known as postmature. Some pregnancies, especially in primiparas, extend beyond the EDD for unknown reasons. Postmature gestation results in the potential for decreased placental perfusion, which places the fetus at risk.

◆ The two most common twin pregnancies are monozygotic and dizygotic. Monozygotic twins result from a single fertilized ovum. These twins are of the same sex and are described as mirror images of each other. Dizygotic twins occur when two ova are fertilized by two separate sperm.

BIBLIOGRAPHY

Boyle, S. J., & Andrews, M. M. (1990). *Transcultural concepts in nursing care* (1st ed.). Philadelphia: J. B. Lippincott.

Campinba-Bacote, J., & Bragg, E. J. (1993). Chemical assessment in maternity care. *The American Journal of Maternal-Child Nursing, 18*(1), 24–28.

Carpenito, L. J. (1993). *Nursing diagnosis: Application to clinical practice* (5th ed.). Philadelphia: J. B. Lippincott.

Eganhouse, D. J. (1992). Fetal monitoring of twins. *Journal of Obstetric, Gynecologic, and Neonatal Nursing, 21*(1), 17–27.

Elmer-Dewitt, P. (1994) The genetic revolution: New technology enables us to improve on nature. How far should we go? *Time, 143*(3), 46–53.

Hite C., & Shannon, M. (1992). Clinical profile of apparently healthy neonates with in utero drug exposure. *Journal of Obstetric, Gynecologic, and Neonatal Nursing, 21*(4), 305–309.

Janke, J. (1990). Prenatal cocaine use: Effects on perinatal outcome. *Journal of Nurse Midwifery, 35*(2), 74–77.

Jones, S., & Headrick, E. (1992). Integration of clinical genetics into assisted reproductive technologies: Implications for nursing practice. *NAACOG Clinical Issues in Perinatal and Woman's Health Nursing, 3*(2), 301–312.

Martin, L. L., & Reeder, S. J. (1990). *Essentials of maternity nursing: Family centered care* (1st ed.). Philadelphia: J. B. Lippincott.

May, K. A., & Mahlmeister, L. R. (1994). *Maternal and neonatal nursing: Family-centered care* (3rd ed.). Philadelphia: J. B. Lippincott.

Moore, K. (1993). *The developing human* (3rd ed.). Philadelphia: W.B. Saunders.

Pillitteri, A. (1992). *Maternal and child health nursing* (1st ed.). Philadelphia: J. B. Lippincott.

Pletsch, P. (1990). Birth defect prevention: Nursing interventions. *Journal of Obstetric, Gynecologic, and Neonatal Nursing, 19*(6), 482–488.

Reeder, S. J., Martin, L. L., & Koniak, D. (1992). *Maternity nursing: Family, newborn, and women's health care* (17th ed.). Philadelphia: J. B. Lippincott.

Scherer, J. C. (1991). *Introductory medical-surgical nursing* (5th ed.). Philadelphia: J. B. Lippincott.

Summers, L., & Price, R. A. (1993). Preconception care: An opportunity to maximize health in pregnancy. *Journal of Nurse-Midwifery, 38*(4), 188–198.

Tabers cyclopedic medical dictionary. (1993). (17th ed.). Philadelphia: F. A. Davis.

Williams, J. K. (1993). New genetic discoveries increase counseling opportunities. *The American Journal of Maternal-Child Nursing, 18*(4), 218–240.

Zacharias, J. (1990). The new genetics. *Journal of Obstetric, Gynecologic, and Neonatal Nursing, 19*(2), 122–133.

CHAPTER 10

Assessment of Fetal Health

◈ OBJECTIVES

When the learning goals of this chapter are met, the reader will be able to :

- ◆ Describe the significance of fundal height measurement.
- ◆ Describe the use of ultrasonography in pregnancy.
- ◆ List the significant results obtained by amniocentesis.
- ◆ Explain the purpose of measuring maternal urine and serum assays.
- ◆ Describe how auscultation of fetal heart tones is accomplished.
- ◆ Describe electronic fetal monitoring.
- ◆ Explain the tests performed in evaluating the fetal heart rate.
- ◆ Discuss the advantages of continuous electronic fetal monitoring during labor.
- ◆ Define fetal blood sampling.
- ◆ State the normal range for fetal blood pH.

TERMINOLOGY

Acceleration

Alpha-fetoprotein

Amniocentesis

Contraction stress test/oxytocin challenge test

Decelerations

Down syndrome

Fetal blood sampling

Fundal height

Funic souffle

Intrauterine growth retardation

Indirect Coombs' test

Lecithin/sphingomyelin ratio

Nonstress test

Uterine souffle

Variability

Vibroacoustic stimulation

At each prenatal visit, the woman's health is monitored and an assessment of fetal well-being is completed. A typical prenatal visit includes a measurement of maternal weight and uterine growth. Fetal activity and fetal heart rate (FHR) are evaluated. Assessments made during prenatal visits are determined by the trimester of pregnancy (see the Assessment Checklist).

During the first trimester, ultrasonography is used to confirm the pregnancy as early as the fourth week. Auscultation of the fetal heart rate is accomplished between the 11th and 12th weeks of gestation. During the second trimester, fundal height is measured to determine fetal growth, and FHR and fetal movement are assessed. Ultrasonography may be ordered to determine the size of the fetus and the placement of the placenta. Blood samples are also drawn from the woman for the analysis of a variety of serum levels. In the third trimester, uterine growth, FHR and fetal movement continue to be evaluated. Ultrasonography may be repeated if there is a question of fetal size or location of the placenta, and an amniotic fluid index may be obtained to determine fetal health.

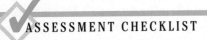

ASSESSMENT CHECKLIST

The Three Trimesters

First Trimester

· Auscultation of fetal heart tones

· Ultrasonography

· Chorionic villus sampling

· Maternal blood samples

Second Trimester

· Fundal height measurement

· Fetal heart tones

· Fetal movement

· Maternal alpha-fetoprotein

· Amniocentesis

Third Trimester

· Fetal heart tones

· Ultrasonography

· Fetal movement

· Amniotic fluid index

· Amniocentesis

Measurement of Fundal Height

Fundal height, as discussed in Chapter 6, is measured to aid in determining gestational age. Fundal height measurements are most accurate between 20 and 31 weeks' gestation. During this time, the height of the fundus measured in centimeters should be the same as the gestational age in weeks. For example, at 22 weeks' gestation, the height of the fundus is 22 cm. If there is less than 2 cm or greater than 6 cm growth in a 4-week period, further assessment is done to determine if there are any underlying problems. Assessment may include ultrasonography, abdominal palpation, or blood work.

Ultrasonography

Ultrasonography uses high-frequency sound waves to produce an image of internal organs or tissues. These ultrasound waves are introduced by a transducer that is passed over the skin. They then pass through soft tissue until they hit tissue of higher density. At this point, the waves are reflected back to the transducer (Fig. 10-1). Using this technique, fetal cardiac activity can be detected as early as 7 weeks' gestation.

It is beneficial for the woman to have a full bladder before beginning ultrasonography studies. The bladder is used as an anatomic landmark and also pushes the uterus out of the pelvic cavity for easier viewing by scanning. The woman is instructed to lie in a supine

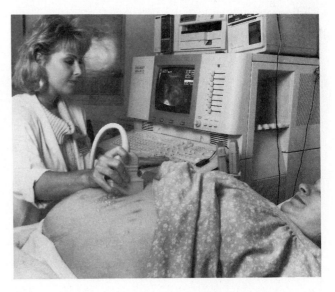

Figure 10-1. *Ultrasound is used in prenatal care.*

position, with the abdomen exposed. A thin layer of conducting gel is applied to the abdomen to reduce friction and increase conductivity before the transducer is slowly passed over the skin. During the last few years, use of the vaginal probe with ultrasound has increased. When it is used, a condom is placed over the probe before it is inserted in the vagina and brought close to the uterus.

Ultrasonography is an objective means of assessing fetal well-being and is performed for a variety of reasons. In the first trimester, it is done to confirm pregnancy, estimate gestational age, evaluate vaginal bleeding, and rule out pelvic abnormalities. In the second trimester, the health care provider can confirm gestational age, determine fetal and placental growth and position, diagnose a multifetal pregnancy, and rule out fetal abnormalities such as hydrocephalus, anencephalus, and hydatidiform mole. In the third trimester, ultrasound can assess fetal position and size, locate the placental implantation site, and rule out cephalopelvic disproportion (see Chapter 13). Ultrasound is used in conjunction with chorionic villus sampling and amniocentesis (discussed in a later section) to ensure safe insertion of a catheter or needle for the withdrawal of tissue or fluid.

There are no known harmful effects resulting from ultrasound scanning, so it is used more readily than other, more invasive procedures to assess fetal status. The earlier in pregnancy that ultrasonography is used, the more accurate the assessment. Ultrasound accuracy in determining pregnancy length in the first trimester is plus or minus 4 days; second trimester, plus or minus 10 days; and third trimester, plus or minus 2 weeks (Fig. 10-2).

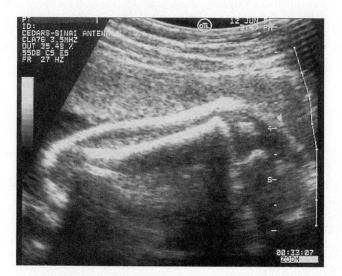

Figure 10-2. *Ultrasound showing normal fetal femur.*

Amniocentesis

Amniocentesis involves the withdrawal of a sample of amniotic fluid surrounding the fetus for analysis. This procedure is typically performed after the 14th week of gestation, when there is sufficient fluid for sampling.

Indications

Generally, an amniocentesis is done to rule out a congenital abnormality called **Down syndrome,** or trisomy 21. It is seen frequently in women older than 40 and in those who already have a child with Down syndrome. Amniocentesis is also indicated when a member of the family has any other genetic defect.

Studies of fetal cells found in amniotic fluid can indicate the sex of the fetus. An open spinal cord defect, such as anencephaly or meningomyelocele, is discovered by assay of the amniotic fluid for **alpha-fetoprotein (AFP).** Alpha-fetoprotein is an antigen carried by the fetus. Elevated levels indicate neural tube defects and low levels may be used to diagnose Down syndrome. All AFP abnormalities are subject to further investigation.

Other indications for amniocentesis include suspicion of **intrauterine growth retardation** (IUGR), which results in fetuses who are small for gestational age (SGA); postmaturity; determination of fetal lung maturity or fetal death; detection of hydramnios; and Rh sensitization.

Abdominal palpation and ultrasonography are used to determine the position of the fetus in preparation for performing an amniocentesis. A sterile needle is inserted through the abdominal and uterine walls into the amniotic fluid (Fig. 10-3). Between 20 and 25 mL fluid are removed and placed in sterile containers for laboratory examination. Use of a local anesthetic before inserting the needle is optional. Possible risks associated with amniocentesis include needle puncture of the fetus, bleeding caused by perforation of the placenta, loss of amniotic fluid, infection, and in rare circumstances, premature labor or spontaneous abortion.

Interpretations

Chromosomal studies (karyotyping) and biochemical analysis are done on the cells found in the amniotic fluid. These cells can then be screened for abnormalities. If there is evidence of a congenital abnormality at this time, the woman may be offered genetic counseling.

The creatinine level in the amniotic fluid is indicative of fetal maturity. As urine is passed from the fetus

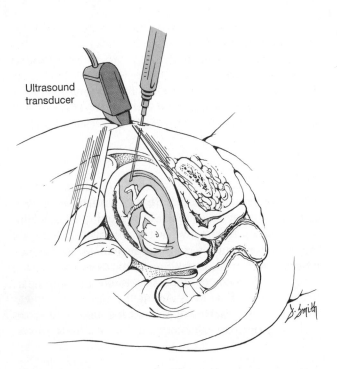

Figure 10-3. Amniocentesis. Amniotic fluid is withdrawn for analysis by a sterile needle inserted through the abdominal and uterine walls.

into the fluid, the creatinine level rises, demonstrating kidney function. At fetal maturity the creatinine level is >1.8 mg/dL.

Amniotic fluid is normally clear in color. If there is a greenish tinge to the fluid, it indicates the presence of meconium. Meconium normally can be found in the fetal gastrointestinal (GI) tract. However, if oxygen delivery to the GI tract in utero becomes inadequate, there is relaxation of the anal sphincter with resulting release of meconium. At term, it is not considered serious or unusual for a fetus in a breech position to have passed meconium as a result of pressure exerted on the bowels and anus. Postmaturity may be another cause of meconium staining resulting from placental degeneration.

The **lecithin/sphingomyelin ratio (L/S ratio) is** used to assess pulmonary maturity in the fetus. When the ratio is 2:1 (at around the 34th week of gestation), it indicates that the fetus's lungs are mature or very nearly so. At this stage, there is less of a chance of respiratory distress occurring at birth. In the last few years, the presence of **phosphatidyl-glycerol (PG)** (a component of a more mature surfactant complex) with a 2:1 L/S ratio has been used to protect against the incidence of false positive L/S tests.

When an emergency arises and an immediate decision about delivery must be made, a Shake test may be done at the bedside. A small amount of amniotic fluid is mixed with saline and ethanol and vigorously shaken. If the bubbles that float are stable and last 15 minutes, fetal lung maturity is assumed.

The level of bilirubin (the orange-colored pigment in bile) in the amniotic fluid is an accurate gauge of the destruction of fetal red blood cells from an Rh-sensitized woman. This is the result of erythroblastosis fetalis, the end result of Rh incompatibility between the woman and fetus.

Chorionic Villus Sampling

For less than 10 years, chorionic villus sampling (CVS) has been used as an innovative way of assessing fetal health. It may be done at as early as 10 weeks' gestation. The procedure can be done intravaginally or transabdominally using a plastic catheter, through which a small number of chorionic villi are aspirated for testing (Fig. 10-4). One advantage of this diagnostic test is that it can be done very early in the pregnancy. It produces results within a matter of days. The risks of spontaneous abortion, damaging the chorionic villi, and infection are considered minimal, at about 5%. CVS is capable of diagnosing many of the same disorders that amniocentesis detects.

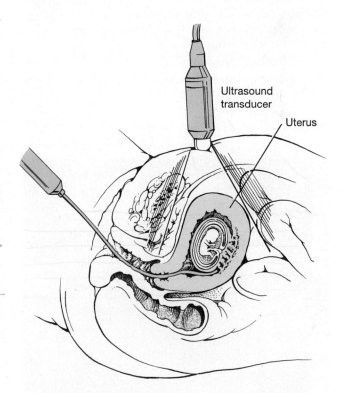

Figure 10-4. Chorionic villus sampling (CVS) of placental and chorionic material with transvaginal catheter and with direct ultrasound guidance.

Maternal Urine and Serum Assays

Maternal urine and serum assays include a urinalysis, complete blood count (CBC), VDRL, indirect Coombs', antibody titers for rubella and hepatitis B, and screening for human immunodeficiency virus (HIV). See Chapter 8 for comprehensive explanations of the tests and the interpretation of test results.

Auscultation of Fetal Heart Rate

Auscultation of the FHR is typically heard as early as 11 to 12 weeks using Doppler velocimetry, and approximately 20 weeks using a fetoscope or Leffscope (Fig. 10-5). The fetal heart rate is rapid and ranges from 110 to 160 beats per minute at term. In early pregnancy the FHR is higher. To avoid error in counting the rate, the pregnant woman's radial pulse is felt at the same time the FHR is auscultated. As soon as the FHR is audible, it is assessed at each prenatal visit.

Other sounds that are audible while listening to the fetal heart tones are the funic souffle and the uterine souffle. The **funic souffle** is a soft, swishing sound made as the blood moves through the umbilical cord. This rate is the same as the FHR. The **uterine souffle** is a soft, swishing sound made by maternal blood as it goes through the large vessels of the uterus. This rate is the same as the maternal pulse rate.

Fetoscope

A fetoscope has a band that fits over the listener's head. This metal band aids in bone conduction of sound to make hearing the fetal heart tones easier. It also frees the hands of the examiner and reduces extraneous noises. There is a weighted end that is placed on the woman's abdomen over the area where the fetal heart beat can be heard most clearly. The fetoscope is not used much in practice today and has largely been replaced by Doppler velocimetry.

Doppler Velocimetry

The Doppler probe is a simple electronic device used to auscultate fetal heart tones (FHT) very early in preg-

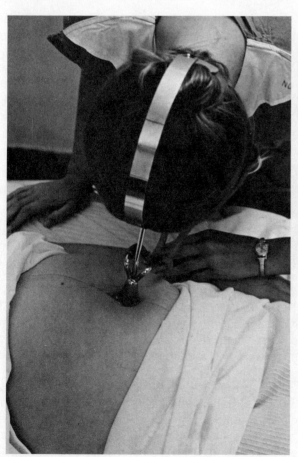

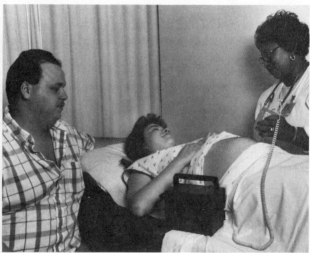

Figure 10-5. (A) Auscultation of the fetal heartbeat using the fetoscope. (B) The fetal heart rate is auscultated by use of Doppler probe.

nancy. This low-energy ultrasound is portable and typically runs on batteries. The FHT is detected by a sensor placed on the woman's abdomen and amplified by a hand-held "speaker." The speaker allows the health care provider, woman, and support person to hear the fetal heartbeat together. This is often an exciting experience and may help to validate the pregnancy at an early stage.

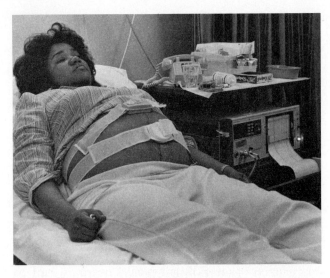

Figure 10-6. *Patient undergoing a nonstress test in the hospital setting. (Photo © Kathy Sloane)*

Electronic Fetal Heart Monitoring

Electronic fetal heart monitoring is used in pregnancy when a problem is suspected or fetal status is uncertain. Very often when a pregnant woman is past her estimated date of delivery (EDD), it will be suggested that she have a FHR tracing done to ensure the adequacy of placental functioning. If a woman complains that fetal movement has decreased, a tracing also will be obtained.

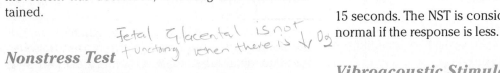

Fetal & placental is not functioning when there is ↓ ↓ O₂

Nonstress Test

A **nonstress test (NST)** is a noninvasive way of assessing fetal well-being. In this test, the FHR reactivity is measured by accelerations in response to fetal movement. A healthy fetus with an adequately functioning placenta will have an **acceleration** in heart rate in response to fetal movement. A fetus whose heart rate does not respond to movement may be suffering from anoxia caused by diminished placental blood flow. ↓ O₂

Diminished placental blood flow may be caused by pregnancy-induced hypertension (PIH), diabetes, placenta previa, abruptio placentae, and postmaturity. There is no danger of a nonstress test injuring the woman or fetus, nor does it initiate premature labor.

The woman is positioned for comfort, usually lying in semi-Fowler's position. Conduction gel is smeared over the abdomen, and an external ultrasound transducer is applied to her abdomen over the area where the FHR is heard the loudest. The tocodynamometer (a device that measures the force of uterine contractions) is applied at the top of the fundus to record any fetal movement (Fig. 10-6). Both monitors are secured with straps and should fit comfortably. The woman is given a push button and told to press it when she feels the fetus move. The nurse will continue to record the tracings for at least 40 minutes to be assured of the results.

The NST is considered reactive and normal when there are two to four FHR accelerations in a 10-minute period in response to movement. These accelerations should increase the rate by 10 to 15 beats and last 10 to

15 seconds. The NST is considered nonreactive and abnormal if the response is less.

Vibroacoustic Stimulation

Vibroacoustic stimulation is used during a NST when the fetus is believed to be "sleeping." An artificial larynx or a fetal acoustic stimulator is applied to the woman's lower abdomen to produce a single, sharp 1- to 2-second sound intended to stimulate an awakened state in the fetus. It may be repeated within a 10-minute period if two accelerations in response to fetal movement have not occurred.

Contraction Stress Test

The **contraction stress test (CST)** is a stress test in which the response of the FHR to contractions is assessed. Often the CST is induced by stimulation of the woman's nipples. This, in turn, stimulates the pituitary gland to release oxytocin, which causes uterine contractions. More often, an intravenous infusion of oxytocin is administered to stimulate uterine contractions. This is known as an **oxytocin challenge test (OCT).** No matter what type of stimulation is used, the desired outcome remains the same, that is, to induce three contractions within a 10-minute period while observing the FHR response.

Oxygen delivery to the fetus is diminished during a contraction. A compromised fetus suffering from placental insufficiency, that is, a fetus whose placenta is not functioning at optimum level, responds with late decelerations. Late **decelerations** refer to decreases in the FHR after the contraction starts. The FHR does not return

BPP is a Better Non stress test

to its prior rate until after the contraction has ended. A healthy fetus does not demonstrate late decelerations.

The woman is positioned on her left side or in semi-Fowler's position, and an ultrasound transducer is placed over the area where the FHR is heard. A tocodynamometer is applied to the fundus to monitor uterine contractions. An initial strip is run to determine the FHR baseline, and then the infusion of oxytocin is initiated. A minimum dose of 0.5 mU/min is begun and increased by 0.5 mU/min every 15 minutes until the desired three contractions are obtained. A 30-minute strip is generally considered sufficient for evaluating fetal response.

When late decelerations occur repeatedly, the test is positive, indicating placental insufficiency. When there are no decelerations for three contractions within the 10-minute period, it is a negative test. At the completion of the test, the infusion is stopped but the monitors remain in place until the contractions have stopped. The OCT/CST are done as early as 32 weeks' gestation and may be repeated as often as twice weekly when indicated.

Biophysical Profile

The biophysical profile consists of five observations that are scored either 0 for abnormal or 2 for normal. A combined score of 8 or 10 is considered reassuring. A total score of 6 must be retested within 24 hours. Scores of 2 or 4 are abnormal and need immediate evaluation. The first observation is a reactive NST. The other observations are made with an ultrasound and include:

1. Gross body movements (3 separate body/limb movements in 30 minutes)
2. Fetal breathing movements (at least one episode lasting continuously for 30 seconds in 30 minutes)
3. Fetal tone (one extension/flexion with return to flexed posture within a 30-minute period)
4. Normal amount of amniotic fluid (at least one pocket greater than 2 cm in two perpendicular planes).

If the amniotic fluid score is 0 and membranes are intact, close observation and further evaluations may be necessary.

Continuous Electronic Fetal Monitoring During Labor

Assessment of the fetal heart rate during labor is usually accomplished by continuous electronic fetal monitoring. Fetal monitoring can detect changes in the FHR in labor that indicate inadequate oxygenation of the fetus. Immediate interventions can be taken in this event. The electronic monitor may be applied externally or internally. This allows for evaluation of the FHR response to uterine contractions.

Electronic fetal monitoring is sometimes used for women who are classified as low risk, but it is used more often for those classified as moderate to high risk. These high-risk women include those with

- Abnormal OCT results
- Multiple gestations
- Placenta previa
- Oxytocin infusions

External fetal monitoring is accomplished by securing a ultrasound transducer and a tocodynamometer to the woman's abdomen (Fig. 10-7). The advantages of external fetal monitoring are that it is noninvasive and can be performed at any time during labor. The disadvantages are that some women find it constricting. Also maternal and fetal movement as well as fetal position affect the quality of the tracing.

Internal fetal monitoring is accomplished through application of an internal fetal spiral electrode (IFSE) directly to the presenting part (head, buttocks, etc.) of the fetus as it is passed through the vagina. The electrode is never attached to the face, fontanelles, sutures, or genitalia. An intrauterine pressure catheter (IUPC) is a catheter that is placed through the vagina into the uterus to measure the intensity of the contractions. Monitoring may be by external, internal, or a combination (such as IFSE and tocodynamometer).

The two major advantages of internal fetal monitoring are: (1) there is minimal interference with fetal tracings from the fetus and the woman and (2) abnormal FHR recordings are more easily recognized. The disad-

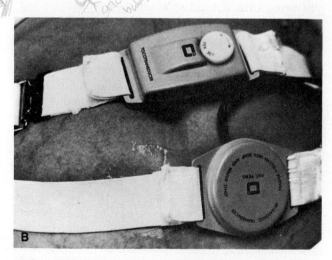

Figure 10-7. *External electronic fetal monitoring devices. The ultrasound transducer (bottom) detects fetal heart sounds. The tocotransducer (top) records the pressure of uterine contractions (Courtesy of BABES INC.)*

vantages are that the membranes must be ruptured for application of the internal monitors, the risk for fetal and maternal infection is greater, and there is the risk of injury to the fetus (such as scalp abscess from IFSE) and to the woman (eg, uterine perforation from IUPC).

The baseline is the FHR recorded between contractions over a period of at least 10 minutes. The normal range for FHR is 110 to 160 beats per minute (bpm) at term. Baseline variability is an indicator of fetal well-being. Variability refers to FHR changes in the baseline from beat to beat (short-term variability) and changes in the baseline over 1 minute (long-term variability). Variability is the single most important characteristic of the FHR. Loss of baseline short-term variability can be a discouraging sign. In the normal, healthy fetus, stimulation caused by a contraction can initiate an increase in baseline variability. Depression of the central nervous system by medications for pain relief may cause a temporary loss of variability.

Tachycardia is a baseline FHR over 160 bpm and can be caused by maternal fever and hypertension, maternal drugs, fetal hypovolemia, and fetal hypoxia. Bradycardia is a baseline FHR below 110 bpm. It is sometimes associated with congenital heart problems of the fetus and prolonged decrease in the supply of oxygen to the fetus.

Accelerations are transient increases in the FHR above baseline. They are generally uniform in shape and occur at the same time in the contraction, and end with the contraction. Accelerations are a reassuring FHR pattern. Decelerations are short-term decreases in FHR below baseline. They are classified as early, variable, and late.

Early decelerations are said to "mirror" a contraction because they start and end with the contraction. Early decelerations typically stay within a normal range for FHR above 110 bpm. A common cause of early decelerations is compression of the fetal head, which stimulates a vagal response of the parasympathetic nervous system. This type of deceleration is usually reassuring, or benign. Variable decelerations are not uniform in shape as they fall and return from baseline abruptly. The FHR may fall as low as 60 bpm but return to normal at the end of the contraction. It is more commonly seen late in labor and caused by compression of the umbilical cord. Variable decelerations are not problematic unless they are prolonged, repetitive, or do not resolve with maternal position changes. Late decelerations are uniform in appearance and have a gradual onset and return to baseline. The deceleration begins at the peak of the contraction and ends after the contraction has ended. Late decelerations are caused by many factors including umbilical cord compression, maternal hypotension or hypertension, hypovolemia, uterine hyperstimulation, abruptio placentae, and placental calcifications or infarcts. Repetitive late decelerations are problematic and require immediate intervention including maternal position change, increasing intravenous fluids, discontinuing oxytocin, oxygen at 8 to 10 L/m by face mask, and notification of the physician or midwife.

Nursing responsibility in identifying and interpreting changes in FHR patterns and initiating appropriate interventions cannot be overemphasized. If undesirable FHR patterns occur, the following interventions are taken:

- The woman is repositioned so that she lies on either side to decrease pressure on the vena cava. The head of the bed is elevated to 30°.
- The oxytocin infusion is discontinued.
- Oxygen is administered by face mask at 8 to 10 L/m.
- The physician or midwife is notified.

See the Nursing Interventions Checklist for a checklist of nursing interventions for continuous electronic fetal monitoring during labor.

✓ NURSING INTERVENTIONS CHECKLIST

Continuous Electronic Fetal Monitoring During Labor

External Monioring

Indications

Recording of baseline fetal heart rate

Assessment of effects of uterine contractions on fetal heart rate

Identification of abnormal fetal heart rate patterns

Analysis of fetal heart rate after administration of analgesia/anesthesia

Assessment of fetal heart rate after rupture of membranes

Identification of accelerations and decelerations

Disadvantages

Distracting to woman while confining movement in bed

Internal Monitoring

Indications

Inability to obtain accurate tracings of baseline fetal heart rate

Increased accuracy of recording fetal heart rate

Allows for more freedom of positional changes for woman while in bed

Disadvantages

Increased potential for infection

Membranes must be ruptured and cervix dilated

Increased risk for hemorrhage

No further ambulation for mother

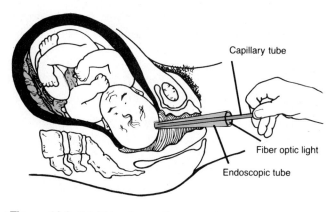

Capillary tube

Fiber optic light

Endoscopic tube

Figure 10-8. *Fetal blood sampling to verify fetal status and assess heart rate pattern as seen on the electronic fetal monitor.*

Fetal Blood Sampling

The fetus with a troubling FHR pattern may become increasingly acidotic. The acidotic fetus suffers from excessive acidity of body fluids. To determine whether the fetus is actually acidotic, fetal blood samples must be drawn and tested.

The sample of blood is drawn from the presenting part, typically the head (Fig. 10-8). The membranes must be ruptured to do this and the cervix dilated 3 to 4 cm. An endoscope is inserted through the cervix, the area cleansed, and the skin pricked so that blood may be collected, after which pressure to the sample site must be held for two contractions. Normal lower ranges for fetal acid/base is pH 7.15 to 7.30, PCO_2 22 to 34, PO_2 7 to 17, and base excess −14.1 to 5.3. A fetal blood pH below 7.2 with a downward trend in values indicates the need for intervention.

Fetal blood sampling gives direct information of fetal physiologic well-being at the time the sample was drawn, but also increases the risk of fetal hemorrhage and infection.

Adolescent Considerations

An adolescent scheduled for an ultrasound, blood work, or an amniocentesis will more than likely have many questions concerning the purpose of the procedures. It requires an informed and skilled nurse to explain the need for these evaluative tests and the potential outcomes in a nonthreatening way.

Cultural Considerations

Cultural beliefs about the necessity for fetal assessment in pregnancy vary widely. Many women believe that ul-

trasound, laboratory assessment of blood, and invasive procedures such as amniocentesis are unnecessary or potentially dangerous. Although there is truth to this for low-risk pregnancies, the benefits can far outweigh the risks for those considered high risk.

Some cultures believe that appropriate care given to the woman in pregnancy is all that is needed to facilitate health in the fetus. The Crow Indians believe that as long as the pregnant woman remains active, fetal circulation and oxygenation will be adequate. Diverse American subcultures perceive pregnancy as a normal physiologic process and therefore do not recognize the need for fetal or maternal assessment.

The nurse caring for a woman whose cultural beliefs do not coincide with her own must present pertinent knowledge to the woman and her family.

The Role of the Nurse

The role of the nurse in assessment of fetal health is more important today than ever before. It is the nurse who spends the most time assessing and counseling the pregnant woman during the antepartum period. It is the nurse who ultimately follows through with the woman during labor, birth, and into the postpartum period.

There are specific nursing diagnoses that help the nurse in planning care for the pregnant woman when fetal assessment is important. The Nursing Diagnoses Checklist highlights some of these nursing diagnoses.

✓ **NURSING DIAGNOSES CHECKLIST**

Nursing Diagnoses Associated with Assessment of Fetal Health

Anxiety, related to unknown status of fetus

Decisional Conflict, related to consenting to amniocentesis

Ineffective Denial, related to impaired fetal health

Fear, related to invasive procedures

Health Seeking Behaviors, impaired related to noncompliance of fetal health assessment

Ineffective Individual Coping, related to outcome of fetal assessment

Risk for Infection, related to fetal blood sampling

Risk for Injury, related to amniocentesis

Knowledge Deficit, related to fetal assessment regimen

Pain, related to invasive diagnostic procedures

SELF-ASSESSMENT

1. Variable decelerations are due to:

- ○ **A.** Uteroplacental insufficiency
- ○ **B.** Head compression
- ○ **C.** Cord compression
- ○ **D.** Maternal hypotension

2. Nursing interventions for late decelerations include all of the following except:

- ○ **A.** Change in maternal position
- ○ **B.** Oxygen administration
- ○ **C.** Notification of physician
- ○ **D.** Increasing infusion rate of oxytocin

3. Meconium in the amniotic fluid may indicate:

- ○ **A.** Hypoxia
- ○ **B.** Congenital anomalies
- ○ **C.** Head compression
- ○ **D.** Maternal temperature

4. Which of the following procedures may be performed following a nonreactive NST?

- ⊙ **A.** Amniocentesis
- ○ **B.** Contraction stress test
- ○ **C.** Vibroacoustic stimulation
- ○ **D.** Ultrasound

5. Which of the following statements regarding the fetal heartbeat is incorrect?

- ○ **A.** The normal rate is 110–160.
- ○ **B.** It can be measured by counting the uterine souffle.
- ○ **C.** It can be detected as early as 11 weeks gestation.
- ○ **D.** It should be assessed at each prenatal visit.

REVIEW AND PREVIEW

In this chapter, we discussed the types and importance of fetal assessment for determining fetal well-being. It has been stressed that maternal observation and fetal monitoring are important in determining interventions for a positive pregnancy outcome. The goal has been to emphasize assessment of fetal health in the provision of appropriate care during the antepartum period.

In the following chapter, we will discuss labor and delivery.

◈ KEY POINTS

◆ Measurement of fundal height determines the adequacy of fetal growth in relation to gestational age. It is done at every prenatal visit, usually after the first trimester, and is a reliable indicator of fetal well-being.

◆ Ultrasonography confirms pregnancy, assesses fetal growth, determines placental position, and rules out multiple abnormalities.

◆ Amniocentesis is an invasive procedure in which a sample of amniotic fluid is obtained to test for or rule out genetic disorders, fetal cell studies, and multiple fetal abnormalities.

◆ Chorionic villi are aspirated during an invasive procedure called chorionic villus sampling and assessed for clues to fetal health. The tissue is microscopically examined for the presence of genetic and chromosomal abnormalities and is done in the first trimester of pregnancy.

◆ Maternal urine and serum assays include urinalysis, CBC, VDRL, indirect Coombs', antibody titers for rubella and hepatitis B, HIV screening, alpha-fetoprotein.

◆ Auscultation of FHR is accomplished by fetoscope or Doppler velocimetry. It is done at each prenatal visit as soon as fetal heart tones are audible. The normal fetal heart rate is 110 to 160 beats per minute.

◆ Electronic fetal heart monitoring in pregnancy includes NST, vibroacoustic stimulation, and CST/OCT. These evaluations are important in assessing fetal response to movement or uterine contractions and are indicative of fetal health.

◆ Continuous electronic fetal heart monitoring during labor displays FHR tolerance during contractions. It is accomplished externally (noninvasive) and internally (invasive).

◆ Fetal blood sampling determines fetal serum pH, pO_2, pCO_2, and base excess levels for assessing fetal well-being. It is an invasive procedure that has risks to the fetus including infection and hemorrhage.

BIBLIOGRAPHY

Boyle, J. S., & Andrews, M. M. (1990). *Transcultural concepts in nursing care.* Philadelphia: J. B. Lippincott.

Carpenito, L. J. (1993). *Nursing diagnosis: Application to clinical practice* (5th ed.). Philadelphia: J. B. Lippincott.

Ewigman, B., Green, J., & Lumley, J. (1993). Ultrasound during pregnancy: A discussion. *Birth, 20*(4), 212–215.

Fischbach, F. (1992). A *Manual of laboratory & diagnostic tests* (4th ed.). Philadelphia: J. B. Lippincott.

Freda, M. C., Mikhail, M., Mazloom, E., Polizzotto, R., Damus, K., & Merkatz, I. (1993). Fetal movement counting: which method?. *The American Journal of Maternal/Child Nursing, 18*(6), 314-321.

Engstrom, J. L., McFarlin, B. L., & Sampson, M. B. (1993). Fundal height measurement: Part 4. Accuracy of clinicians' identification of the uterine fundus during pregnancy. *Journal of Nurse-Midwifery, 38*(6), 318–323.

Engstrom, J. L., & Work, B. A. (1992). Prenatal prediction of small- and large-for-gestational age neonates. *Journal of Obstetric, Gynecologic, and Neonatal Nursing, 21*(6), 486-496.

Gebauer, C. L, & Lowe, N. K. (1993). The biophysical profile: Antepartal assessment of fetal well-being. *Journal of Obstetric, Gynecologic, and Neonatal Nursing, 22*(2), 115–127.

Gregor, C. L. (1992). Obstetric ultrasound: Who should perform sonograms?. *Birth, 19*(2), 92–99.

May, K. A., & Mahlmeister, L. R. (1994). *Maternal and neonatal nursing: Family-centered care* (3rd ed.). Philadelphia: J. B. Lippincott.

Pilliteri, A. (1992). *Maternal and child health nursing: Care of the childbearing and childrearing family* (1st ed.). Philadelphia: J. B. Lippincott.

Reeder, S. J., Martin, L. L., & Koniak, D. (1992). *Maternity nursing: Family, newborn, and women's health care* (17th ed.). Philadelphia: J. B. Lippincott.

Rosdahl, C. B. (1991). *Textbook of basic nursing* (5th ed.). Philadelphia: J. B. Lippincott.

Sala, D. J., Moise, K. J., Weber, V. E., & Cordella-Simon, L. (1992). Maternal blood donation for intrauterine transfusion, *Journal of Obstetric, Gynecologic, and Neonatal Nursing, 21*(5), 365–376.

Wayland, J., & Tate, S. (1993). Maternal-fetal attachment and perceived relationships with important others in adolescents. *Birth, 20*(4), 198–203.

Williams, J. K. (1993). New genetic discoveries increase counseling opportunities. *The American Journal of Maternal/Child Nursing, 18*(4), 218–240.

The Family in the Intrapartum Period

CHAPTER 11

The Process of Labor and Delivery

◆ OBJECTIVES

When the learning goals of this chapter are met, the reader will be able to:

◆ List the four forces of labor.

◆ Describe the onset of labor.

◆ List at least five signs and symptoms of labor.

◆ Differentiate true from false labor.

◆ Discuss factors that influence labor.

◆ List and define the four stages of labor.

◆ Differentiate between cervical effacement and cervical dilatation.

◆ Describe the two phases of the first stage of labor.

◆ Distinguish between fetal position, fetal lie, and fetal presentation giving examples of each.

◆ Define the mechanisms of labor.

TERMINOLOGY

Active phase

Descent

Dilatation

Effacement

Expulsion

Extension

False labor

Fetal presentation

Fetal position

Flexion

Internal rotation

Latent phase

Restitution

Transition phase

True labor

The process of labor and childbirth brings about the event that the woman has been anticipating throughout her pregnancy. This is a time of high expectations and much anxiety for the laboring woman and her support person. *Labor* is a very appropriate term for this process, because the woman must work very hard to accomplish the end result of childbirth. This chapter focuses on the physical and psychosocial aspects of the forces, onset, and stages of normal labor to provide the nurse with the basic knowledge needed to successfully carry out nursing care of the woman and her child.

Labor is defined as the rhythmic contraction and relaxation of the uterine muscles in the process of expelling from the uterus the products of conception, the neonate and the placenta. The precise mechanism that causes the onset of labor is not completely understood. A number of theories have been proposed. Four common theories include the uterine stretch theory, the pressure or oxytocin stimulation theory, the progesterone deprivation theory, and the prostaglandin cascade theory.

The *uterine stretch theory* embraces the theory that the full uterus will automatically empty itself. The *pressure* or *oxytocin stimulation theory* supports the idea that pressure from the descending fetus stimulates an increase in the secretion of oxytocin by the posterior pituitary gland of the mother. This increase in oxytocin stimulates uterine contractions, and labor begins. The *progesterone deprivation theory* is somewhat controversial. Progesterone is essential to the maintenance of pregnancy. This theory is founded on the concept that labor begins when unknown physiologic responses result in the decrease of progesterone and the increase of estrogen in the woman. The *prostaglandin theory* is based on the fact that prostaglandin, which can cause uterine contractions, is found at high levels in the amniotic fluid and blood of laboring women. The increased prostaglandin is thought to be a result of interaction between the fetal adrenal gland and the uterus. No matter what the initial cause of labor, the fact remains that once started it is difficult to stop this natural process.

Forces of Labor

The forces of labor are commonly referred to as the "Four Ps." They are: the passage, the passenger, the powers, and the psyche. These important factors must work together for labor to progress normally. An alteration in any one or a combination of the forces can alter the outcome of labor.

Passage

The **passage** refers to the true pelvis (see Chapter 2). It is described by its structure, type, and diameters. The bony canal of the pelvis is divided into three components: the inlet; the outlet; and the midpelvis, or pelvic cavity (Fig. 11-1). The inlet is the entrance to the true pelvis. It is at the level of the linea terminalis, the division between the true pelvis and the false pelvis. The outlet is the space between the symphysis pubis in the front, the ischial tuberosities on either side and the coccyx in the back.

Pelvic Types

There are several types of pelves: the gynecoid (female), android (male), anthropoid (oval), and platypelloid (flat) pelves (Fig. 11-2). Each type of pelvis is characterized by its shape and significant bony structures. The type of pelvis determines the position and ease of descent of the fetus. The gynecoid pelvis is considered the most favorable to childbirth. However, mixed or intermediate types are common, and most women have a combination of two types.

Pelvic Structure

The structure of the female pelvis is very different from that of the male. The most obvious dissimilarity is a wider suprapubic arch in women. The female pelvis is shallow, broader, and more spacious, whereas the male pelvis is deep and compact. These differences develop at puberty, and make the female pelvis more conducive to delivery.

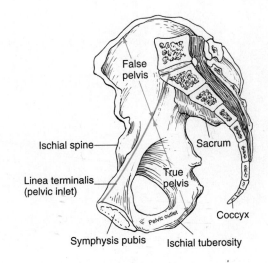

Figure 11-1. *Pelvic cavity showing planes of the inlet and the outlet.*

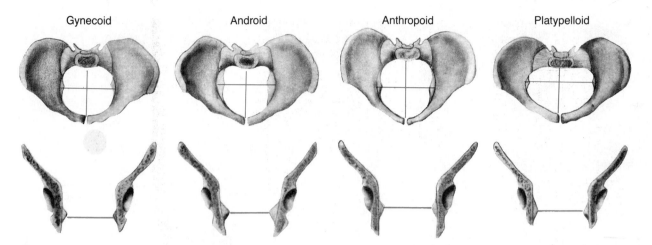

Gynecoid   Android   Anthropoid   Platypelloid

Figure 11-2. *The four main pelvic types. The lines are drawn to illustrate the widest diameters.*

Pelvic Diameters

Pelvic diameters are measured during a prenatal visit by the physician or midwife (see Chapter 6). The procedure is called *pelvimetry*. These measurements may be repeated when the woman is admitted to the birthing area, if the birth attendant chooses. The measurements help to determine the amount of space that is available for the fetus to pass through the mother's pelvic structure. The diagonal conjugate, obstetric conjugate, and the biischial diameter are measured manually. The term *conjugate* means paired, or working together, and refers to measurements taken between two bony areas. The diagonal conjugate is the measurement from the symphysis to the promontory of the sacrum. The obstetric conjugate represents the smallest diameter of the inlet through which the fetus must pass (Fig. 11-3). The biischial diameter describes the transverse measurement of the outlet. It is determined by placing a closed fist against the perineum to palpate the ischial tuberosities.

Passenger

The fetus is the passenger. The progress of labor is influenced by the fetal head, fetal lie, fetal attitude, fetal station, fetal presentation, and fetal position. Difficulties during childbirth may arise because of deviations in one or more of these aspects even though the pelvis is adequate in size.

Fetal Head

Because the fetal head is the largest part of the fetus to be delivered, its size greatly influences the ease or difficulty of childbirth. Typically, the rest of the fetal body follows with little difficulty, although the shoulders may sometimes present problems. The fetal head is formed

by eight cranial bones. Four of these, the two parietal, the occipital, and the frontal bones, are important from an obstetric point of view (Fig. 11-4).

These bones are not fused at birth. They are separated by membranous tissue called sutures, which permit overlapping of the bones during birth to decrease the size of the skull. This overlapping process is called molding. Molding gives the newborn's head a mis-

Antidote for mgso4 — Calcium gluconate

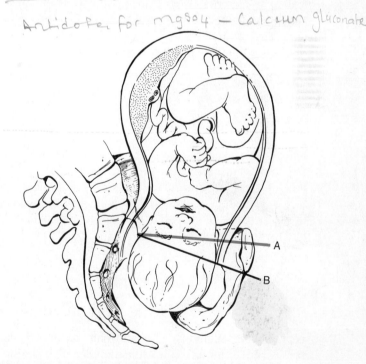

Figure 11-3. (A) *Obstetric conjugate. This important diameter is the shortest anteroposterior distance between the sacral promontory and symphysis pubis.* **(B)** *Diagonal conjugate. Because the obstetric conjugate cannot be measured directly, its length is estimated by measuring the diagonal conjugate, which is the distance between the sacral promontory and the lower border of the symphysis pubis.*

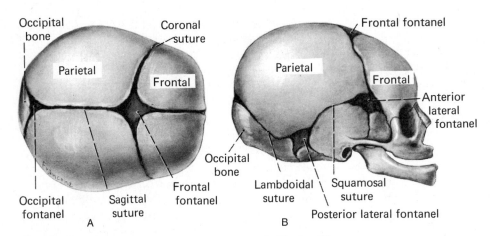

Figure 11-4. *Fetal skull showing fontanels, bones, and sutures. (A) Superior view. (B) Lateral view.*

shapen appearance that usually disappears within a day or two. After a long labor, the newborn's head may show evidence of molding for several days after birth.

Fetal Lie

The fetal lie refers to the relationship of the spine of the fetus to the spine of the mother. The two most frequently discussed lies are longitudinal and transverse. The longitudinal lie is the most common. This occurs when the fetal and maternal spines lie parallel to each other. Transverse lie occurs when the fetal spine lies horizontal to the maternal spine. That is the fetal spine is more or less at a right angle to the maternal spine.

Fetal Attitude

The fetal attitude describes the relationship of fetal parts to one another. The most common attitude of the fetus is a tucked position. The head is bowed with the chin against the chest, the arms are folded against the chest, the spine is curved forward, and the legs are flexed against the abdomen. This typical attitude effectively decreases the length of the fetus to approximately half its stretched-out length.

Fetal Station and Engagement

As the fetus descends into the pelvis, an estimation of the level of the presenting part (the head in a cephalic presentation) in relationship to the ischial spines is determined. This estimation is called station. Station is measured in centimeters. Above the imaginary line drawn between the ischial spines, station is expressed in minus terms; below this line, station is expressed in plus terms. For example, if the head of the fetus is 1 cm above the ischial spines, the fetus is said to be at station −1. Conversely, if the head of the fetus is 1 cm below the ischial spines, it is said to be at

station +1. When the head is at the ischial spines, it is at station 0. Stations range from −4 to −1 and +1 to +4 (Fig. 11-5).

Engagement is the term used when the widest diameter of the presenting part is at the level of the ischial spines. In cephalic presentation, this is the biparietal diameter. In breech presentation, it is the intertrochanteric diameter. When lightening occurs (discussed in first stage of labor), engagement has taken place.

Fetal Presentation

In 95% of births, the fetal head enters the birth canal first. A head-first presentation is called cephalic presen-

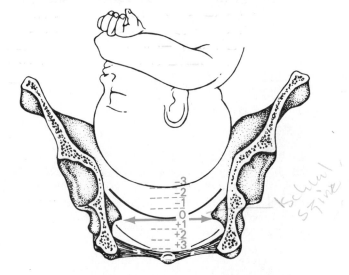

Figure 11-5. *Stations of the fetal head:*
−3 station—vertex is 3 cm above the spines.
−2 station—vertex is 2 cm above the spines.
−1 station—vertex is 1 cm above the spines.
0 station—vertex is at the level of the spines.
+1 station—vertex is 1 cm below the spines.
+2 station—vertex is 2 cm below the spines.
+3 station—vertex is 3 cm below the spines.

tation. Cephalic presentations are further classified as vertex and face. Vertex is the most common cephalic presentation. In it, the head is tucked, with the chin on chest and the occipital bone leading. In face presentations (which occur more rarely), the head is flexed, with the occipital bone touching the back and the chin leading. Additional presentations include breech, when the buttocks enter the birth canal first, and shoulder presentations, seen when there is a transverse lie (Fig. 11-6).

Fetal Positions

Fetal position indicates the relationship of the fetal presenting part to the maternal pelvis. The maternal pelvis is divided into four quadrants, identified as right or left and posterior or anterior. The left or right quadrant is relative to the left or right side of the woman's body. Posterior indicates the presenting part is positioned toward the woman's sacrum, or back. Anterior indicates the presenting part is positioned toward the woman's symphysis pubis, or front. In the case in which the presenting part is midway between the front and back of the woman, the term *transverse* is used instead of anterior or posterior.

Fetal position is designated by three letters. The first letter indicates left or right, the second letter indicates the presenting part, such as occiput or sacrum, and the third letter indicates anterior, posterior, or transverse. Thus, LOA is the abbreviation that signifies the fetus is to the *L*eft, the *O*cciput is the presenting part, and it is *A*nterior, or toward the maternal symphysis. LOA is the most common position fetal position. Frequently during labor the fetus is turned to an anterior position by the

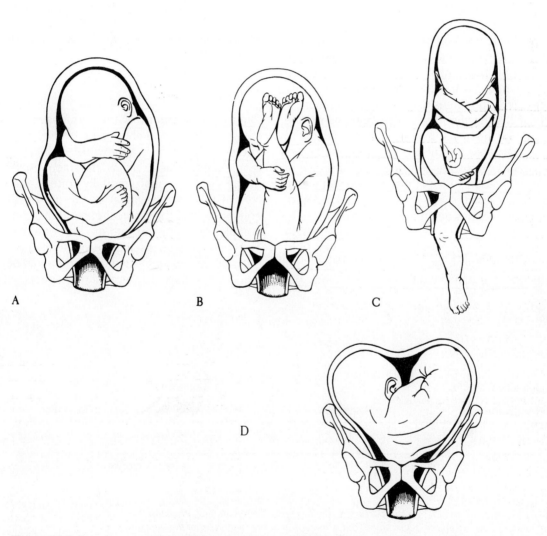

A B C

D

Figure 11-6. *Breech presentation. **(A)** Complete breech. **(B)** Frank breech. **(C)** Footling breech. **(D)** Transverse or shoulder presentation. (Used with permission of Ross Products Division, Abbott Laboratories, Columbus, OH 43216, from* Clinical Education Aid #18, *© 1995 Ross Products Division, Abbott Laboratories.)*

forces of labor. Occiput anterior is the most favorable to childbirth.

Powers

The primary power in normal labor and childbirth are the contractions of the uterus. With these contractions, cervical effacement and dilatation also occur. Secondary power is provided by the bearing-down efforts of the mother during the second stage of labor.

Uterine Contractions

The uterus is a powerful muscular organ. The muscles of the uterus are smooth muscles and function involuntarily. The contractions usually are rhythmic, increasing in intensity during the course of labor. The muscles of the upper portion of the uterus, the fundus, never completely relax. These muscles hold their shortened length to maintain the downward pressure achieved with the contraction. Each contraction has three phases: the increment (incline or increasing intensity), the acme (peak), and the decrement (decline or decreasing intensity). Uterine contractions are assessed for frequency, duration, and intensity.

Frequency is the time from the beginning of one contraction until the beginning of the next contraction. Frequency is reported in minutes. Frequency indicates how often contractions are occurring. For instance, a frequency of 5 minutes means that the woman's contractions are occurring every 5 minutes. As labor progresses, the contractions occur more frequently.

Duration refers to the length of the contraction from the beginning of the contraction to the end of it. Duration is reported in seconds (Fig. 11-7). When labor begins, contractions may last only 15 to 20 seconds, but as labor progresses the duration extends to 60 to 90 seconds.

Intensity describes the peak strength of the contraction. Mild, moderate, or strong contractions are confirmed by palpation. If external electronic fetal monitoring is used, the frequency, duration, and intensity of uterine contractions are recorded by a tokodynamometer placed on the fundus of the uterus. The tokodynamometer is standard equipment on the external electronic fetal monitor.

Two points about contractions are very important. First, the duration of contractions lasting longer than 90 seconds must be reported at once. Vasoconstriction that occurs during the contraction seriously reduces the amount of oxygen available to the fetus. The placenta can supply sufficient oxygen to the fetus for only 90 seconds without the ability to refresh the blood supply through the uterine circulation. Second, contractions that occur less than 1 minute apart do not provide enough rest to the uterine muscle between contractions. This may lead to rupture of the uterine muscle.

Cervical Effacement and Dilatation

Cervical **effacement** is the term used for the softening, thinning, and shortening of the cervical canal. The cervical canal is approximately 2 cm (0.8 in.) at term. As effacement begins, the internal os (opening) of the cervical canal gradually softens and becomes part of the lower segment of the uterus. Effacement continues until the cervical canal thins, shortens, and completely disappears into the lower uterine segment. The cervical canal is said to be obliterated (wiped out). Cervical effacement occurs in primiparas before dilatation takes place. However, in multiparas, effacement

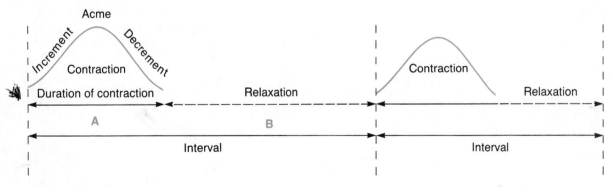

Figure 11-7. The interval and the duration of uterine contractions. The frequency of contractions is the interval timed from the beginning of one contraction to the beginning of the next contraction. The interval consists of two parts: **(A)** the duration of the contraction and **(B)** the period of relaxation. The broken line indicates an indeterminate period, because the time **(B)** is usually of longer duration than the actual contraction **(A)**.

and dilatation usually occur at the same time. Cervical effacement is measured in percentages. When no effacement has occurred, effacement is said to be 0%. When the cervical canal is approximately 1 cm (0.4 in.) in length, effacement is 50%. Completion of effacement is 100% when no rim (edge) of the cervical canal can be felt.

Cervical **dilatation** is the increase in the size of the external os of the cervical canal from an opening of just a few mm to an opening of 10 cm (4 in.) in full dilatation. This is necessary to allow the passage of the fetus. Cervical effacement and dilatation are determined throughout labor by palpating with a fingertip during vaginal examinations. The force of amniotic sac pushing against the cervix aid in dilation of the cervix. After the membranes have ruptured, the fetal presenting part continues to exert pressure to enlarge the cervical os (Fig. 11-8).

Maternal Expulsive Forces

After full cervical effacement and dilatation, the laboring woman is encouraged to "bear down." This secondary power uses the force of her abdominal muscles to intensify the effect of the uterine contractions. To avoid exhaustion and cervical edema, the woman is discouraged from pushing until effacement and dilatation is complete. This occurs in the second stage of labor.

Psyche

The psyche refers to both the conscious and the unconscious mental force of the woman, including thought, judgment, and emotion. The psyche factor can greatly effect the progress of the labor. The woman's psyche is influenced by a number of factors, including psychologic state, support systems available to her, whether she has had any childbirth preparation, past experiences, and coping strategies.

Psychologic State

The woman may have a high level of excitement and anxiety when she enters the facility in labor. For a primipara, the unknown experience may contribute to her apprehension. Some of her anxiety may be caused by the threat to her self-image that the birth of a baby may represent. She also may fear that she will be unable to successfully do her part in the labor process. In addition, she may have unrealistic expectations of herself and her own behavior, formed in part from talking with friends and relatives or from watching television. Maternal anxiety can cause physical changes that may de-

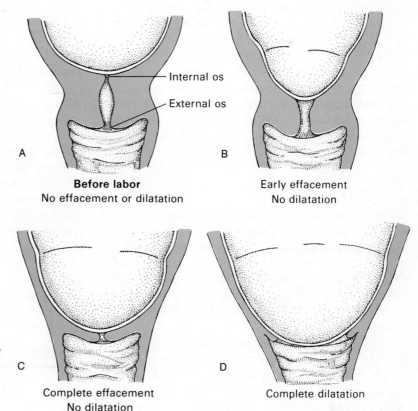

Figure 11-8. Stages in cervical effacement and dilatation. **(A)** Before labor; no effacement or dilatation. **(B)** Early effacement, no dilatation. **(C)** Complete effacement, no dilatation. **(D)** Complete dilatation.

A — Internal os — External os
Before labor
No effacement or dilatation

B
Early effacement
No dilatation

C
Complete effacement
No dilatation

D
Complete dilatation

crease uterine activity, causing labor to be longer. A supportive, sensitive nurse can help the woman become more comfortable and relaxed.

Support Systems

The role of the woman's support person is especially important during labor. The support person's level of anxiety, apparent understanding of labor routines, and efforts to comfort and reassure the laboring woman are evaluated. This evaluation helps the nurse determine the role that the support person is able to assume. The nurse must be prepared to provide additional support to the laboring woman as needed.

Childbirth Preparation

The woman and her support person may have attended childbirth preparation classes to prepare for the event (see Chapter 7 for full discussion). However, when faced with the actual situation, either or both of them may have difficulty recalling techniques for breathing, relaxation, and management of pain. Each birth is different, and unexpected events may occur for which they are not prepared. Ongoing nursing assessment helps to identify when the woman and the support person are experiencing increased anxiety. The nurse can intervene to help alleviate these anxieties.

Past Experiences

The multipara may remember a difficult situation and be very apprehensive about the current labor and childbirth experience. Conversely, if she had an easy previous labor, she may fear that this one will not be easy. Often these attitudes influence her approach to the current labor.

Coping Strategies

Many factors may play a part in the woman's coping strategies (how she handles the experience) during labor. Her self-confidence, her relationship with the baby's father, her attitude about the anticipated birth, and the emotional support she has from her family all contribute to her ability to summon the strength she needs to gain control and work in harmony with her uterine contractions.

Maternal behavior changes throughout the course of labor. Early in labor, the mother may be excited and perhaps mildly apprehensive. She may communicate freely or remain quiet. She usually follows instructions easily. As contractions increase in intensity, the woman

becomes more serious. She may be apprehensive and require encouragement and companionship. Additional relaxation techniques such as back rubs and position changes may be needed. During this time, the woman may have more difficulty following instructions. As birth nears, she may feel that labor will never end. She may question her ability to cope with contractions. At this time she may have difficulty following instructions. Physical symptoms such as shaking, nausea, vomiting, and increased pelvic pressure typically occur.

◆ Onset of Labor

In the several weeks before labor begins, the woman may experience physical changes that alert her that labor is approaching. She becomes sensitive to each change in her body, anticipating the beginning of labor.

Signs and Symptoms

The signs and symptoms that occur in the last few weeks of gestation are considered premonitory (warning) signs. The signs are lightening, cervical changes, weight loss, and backache. In addition, signs of false labor may need to be differentiated from those of true labor.

Lightening

Approximately 10 to 14 days before labor begins, primiparas may notice that the fetus has moved down into the pelvis. Many women say that the baby has "dropped." This is actually the settling of the fetus into the brim of the pelvis. It is called lightening. The woman experiences a relief of the pressure against the diaphragm and is able to breathe more easily. However, the uterus now presses against the bladder, causing frequent urination. The increased pressure in the pelvis may cause maternal leg cramps or backache. This discomfort is caused by pressure on the sciatic nerve. Multiparas may not experience lightening and the associated symptoms until the onset of labor.

Cervical Changes

The cervix undergoes a number of changes before the onset of actual labor. The cervix softens because of increased vascularity, edema, and increased production (hyperplasia) of cervical glands. During pregnancy, the feel of the cervix is compared to the feel of the ear lobe. As labor approaches, the cervix becomes much softer, preparing for effacement. At this time, the cervix is said to feel as soft as the lower lip. This softening is referred to as ripening of the cervix. It is at this point that effacement begins in primiparas; dilatation also may begin. It is not unusual for the woman's cervix to be dilated 1 cm or more before labor begins. These are signs that can be detected through vaginal examination, but are not detected by the woman.

One cervical change that can be detected by the woman is show or "bloody show." Shortly before the onset of actual labor, the pregnant woman may have a small amount of pink-tinged or blood-tinged vaginal discharge. This discharge, called show, consists of the mucus plug from the cervical canal mixed with a small amount of blood. The blood is from tiny capillaries located in the cervix. These capillaries rupture as the uterus changes and prepares for labor. Show may be seen a few hours or a few days before the onset of labor.

Infrequently, the woman may experience spontaneous rupture of the membranes (SROM) before the onset of regular uterine contractions. The woman may report that she has had a small trickle or a large gush of fluid. Most women reaching full term will enter spontaneous labor within 24 hours of rupture. The woman is instructed to seek prompt evaluation if the membranes rupture.

Weight Loss

It is not unusual for the pregnant woman to experience a 1- to 3-pound weight loss before labor begins. The woman may report gastrointestinal disturbances such as diarrhea, nausea, vomiting, and indigestion. The cause of these gastrointestinal alterations is not known.

Backache

Persistent backache can occur during pregnancy. It usually is caused by the redistribution of maternal weight. Backache is most common after lightening occurs. The body's center of gravity shifts forward, with relaxation of the abdominal muscles and shortening of the muscles of the back. An awkward gait results and contributes to low backache. Low-back pain may be worsened by sciatic nerve pressure. Low dull backache accompanied by mild cramping are characteristic of the backache experienced at the onset of labor.

Late in pregnancy, many women develop an overall feeling of fatigue. This may be relieved 24 to 48 hours before the onset of labor when the woman has a sudden burst of energy. The woman may feel compelled to accomplish multiple tasks before the birth of the newborn, so-called nesting behaviors. Most women do not experience this phenomenon. It is important to encourage the woman to get adequate rest before the onset of labor.

True Versus False Labor

False labor is the misinterpretation by the woman of Braxton Hicks contractions, which become stronger in the last week or so before labor begins. Extremely strong Braxton Hicks contractions are experienced for a variable period toward the end of pregnancy. These intermittent contractions actually occur throughout pregnancy, but become more uncomfortable for the woman as pregnancy reaches full term. Although they may be painful, these contractions are usually short in duration and irregular in timing. They do not increase in intensity and can normally be relieved by walking. These false labor contractions start in the abdomen and do not radiate elsewhere. The cervical changes of effacement and dilatation do not result from false labor.

True labor, however, consists of contractions that increase in regularity, frequency, intensity, and duration. The contractions of true labor begin in the back and radiate to the abdomen. True labor contractions increase with ambulation. The effacement and dilatation of the cervix results from true labor contractions.

When false labor contractions become so strong that they are misinterpreted, true labor is probably not far away. Display 11-1 highlights the characteristics that differentiate false labor from true labor.

DISPLAY 11-1
True Versus False Labor

True Labor	· Contractions regular
	· Uterine contractions increase in intensity, frequency, and duration
	· Felt in lower back and radiates around to abdomen
	· Effacement and dilatation of the cervix
	· Intensify with walking
False Labor	· Contractions irregular
	· No increase in intensity, frequency, or duration of contractions
	· Felt in abdomen only
	· Relieved by walking
	· No cervical change

Stages of Labor

Labor starts when uterine contractions occur at regular intervals and cause cervical effacement and dilatation. Labor is divided into four stages, which describe the major physical changes that occur. The first stage is the stage of effacement and dilatation. The cervix dilates to 10 cm by the end of the first stage of labor. The second stage is the stage of **expulsion**, or birth, of the neonate. The third stage is the expulsion of the placenta. Recovery is the fourth stage. The average length of the first and second stages of labor differs for primiparas and multiparas. The third and fourth stages are not affected by parity (Fig. 11-9).

First Stage: Effacement and Dilatation

Effacement and dilatation, which are assessed throughout labor, have already been defined. The first stage of labor begins with the first regular contractions and ends when the cervix is fully dilated at 10 cm. The first stage of labor is subdivided into three phases: latent, active, and transition.

Latent Phase

The **latent phase**, the longest phase of first stage of labor, is defined as the period during which the cervix dilates from 0 cm to 3 to 4 cm. In the beginning of the latent phase, contractions may be somewhat irregular. The frequency of contractions can vary from 10 to 20 minutes apart to 5 to 10 minutes apart. Contractions are mild and last approximately 15 to 30 seconds (duration). The woman may experience abdominal cramping, low dull backache, and there may be light bloody show. The woman may ambulate with ease through this phase, even during contractions. Many women spend this time at home. The latent phase may average 8 or more hours in length, with an upper limit of 20 hours in the primipara. In the multipara, the phase lasts an average of 5 hours, with an upper limit of 14 hours.

Active Phase

The **active phase** of the first stage of labor begins when the cervix is 4 cm dilated and lasts through 7 cm of dilatation. Contractions become more frequent, occurring every 3 to 5 minutes. Contractions are moderate in intensity, and they range in duration from 30 to 60 seconds. The woman's level of discomfort with contractions is mild to moderate at the beginning of the active phase. By the end of the active phase, the discomfort level is moderate to severe. Membranes may rupture during this time, if they have not already ruptured. In some women, membranes may not rupture until the second stage of labor. Early in the active phase, the woman can continue to ambulate with little difficulty, but by the end of this phase, ambulation becomes difficult or impossible during contractions. Many women wish to rest in a sitting or reclining position by the end of this phase.

Transition Phase

The **transition phase** is the final phase of first stage. During this phase, the cervix dilates rapidly from 8 to 10 cm. Frequency of contractions is every 2 to 3 minutes. They are moderate to strong in intensity and 60 to 90 seconds in duration. The woman experiences a moderate to severe level of discomfort with contractions. Bloody show increases. The woman may have a strong

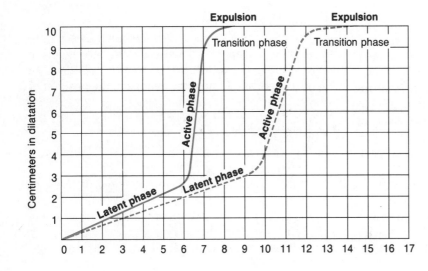

Figure 11-9. *Graphic analysis of labor using Friedman's curve. The mean labor duration for primagravidas is shown by the dotted line, and the mean for multigravidas is shown by the solid line.*

desire to bear down during this phase because the presenting part of the fetus is low in her pelvis. The woman tends to focus on herself, withdrawing from those around her. She may experience hiccoughs, nausea, vomiting, diaphoresis, involuntary shaking, and leg cramping. At the end of transition, the urge to bear down may seem irresistible. When cervical effacement is 100% and dilatation is 10 cm, the woman moves into the second stage of labor.

Second Stage: Expulsion

During the second stage of labor, the fetus passes through the pelvis and emerges from the vaginal opening. This is accomplished by the combined efforts of the uterine contractions and maternal expulsive forces. When the cervix is completely dilated, the woman experiences intense pressure on the internal perineum from the presenting part. This feeling is similar to that of defecation. This may be accompanied by bloody show. Contractions are usually very strong and may occur as often as every 1 to 2 minutes, lasting 60 to 90 seconds each. If the membranes have not previously ruptured, spontaneous rupture often happens at the beginning of the second stage. If not, they may be ruptured artificially at this time.

Crowning

Crowning occurs when the fetal head appears at the vaginal opening. It signals the approach of the end of the second stage. The perineum bulges as contractions and maternal pushing force the fetal head to descend. Eventually, the fetal head is visible in the opening. It advances with each uterine contraction and pushing effort of the woman and may disappear between contractions (Fig. 11-10).

Mechanisms of Labor

The presenting part of the fetus undergoes positional changes as it passes through the birth canal. These positional changes, known as the mechanisms, or cardinal movements, of labor, are descent, flexion, internal rotation, extension, external rotation, restitution, and expulsion. More than one of these movements may be occurring at the same time. Figure 11-11 presents the movements with an accompanying drawing of the maternal pelvic bones in relation to the bones of the fetal head. Careful examination of the drawings provides an increased understanding of the adaptive movements made by the fetus in adjusting to the smallest diameter of the maternal pelvis. In this way, the fetus meets with the least amount of physical resistance.

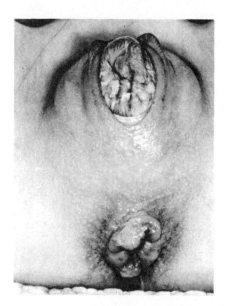

Figure 11-10. *Crowning with extreme bulging of the perineum showing a distended and an everted (turned outside) anus.*

Descent
Descent is the downward movement of the presenting part of the fetus. Physical forces that act independently or together to cause descent include pressure from the amniotic fluid, uterine pressure on the fetal buttocks (in a cephalic presentation), contraction of the maternal abdominal muscles, and positioning of the fetal body.

Flexion
Flexion ordinarily occurs as the descending head contacts and meets resistance from the pelvic wall, the cervix, or the pelvic floor. In flexion, the fetal head flexes with the chin resting on the sternum. This presents the smallest possible diameter to the pelvis.

Internal Rotation
The fetal head usually enters the pelvis in the transverse position. **Internal rotation** is the movement of the head from this position to the anterior position (See Fig. 11-11A, B, and C: note the change in the position of the fetal head in relation to the maternal pelvic bones). After internal rotation, the occiput rests beneath the woman's symphysis pubis.

Extension
At the completion of internal rotation, the base of the occiput passes under the symphysis pubis, causing **extension** of the head. It is during this time that crowning occurs. As extension continues, the occiput appears first, followed by the forehead, nose, mouth, and chin.

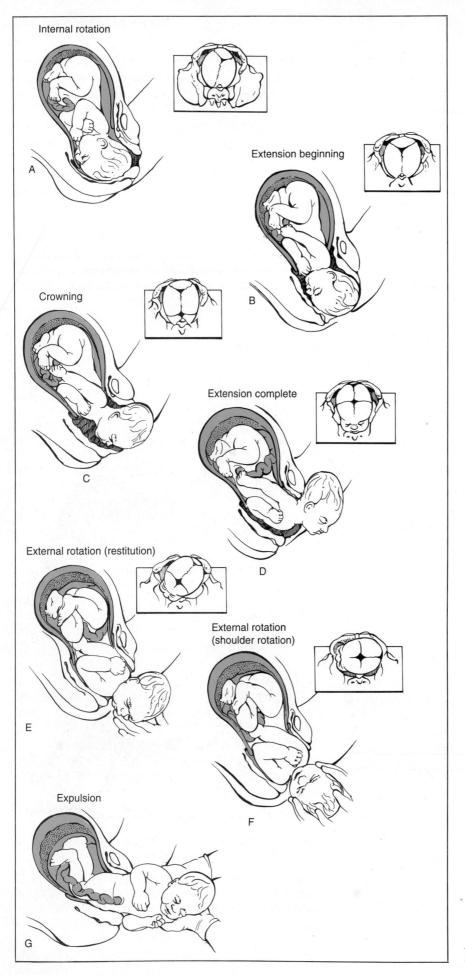

Figure 11-11. *Mechanisms of normal labor and cardinal positions.*

Extension is complete when the entire head has been expelled.

External Rotation (Restitution)

When the head appears, it is slightly twisted in relation to the shoulders. **Restitution** is achieved when the head rotates to alignment with the shoulders. This restitution of the head is the first step to *external rotation*. External rotation continues as the shoulders rotate to an anteroposterior (front to back) position to take advantage of the direction of the widest diameter of the maternal pelvic outlet.

Expulsion

Expulsion occurs as the anterior shoulder is born, followed by the posterior shoulder and the rest of the body. The rest of the body follows very quickly after the head and shoulders are born.

The second stage of labor concludes with the birth of the neonate. Display 11-2 presents a list summarizing the mechanisms of labor.

Third Stage: Placental

The third stage of labor begins with the birth of the neonate and ends with the expulsion of the placenta. The average length of the *placental stage* is 5 to 30 minutes. There is an increased risk for complications if it takes longer than 30 minutes for the placenta to be expelled. However, efforts to shorten this stage, such as twisting or tugging on the umbilical cord, can cause serious complications and should be avoided.

Placental separation from the uterine wall occurs as the result of strong contractions. As the uterine size decreases after the birth of the neonate, the placenta folds, causing it to buckle off the uterine wall. Additional

bleeding causes further separation of the placenta from the uterine wall. Signs of placental separation include a change in the shape of the uterus to a globular shape, the rising uterus in the abdomen, increased length of the umbilical cord, and a gush of blood from the vagina. The woman is encouraged to bear down to promote expulsion of the placenta as these signs occur.

Two types of expulsion of the placenta have been identified. The most common mechanism, occurring in approximately 80% of deliveries, is the Schultze mechanism. In this mechanism, the central portion of the placenta releases first and the shiny fetal side of the placenta appears first. The Duncan mechanism occurs in the remaining 20% of deliveries. Separation takes place along the edges of the placenta first. The placenta is expelled sideways with the rough, dull ma-

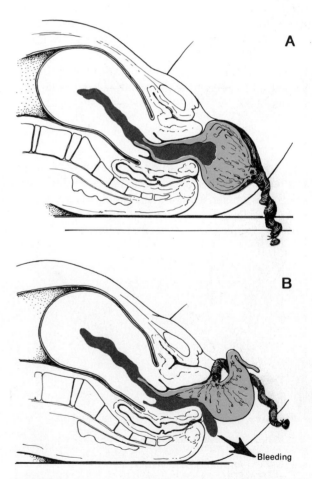

Figure 11-12. *Expulsion of the placenta by* **(A)** *Schultze mechanism, whereby the placenta is turned inside out within the vagina and is delivered with the glistening fetal surfaces to the outside, and by* **(B)** *the Duncan mechanism, whereby the placenta is rolled up in the vagina and is delivered with the maternal surface to the outside.*

DISPLAY 11-2
Second Stage of Labor

Effacement: 100%

Dilatation: 10 cm

Contractions

    Intensity—strong

    Frequency—every 1 to 3 minutes

    Duration—60 to 90 seconds

Length of stage

    Primipara—1 hour

    Multipara—30 minutes

    Outer limits—2 hours

DISPLAY 11-3
Third Stage of Labor

Placental delivery occurs in 5 to 30 minutes

Placental separation

    Fundus firmer and globular in shape

    Uterus rises in abdomen

    Umbilical cord lengthens as it extends from the vagina

    Increase in vaginal bleeding, often gushing

Bleeding may range between 250 mL and 500 mL

---

ternal side appearing first. They can be remembered by shiny Schultze (shiny fetal side appearing first) and dirty Duncan (rough, dull maternal side appearing first). Figure 11-12 illustrates both mechanisms. Contraction of the uterus after the expulsion of the placenta aids in the control of bleeding by helping to clamp the numerous small blood vessels. Normal blood loss during third stage of labor varies from 250 to 500 mL. The third stage of labor is summarized in Display 11-3.

Fourth Stage: Recovery

The first few hours (up to 4 hours) after birth are considered the fourth stage of labor. This is a period during which the woman's physiologic stability is restored. This stage of recovery is one in which there are risks of hemorrhage, hypotension, urinary retention, and reaction to

---

DISPLAY 11-4
Fourth Stage of Labor

Physiologic Characteristics

Fundus in the midline at the umbilicus

Perineal tenderness

Intermittent menstrual-type cramps

Vaginal bleeding bright red, with few small clots

May be insensitive to fullness of bladder

Psychologic Characteristics

Demonstrates elation about birth of baby

Touching of neonate progresses from fingertip to full embracing

Makes effort to have eye contact with neonate

Reaches actively for neonate

---

anesthesia if administered. The woman's body must begin to adapt to a nonpregnant state. Many psychologic changes also occur during this time. The early hours of this stage are very important in the beginning of the parent–child interactions and building of family relationships. Display 11-4 lists physical and psychologic characteristic of the fourth stage of labor.

Adolescent Considerations

The adolescent is still completing her own physical and psychologic growth. This may contribute to inadequate forces of labor. The adolescent's smaller size may cause problems in the passage. The psychologic aspects and insecurities of the adolescent may contribute to decreased or slowed uterine contractions. This increases the length of labor. In addition, the adolescent may be more concerned about her own self-image than the ultimate outcome of the labor.

The adolescent may lack a good support system during her labor. She may not have participated in childbirth preparation classes. The nurse needs to assess her knowledge to determine the additional support she will need during the first stage of labor. The adolescent may need complete information about her progress through labor. Sensitive nursing care is essential with the adolescent.

Cultural Considerations

When a woman who cannot speak or understand the language is admitted to a birthing unit, serious barriers in communication may exist. Frequently, the woman of another culture has been taught to suffer pain without complaining. This can obstruct the progress of first-stage labor. The nurse must be sensitive to the particular cultural attitudes of the woman.

The woman's sense of privacy and modesty is another primary concern. She may be sensitive or offended when she has to put on a hospital gown, or when she does not have the privacy she needs. Cultural patterns that establish the appropriate support person vary from one group to another. The woman should be permitted to have the support person of her choice with her.

The Role of the Nurse

The nurse must have a complete understanding of each of the four stages of labor to care for the woman in labor and childbirth. Understanding the importance of the forces of labor helps the nurse assess the woman and

SELF-ASSESSMENT

1. A fetus is considered engaged when the presenting part is level with:

- ☒ **A.** The ischial spines
- ○ **B.** The pelvic inlet
- ○ **C.** The pelvic outlet
- ○ **D.** The diagonal conjugate

2. How would you answer a patient who asks what it means that her baby is in a longitudinal lie?

- ○ **A.** The baby's head is the presenting part
- ○ **B.** The baby's buttocks is the presenting part
- ☒ **C.** The baby's spine is parallel to the mother's spine
- ○ **D.** The baby's spine is horizontal to the mother's spine

3. Which of the following contraction patterns should be immediately reported to a physician?

- ○ **A.** Every 2 minutes, lasting 90 seconds
- ☒ **B.** Every 4 minutes, lasting 110 seconds
- ○ **C.** Every 3 minutes, lasting 60 seconds
- ○ **D.** Every 7 minutes, lasting 15 seconds

4. Common subjective symptoms following lightening include all of the following EXCEPT:

- ○ **A.** Leg cramps
- ○ **B.** Frequent urination
- ○ **C.** Backache
- ☒ **D.** Dysuria

5. A woman at 38 weeks' gestation reports having a blood-tinged mucous discharge. The nurse should advise her to:

- ○ **A.** Immediately contact the physician
- ☒ **B.** Watch for signs of labor
- ○ **C.** Avoid strenuous activity
- ○ **D.** Count the number of times the fetus moves during the next 4 hours

DFIE

D— Descent — movement of the presenting part

F— Flexion — descending head meets resistance from the pelvic wall

I— Internal Rotation — is the movement when fetal head of the head from this position to the Anterior position

E— Extention — base of the occiput passes under the symphsis pubis causing extention of the head

E— External Rotation — when the rotation to align c̄ the shoulders

E— Explosion — when anterior shodder is born followed by posterior

identify any aspects that must be reported. Signs and symptoms of the onset of labor alert the nurse to the progress of the beginning of labor.

With accurate knowledge of the first stage of labor, the nurse can assess the progress of labor, assess the woman's need for pain relief, and assist her and her support person throughout the long latent phase, into the active phase, and through the transition to the sec-ond stage of labor. In the second and third stages of la-bor, the nurse can help detect the needs of the mother as the baby is born and the placenta is expelled. In the fourth stage of labor, the nurse has many responsibili-ties to assess and evaluate the woman's condition. The nurse's knowledge of the physical and psychologic con-siderations provide the basis for planning and imple-menting individualized nursing care.

REVIEW AND PREVIEW

In this chapter, the process of labor and childbirth were dis-cussed. The signs and symptoms of the onset of labor were pre-sented, including lightening, cervical changes, weight loss, and backache. The differentiation between true and false labor were examined. The progress that occurs from the latent to the active to the transition phases in the first stage of labor were presented, including the criteria used to determine when the woman is mov-ing from one phase to another. The discussion of the second stage of labor touched on the mechanisms of labor, including crowning and birth of the neonate. The adaptations of the fetus to the ma-ternal pelvic openings completed the discussion of the second stage of labor.

The third stage of labor, the placental stage, included signs that indicate the placenta is about to be expelled. The two placenta expulsion mechanisms, Schultze and Duncan, were addressed. Fi-nally, the concerns of the fourth stage of labor, recovery, were pre-sented. The adaptation of the woman's body to a nonpregnant state is begun.

In the next chapter, the physiologic and psychologic consid-erations presented in this chapter will provide the framework for the nursing care of the family having a baby. The importance of sensitive, empathetic, knowledgeable nursing care in the assess-ment, intervention, and implementation will be stressed in caring for the woman with an uncomplicated labor and childbirth experi-ence.

◈ KEY POINTS

◆ The forces of labor are the passenger, the passage, the pow-ers, and the psyche.
◆ The onset of labor is determined by assessing effacement and dilatation of the cervix.
◆ Signs and symptoms of impending labor are lightening, cervi-cal changes, rupture of membranes, gastrointestinal distur-bances, persistent backache, and nesting behaviors.
◆ In true labor, uterine contractions increase in intensity, fre-quency, and duration, and the cervix effaces and dilates.
◆ In false labor, there are no cervical changes, and contractions are irregular.
◆ Factors influencing labor include the woman's psychologic state, support system, childbirth preparation, past experi-ences, and coping strategies.

◆ There are four stages of labor: first, effacement and dilata-tion; second, expulsion; third, placental; fourth, recovery.
◆ Cervical effacement is the obliteration of the cervical canal; cervical dilatation is the gradual enlargement of the exter-nal cervical os.
◆ The three phases of the first stage of labor are latent, active, and transition.
◆ Fetal position is the relationship of the fetal presenting part to the maternal pelvis; fetal lie is the relationship of the fetus to the maternal spinal column; fetal presentation is the fetal part that enters the pelvis first.
◆ The mechanisms of labor are descent, presenting part en-gages the pelvis; flexion, fetal chin rests on sternum; internal rotation, fetal head rotates from transverse position to ante-rior or posterior position; extension, fetal head extends to-ward vulvar opening; external rotation (restitution), at birth, fetal head rotates to align with shoulders; and expulsion, birth of neonate.

BIBLIOGRAPHY

Cunningham, F. G., MacDonald, P. C., Gant, N. F., Leveno, K. J., & Gilstrap, L. C. (1993). *Williams obstetrics* (19th ed.). Norwalk, CT: Appleton-Lange.

Khazoyan, C. M. & Anderson, N. L. R. (1994). Latinas' expectations from their partners during childbirth. *Maternal Child Nursing 19*: 226–229.

Knupple, R. A., & Drukker, J. E. (1993). *High-risk pregnancy: A team ap-proach* (2nd ed). Philadelphia: W. B. Saunders.

Koniak-Griffin, D. (1993). Maternal role attainment. *Image, Journal of Nursing Scholarship 25* (3), 257–262 .

May, K. A., & Mahlmeister, L. R. (1994). *Comprehensive maternity nursing, nursing process, and the childbearing family* (3rd ed) Philadelphia: J. B. Lippincott.

Miller, B. F., & Keane, O. B. (1992). *Encyclopedia and dictionary of med-icine, nursing, and applied health* (5th ed.). Philadelphia: W. B. Saunders.

Quirk, J. G. (1992). *Perinatal Educational Resource and Learning System— PERLS.* Little Rock: University of Arkansas for Medical Sciences.

Reeder, S. J., & Martin, L. L. (1991). *Essentials of maternity nursing: Family centered care.* Philadelphia: J. B. Lippincott.

Reeder, S. J., Martin, L. L., & Koniak, D. (1992). *Maternity nursing: Family, newborn, and women's health care* (17th ed.). Philadelphia: J. B. Lip-pincott.

Scherer, J. C. (1992). *Introductory clinical pharmacology* (4th ed.). Philadelphia: J. B. Lippincott.

CHAPTER 12

Nursing Care During Normal Labor and Childbirth

◆ OBJECTIVES

When the learning goals of this chapter are met, the reader will be able to:

◆ Discuss the admission process, including the routine procedures the nurse performs.
◆ List the important information the nurse collects during the admission assessment.
◆ Explain the reason for pain relief in labor and birth and identify the two types of pain relief approaches that are used.
◆ List the nonmedicated comfort measures that are available to women during labor and childbirth.
◆ Describe how the nurse provides physical and psychosocial support during the first stage of labor.
◆ Discuss the nurse's role during the second stage of labor.
◆ Describe the care of the neonate immediately after birth.
◆ Explain the events that signify the third stage of labor, and list the primary concerns of the physical supportive care for the woman.
◆ Define the fourth stage of labor.
◆ Discuss cultural considerations and their significance for families during labor and birth.

TERMINOLOGY

Amniotomy	Ferning
Analgesia	Local infiltration
Anesthesia	Nitrazine paper
Apgar score	Nuchal cord
Ataractic	Paracervical block
Barbiturates	Pudendal block
Epidural	Spinal block
Episiotomy	

The process of labor and birth can be an incredibly exciting and rewarding experience for families and nurses. Maternal-newborn nursing care focuses on providing support, comfort, and safety for the woman and the neonate during childbirth. Routine admission procedures prepare the woman for labor and birth. During the admission process, the nurse helps the family feel welcome and becomes familiar with the woman and her needs and preferences. Establishing an open, accepting approach encourages the woman and her family to discuss their concerns and develop trust in the nurse. The nurse explains procedures and prepares the woman for the labor and birth process.

This chapter discusses the role of the nurse during admission and the four stages of labor. Physical and emotional support are stressed. The nurse can use methods of pain relief, such as comfort measures and medications, and can provide information about regional anesthesia, to promote a positive childbirth experience. A variety of nursing assessment activities supply the nurse with necessary information about the health and well-being of the woman and the neonate. Nursing care is based on the needs of the woman and her family. Individual cultural beliefs and practices are considered as the plan of care is developed and implemented.

Admission Care and Procedures

Each health care facility has its own set of standard admission procedures that establish the guidelines for care. When a woman reaches the labor and delivery area in active labor, an identification bracelet is placed on her wrist. The time and date are noted in the record. The woman, her support person, and family receive explanations about visiting hours, the location of the call bell system, how to control the bed, and the location of the bathroom. It is appropriate to introduce the woman and her companion to the health care team members who will participate in her care and the care of the neonate. The health care team members vary from one facility to another. Included are the nursing personnel, the birth attendant (obstetrician or midwife), and possibly an anesthesiologist.

The nurse provides privacy for the woman and asks her to change into a gown. The support person is made comfortable in an appropriate area. Personal valuables are handled according to the facility's policy. The woman's prenatal records are requested to determine the type and frequency of prenatal care. The nurse dou-

ble-checks this information and confirms with her the expected date of delivery (EDD), parity, health care providers, and her preferred method of infant feeding. If the woman has not received any prenatal care, the nurse performs a full antepartum assessment (see Chapter 6).

The initial assessment includes obtaining baseline data and ruling out high-risk situations. The nurse begins by checking the woman's vital signs. Contractions are assessed to determine their frequency, duration, and intensity. The nurse questions the woman to determine the time that labor began, the activity level of the fetus, and whether her membranes (bag of waters) have ruptured. If the membranes have ruptured, the nurse further determines the time they ruptured and the character and color of the fluid. The fetus is evaluated by determining the rate and location of the fetal heart tones. The nurse uses external electronic fetal monitoring to obtain a baseline 20- to 30-minute monitor strip of fetal heart tones and contractions (see Chapter 10).

While the woman is being monitored, the nurse documents the time the woman last ate and what type of food she ate. Fluids and ice chips may be offered according to protocol. After the external monitoring is completed, a vaginal examination is generally performed as long as there is no vaginal bleeding and the membranes are intact. The degree of dilatation and effacement of the cervix is noted (see Chapter 11). If the policy of the facility allows the practice, a nurse may perform the examination. The woman may be encouraged to walk, if the assessment thus far is normal and she is in early labor. The health care provider is notified about the admission, and appropriate orders are documented. Intravenous fluids, enemas, and perineal shaves may be ordered or may be part of the facility's protocol.

Assessment

To plan appropriate care, the health status of the woman and fetus are determined, including any apparent maternal-newborn problems. On admission, baseline information is gathered to assess the woman's health condition and stage of labor and to rule out complications. See the Assessment Checklist for a summary of the activities that occur during admission.

History

A history of medical and obstetric information about the woman and her family is obtained from the

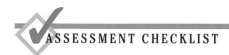

ASSESSMENT CHECKLIST

Admission Care and Procedures

History

Medical and obstetric history of woman and family

Blood type and Rh factor

Allergies to food and medication

Physical Assessment

Head to toe

Swelling of hands, face, and ankles

Weight

Fundal height

Hydration

Elimination patterns

Epigastric problems

Respiratory difficulties

Reflexes

Headaches/visual disturbances

Oxygenation status

Abdominal palpation

Psychosocial Assessment

Prenatal education

Labor partner effectiveness

Self-confidence

Response to labor

Coping strategies

Neonatal feeding choice

Laboratory Tests

CBC

Blood type

Rh factor

Indirect Coombs'

Urinalysis

VDRL

Glucose

Hepatitis

Sickle cell preparation (according to policy)

Maternal Assessments

Vital signs

Contraction frequency, duration, intensity

Status of membranes

Vaginal bleeding

Fetal Assessments

Fetal heart tones (FHT)

Presentation

Progress of Labor

Degree of dilatation and effacement

Fetal station

---

woman's records and the admission interview. The nurse discusses any medical problems that may influence the course of labor and birth, including past birthing experiences. Any other pertinent information the woman offers is communicated to the health care team and documented in the patient record. The interview gives the nurse a chance to talk with the woman to identify any important predisposing factors.

Psychosocial Assessment

The emotional, or psychosocial, needs of the woman are just as essential as her physical requirements. Accurate assessment of the woman's ability to cope with the childbirth experience is more challenging than measuring vital signs. The nurse provides opportunities for the woman and her support person to ask questions and review various relaxation and breathing techniques. If they lack preparation, the nurse explains, in an unhur-

ried manner, ways the labor coach can support the woman (Fig. 12-1). Generally, continual reinforcement about ways to improve the woman's comfort level are appreciated by everyone. The nurse's caring, compassionate approach, with positive feedback and a "you can do it" attitude, sets the tone. The nurse assesses the support person's expectations and ability and willingness to participate. By offering guidance and suggestions, the nurse encourages continual sharing of information.

The woman's response to labor and her coping strategies are essential clues in establishing appropriate nursing diagnoses. Nursing interventions are directed at assisting the woman and her support person to cope with the labor process. The nurse is available for support and allows the support person to lead as long as the woman remains relaxed and follows her partner's directions. If the woman is unable to relax and breathe effectively with contractions, the nurse takes a more ac-

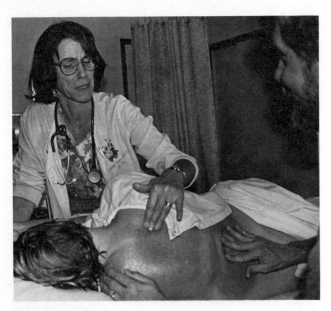

Figure 12-1. *The first stage of labor is generally the best time to reinforce or teach support measures to the woman and her partner.*

tive approach. The nurse keeps the family informed about the progress of labor.

The nurse evaluates the woman's infant feeding preference, including possible indecision about whether she will breast- or bottle-feed her newborn. This uncertainty, along with family pressure about infant feeding, may create anxiety for the woman. The nurse provides information to the mother about the advantages and disadvantages of each method.

Laboratory Tests

The nurse reviews the prenatal and intrapartum laboratory test results. In particular, the nurse evaluates the findings of the complete blood count (CBC), blood type, Rh factor, indirect Coombs', urinalysis, Venereal Disease Research Laboratory tests (VDRL), glucose screen, hepatitis screen, and sickle cell preparation. Sickle cell preparation is performed according to facility protocol. Results from these tests may indicate potential or actual presence of anemia, diabetes, fetal hemolytic disease (eg, erythroblastosis fetalis), infection, bleeding problems, active sexually transmitted diseases (STDs), and compromised oxygen-carrying capacity of the blood. (See Appendix D.)

Maternal Status

The woman's condition has a major impact on the outcome of labor and fetal well-being. Assessment of the woman's status includes measurement of vital signs, de-

termination of frequency, duration, and intensity of contractions, membrane status, and presence of vaginal bleeding.

Vital Signs

The nurse measures and records the woman's blood pressure, pulse, respiratory rate, and temperature. A comparison with baseline vital signs from the prenatal record is completed; abnormal variations are noted and reported. An increase in temperature may suggest infection; elevated blood pressure may indicate anxiety or preeclampsia; and changes in pulse and respiratory rates may imply that other physiologic difficulties are occurring.

Contractions

The duration, frequency, and intensity of contractions give the nurse information about the progress of labor. A typical pattern documented in normal labor indicates that progress is occurring in a timely fashion. Normally, contractions progress from 30 to 90 seconds in duration, occur from 15 to 2 minutes apart in frequency, and intensify as labor accelerates.

Membrane Status

The woman is questioned to determine whether her membranes have ruptured. The nurse explains that a small amount of trickling of fluid may indicate that the membranes have ruptured. Women are often unsure if their membranes have ruptured or whether what they felt was leaking urine caused by pressure of the fetus on the bladder. To confirm if there was spontaneous rupture of the membranes (SROM), the nurse performs a nitrazine paper test. **Nitrazine paper** is a small strip of paper that is sensitive to pH. It turns blue when moistened by amniotic fluid. The sample of fluid can be obtain by touching the paper strip against woman's moist vaginal tissue. In another test, a small amount of fluid is placed on a slide and viewed under a microscope. Amniotic fluid displays a characteristic frondlike pattern called **ferning**. The nurse documents the woman's response to the question about ruptured membranes, including the time, appearance, and amount of the amniotic fluid released, if the membranes did indeed rupture. If the membranes remain intact, the birth attendant may allow them to rupture naturally or may decide to perform an amniotomy.

An **amniotomy** is the artificial rupture of the membranes (AROM). The amniotomy is performed during a vaginal exam. The attendant uses a special sterile plastic hooklike device to pierce the membranes without harming the fetus. Whenever the membranes rupture, the time of rupture, color, and odor of the amniotic fluid are recorded. Amniotic fluid is normally clear or pale amber with a slightly fleshy odor. Whenever the membranes rupture, whether spontaneously or artificially, the fetal heart rate (FHR) is assessed and documented to detect the possibility of prolapsed cord (see Chapter 13).

Bleeding

The presence of vaginal bleeding is carefully assessed for amount, color, and potential signs of hemorrhage. Bloody show and small amounts of vaginal bleeding during the first stage of labor are considered normal. This bleeding comes from small capillaries, which rupture as the mucus plug is expelled and the cervical os changes. Moderate to large amounts of bleeding should be reported immediately so that its cause can be determined. Vaginal examinations are not performed if bleeding is moderate to heavy in amount.

Fetal Assessment

Fetal assessment begins soon after the woman is admitted. The fetal heart rate (FHR) is traced during electronic fetal monitoring (EFM), or by intermittent fetoscope or Doppler probe. A baseline monitor strip is obtained for evaluation of fetal heart rate patterns and for later comparison. Normal fetal heart rate is between 120 and 160 beats per minute. Decelerations, or lowering, of the heart rate are reported and analyzed for signs of fetal distress. The FHR is evaluated in relationship to the uterine contractions (see Chapter 10). In early labor, the woman may walk about with hourly assessments of the fetus. As labor progresses, fetal assessments are made every 15 to 30 minutes. Tracings using the EFM are often continued throughout the second stage of labor (see later discussion).

Progress of Labor

The pattern of labor is evaluated to determine how far it has progressed over a given period. A vaginal examination is performed to assess the dilatation and effacement of the cervix and the station of the presenting part. The examiner performs the vaginal examination with a sterile lubricated gloved hand. The examiner's fingers are inserted into the vagina, and the cervix is palpated to calculate effacement and dilatation (Fig. 12-2).

The station of the presenting part of the fetus is measured in relation to the maternal ischial spines (see Chapter 11). The potential for a prolapsed cord is increased when the presenting part is not yet engaged. Chapter 13 discusses prolapsed cord and other complications during labor and childbirth.

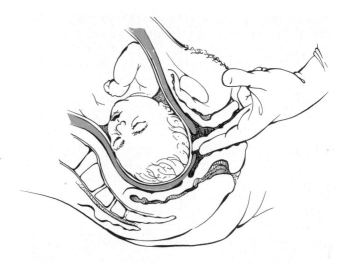

Figure 12-2. *The vaginal examination provides important information about the progress of labor, including the cervical effacement and dilatation.*

Preparation According to Facility Protocol

Preparation of the woman varies from one facility to the next. The nurse is expected to be familiar with the facility protocols and follow the established guidelines. Orders from birth attendants may vary from the standard protocols but still be within acceptable practice limits. Examples of acceptable practices ordered by birth attendants include small snacklike nourishments, lukewarm bathing (if the membranes are intact), and showering.

Pain Management in Labor and Birth

An important part of nursing care in labor and birth is pain management. The alleviation or reduction of pain can be accomplished with nonpharmacologic and pharmacologic approaches, or a combination of both. Pain management is aimed at reducing stress and anxiety. The objective of pain management is to provide maximum relief while maintaining maximum safety for the woman and fetus. When these goals are achieved, the chances of providing a positive family experience during labor and childbirth are increased.

Causes of Pain During Labor and Birth

There are different causes of pain in each stage of labor. During the first stage of labor, uterine contractions force the cervix to dilate and efface. This change in the cervical os is accomplished by stretching and pulling of the associated muscles. The entire uterus contracts during labor in an effort to expand its lower segment for the birth of the fetus; and the vaginal canal stretches to accommodate passage of the fetus. Stretching of the uterus, cervix, and birth canal produces the pain most commonly experienced during labor. Fetal presentation also can add to discomfort when the head is in a posterior position, such as ROP (right occiput posterior) or LOP (left occiput posterior), as described in Chapter 11. The fetal head pressing against the woman's spine adds to back strain and discomfort.

In the second stage of labor, tremendous pressure is exerted on the perineum as the fetus is pushed forward. The result is extreme stretching of the vaginal canal and opening. The intensity of uterine contractions increase markedly here, adding to the degree of discomfort. If an **episiotomy** (surgical incision into the perineum) is performed, the woman may experience associated uneasiness when local anesthetic is injected into the perineum. Lacerations in the cervix or vagina during the second stage of labor increase the woman's sensation of pain.

The third stage of labor is a relatively relaxed time for the woman, with the exception of a few strong uterine contractions that occur just before the placenta is delivered. The use of fundal pressure to assist in the expulsion of the placenta typically causes discomfort (Fig. 12-3).

Repair of the episiotomy or lacerations takes place during the third or fourth stage of labor. Injection of extra local anesthetic at the repair site is felt by many women. The woman may have an exaggeration of discomfort in the fourth stage. This is because she may have been sensitized to the extreme amount of discomfort she experienced during labor, and now feels pain in magnified proportions.

A cycle of responses known as the fear–tension–pain syndrome may be assessed at any stage of labor. If the woman fears the outcome of labor or the pain she feels, she becomes more tense; as tension increases, muscles contract and pain increases. As pain increases, fear increases, and so on, leading to a vicious cycle. Pain relief is critical to breaking the cycle (Table 12-1).

Comfort Measures

There are many nonpharmacologic comfort measures that promote pain management and are very effective in decreasing the need for administering analgesics. Proper position and frequent changes in positioning are key factors in increasing comfort in labor. Many women often find showering during labor helps to reduce pain and foster comfort. Physical touch can be very soothing to the woman in labor during the early phase of labor. Back rubs, back supports, and gentle abdominal massage (effleurage) aid in relaxing muscles and decreasing pain. Many women state that a cool cloth applied to the forehead between contractions is very refreshing.

Distraction is an effective method of pain reduction. Playing music that the woman finds relaxing, watching television, or talking on the phone are all ways of drawing attention away from the woman's discomfort. Guided imagery, a relatively new form of relaxation, refocuses attention from pain toward more pleasant thoughts. The nurse encourages the woman to concentrate on a particular place or moment in her life that induces feelings of calmness or interest. This peaceful memory serves to distract attention from the discomfort of labor contractions. Meditation is often used. In this method the woman has a focal point, such as a favorite photo or other object. During contractions she concentrates on the focal point while using her breathing patterns. Along with relaxation and proper breathing, some professionals report hypnotherapy during labor is helpful in reducing pain.

There are times when nonpharmacologic methods of pain relief need to be combined with pharmacologic management. Regardless of the choice of pain relief method, the nurse provides support to the woman who is ultimately responsible for choosing the method of pain control. The nurse can provide reassurance to the woman and her partner that pharmacologic methods

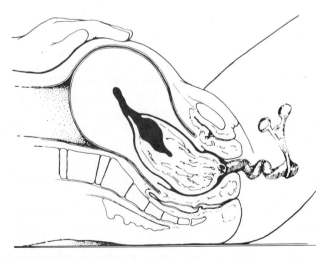

Figure 12-3. *The birth attendant may apply gentle fundal pressure to promote placental separation and delivery. The woman may experience pain and discomfort during the third stage of labor.*

Table 12-1. *Pain Responses in Labor*

Stage of Labor	Cause of Pain	Where Pain Is Experienced	Physiologic and Psychologic Response
First Stage	Cervical stretching Pressure on bladder and urethra Distention of the lower uterine segment Pressure on the nerve ganglia around the uterus and vagina	Lower abdomen, lower lumbar spine, and upper sacrum. Also may be felt in the upper thighs and umbilical region.	Anxiety causes stress resulting in: Hyperventilation, increased oxygen consumption, increased autonomic activity. Increased autonomic activity may result in: Increased peripheral resistance, increased cardiac output, and blood pressure. Impaired uterine contractions. Metabolic acidemia may result from respiratory alkalosis as a result of hyperventilation and increased fatty acids from lipolysis. Fetal acidosis may result from: Decreased placental perfusion and maternal metabolic acidemia. Woman may have increased gastric acidity.
Second Stage	Stretching of the vagina and perineum	Vagina and pelvic floor	See above. The muscles of the pelvic floor may tighten, obstructing the descent of the fetus.
Third Stage	Episiotomy, lacerations of the birth canal, hematomas, and edema. Uterine contractions in expulsion of the placenta	Vaginal and perineal region; contractions felt in the abdominal region.	Anxiety of additional pain may result in woman's lack of cooperation in expelling the placenta.
Fourth Stage	Repair of episiotomy, lacerations	Vaginal and perineal region.	May interfere with the woman's interaction with the neonate. May cause anger and resentment toward infant and family members. Woman may be very fatigued.

From: May, K. A. & Mahlmeister, L. R. (1994). *Maternal & neonatal care: Family-centered care* (3rd ed.). Philadelphia: J. B. Lippincott.

[handwritten margin notes: Fear → Pain → Tension — Dr Grantly Dick Read Theory.]

are safe and acceptable when they are carefully administered and monitored.

Pain Medication

Pain medication in labor can assist the woman to maintain control and actively participate in the birth experience. Typically, the dosage ordered is enough to take the "edge" off, so that adequate relaxation and breathing can be realized. There are many forms of pain medication used in labor, including analgesics, barbiturates, ataractic, and regional anesthesia. All forms of pain medications cross the placental barrier and must be given with appropriate judgment to prevent fetal or maternal complications. The woman will be able to determine her choice for pain relief if she is provided easy-to-understand information. Herbal pain remedies may be used in some cultures to reduce pain and dis-

Table 12-2. *Analgesics Commonly Used During Labor*

Drug	Maternal Side Effects	Fetal/Neonatal Side Effects	Nursing Implications
Analgesics Morphine sulfate Meperidine hydrochloride (Demerol) Fentanyl (Sublimaze) Nalbuphine Nubain	All cause CNS depression, especially respiratory; and nausea and vomiting. All except morphine cause hypotension. Fentanyl and Nalbuphine cause blurred vision. Nalbuphine also causes dry mouth and diaphoresis; may precipitate withdrawal in narcotic-dependent women.	All cause transient decrease in FHR variability. Morphine, meperidine, and fentanyl cause CNS depression. Nalbuphine causes respiratory depression.	Morphine not commonly used in labor; more commonly used to induce speed in the onset of labor. Meperidine is the most commonly used narcotic in labor. Best administered at least 2 hours before birth to decrease CNS depression in neonate. Fentanyl is short-acting for use in late active phase. Must watch for respiratory depression; be prepared to administer narcotic antagonist for depression noted in woman or neonate. Nalbuphine not to be administered to narcotic-dependent woman. Narcan may need to be administered to neonate for CNS depression.
Barbiturates Sodium secobarbital (Seconal) Sodium pentobarbital (Nembutal) Sodium phenobarbital (Luminal)	Reduced tension, release of inhibitions; lethargy, hypotension, decreased sensory perception; restlessness in presence of pain or as an idiosyncrasy.	CNS depression; neonatal hypotonia; delay in establishing feeding.	Used to induce sedation in prolonged latent phase of labor. *There is no available antagonist.* Will cause restlessness in woman in pain; avoid use in active labor.
Ataractics Promazine (Sparine) Promethazine (Phenergan) Hydroxyzine (Vistaril)	Potentiates narcotic effects; antiemetic. Use with analgesic; may produce pseudo-hypnotic effect. Hydroxyzine may cause pain at IM site.	Potentiates CNS depression.	Monitor all closely; use safety measures for medicated woman. Administer promethazine deep IM. Administer hydroxyzine deep IM using z-track technique; alert care provider if spasmodic eye or neck movements noted.

Adapted from May, K. A. & Mahlmeister, L. R. (1994). *Maternal & neonatal care: Family-centered care* (3rd ed.). Philadelphia. J. B. Lippincott, Table 24-2, p. 607.

comfort. Ideally, options should be discussed during early labor when the woman is better able to concentrate.

Analgesia

Analgesia is the relief of pain without the loss of consciousness. A variety of options are available, including analgesics, barbiturates, ataractics, and tranquilizers. Table 12-2 presents a comparison of drugs commonly used for analgesia in obstetrics.

Anesthesia

Anesthesia is the loss of feeling or sensation. Pain management during labor can be achieved with either local, regional, or general anesthesia. The benefit of all of these methods, except general anesthesia, is that the woman remains awake and can participate in the birth of her neonate. The side effects of the various methods are considered. Some situations require general anesthesia, but this method is reserved for emergency situations and is not deemed a form of pain management. Table 12-3 provides an overview of the various types of anesthesia used in labor and birth.

Nurses educate families about the advantages and disadvantages of pain management options. Nursing care provides physical and psychosocial support and comfort measures during the four stages of labor. See the Nursing Interventions Checklist on page 200 for pain management during labor and birth.

Nursing Care During the First Stage of Labor

The first stage of labor is also called the stage of effacement and dilatation. It starts with the onset of true labor and is complete when the cervix reaches 10 cm (full dilatation) and 100% effacement. A nursing care plan is established (See Nursing Care Plan: The Pregnant Woman in the First Stage of Labor on page 201). Nursing care during the first stage of labor includes ongoing assessment and physical and psychosocial support of the woman and her partner.

Ongoing Assessment

As the cervix dilates and effaces, the nurse continually assesses maternal contractions. Maternal vital signs, level of anxiety, knowledge deficits, and the ability to relax during labor are monitored. Fetal status is determined by auscultating or recording the fetal heart rate at various intervals. These assessment activities take place regularly to confirm that labor is continuing in a normal fashion. Early recognition of deviations from normal allow the health care team to intervene and ensure the health and well-being of the woman and the fetus.

Physical Support

Under normal circumstances, maternal vital signs are recorded at least every hour during early labor. Temperature measurements are taken every 2 to 4 hours if the findings are normal. During transition, the last phase of the first stage of labor, the vital signs are taken every 30 minutes.

Uterine contractions are monitored every hour as long as the woman feels comfortable enough to sit or walk around. This is true as long as there are no contraindications, such as vaginal bleeding. As transition approaches, most women prefer a reclining position. At this time, continuous contraction and fetal monitoring can be easily performed. The frequency of vaginal examinations depends on the signals from the woman. Generally, cervical dilatation and effacement are assessed hourly during active labor.

In low-risk situations, the FHR is assessed every hour in the latent phase and every 30 minutes in the active phase of first-stage labor. In high-risk situations, the FHR is assessed every 30 minutes in the latent phase and every 15 minutes in the active phase. Changes in maternal vital signs require more frequent assessment of the FHR to determine the presence of decelerations (see Chapter 10). The FHR and response to contractions is measured continuously or every 15 minutes during transition.

Comfort measures during the first stage of labor include position changes, such as a left side-lying position to improve maternal–placental circulation, elevation of the head of the bed, or using several pillows for support of the woman's back and legs. The nurse changes the bed linens and pads as needed to provide a clean dry bed for comfort. The woman may appreciate ice chips to suck or a cool cloth to her forehead. Lower back and abdominal massages may be helpful.

During the early phase of the first stage of labor, the nurse suggests helpful comfort measures the support person may use. The woman and her partner are often best able to hear and understand new information at this time.

The woman is encouraged to empty her bladder at frequent intervals. A full bladder increases discomfort and may require catheterization as labor progresses. Regional anesthesia also may decrease the woman's perception of the need to void. Perineal care after voiding and as needed provides an improved sense of comfort for the woman. The nurse provides privacy when the perineum is cleansed. Many women express an interest in showering during labor. The warm water may improve her ability to relax and improve the action of the uterine contractions.

During transition, the woman may become overwhelmed by the strong, rapid contractions. A feeling of panic may come over her. The nurse needs to stay with the laboring woman and her partner during this stressful time. The woman may experience diaphoresis, nausea, and vomiting, or she may have chills and shaking. The nurse provides a cool cloth, a fan, and ice chips for diaphoresis. A blanket is comforting if she is chilling, and holding her limbs may help control the shaking. The nurse can give the woman an emesis basin and reassure her that the nausea and vomiting are not unusual. If the woman is upset that she

Table 12-3. *Types of Anesthesia Used During Labor and Birth*

Type	Site	When Administered	Purpose	Effects	Side Effects
Pudendal block (Figure 12-4A)	Around pudendal nerve	Late second stage	For episiotomy and repairs	Produces perineal anesthesia, results in relaxation; hastens descent and birth	None known
Local infiltration (Figure 12-4B)	Into perineal tissues	Late third stage	For episiotomy and repairs	Small area anesthetized for short period	None known
Paracervical block (Figure 12-4C)	Intravaginally into the rim of the cervix	Active phase of first stage	Local relief of pain	Pain relief at site of injection (used infrequently)	High risk of maternal hypotension, fetal bradycardia and distress
Spinal block	Injected directly into spinal fluid in spinal canal	Late in second stage in vaginal birth; also used as anesthesia for cesarean birth	Vaginal or cesarean births	Peaks immediately; lasts up to 6 hours. Must be carefully placed to avoid anesthesia above the level of the uterus; maternal hypotension, and fetal hypoxia.	Maternal hypotension, post administration spinal headache. Woman may be kept flat for 6 hours postpartum. Adequate hydration may help alleviate.
Epidural (Figure 12-5)	Injected into the epidural space of spine using flexible catheter.	Usually when cervix is dilated 4 to 6 cm	Vaginal or cesarean births	Provides continuous pain relief during labor, birth and repair of episiotomy. Narcotics such as fentanyl or morphine can be added to increase duration. Can be left in place for patient-controlled analgesia postpartum	Maternal hypotension and fetal bradycardia. Spinal headaches rare
General anesthesia	Administered intravenously by anesthesiologist	Minimal anesthesia before fetus removed. Woman further anesthetized for completion of procedure.	Cesarean birth. No longer used for vaginal births	Woman completely anesthetized	High risk of circulatory and respiratory depression in fetus. Neonate sluggish at birth. High risk of maternal aspiration resulting in severe pneumonitis from acidic gastric contents. If necessary in emergency, sodium citrate administered preoperatively to neutralize stomach pH

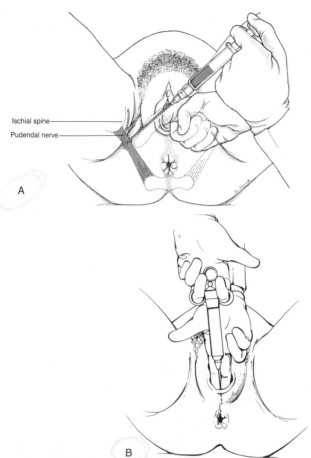

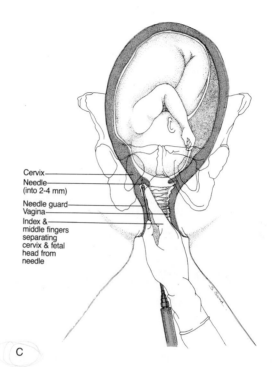

Figure 12-4. *Sites for anesthesia:* **(A)** *The pudendal block.* **(B)** *Local infiltration.* **(C)** *The paracervical block.*

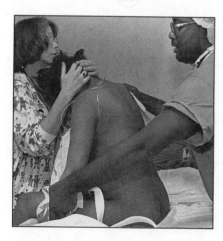

Figure 12-5. *The nurse assists the woman into the correct position for insertion of the epidural catheter into the epidural space.*

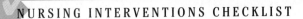

NURSING INTERVENTIONS CHECKLIST

Pain Management in Labor and Birth

Causes

First Stage

Uterine contractions

Dilatation and effacement of cervix

Stretching of vaginal canal

Fetal presentation

Second Stage

Perineal pressure

Strong uterine contractions

Episiotomy

Lacerations

Third Stage

Uterine contractions

Fundal pressure

Fourth Stage

Repair of episiotomy

Interventions

Nonpharmacologic

Relaxation and breathing

Position changes

Showering

Back support

Back rub

Abdominal massage

Cool cloth to forehead

Distraction

Hypnosis

Pharmacologic

Analgesics

    Demeraol, morphine sulfate

Barbiturates

    Seconal, Nembutal

Ataractic

    Sparine, Phenergen

    Vistaril

Regional anesthesia

    Spinal block

    Epidural

    Paracervical

    Pudendal block

    Local infiltration

is hiccoughing, burping, or expelling flatus, the nurse can reassure her that this is common and beyond her control. Some women have an urge to push before full dilatation of the cervix. The nurse must urge her not to push, but to blow the contractions away. Calm reassurance by the nurse is helpful during this stressful time.

Psychosocial Support

The woman may experience feelings of frustration, exhaustion, disappointment, and abandonment as contractions increase in frequency and intensity. The support person may experience feelings of inadequacy in providing measures to alleviate the woman's pain and discomfort.

Understanding and empathy expressed by the nurse can help to calm the unstable emotions of the woman and her partner. It is crucial that the woman, family, and partner be kept informed about the progress of labor. Reminders that the woman is doing a great job handling the contractions and the fetus is stable reinforces a positive attitude in the woman. Praise and positive feedback sustain the woman and give her the desire to see labor through until the end. See the Nursing Interventions Checklist for care during the first stage of labor.

NURSING CARE PLAN
For the Pregnant Woman in the First Stage of Labor

ASSESSMENT: Complaints of painful uterine contractions
Spontaneous rupture of membranes
Bloody show
EDD demonstrates 40 weeks' gestation

NURSING DIAGNOSIS #1: Pain, related to regular uterine contractions

EXPECTED OUTCOME: The woman will verbalize a tolerance of pain as evidenced by increased ability to relax and breath appropriately during contractions.

Nursing Interventions	*Rationale*
1. Demonstrate and evaluate the woman's and support person's breathing techniques.	1. To analyze if appropriate breathing is being done.
2. Change positions frequently and support back and legs with pillows.	2. Changing positions often increases comfort level.
3. Encourage showering.	3. Warm water relaxes abdominal muscles and reduces pain.
4. Medicate with analgesics as needed.	4. Decreases sensation to pain.

EVALUATION: The woman experiencing pain with uterine contractions verbalized an ability to tolerate pain.

NURSING DIAGNOSIS #2: Anxiety, related to unknown outcome of labor experience

EXPECTED OUTCOME: The woman will express a reduction of anxiety after teaching and reassurance by the nurse.

Nursing Interventions	*Rationale*
1. Offer support and reassurance that a positive outcome is anticipated.	1. Anxiety decreases with positive attitudes by staff.
2. Evaluate existing knowledge of labor and childbirth.	2. To provide individualized teaching based on needs and learning ability.
3. Discuss normal and probable events of an uncomplicated labor and childbirth.	3. Familiarity with what should be expected decreases fear and anxiety.

EVALUATION: The woman with a knowledge deficit stated what is expected in normal labor and childbirth, and what she can anticipate as she progresses.

Nursing Care During the Second Stage of Labor

The second stage of labor is defined as complete effacement and dilatation of the cervix, ending with the birth of the neonate. During this stage, nursing care shifts to supporting the woman as she actively participates in bearing down, pushing the fetus downward through the dilated cervix. Ongoing assessment and physical and psychosocial support are required. The nurse assists in positioning and preparing the woman for childbirth. If an episiotomy is performed, the nurse supports the woman and helps the birth attendant. All maternal-newborn care is documented in the record.

Ongoing Assessments

A vaginal examination is performed if the woman experiences tremendous perineal pressure and a strong urge to push or bear down during contractions. The woman must be discouraged from pushing before full cervical dilatation to avoid edema of the cervix. When the cervix is fully effaced and dilated, the woman is encouraged to push and bear down.

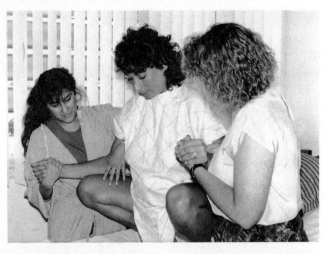

NURSING INTERVENTIONS CHECKLIST

Care During the First Stage of Labor

Physical Support

Record maternal contractions, FHT, and maternal vital signs

Encourage ambulation or sitting out of bed

Encourage position changes, such as side-lying

Elevate head of bed

Massage back and abdomen

Apply cool cloth to forehead

Showers as desired

Keep bed clean, dry, and wrinkle-free

Cleanse perineal area frequently

Assist with breathing and relaxation

Provide sips of fluids or ice chips PO PRN

Give praise and encouragement

Figure 12-6. *The woman may be extremely worn out by the time she needs to participate actively in pushing activities. The nurse or the support person assists the woman so she can maintain the proper position during bearing-down efforts.*

Physical Support

The nurse already should have discussed effective pushing techniques with the woman and her partner during the first stage of labor. It is essential to reinforce the importance of appropriate pushing during this stage. The woman is reminded to place her chin on her chest, curl forward, and put her hands around her knees, drawing them upward and apart during pushing efforts.

The nurse tells the woman to take two deep breaths as she feels the contraction begin. A third breath is inhaled deeply and held. The support person or nurse can assist the woman into the bearing down position (Fig. 12-6). The woman pushes down in an effort to move the fetus toward the perineum to the count of 10. Then she quickly exhales and repeats the cycle two or three times until the contraction ends. Two cleansing breaths follow the pushing activities, providing oxygenation to the fetus.

Physical comfort during the second stage of labor is harder to achieve. Measures used in the first stage can be tried; however, the intense work required to push the fetus out of the birth canal may overpower the effectiveness of the comfort measures. Bloody show may increase in the second stage of labor; however, most women do not desire perineal care at this time. The woman most often remains in bed during bearing-down activities. Placing dry, clean pads under the woman's buttocks may improve comfort.

Comfort measure used earlier may still be helpful. The woman and support person are encouraged to rest between contractions. Some women feel more comfortable if they remove their clothing.

Psychosocial Support

The woman may express anxiety as the fetal head descends into the birth canal. The pressure of the presenting part on the perineum has been described as an intense feeling, almost a sense of "bursting." The nurse reassures the woman that her experience is proceeding normally and that the perineal muscles are able to stretch. She may also be reassured that the birth attendant will perform an episiotomy to prevent tearing, if necessary.

The nurse provides additional support and teaching when the woman's pushing efforts are ineffective. Helping the woman correctly assume the bearing-down position or offering alternative positioning may be useful. The woman may prefer to squat or get up on all fours for some of the pushing activities. The nurse may insert two sterile gloved fingers into the base of the vagina and instruct the woman to try and push her fingers out. This approach may redirect the woman's efforts and result in more effective bearing-down techniques.

Birthing Alternatives and Positions

In the past, most women were placed in a supine lithotomy position with their feet in stirrups on a delivery table. The head of the table may have been elevated slightly. This position limited the woman's ability to push effectively.

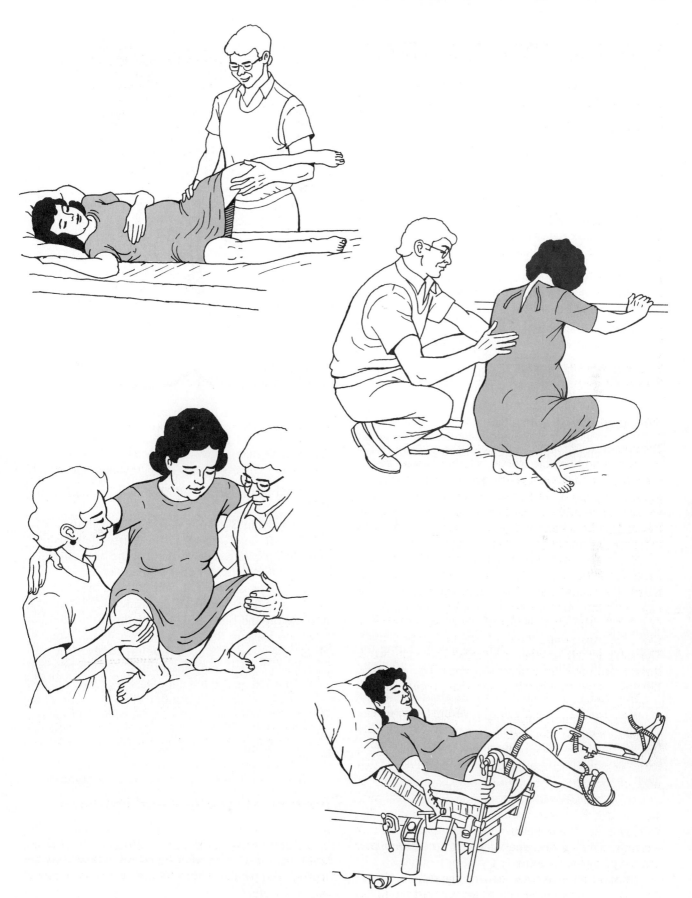

Figure 12-7. *A variety of positions may be used during the second stage of labor, as the woman works to push the fetus downwards towards the vaginal opening.*

Modern practice provides proven positioning alternatives. Birthing chairs and stools are available. The woman may prefer to squat in her bed. Assuming a side-lying position in bed with the support person holding the woman's uppermost leg facilitates pushing. Different positions are tried and changed according to the needs of the woman (Fig. 12-7). Using the same bed for labor, birth, and recovery reduces the need to move the woman to another location before the arrival of the neonate.

Preparation for Birth

If circumstances dictate the need for advanced equipment or pediatric support, the woman may be moved to a specially equipped room. Alternative positioning devices such as the birthing chair or bed may be located in a separate area.

Privacy is maintained as the woman is prepared for childbirth. The perineum is cleansed with an antiseptic solution from front to back. Lighting is checked to ensure clear visualization of the birth process. A large standing mirror may be offered so that the woman and her partner can watch the birth of the neonate. The support person is made comfortable by the woman's side. Stools or chairs are recommended for the observers. All emergency and routine equipment are prepared.

Episiotomy

An episiotomy is the surgical incision into the perineum to enlarge the vaginal opening. An episiotomy may be performed by the birth attendant just before birth. It allows birth of the presenting part with minimal trauma to the perineum. A central (straight back) or medialateral (off center to the right or left) episiotomy widens the birth canal and may reduce perineal lacerations during childbirth (Fig. 12-8). The use of perineal massage and gentle manual stretching of the perineum during the second stage of labor may reduce the need for an episiotomy.

The woman is assured that a local anesthetic administered at the perineal site will prevent her from feeling the incision or the repair. The nurse explains the procedure and assesses the woman's need for additional pain medication or anesthetic once birth of the neonate has occurred.

Birth

The urge to push is overwhelming as the presenting part nears the vaginal opening. Blowing or panting breaths are needed to reduce the likelihood of a rapid birth and

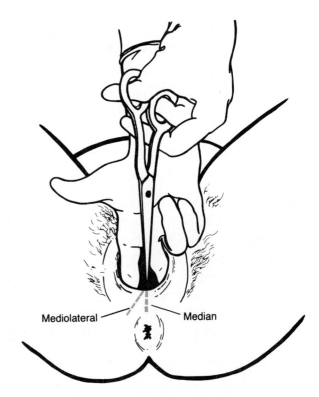

Figure 12-8. *A median or mediolateral incision are most commonly chosen if the woman requires an episiotomy.*

potential lacerations to the perineum. Slow, deliberate, controlled bearing-down efforts are encouraged at this time.

The woman is instructed to avoid pushing as soon as the fetal head emerges. The nurse demonstrates panting or blowing at this instant, as the birth attendant suctions the mouth and nose of the neonate. A special suction device is used if the fetus passed meconium in utero, as indicated by meconium-stained amniotic fluid. Before the body is delivered, the birth attendant checks to be sure the umbilical cord is not wrapped around the newborn's neck (**nuchal cord**). If the newborn has a nuchal cord, the birth attendant must slip the cord from around the neonate's neck to avoid constriction of the airway and suffocation. The birth of the neonate is completed as the birth attendant encourages the woman to bear down slowly. In a vertex presentation (head first), the anterior shoulder is followed by the rest of the body as the neonate emerges quickly into the world. The second stage of labor comes to an end.

Documentation

Maternal contractions, vital signs, and temperature are noted in the patient record. The woman's responses to

✔ NURSING INTERVENTIONS CHECKLIST

Care During the Second Stage of Labor

Assist in assuming proper position for pushing

Apply cool cloth to forehead between contractions

Reposition frequently to promote bearing-down efforts

Increase verbal praise and encouragement

Provide support during episiotomy

Assist in choosing desired birthing position

Assist in choosing desired birthing environment

Prepare for childbirth

Assist in birth

Nursing documentation

labor and pain management techniques also are documented. Procedures and activities are included on facility-specific flow charts or appropriate forms. The fetal monitor strip, which contains information about vaginal examinations, rupture of membranes, and any special procedures such as administration of oxygen to the woman, is included as well. The birth attendant's name, the date, time of birth, presentation and sex of the neonate are recorded. The type of birth (vaginal or cesarean) is included with information about any special circumstances, such as the use of forceps or vacuum extractor. During ongoing assessments, the health status of the mother and neonate are accurately documented. See the Nursing Interventions Checklist for care during the second stage of labor.

Nursing Care During the Third Stage of Labor

The third stage of labor (placental stage) follows the birth of the neonate and ends with the expulsion (delivery) of the placenta. The nurse, working with the birth attendant, inspects the placenta to ensure it has been completely delivered and no fragments are missing.

The nurse assesses the health status of the mother and the neonate immediately after birth as the mother and the support person meet the newborn for the first time. This is a highly charged emotional experience every time.

Immediate Assessment

Immediately after birth, the nurse determines how well the neonate is adjusting to extrauterine life (see later discussion on Apgar score). The newborn also is inspected for any obvious physical deformities that may indicate immediate or future problems. These assessments are performed with minimal disruption to the bonding experience between the newborn and the couple. The birth attendant typically places the newborn on the woman's abdomen after birth. The umbilical cord is clamped in two places, and the birth attendant or support person cuts the cord. Repair of the episiotomy is initiated, using adequate anesthetic to reduce pain. The nurse continually assesses the woman's response to childbirth, including signs of potential hemorrhage. These signs include hypotension; rapid, thready pulse, and a uterine fundus that is not firm and is above the midline. Bonding activities are encouraged throughout the third and fourth stage of labor.

Placental Assessment

On delivery, the placenta is assessed for size, color, and composition, and to determine whether it is completely intact. The birth attendant inspects for the presence of all cotyledons (placental lobes), and the texture of the placenta on the maternal side. The membranes are examined to see if any fragments have been left behind. The insertion site (the point at which the cord is attached to the placenta) and length of the umbilical cord are checked. Normally, there are two arteries and one vein in the umbilical cord (Fig. 12-9). Any signs of abruption or infarction are noted. These signs include very dark red or yellowish white areas appearing on the maternal side of the placenta. The time of placental delivery and findings are recorded.

Physical Support of the Neonate

The neonate is placed in the Trendelenburg position (head down slightly) either on the mother's abdomen or in a nearby heated crib-unit. This promotes drainage of secretions. Suctioning of the nose and mouth may be repeated as needed. Immediately after birth, the newborn is dried energetically to maintain warmth and provide stimulation for lung expansion through crying. Warm dry towels or blankets are wrapped around the neonate. Vital assessments of the neonate are made immediately after birth.

Respiratory effort, heart rate, color, muscle tone, and irritability indicate the neonate's ability to with-

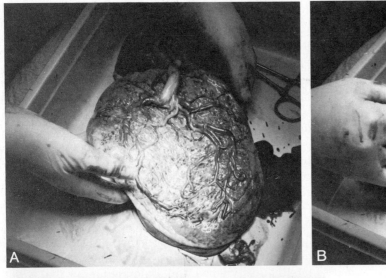
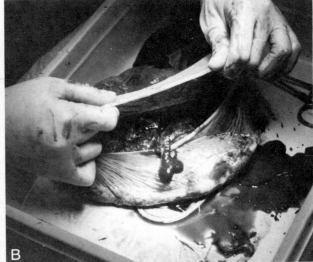
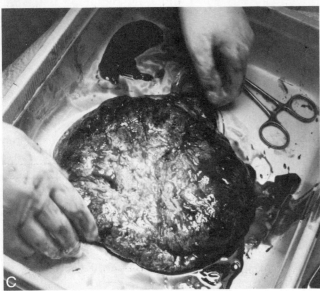

Figure 12-9. *The placenta is inspected for completeness. (**A**) Fetal surface. (**B**) The placenta is carefully turned inside out. (**C**) Maternal surface.*

stand the new extrauterine environment. The nurse examines the neonate's physical characteristics, observing carefully for any physical abnormalities. The head, mouth, nose, back, and extremities are examined. The amounts of vernix caseosa (cheesy substance covering the skin) and lanugo, the fine downy hair found on the back and shoulders, help determine the neonate's age. As the neonate's gestational age increases, lanugo decreases. Usually there is a thick covering of vernix caseosa between 36 and 38 weeks' gestation, but by 40 weeks it is usually found only in the folds of the axilla and groin.

Before the newborn and mother are separated, it is essential that each be fitted with matching identification bracelets. The mother's bracelet is placed on her wrist; the newborn wears one or two bracelets on the ankle or the wrist. The newborn's footprints are taken as a means of further identification, along with the mother's index finger or thumbprint.

Apgar Score

In 1952, Dr. Virginia Apgar developed the Apgar scoring system as a means of assessing the physical condition of the neonate immediately after birth. The **Apgar score** is determined at 1 and 5 minutes. The score serves as a guide for determining the resuscitative needs of the newborn (Fig. 12-10). The total score ranges from 0 to 10, based on five indicators of the health status of the neonate. The heart rate, respiratory effort, muscle tone, reflex irritability, and color of the

APGAR SCORING CHART

Sign	0	1	2	1 min	5 min
Heart rate	Absent	Below 100	Above 100	_____	_____
Respiratory rate	Absent	Slow, irregular	Good crying	_____	_____
Muscle tone	Limp	Some flexion of extremities	Active motion	_____	_____
Reflex irritability - response to catheter in nostril or - slap to sole of foot	No response No response	Grimace Grimace	Cough or sneeze Cry and withdrawal of foot	_____	_____
Color	Blue, pale	Body pink, extremities blue	Completely pink	_____	_____

(Developed by Dr. Virginia Apgar)

Figure 12-10. *Apgar scoring system. Assessments of the neonate are made at 1 and 5 minutes after birth.*

[handwritten: tachycardia sign of Hypovolemia]
[handwritten: 250 to 500ml Average blood loss during childbirth]

neonate are each rated from 0 to 2. Figure 12-10 provides a quick reference for calculating the newborn's Apgar score at 1 and 5 minutes. A score of 8 to 10 indicates a neonate in good condition, whereas a neonate with a score of 7 or lower may require special attention. A neonatal score below 4 signifies serious respiratory and cardiovascular depression. Resuscitative intervention must be initiated immediately. See the Nursing Interventions Checklist for immediate care of the newborn.

✔ NURSING INTERVENTIONS CHECKLIST

Immediate Care of the Newborn

· Place in Trendelenburg position
· Keep warm
· Provide oral and nasopharyngeal suctioning with bulb syringe
· Dry and stimulate to cry
· APGAR score (Fig. 12-10)
· Apply umbilical cord clamp
· Assess for physical abnormalities
· Assess for vernix caseosa and lanugo
· Apply identification bands to wrist and ankle
· Take footprints

Physical Support of the Woman

A large amount of fluid volume is lost during childbirth. This fluid loss results from diaphoresis, hyperventilation, reduced fluid intake, polyuria, and blood loss.

Immediate care of the woman after childbirth is aimed at the prevention of complications. The maternal blood pressure is assessed for return to prelabor levels. Pulse and respirations normally return to prepregnancy rates. The uterine fundus is palpated and gently massaged to reduce uterine bleeding. The level of the fundus is usually at the level of the umbilicus or one finger's breadth below after birth. It should be located in the midline. A full bladder may push the uterus to the side and reduce the normal contractions and clamping down of the uterus. The woman is encouraged to empty her bladder when this occurs. Vaginal discharge, lochia rubra, is bright red and small to moderate in amount. There should not be any blood clots.

Excessive bleeding after delivery of the placenta most often results from relaxation of the uterus. To promote uterine contractions and reduce the risk of postpartum hemorrhage, the woman is often given a uterine tonic. A uterine tonic is a drug that stimulates contraction of the uterine muscles. Oxytocics most commonly used are oxytocin and ergonovine. The administration of oxytocin (Pitocin and Syntocinon) may be ordered by the birth attendant to promote hemostasis. Oxytocin can be added to the intravenous fluids or administered as an intramuscular injection after childbirth. The normal dose is 10 to 40 IU/L intravenous fluid infused at a rate of 10 to 40 mU/min or 10 to 20 IU given intramuscularly. Ergonovine maleate (Ergotrate) or methylergonovine maleate (Methergine) may be

[handwritten: If the Pt has ↑ B/P No Methergine]

✔ NURSING INTERVENTIONS CHECKLIST

Care During the Third Stage of Labor

- Assess for signs of excessive bleeding
- Assist with delivery of placenta
- Assist with assessing placenta for intactness
- Administer ordered oxytocin medication

✔ NURSING INTERVENTIONS CHECKLIST

Care of the Woman During Fourth Stage of Labor

Immediate Care

- Blood pressure, pulse, respirations
- Palpation and massage of uterine fundus
- Assessment of vaginal lochia
- Assessment of episiotomy
- Keep warm with blankets
- Administer IV or IM oxytocin
- Assess and encourage maternal–infant attachments
- Assist with breastfeeding, if desired

Continuing Care

- Settle in postpartum room
- Continue vital sign, fundal, and lochia assessments
- Encourage rest and sleep
- Provide fluids and light meals if desired
- Encourage to empty bladder as soon as possible
- Assess episiotomy

given intramuscularly after the placenta is expelled. The normal dose of either of these medications is 0.2 mg. intramuscularly. Uterine massage and manual nipple stimulation or breast feeding also promote uterine tone and minimize bleeding. See the Nursing Interventions Checklist for care during the third stage of labor.

The woman may experience chills and have uncontrollable shaking after childbirth. The nurse provides the woman with a warm blanket and the reassures her these effects are normal responses to labor and birth. Excessive perspiration during labor cools the body and leads to a lower basal body temperature after childbirth. This may contribute to the shaking and chills she is experiencing. Some theories suggest that the tremendous hormonal shifts that accompany birth may contribute to the woman's response.

The nurse performs maternal assessments every 15 minutes for the first hour, every 30 minutes for the next 1 to 2 hours, and then every 4 hours for the first day. If the woman remains in the facility for more than 24 hours, the following are monitored every shift: vital signs, condition of the episiotomy site, fundal height, and lochia. Under normal circumstances, the perineum shows minimal signs of edema and bruising. If an episiotomy was performed, the sutures are intact and do not appear inflamed. Any abnormal findings or complications necessitate more frequent assessment. Findings are documented and reported appropriately. See the Nursing Interventions Checklist for a checklist for immediate care of the woman in the fourth stage of labor.

Psychosocial Support

During the first hour after birth, the neonate is very alert and able to receive stimulus. Attachments and relationships begin to form at this time. If the mother wishes to breast-feed the newborn right away, the nurse provides clean, dry linens and a gown and helps the woman assume a comfortable position. The nurse encourages the mother and her partner to hold the newborn, stroke its

body, talk softly, and look into the newborn's eyes. Other members of the family will be invited to share in the bonding experience shortly thereafter. The new family is given ample time to get acquainted.

Some alternative birth methods prefer little or no intervention for the mother and baby. For example, the LeBoyer method of childbirth advocates dimming the lights in the birthing room and placing the newborn in a tub of warm water immediately after birth. This situation is thought to be comforting to the newborn because it simulates intrauterine life. In the Bradley method of childbirth, as little intervention as possible is advocated. It is important to consider and respect the childbearing families' wishes and plans when possible. Alternative methods of childbirth require more planning and flexibility on the part of the nurse to adequately monitor the newborn's status.

Nursing Care During the Fourth Stage of Labor

The fourth stage of labor begins immediately after the delivery of the placenta and ends when the woman's physical condition is stabilized. This is a critical time during which the well-being of the neonate and mother are carefully monitored.

Physical Support

The nurse in the labor and birthing area continues to assess the woman's physical and psychosocial well-being as described during the third stage of labor. Typically, the woman's condition stabilizes within 1 to 2 hours. The neonate generally remains with the family during the first couple of hours after birth. Neonatal care and nursing assessment are discussed in detail in Chapters 17 and 18.

In an acute care facility, the woman is usually transferred to the postpartum unit once her condition is stable. The nurse communicates the course of labor and birth to the staff who will be assuming the mother's postpartum care. This ensures continuity of care and helps familiarize the nursing staff with the woman and her family. Any special circumstances or needs are documented and communicated to the postpartum staff. The postpartum staff encourages rest and sleep as much as possible. Examples of measures that promote comfort include: oral fluids and light nourishment, perineal care, ice packs to the perineum and episiotomy, a soothing back rub, and a quiet, darkened room. The woman usually is encouraged to walk to a nearby bathroom to empty her bladder at this time. The nurse administers medications as ordered by the birth attendant to promote pain relief for the woman.

Psychosocial Support

The family's early reactions to the neonate are often revealing signs of their hopes and desire for future relationships. Difficult labor or long, tiring, labor may interfere with the family's ability to get to know the newborn in a positive manner. The nurse needs to provide supportive care that encourages family attachments. The nurse carefully monitors the family throughout the postpartum period to determine their ability to form attachments and incorporate the new member into the family.

◆ Adolescent Considerations

Labor and childbirth can be frightening and overwhelming to adolescent women and their partners. They may not be prepared for the related physical and emotional challenges. Immaturity, lack of life experience, and lack of self-confidence may further compound the situation. The adolescent's self-esteem may be significantly impacted either positively or negatively from the pregnancy and birthing experience. Careful explanation and up-to-the-minute reporting about various activities help reduce the adolescent's level of fear and stress. The nurse may stand in as the support person, bolstering the teen's confidence and ability to handle labor, while providing direct nursing care. The nurse encourages and guides the adolescent to engage in bonding activities during the fourth stage of labor.

◆ Cultural Considerations

It is important for the nurse caring for childbearing families to consider the members' cultural beliefs and practices. Special consideration of the family's needs allow the nurse to integrate these issues into the nursing care plan.

Women from North America have traditionally given birth on a delivery table with their legs in stirrups. Over the past few decades, less traditional approaches involving the use of chairs, stools, and other nontraditional settings have been advocated, providing many options from which the woman can choose. Other cultures may not encourage this type of choice and independence. For example, Vietnamese women do not inquire about their birthing options, rather they respond "yes" to most questions because to say "no" is considered disrespectful.

◆ The Role of the Nurse

The nurse is responsible for a wide range of activities during labor and childbirth. The nurse sets the tone of the birthing experience during the initial contact with the woman in labor and her family. Physical and psychosocial needs of childbearing families are constantly changing during each stage of labor. The knowledgeable nurse anticipates each stage of labor and is prepared to intervene as needed in a supportive role. The nurse is sensitive to the needs of the woman, the baby, the support person, and the family throughout this special experience.

Successful birthing outcomes include the health and well-being of the woman and the safe birth of the neonate. The nurse can promote a smooth transition with guidance, supportive care, and parent education. The family members' ability to adapt and incorporate the birthing experience into their lives will be enhanced by the skilled nurse's ability to provide complete, compassionate nursing care.

REVIEW AND PREVIEW

This chapter presented the nursing care of families during normal labor and birth. A review of admission procedures and care, including detailed assessment throughout the four stages of labor, were addressed. In the discussion of pain management, the emphasis was placed on nonpharmacologic interventions followed by pharmacologic interventions. This information equips the nurse with a variety of techniques and approaches for relieving the pain and discomfort associated with labor. Adolescent and cultural considerations were included to emphasize the need to modify care to meet the individual needs of a variety of families.

The following chapter addresses a variety of complications that may occur during labor and birth. The nursing assessment and management of each complication will be presented. Operative procedures and emergency childbirth will be described. Families at risk require specialized nursing care that builds on the nurse's knowledge of care in normal labor and birth.

◉ KEY POINTS

◆ When a woman in labor is admitted to the birthing unit, the nurse makes her and her family feel welcome. The nurse applies an identification bracelet and provides an orientation. This is followed by a review of patient records, a history, physical, psychosocial assessment, contraction and fetal monitoring, and possibly a vaginal examination.

◆ The nurse is responsible for obtaining important assessment information such as laboratory test findings, maternal vital signs, fetal heart rate, position and presentation, and a 20- to 30-minute electronic fetal monitor strip. Additionally, the nurse determines the membrane status, presence of any bleeding, and identifies any complications or risk factors.

◆ Pain relief in labor serves to reduce maternal stress and discomfort and promote the safe birth of a healthy neonate. Pain management is achieved with nonpharmacologic or pharmacologic measures.

◆ Common nonpharmacologic pain relief comfort measures include proper positioning, walking, showering, back rubs, back support, gentle abdominal massage, cool cloths, relaxation techniques, distraction, music, television, guided imagery, and hypnosis.

◆ During the first stage of labor (dilating stage), the nurse assesses maternal and fetal conditions hourly, unless circumstances dictate more frequent observations. Maternal vital signs, uterine contractions, FHR, and the response to labor are evaluated. Vaginal examinations are typically performed hourly, but the schedule may vary depending on the woman's condition. The facility's policy determines who performs the vaginal examination. The nurse helps the family cope with the wide range of emotions they may experience.

◆ Nursing care during the second stage of labor includes assisting with pushing techniques, encouraging rest between contractions, offering ice chips or sips of fluid, and preparing and assisting with the actual birth. Safe birth and health promotion for the mother and neonate are determined by ongoing assessments of the woman and the neonate.

◆ Immediate care of the newborn after birth includes providing warmth through drying activities, stimulation, Apgar scoring, physical assessment, and proper identification procedures.

◆ The third stage of labor occurs after the neonate is born and ends when the placenta separates and is expelled. The nurse may assist in assessing the placenta watches the woman for signs of hemorrhage, administers oxytocics as ordered, and continues to observe the condition of the neonate.

◆ The fourth stage of labor describes the period after the placenta is delivered up to the time the woman's condition is stabilized. This process takes from 1 to 2 hours after placental expulsion. However, the woman is closely observed for the first 4 hours after birth.

◆ The family's cultural background may play an important role in the various stages of childbirth. The process of labor and pain management may be influenced by the individual's personal beliefs. The nurse needs to discuss the woman and family's personal preferences and cultural practices that may become significant during labor and childbirth.

BIBLIOGRAPHY

Biancuzzo, M. (1993). Six myths of maternal posture during labor. *Maternal Child Nursing*, *18*(5), 264–269.

Byrne, M. W., & Lerner, H. M. (1992). Communicating with addicted women in labor. *Maternal Child Nursing*, *17*(1), 22–26.

Chapman, L. (1992). Expectant father's roles during labor and birth. *Journal of Obstetric, Gynecologic, and Neonatal Nursing*, *21*(2), 114–120.

Cosner, K. R., & deJong, E. (1993). Physiologic second-stage labor. *The Journal of Maternal Child Nursing*, *18*(1), 38–43.

Fischbach, F. (1992). *A manual of laboratory and diagnostic tests* (4th ed.). Philadelphia: J. B. Lippincott.

Fleming, B. W., Munton, M. T., Clarke, B. A., & Strauss, S. S. (1993). Assessing and promoting positive parenting in adolescent mothers. *The American Journal of Maternal-Child Nursing*, *18*(1), 32–37.

Isenor, L., & Penny-MacGillivray, T. (1993). Intravenous meperidine infusion for obstetric analgesia. *Journal of Obstetric, Gynecologic, and Neonatal Nursing*, *22*(4), 349–356.

Kennell, J., Klaus, M., McGrath, S., Robertson, S., & Hinkley, C. (1991). Continuous emotional support during labor in a US hospital. *Journal of the American Medical Association*, *262*(17), 2197.

Martin, L. L., & Reeder, S. J. (1990). *Essentials of Maternity Nursing: Family Centered Care* (1st ed.). Philadelphia: J. B. Lippincott.

May, K. A., & Mahlmeister, L. R. (1994). *Maternal & Neonatal Nursing: Family-Centered Care* (3rd ed). Philadelphia: J.B. Lippincott.

McIntosh, D., & Rayburn, W. (1991). Patient controlled analgesia in obstetrics and gynecology. *Obstetrics and Gynecology*, *78*(6), 1129.

SELF-ASSESSMENT

1. A woman in the transitional stage of labor is most likely to exhibit which of the following behaviors?

- ○ **A.** Excited to talk about the pending delivery
- ○ **B.** Using cleansing breaths before and after contractions
- ○ **C.** Asking to take a shower
- ⊗ **D.** Agitated and overwhelmed

2. A woman who is 9 centimeters dilated expresses the urge to push. What should be the nurse's initial response?

- ○ **A.** Immediately notify the physician
- ○ **B.** Prepare for delivery
- ⊗ **C.** Discourage her from pushing
- ○ **D.** Teach her to push effectively

3. Upon assessment at 1 minute of life, the nurse notes the following: blue extremities and pink body, heart rate 110, irregular breathing, no response to suction catheter, and slight flexion of the extremities. What is the infant's Apgar score?

- ○ **A.** 4
- ⊗ **B.** 5
- ○ **C.** 6
- ○ **D.** 7

4. What color will Nitrazine paper turn when it comes in contact with amniotic fluid?

- ○ **A.** Green
- ○ **B.** Red
- ⊗ **C.** Blue
- ○ **D.** Yellow

5. Several hours after delivery, the nurse palpates a patient's uterus 1 finger-breadth above the umbilicus and displaced to the left. This finding is most likely the result of:

- ⊗ **A.** A distended bladder
- ○ **B.** Retained placental fragments
- ○ **C.** Blood clots
- ○ **D.** Overdistension from a large infant

McRae, M. J. (1993). Litigation, electronic fetal monitoring, and the obstetric nurse. *Journal of Obstetric, Gynecologic, and Neonatal Nursing, 22*(5), 410–419.

NAACOG. (1992). *Nursing Responsibilities in Implementing Intrapartum Fetal Heart Rate Monitoring*, Position Statement. Washington, DC: Author.

Reeder, S. J., Martin, L. L., & Koniak, D. (1992). *Maternity nursing: Family, newborn, and women's health care* (17th ed.). Philadelphia: J. B. Lippincott.

Rosdahl, C. B. (1991). *Textbook of basic nursing* (5th ed.). Philadelphia: J. B. Lippincott.

Taylor, T. (1993). Epidural anesthesia in the maternity patient. *The American Journal of Maternal-Child Nursing, 18*(2), 86–93.

Waldenstrom, V., & Axel-Nilsson, C. (1992). Warm tub bath after spontaneous rupture of the membranes. *Birth, 19*(2), 57–63.

Wild, L., & Coyne, C. (1992). Epidural analgesia. *American Journal of Nursing, 92*(4):26.

CHAPTER 13

Nursing Care in the Complicated Intrapartum Period

◈ OBJECTIVES

When the learning goals of this chapter are met, the reader will be able to:

◆ Define preterm labor and list 10 contributing factors.
◆ Define induction of labor and identify three common methods.
◆ Explain dystocia and identify its causes.
◆ Describe how fetal position affects progress in labor and birth.
◆ Differentiate between PROM and PPROM.
◆ Define hydramnios; state how it affects labor.
◆ List the dangers associated with prolapsed cord.
◆ Describe nursing interventions in prolapsed cord.
◆ Define cesarean birth and list five reasons for this procedure.
◆ Describe the nurse's role in emergency delivery.

TERMINOLOGY

Cesarean birth	Prolapsed cord
Dystocia	Prostaglandin gel
Forceps delivery	Tocolysis
Hydramnios	Uterine inversion
Induction of labor	Uterine rupture
Oxytocin induction	Vacuum extraction
Preterm labor	VBAC

Most women experience a normal antepartum and intrapartum course. They complete labor and childbirth with no significant complications. However, some approach labor with risk factors that place the woman or her fetus in danger of a poor perinatal outcome. Still other women develop complications during labor and childbirth. Complications that occur during the intrapartum period may be serious enough to produce an unfavorable outcome for the woman or the neonate. The nurse must make every effort to keep the woman and her family informed. In this very upsetting time, an understanding, empathetic nurse makes an important contribution to relieving the stress and anxiety of the woman and her family.

Families at Risk

Various physical, emotional, or cultural factors can place pregnancies in potential danger. These are frequently identified in the antepartum period (see Chapter 8). Identification of families at risk enables the nurse to plan appropriate nursing interventions to prevent or reduce complications during labor and childbirth.

Preterm Labor

Preterm labor is defined as the onset of regular uterine contractions resulting in cervical dilatation and effacement after 20 weeks and before 37 weeks of pregnancy are completed.

Preterm birth has great significance for society because it accounts for most perinatal deaths not resulting from congenital anomalies. Preterm infants have a 120-times greater chance of neonatal mortality than infants born at term. In addition, there is an exceptional increase in neonatal complications as a result of prematurity. Some of these complications are respiratory distress, hyperbilirubinemia, and infection. Neurologic complications such as neonatal seizures and cerebral palsy are 22 times more common in the preterm infant. The incidence of preterm birth in the United States is approximately 9% across all women, with the average rate equaling 8% for white women and 16% to 17% in African American women. The financial cost of caring for an extremely premature neonate is staggering. It can easily exceed $100,000 for an admission to the intensive care nursery.

Contributing Factors

The exact cause of preterm labor is unclear. As a result, there is no assessment tool that can identify with com-plete accuracy the patient who will have preterm labor. However, there are many factors that increase the risk of preterm labor (see Chapter 6). All women must be carefully assessed for these risk factors. The woman is assessed during her initial prenatal visit, and assessments continue through each visit thereafter.

Prevention of preterm labor is directed at improving the woman's general health. This involves encouraging early prenatal care, improving nutrition, and counseling against cigarette smoking and the use of alcohol and other substances.

Assessment

There are seven warning signs of preterm labor for which nursing personnel and women must be alert. These signs are regular uterine contractions, frequently painless; abdominal cramping, occasionally with diarrhea; menstrual-like cramps; low backache; pelvic pressure; change in vaginal discharge; or bloody vaginal discharge. Many of these signs may be difficult to differentiate from false labor (see Chapter 11), but they should not be ignored. The woman experiencing one or more of these warning signs must seek immediate medical evaluation.

All women with suggested preterm labor should be evaluated in an inpatient setting. The woman is monitored with electronic fetal monitoring. This determines the status of the fetus and the frequency, duration, and intensity of the uterine contractions. The nursing assessment includes determining the presence of intact or ruptured membranes. To determine if the woman's membranes have ruptured, a nitrazine paper test or examination of vaginal discharge for ferning is performed. When membranes rupture early in pregnancy, it is called preterm premature rupture of membranes (PPROM). This is differentiated from membranes that rupture before uterine contractions begin in a woman whose pregnancy is full term (PROM). The uterus is palpated to determine the strength of contractions. Additionally, if membranes are intact, a gentle, cervical examination is performed to establish dilatation and effacement. If membranes have ruptured, little can be done to stop the labor.

Management

Nursing care of the woman experiencing possible preterm labor includes maintaining her on bed rest in the left lateral position. This position provides the best circulatory supply to the placenta and fetus. The woman may receive either oral or intravenous hydration. Sedation is frequently ordered by the physician to help her rest. The nurse institutes appropriate safety measures. Monitoring of external fetal heart rate and uterine activity are initiated. A sterile urine specimen and cervical culture may be obtained to assess for the presence of urinary tract or cervical infections. This is because of the reported correlation between these infections and preterm labor. The nurse encourages the woman to relax and provides the opportunity for the woman and her family to ask questions. Explanations in understandable terminology and realistic reassurance regarding the welfare of the woman and fetus are provided.

For some women with regular contractions, uterine activity may stop with bed rest and hydration. If cervical change does not occur and the membranes are not ruptured, the woman may be discharged. She is taught how to palpate her fundus. This helps her recognize the rhythmic tightening and relaxing of the uterus as contractions. The nurse reviews with her the signs and

---

DISPLAY 13-1
Warning Signs and Symptoms of Preterm Labor

Regular uterine contractions—frequently painless

Abdominal cramping—occasionally with diarrhea

Menstrual-like cramps

Low backache

Pelvic pressure

Change in vaginal discharge

Bloody vaginal discharge

---

symptoms of possible preterm labor about which she should be aware. She is advised to seek medical attention immediately if she has any of these signs or symptoms (see Display 13-1). Additionally, the woman may

---

Table 13-1. *Tocolytic Drugs Used to Inhibit Preterm Labor*

Drug	Action	Major Side Effects	Minor Side Effects	Contraindications
ß-adrenergic agonists Ritodine (Yutopar) Terbutaline (Brethine)	Relaxes uterine smooth muscle	*Maternal* Widening of pulse pressure Tachycardia Dysrhythmias Pulmonary edema Myocardial ischemia Hyperglycemia Hypokalemia *Neonatal* Tachycardia Dysrhythmias Hypoglycemia Hypocalcemia Hypotension Ileus Intraventricular hemorrhage	*Maternal* Nausea and vomiting Tremors Headache Erythema Nervousness Jitteriness Anxiety	Hypertension Undiagnosed vaginal bleeding Hyperthyroidism Maternal cardiac disease Diabetes mellitus
Magnesium sulfate	Depresses uterine contractility	*Maternal* CNS depression Pulmonary edema Respiratory depression Cardiac arrest *Neonatal* Hypotonia Respiratory depression	*Maternal* Flushing Headache Nausea Vomiting Dizziness Dry mouth Lethargy Blurred vision *Neonatal* Drowsiness	

NURSING CARE PLAN
for the Woman Experiencing Preterm Labor

ASSESSMENT: Date 3-20-95. LMP 8-5-94, EDD 5-25-95, gestational age by dates 32 weeks. States she has contractions every 7–10 minutes, lasting 30–40 seconds, and moderate in intensity. Denies ROM. Vaginal exam: cervix 2–3 cm; 50% effaced; –2 station.
Medical diagnosis: preterm labor

NURSING DIAGNOSIS #1: Risk for Injury, fetal, related to preterm labor

EXPECTED OUTCOME: The fetus will not experience injury from preterm labor

Nursing Interventions	*Rationale*
1. Monitor maternal vital signs and fetal heart rate by external monitoring.	1. Changes in baseline values may indicate latent problems or complications of therapy.
2. Maintain bed rest in left lateral position.	2. Improves maternal venous return and placental blood flow.
3. Infuse intravenous tocolytic agent as prescribed.	3. Stops or slows preterm contractions.

EVALUATION: The fetus of the woman experiencing preterm labor will be uninjured as evidenced by stable fetal heart rate and maternal vital signs.

NURSING DIAGNOSIS #2: Anxiety, related to unknown neonatal outcome

EXPECTED OUTCOME: Anxiety will be minimized, as evidenced by the woman's verbalization of understanding

Nursing Interventions	*Rationale*
1. Encourage expression of fear and anxiety.	1. Verbalization outlines need for education of the woman.
2. Provide discussion of plan of care and potential outcomes.	2. Increasing the woman's knowledge and offering realistic assurances decreases fear.

EVALUATION: The woman in preterm labor has decreased anxiety, as evidenced by verbal expression and positive response to care.

be instructed to maintain periods of bed rest and to avoid sexual intercourse.

The diagnosis of preterm labor is made when uterine contractions are documented at a frequency of four contractions in 20 minutes or eight in 60 minutes accompanied by cervical effacement of 80%, or dilatation of 2 or more centimeters. Stopping preterm labor before advanced cervical dilatation of 4 to 5 cm is the primary goal of intervention. This effort is undertaken with the use of **tocolysis**, drug therapy directed at stopping uterine activity. The most commonly used tocolytics in the United States include the β-adrenergic agonists (ritodrine hydrochloride and terbutaline) and magnesium sulfate.

Ritodrine (Yutopar) and terbutaline (Brethine) act to reduce uterine activity by the relaxation of uterine smooth muscle. Ritodrine is the only one of these two drugs approved for use in preterm labor. It usually is given first as an intravenous infusion on a volume-

controlled pump, followed by oral administration after uterine activity has ceased. Intravenous medication is usually continued until several hours after contractions have stopped, or until advanced cervical dilation has occurred. Terbutaline is used in the United States on an experimental basis for preterm labor. It also may be given intravenously, but the subcutaneous and oral routes are more common.

The effects of these drugs are not specific to the uterus. Other body systems, such as the heart and lungs, are affected as well. Serious complications are more common with the intravenous route of administration. If a major side effect occurs, the medication is discontinued. The minor side effects may be upsetting to the woman, but they can usually be tolerated with encouragement by nursing personnel.

Magnesium sulfate may be used in the place of intravenous β-adrenergic medications for tocolysis. It is thought to reduce uterine activity by depressing the contractility of uterine smooth muscle. Magnesium sulfate can only be given by the intravenous route. It is best maintained on a volume-controlled pump. The drug is continued for several hours after contractions have stopped or until the advanced cervical dilatation occurs. If successful, the patient is started on an oral medication for maintenance, usually ritodrine or terbutaline. The risk of cardiovascular complications is much less with magnesium sulfate than with ritodrine. Magnesium toxicity may occur if renal function is impaired, so monitoring of urine output is necessary. Calcium gluconate 10% is administered as an antidote if needed. The patellar jerk reflex is assessed frequently to observe for signs of central nervous system depression. Table 13-1 presents the major and minor side effects and contraindications for these drugs.

The woman is prepared for childbirth if the efforts to stop labor are not successful. If the woman is in a community facility, she may be transported to a major medical center for the birth of her neonate. The birth attendant makes the decision to transport the woman. Some determining factors include the length of the

---

DISPLAY 13-2
Preterm Labor: Nursing Assessments and Interventions

Assessment

Between 20 and 37 completed weeks' gestation

Regular uterine contractions:

(4 in 20 minutes or 8 in 60 minutes) with cervical change

Effacement–80%

Cervical dilatation–2 cm.

Monitor

External fetal heart rate and uterine activity

Care

Bedrest

Sedation or antibiotics as indicated

Hydration

Safety measures

Reassurance

Medication

Magnesium sulfate

ß-adrenergic agonists

Ritodrine hydrochloride

Terbutaline

---

pregnancy, the advancement of labor, and how quickly the transport can be completed. The woman and her family must be included in these decisions and kept fully informed. See Nursing Care Plan for the Woman Experiencing Preterm Labor. Display 13-2 presents nursing assessments and interventions for preterm labor.

Induction of Labor

The **induction of labor** is the stimulation of the uterus to cause contractions before the spontaneous onset of labor. Induction of labor has some risk for the woman and the fetus. Some of these risks include fetal distress, uterine rupture, amniotic fluid embolus, precipitate labor, lacerations of the cervix, and postpartum hemorrhage. These risks are minimized when induction is performed in a safe manner.

Reasons for Induction

The induction of labor may be performed in instances when there is a clear indication for delivery and when the delay of delivery would place the woman or fetus at significant risk. Induction of labor should not be performed simply for the convenience of the woman or the physician. Maternal indications for induction include chorioamnionitis, medical disorders (eg, chronic hypertension, insulin-dependent diabetes mellitus), pregnancy-induced hypertension, premature rupture of membranes, and postmature pregnancy (42 weeks). Fetal indications include fetal demise (death of the fetus), intrauterine growth retardation (IUGR), and suggested fetal jeopardy. Before inducing, a thorough pelvic examination is performed to determine clinical pelvimetry, fetal presentation, estimated fetal weight, station of the presenting part, and cervical dilation and effacement (see Chapter 11).

Methods of Induction

Induction of labor is most often attempted by amniotomy, oxytocin infusion, and prostaglandin gel/suppository administration. The physiologic readiness of the woman and the fetus are assessed before induction of labor is started. Tests are performed to determine the condition of the fetus as well as the gestational age and lung maturity of the fetus. The woman's cervix is examined for ripening (the softness, amount of effacement, and dilatation). The station of the fetus is also evaluated (see Chapter 11). The fetus should be at engagement to avoid the possibility of prolapsed cord (discussed later in this chapter).

Amniotomy

Amniotomy is the artificial rupture of membranes, often abbreviated AROM. This surgical induction of labor is performed only when delivery is desired, and when the fetal presenting part is well down against the cervix. Rupturing membranes too early can cause prolonged rupture of the membranes. Prolonged rupture predisposes mother and fetus to the development of intrauterine infections. Vaginal examinations are kept to a minimum after the membranes are ruptured to reduce this risk. Amniotomy, performed by the birth attendant, is accomplished with the use of a sterile amnihook, and allows the amniotic fluid to escape (Fig. 13-1). Uterine contractions are thought to result from an increase in the release of plasma prostaglandins that occurs at the time of rupture.

When artificial rupture of membranes is performed, the nurse documents the time and the character, odor, and amount of the amniotic fluid. The fetal heart rate is assessed and documented at the time of the rupture and again in 15 minutes.

Oxytocin Induction and Augmentation

As stated earlier, induction of labor is initiated before the onset of spontaneous labor. Augmentation refers to stimulation of uterine contractions in the presence of spontaneous contractions and confirmed labor. A clear indication for delivery is necessary before initiating induction or augmentation. Drugs approved in the United States for these uses are Pitocin or Syntocinon, a synthetic form of the hormone oxytocin, which initiates or intensifies uterine contractions.

Before oxytocin administration a vaginal examination is performed to assess cervical dilatation and effacement, as well as fetal presentation and position. The woman's vital signs are assessed and recorded, and fetal well-being is confirmed. Continuous electronic fetal and uterine activity monitoring usually is initiated before and continued during the oxytocin infusion.

Uterine hyperstimulation (contractions less than 2 minutes apart) or uterine tetany (loss of relaxation between contractions) may occur with the use of oxytocin. Serious complications can result, including abruptio placentae (see Chapter 8), uterine rupture, amniotic fluid embolus, cervical lacerations, and fetal hypoxia. Other reported complications include maternal hypotension, fluid overload, and water intoxication. An experienced nurse must care for the woman.

There are a number of protocols available for preparation of an oxytocin infusion. One commonly used protocol involves adding 10 units oxytocin to 1000 mL intravenous fluid. This solution is piggy-backed into the mainline intravenous fluid and the rate maintained by volume-controlled pump. The lowest possible dose is generally used to begin the infusion. It is then gradually increased until uterine contractions occur every 2 to 3 minutes, last 45 to 60 seconds, and are moderate to strong in intensity.

Oxytocin is capable of producing strong uterine contractions in a short time with even minimal dosages, and response of an individual woman is difficult to predict. The woman should be closely observed during administration for changes in vital signs and urine output. Frequent assessments of the fetal heart rate and uterine activity are necessary. One-on-one care provided by a skilled nurse is essential. A physician qualified to intervene must be immediately available during the administration. The infusion should be discontinued if the fetus demonstrates signs of stress (fetal heart rate decreases

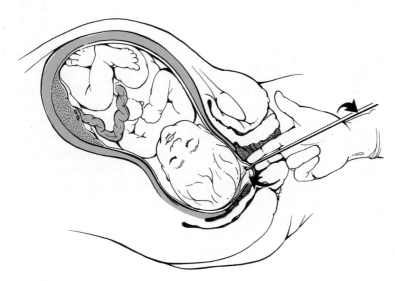

Figure 13-1. Amniotomy (artificial rupture of the membranes). A sharp point on one side of the plastic amnihook punctures the amniotic sac. It is sterile when used.

to 60 beats/min), or if uterine hyperstimulation or tetany occurs.

Prostaglandin Gel

The induction of labor may enhanced by a favorable cervix, one that is soft, partially effaced, and dilated. At times, the induction of labor may be required when the cervix is not favorable, and mechanical methods of cervical ripening may be initiated. One such method is the placement of prostaglandin E_2 (PGE_2) gel into the vagina. *Prostaglandin E_2 gel* (or suppository) is a product made from a hormone produced by the cervix and placental trophoblastic tissue. When inserted into the vagina, it causes biochemical responses in the cervix, resulting in cervical change and uterine contractions. Side effects of prostaglandin therapy include nausea, vomiting, fever, and elevated uterine baseline tone. Side effects are more common with higher doses.

The woman may be placed in a modified Trendelenburg position for an hour or two after insertion to decrease the possibility of leakage. Electronic fetal monitoring is conducted for 1 or 2 hours after insertion to evaluate fetal well-being.

Other methods of induction have been used in the past. However, these three methods are currently the most frequently used.

◆ Dystocia

Dystocia, or difficult labor, is the term used to describe labor that progresses at a slower than normal rate. Dystocia may occur as the result of a single problem or a combination of problems with the powers, passage, passenger, or psyche (see Chapter 11).

Difficulties with the powers, or uterine dysfunction, may occur during the first stage of labor when either the intensity or regularity of contractions are insufficient to effect cervical change. Dystocia in the second stage of labor may occur as a result of inadequate uterine activity or expulsive forces. Passage difficulties occur when the size or shape of the bony pelvis, or unusual configurations of the reproductive tract, prevent descent and eventual delivery of the fetus. Problems with the passenger that may cause dystocia include fetal abnormalities, variations in size, malpresentations, and malpositions. Additionally, the woman's psyche can influence the normal course of labor. The woman's anxiety or lack of preparation can act alone or together with other factors to slow or stop labor. The Assessment Checklist presents the forces that need to be assessed in dystocia.

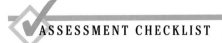

✓ ASSESSMENT CHECKLIST

> *Dystocia*
>
> *Powers*
> Uterine dysfunction
>
> *Passenger*
> Fetal abnormalities
> Variations in size
> Malpresentations
> Malpositions
>
> *Passage*
> Pelvic shape or size
> Unusual configuration
>
> *Psyche*
> Maternal anxiety

Uterine Dysfunction

Uterine dysfunction is defined as uterine contractions that cause cervical change at a slower rate than expected. Uterine dysfunction can occur during the latent or active phase of the first stage of labor. The dysfunction is described as either hypertonic or hypotonic. Hypertonic uterine dysfunction causes upper and lower uterine segments to contract, uncoordinated and ineffective uterine contractions, and increased pain. Hypotonic uterine dysfunction causes a decrease in contraction intensity, duration, frequency, and the slowing or stopping of dilatation. *babi*   *Too strong*   *Slow contractions*

Assessment

The nurse must be skilled and knowledgeable to accurately assess the intensity of contractions. This is performed by indenting the fundus of the uterus with the fingertips at the acme of the contractions (see Chapter 11). At the peak of a strong contraction the uterine wall cannot be indented. At the acme of a contraction of moderate intensity, the uterine wall can be slightly indented. At the peak of a mild contraction, the uterine wall can be indented easily (Fig. 13-2). The timing of contractions (duration and frequency) can be accurately assessed by palpation or with the use of the external uterine activity monitor (tokodynamometer; see Chapter 11). Contraction intensity and baseline tone can only be precisely assessed with an intrauterine

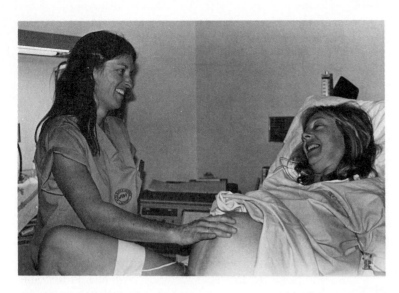

Figure 13-2. The nurse palpates the woman's uterine fundus to determine the intensity of the uterine contraction. The nurse's fingertips are placed at the top of the fundus; pressure is exerted on the uterine wall to assess its firmness. (Photo © Kathy Sloane, Courtesy of Alta Bates Medical Center.)

pressure catheter. The intrauterine pressure catheter is placed through the cervix into the uterus by the birth attendant. The membranes must be ruptured before the internal catheter is used (Fig. 13-3).

Management

With normal effective uterine contractions, the fundus and upper uterine segment contract while the lower uterine segment, including the cervix, relaxes. In hypertonic uterine dysfunction, uncoordinated uterine action occurs, with both segments of the uterus contracting at the same time. This distorts the normal distribution of the contractions, is very painful, and is ineffective at producing dilatation. Between contractions, the uterine muscle does not relax to the normal degree.

Nursing care of the woman with hypertonic uterine dysfunction includes rest and increased fluid intake. Sedation may be prescribed to allow her to rest. Safety precautions for the sedated woman are implemented. An intravenous infusion is often administered to maintain hydration and electrolyte balance. Normal labor usually resumes after a period of rest and hydration.

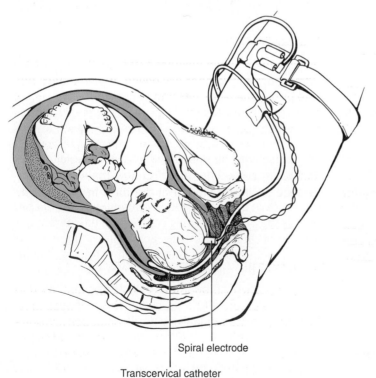

Spiral electrode

Transcervical catheter

Figure 13-3. The intrauterine pressure catheter in place in the uterus. The internal (direct) fetal monitor is also in place, attached to the scalp of the fetus. This method provides the greatest accuracy for uterine activity and fetal well-being.

In hypotonic uterine dysfunction, regular uterine contractions have been effective in dilating the cervix to at least 4 cm. After reaching this level, the contractions decrease in frequency, intensity, or duration. This reduction in uterine activity slows or stops the progress of cervical dilatation.

When hypotonic uterine dysfunction is suggested, pelvimetry is performed to assess for pelvic contracture. Assessments for abnormal fetal position, or other abnormalities, also are performed to determine if any of these contribute to the slowing of labor. If the passage and passenger are not the cause, labor may be augmented by amniotomy or oxytocin as discussed earlier.

Persistent Occiput Posterior Position

The persistent occiput posterior position is a problem with the passenger. This position occurs in approximately 25% of all labors. In the occiput posterior position, the occiput (the back of the fetus' head) is in the right (ROP) or left posterior (LOP) position (see Chapter 11). In either of these positions, the fetus makes a slow descent into the pelvis. The head of the fetus does not flex enough to present its smaller aspect to move through the pelvic outlet. This prolongs the labor.

Assessment

The position of the fetus is assessed through vaginal examinations and abdominal assessment. The labor is frequently long. The woman experiences quite a lot of back pain. This is commonly referred to as "back labor." The active phase of first stage of labor is usually prolonged. The extended time in labor causes the woman to become very tired, frustrated, and may lead to dehydration. If childbirth occurs without rotation to an anterior position, the woman may have severe perineal lacerations.

Management

The extended time in labor and the persistent back pain is often very discouraging to the woman and her labor partner. Back rubs, sacral pressure, and position changes may provide some comfort. Analgesia also can be administered within the guidelines of the birth attendant.

Breech Presentation

In approximately 3% of all gestations, the presenting part of the fetus is breech. This presentation is associated with a number of maternal and fetal complications, including multifetal pregnancy, fetal anomalies, hydramnios, placenta previa, prematurity, and grand multiparity (six or more viable pregnancies). Three types of breech presentations occur (see Chapter 11). Many breech presentations are delivered by cesarean birth. In vaginal birth, dystocia often occurs because the fetal buttocks are soft and do not dilate the cervix as well as the head does. Risks to the fetus in vaginal birth include aspiration of amniotic fluid, entrapment of the aftercoming head, fractures from manipulation during delivery, and prolapsed cord (discussed later in this chapter).

Assessment

Most breech presentations are identified during the second trimester. However, many of these turn to become vertex presentations before birth. Breech presentations occur more frequently when fetal weight is low, especially in preterm or multifetal pregnancies.

When breech presentation is confirmed, usually during a prenatal visit in late pregnancy, a decision is made concerning the best method of birth. Fetal size, pelvic adequacy, and fetal anomalies are some of the factors that determine the preferred birth method.

Occasionally labor begins before breech presentation is discovered. Assessment of the adequacy of the woman's pelvis and the size and position of the fetus must be made at that time to decide the preferred method of birth. Ultrasonography is used to aid in gathering the necessary information.

Management

Nursing intervention includes preparing the woman for ultrasonography if labor has begun. If membranes rupture during the labor, the nurse must carefully examine the vaginal discharge for the presence of meconium. Its presence must be reported immediately. Meconium is common in breech births because of the pressure on the buttocks of the fetus. However, it also may mean that the fetus is in distress. Neonatal attendants may be required to be present at the birth in that circumstance. The condition of the fetus is carefully monitored throughout the birth.

Cephalopelvic Disproportion

Cephalopelvic disproportion (CPD) is the term used to describe a problem with the size of the fetal head in relationship to the woman's pelvis. Cephalopelvic disproportion can be absolute or relative. Absolute CPD exists when a safe vaginal birth is impossible. Relative CPD occurs when the fetal head is positioned in such a way

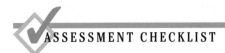

CPD

Absolute CPD:

Size of the fetal head in comparison with maternal pelvis prevents vaginal delivery

Relative CPD:

Fetal head is positioned in such a way that vaginal delivery will be difficult or impossible

Failure to progress:

General description of a lack of cervical change and fetal descent during the active phase of first stage of labor

that vaginal delivery will be difficult or impossible. The term *failure to progress* has been used to describe in general terms the lack of cervical change and fetal descent during the active phase of labor. These are summarized in the Assessment Checklist.

Assessment

During prenatal examinations, the differences between the size of the pelvis and the fetus are frequently detected. If there is a reasonable expectation that a successful vaginal birth might be possible, the woman may have a "trial labor." The uterine contractions may be strong enough to push the head of the fetus through the pelvis, and a vaginal birth proceeds. All four of the forces of labor (see Chapter 11) are factors in determining whether a vaginal birth can be successful. When absolute CPD is apparent, a cesarean birth is planned.

Management

If a cesarean birth becomes necessary, the nurse takes a positive attitude about the turn of events. Stressing the importance of the safety of the baby, the nurse can help the woman and her labor partner accept the need for the operative procedure.

Other Conditions Affecting the Onset of Labor

Several other factors may cause the onset of labor to begin earlier than desired. Two of the factors include prob-

lems with amniotic fluid, PROM, and hydramnios (excessive amniotic fluid). The third factor discussed here is multiple pregnancies (multifetal pregnancies). Each affect the onset of labor in their own way.

Premature Rupture of Membranes

Most women experience spontaneous rupture of the membranes during active labor (Chapter 11). However, rupture of amniotic fluid may occur before the onset of labor. When this happens at later than 37 weeks of pregnancy, it is referred to as **premature rupture of the membranes (PROM)**. When it occurs at less than 37 weeks, it is termed preterm premature rupture of the membranes (PPROM). This discussion centers on rupture of membranes after the 37th week of pregnancy.

Before 20 wks

Assessment

Any woman who states she has had a "loss of fluid" must be evaluated for PROM. An examination with a sterile speculum is performed to observe for amniotic fluid in the vagina or leaking from the cervix. A sample of fluid is obtained for testing by means of the nitrazine or fern test (see Chapter 11). If amniotic fluid is present, the nurse notes the character, color, and odor of the fluid. Nursing assessment includes a careful review with the woman to determine the time the membranes ruptured and the amount and character of the expelled fluid. In addition, fetal heart tones are monitored to assure fetal well-being.

Cervical cultures may be taken to evaluate for the presence of infections, such as group B streptococcus and trichomoniasis. Cervical dilatation is determined by an examination. The presence of prolapsed cord is also ruled out. Ultrasonography may be performed to confirm a reduced amount of fluid around the fetus. To reduce the possibility of introduction of infection, digital examination is avoided until the woman is in active labor.

Management

Management of the woman with PROM is somewhat controversial and varies from one birth attendant to another. Some wait several days to allow labor to start spontaneously while carefully observing the woman for signs of intrauterine infection (chorioamnionitis). Other birth attendants may wait only 6 to 12 hours before inducing labor. Fetal heart tones are monitored periodically throughout this time.

The woman is admitted to the labor unit for observation and evaluation. The nurse has assesses for signs of infection such as fever, tachycardia of the woman or fetus, the woman's elevated white blood cell count, or presence of fundal tenderness. Monitoring the status of the fetus and reducing potential risk factors for introducing infection must be ongoing. In addition, the nurse must support the woman and her family throughout this time. Nursing interventions to promote labor and provide comfort are initiated. If infection is determined to be present, antibiotics are administered and labor is induced.

Hydramnios

Hydramnios (also called polyhydramnios) is the accumulation of more than 2000 mL amniotic fluid. Amniotic fluid normally increases during pregnancy until it peaks at approximately 34 weeks. The volume is approximately 980 mL at that time. From that time until 40 weeks, there is a decrease of 150 to 830 mL. Review Chapter 9 for the functions of amniotic fluid. During pregnancy, the fetus swallows and voids amniotic fluid. In late pregnancy, this swallowing and voiding exchange is approximately 400 to 500 mL/day. Any fetal anomaly that may upset this exchange can cause an excess accumulation of amniotic fluid. These congenital anomalies may include neural tube or gastrointestinal tract defects. Conditions of the woman that are contributing factors include diabetes mellitus, Rh isoimmunization, and multiple pregnancies.

It can cause a prolapse cord
Less than 500cc Oligohydramnios. -IUGR
Dehydration

Assessment

The usual first indication of hydramnios is uterine enlargement greater than expected for the length of the pregnancy and excessive weight gain of the woman. On abdominal palpation, fetal parts may be difficult to detect. The fetal heart may be difficult to auscultate. An ultrasound examination confirms the extent of the hydramnios. As the result of severe hydramnios, the woman may have abdominal discomfort, difficulty ambulating or moving about, edema, dyspnea, or varicosities of the lower extremities or vulva.

Management

A series of amniocentesis may be performed to drain excess amniotic fluid before the onset of labor. When membranes rupture, there is a increased danger of prolapsed cord. Nursing interventions are directed to increasing the woman's comfort level. Respiratory discomfort is common, because of the excessive pressure placed on the diaphragm by the extra fluid and enlarged uterus. Ambulation may be reduced or prohibited because of the danger of prolapse cord should the membranes rupture during ambulation.

Multiple Gestations

Multifetal pregnancy predisposes the woman and fetuses to an increased risk of complications throughout the antepartum and intrapartum periods. The atmosphere of a multifetal birth is charged with excitement and anticipation.

Assessment

Approximately 50% of twins are born before 37 weeks' gestation. Intrauterine growth retardation also is a concern because of limited space available to the fetuses. Other potential fetal complications for which the nurse must be alert include congenital anomalies, placental abnormalities, cord accidents (nuchal cord, prolapsed cord), and malpresentations. In addition, maternal pregnancy-induced hypertension, hydramnios, and significant anemia may occur. These factors all must be considered during assessment.

Management

As a result of malpresentation or prematurity, many twin gestations, and all triplet or greater gestations, require delivery by cesarean birth. The decision to allow the woman to attempt vaginal birth is made based on gestational age and fetal presentation. The vaginal birth of vertex–vertex twins is considered to be safe. In other presentations, such as breech–vertex, cesarean birth is generally necessary (Fig. 13-4).

In the event vaginal birth of a twin pregnancy is planned, continuous fetal and uterine activity monitoring is used during labor and birth. There is no contraindication to anesthesia or analgesia. Oxytocin augmentation may be used if indicated. There is an increased risk for uterine rupture (discussed later in this chapter) or postpartum hemorrhage as a result of uterine overdistension. Vaginal birth of a twin pregnancy should take place only in a facility with the ability to perform emergency cesarean birth and provide adequate neonatal support.

The nurse must monitor the condition of the woman and both fetuses throughout the labor and birth. As each neonate is born, careful identification must be performed. A second nurse is needed to help with the second neonate, especially if they are born in rapid succession. Resuscitation is administered to the neonates as needed. Equipment for this possibility is kept close at hand for emergency use.

When cesarean birth is determined to be appropriate, routine cesarean birth preparation is performed. Two neonatal nurses and a neonatologist or pediatrician frequently are in attendance at the birth. They care

Amniotic Fluid Embolism — Can be Caused by hypertonic Labor Contraction
May be caused by Oxytocin therels a tear in the fluid
And it gets into the mothers Circulation

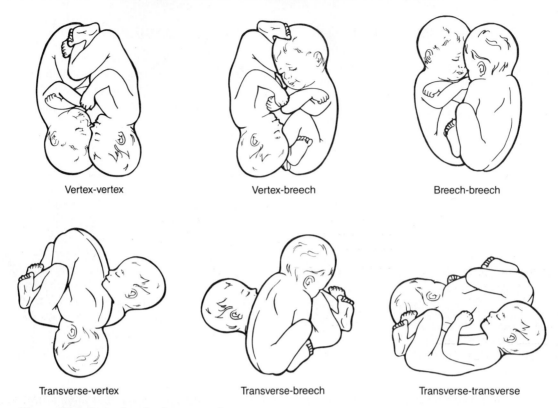

Vertex-vertex   Vertex-breech   Breech-breech

Transverse-vertex   Transverse-breech   Transverse-transverse

Figure 13-4. *Examples of twin presentations.*

for the neonates immediately after birth. A double set of equipment must be available to care for the neonates.

Complications During the Childbirth Process

During the process of birth, problems can occur that seriously threaten the health of the fetus or the mother. Several of these are fetal cord prolapse, uterine rupture, and uterine inversion.

Prolapse of the Umbilical Cord

Prolapse of the umbilical cord (**prolapsed cord**) is the dropping or slipping down of the umbilical cord into the pelvic outlet ahead of the presenting part. It occurs most often in early labor when the fetal presenting part is not engaged in the pelvic inlet (see Chapter 11). When membranes rupture, either spontaneously or artificially, amniotic fluid carries a loop of the umbilical cord into the pelvis or cervix. The fetal presenting part may partially or completely compress the umbilical cord and reduce or stop the flow of blood to the fetus (Fig. 13-5).

Factors that contribute to the possibility of prolapsed cord include rupture of the membranes before engagement, prematurity (because of the small size of the fetus), hydramnios, multifetal gestation, abnormally long umbilical cord, and abnormal fetal position.

Assessment

At times a prolapsed cord can be easily identified by palpation of the cord in the cervix or vagina. More often, the first indication of cord prolapse is a change in the fetal heart rate with the development of bradycardia or decelerations. When membranes rupture, whether spontaneously or artificially, the nurse assesses the fetal heart rate immediately and again in 15 minutes for signs of bradycardia or decelerations.

Management

Prolapsed cord is an emergency situation. It demands an immediate response from the nurse. This requires repositioning the woman to relieve the pressure of the presenting part against the cord. The woman is placed in the Trendelenburg position with her head lower than her hips or in a knee–chest position (Fig. 13-6). Placing three pillows under the woman's hips helps relieve the pressure if she cannot be easily placed in Trendelenburg's position. In some instances, the presenting part can be pushed away from the cord by inserting a sterile

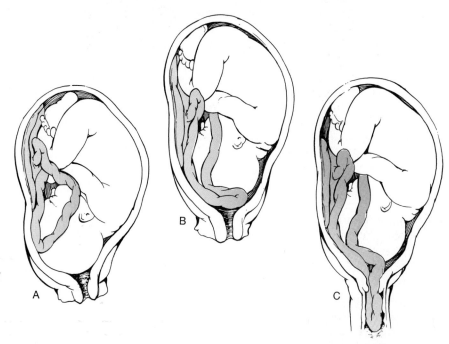

Figure 13-5. Prolapse of the cord. As the head comes down, the compression of the cord between the fetal skull and the pelvic brim will shut off circulation completely. **(A)** Occult prolapse. **(B)** Cord prolapse in front of head. **(C)** Cord prolapse into vagina.

gloved hand into the vagina. Delivery of the neonate must be accomplished as quickly as possible. In some facilities, 500 to 1000 mL normal saline is instilled into the woman's bladder through an indwelling catheter in an attempt to elevate the presenting part. Unless the cervix is sufficiently dilated, a cesarean birth is necessary.

Uterine Rupture

Fortunately, **uterine rupture**, catastrophic rupture of the uterine muscle, occurs very rarely. However, when it does occur it carries a significant risk for fetal or neonatal mortality. The woman is also at risk for hypotension, hypovolemia, infection, and death.

The most common cause of uterine rupture is dehiscence (separation) of a previous uterine scar. The risk is much greater with a vertical scar, such as those

seen with a previous classical cesarean birth scar. Uterine rupture has also been associated with improper use of oxytocin. Other causes include maternal abdominal trauma, prolonged labor, fetal malpresentations or malpositions, large fetal size, and traumatic birth.

Assessment

The woman with a suspected uterine rupture may have a variety of signs and symptoms dependent on the extent of the injury. The rupture may be small without signs. It may not be diagnosed until cesarean birth is in progress. Often signs and symptoms become more evident over a period of hours. These include abdominal pain and tenderness, loss of fetal heart rate, vaginal bleeding, and signs of shock in the woman. At other times the onset may be more dramatic, with sudden, intense abdominal pain, loss of uterine contractions, and

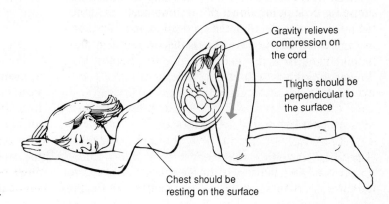

Gravity relieves compression on the cord

Thighs should be perpendicular to the surface

Chest should be resting on the surface

Figure 13-6. Woman assumes a knee–chest position to relieve pressure on the cord when cord is prolapsed.

fetal death. The fetus may be palpable outside of the uterus.

Management

Uterine rupture requires immediate delivery, usually cesarean. The woman may require blood transfusions, antibiotics, and fluid replacement. It is sometimes possible to repair a ruptured uterus surgically, but many require hysterectomy.

Uterine Inversion

Uterine inversion is the partial or complete turning inside-out of the uterus. It may occur in the third or fourth stage of labor and has serious implications for the woman. There is pronounced vaginal bleeding, which reaches hemorrhagic proportions almost immediately. Uterine inversion is associated with abnormal placental implantation, precipitous (very rapid) births, excessive pulling of the umbilical cord for delivery of the placenta, and fundal pressure or kneading during the birth process.

Assessment

Assessment of uterine inversion is made during or just after delivery of the placenta. Partial inversion occurs when the fundus enters the uterine cavity without extending through the cervical os. Discovery of a partial inversion usually is made after the woman is transferred to the recovery or postpartum unit. Complete uterine inversion happens when the entire uterus turns on itself and extends beyond the cervical os. Complete inversion generally is visualized at the time of placental delivery. Bleeding associated with uterine inversion must be controlled quickly to avoid hypovolemic shock and possible death.

Management

Management of uterine inversion consists of manually reinverting the uterus to its normal position. This may need to be done under anesthesia. The nurse must stay with the woman continuously and summon help immediately when uterine inversion is discovered. The birth attendant replaces the uterus into position. Surgery may be necessary.

◆ Operative Procedures

Operative obstetrics are specific procedures undertaken to achieve delivery of the fetus. Two operative procedures used to assist in a vaginal birth are forceps delivery and vacuum extractions. The most common surgical operative procedure to achieve delivery is cesarean birth.

Forceps Delivery

Forceps are instruments used to help deliver the fetus in a vaginal delivery. They are like large metal tongs that can be separated and applied one side at a time. In this way, forceps are applied to the fetal head, and traction is exerted. When forceps are used, the second stage of labor is shortened. Forceps also are used to rotate the fetal head from an undesirable position to one more conducive to delivery (Fig. 13-7).

Each pair of forceps has a right and left blade. The blades are curved to conform to the fetal head and maternal pelvis. There are specific forceps designed for specific maternal and fetal indications. Forceps deliveries are classified according to the level and position of the head in relationship to the maternal pelvis outlet as outlet forceps or low forceps, midforceps, or high forceps. Forceps used to guide and control the head after it is visible or nearly visible at the vaginal opening the are called outlet or low forceps. Midforceps are those applied when the head of the fetus is engaged, but is higher than station +2. High forceps, no longer in use because of danger to the woman or fetus, were applied when the head was above engagement.

Conditions that may indicate the need for forceps delivery are prolonged second stage, cardiac disease of the woman, or exhaustion. The most common fetal indication is fetal heart rate abnormalities.

The birth attendant makes the decision to use forceps. The nurse supports the woman, keeping her informed about what is happening. Injuries may occur to the tissues of the woman's vagina and cervix or the episiotomy may extend into the rectal tissues. The woman may be at a greater risk for infection from these injuries. Careful observations for infections is an essential part of postpartum nursing care after forceps delivery. The neonate may have some bruising on the head or face, which will disappear in a few days. There also is a possibility of neurologic damage as a result of skull fracture and intracranial hemorrhage.

Vacuum Extraction

Vacuum extraction involves applying a cup, called a vacuum extractor, to the fetal head and withdrawing air from the cup. This creates a vacuum within the cup, securing it to the fetal head. Traction is then applied to deliver the fetal head. The cups come in various sizes, and the largest one that can be applied easily is used (Fig. 13-8). This procedure is an alternative to forceps delivery. The indications for vacuum extraction are the same as for forceps deliveries.

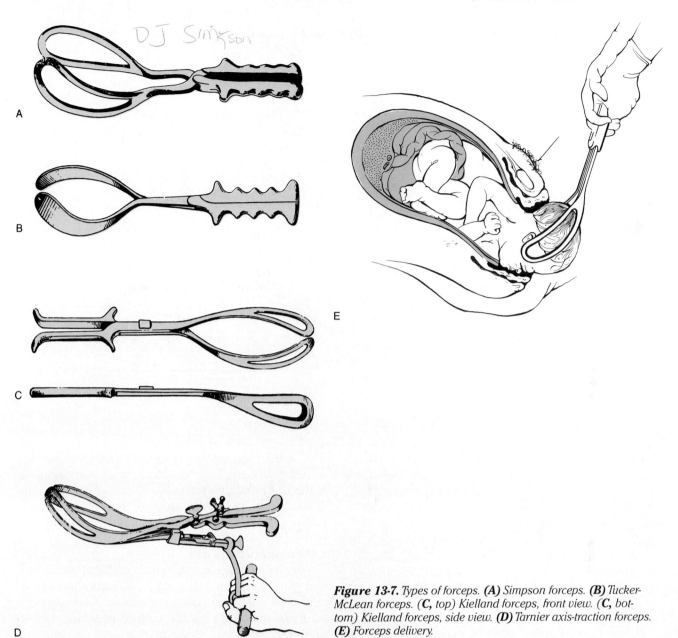

Figure 13-7. *Types of forceps.* **(A)** *Simpson forceps.* **(B)** *Tucker-McLean forceps.* **(C,** *top) Kielland forceps, front view.* **(C,** *bottom) Kielland forceps, side view.* **(D)** *Tarnier axis-traction forceps.* **(E)** *Forceps delivery.*

There are no apparent risks to the woman in a vacuum extraction delivery. Disadvantages to the fetus include bruising or edema of the fetal scalp. There is an increased risk for cephalhematoma (bleeding between the periosteum and the bone in the fetal skull) or lacerations of the scalp. The nurse explains to the family that the injuries to the neonate's head are temporary. There are no long-term effects from these injuries.

Cesarean Birth

Cesarean birth (also called cesarean section) is a surgical procedure in which birth is accomplished through an incision into the abdomen and uterus of the woman. Two types of incisions are used to perform the procedure, classical and low segment (bikini). The classical incision is a vertical incision into the body of the uterus. This type of incision can be performed quickly. It may be selected when an emergency exists, such as maternal hemorrhage or prolapsed cord. It also may be necessary for the delivery of a very early preterm fetus. The skin incision for the low segment delivery is made transversely on the mons pubis. The lower segment of the uterus is cut horizontally. The external incision is later covered by pubic hair; therefore, it is called a bikini cut. This type of incision reduces the risk of bleeding and is easier to repair (Fig. 13-9). The number of cesarean births has increased in the United

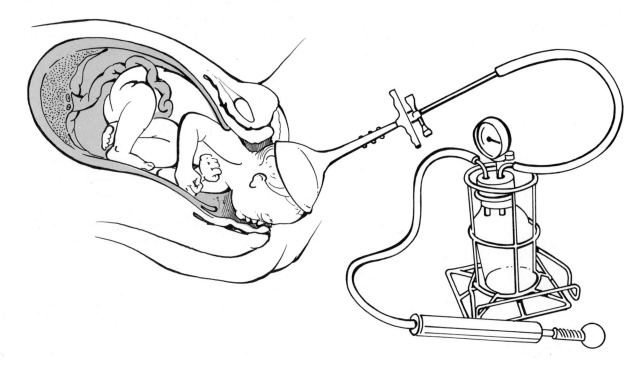

Figure 13-8. *Vacuum extractor with suction cup applied to the scalp of the fetus.*

States in recent years. Factors thought to contribute to this increase include increased electronic fetal monitoring, an increased number of high-risk pregnancies carried to term, and changing criteria for managing breech births. A surgical procedure results in more risks to the woman and the fetus. These risks must be balanced against the anticipated risks in a vaginal birth when the decision is made to perform the cesarean procedure.

Assessment

A cesarean birth is performed when vaginal delivery is not possible or not safe. The most common indications for cesarean birth include CPD, labor disorders, malpresentations, fetal distress, and previous cesarean birth. An emergency cesarean is performed when immediate delivery is necessary to prevent maternal or fetal morbidity or mortality. An elective cesarean is one that is planned ahead of time when a vaginal delivery is determined to be unwise.

Prenatal assessment determines the need for an elective cesarean birth. Prenatal stress testing, electronic fetal monitoring (EFM), and ultrasonography contribute to forming an accurate picture of possible birth problems. During labor, EFM, internal uterine transducers, and fetal scalp blood pH contribute to making the decision to perform a cesarean.

Management

Care for the woman who is undergoing a cesarean birth procedure falls into three phases, preoperative, intraoper-

ative, and postoperative. During each phase the needs of the fetus also are addressed. The surgery may take place in the labor and delivery unit or in the operating room, depending on the facility. Much of the woman's care is similar to that for any abdominal surgery procedure.

Preoperative Care

In an elective (planned) cesarean birth, the woman and her labor partner often have the opportunity to attend cesarean birth preparation classes. These are helpful in orienting the couple to the procedure and in answering questions. However, there may be little opportunity to do much preoperative teaching with the woman having an emergency cesarean. As much information as possible must be provided to the woman, even when the decision to perform a cesarean birth is made during labor.

Routine preoperative teaching, including early ambulation and coughing and deep breathing postoperatively, is included in preoperative teaching. This includes where the procedure will take place, the anesthesia planned, approximately how long it will take, when the neonate will return to the nursery, the woman's recovery period, and when she will return to her postpartum room.

The woman undergoing cesarean birth has an indwelling urinary catheter inserted into the bladder to keep it empty during surgery. This reduces the risk of injury to the bladder when the incision is made. The catheter may be inserted in the operating room just before surgery begins, if the physician chooses. The ab-

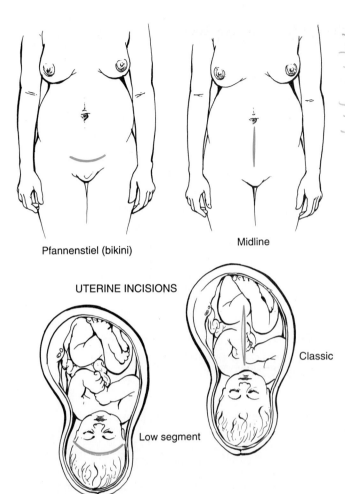

Pfannenstiel (bikini) Midline

UTERINE INCISIONS

Classic

Low segment

Figure 13-9. Cesarean birth incisions.

domen is shaved. It is cleansed with antiseptic solution immediately before the skin incision is made. The woman is NPO (nulla per os; allowed nothing to eat by mouth). An intravenous infusion through a wide-bore catheter is started. Preoperative narcotics are rarely ordered to avoid neonatal respiratory depression. An anticholinergic (atropine) may be administered to dry secretions. An antacid to neutralize stomach acids may be administered to prevent pneumonia in case of vomiting and aspiration during surgery. The woman's vital signs and the fetal heart rate are monitored at least every 4 hours before surgery. The support person who is going to surgery with the woman needs instructions about changing into scrub clothes and the role that he or she is expected to take.

Intraoperative Care

The type of anesthesia selected for cesarean birth depends on many factors. If the surgery is elective, regional anesthesia, epidural or spinal, is often adminis-

tered. One of the most common complications of this type of anesthesia is hypotension in the woman. Placing the woman in a left lateral position and providing adequate hydration with intravenous fluids are often helpful in combating anesthesia-induced hypotension. Severe postpartum headaches are occasionally experienced with spinal anesthesia.

General anesthesia is most often administered in emergency situations, or when regional anesthesia is contraindicated. One of the most serious complications encountered with the use of general anesthesia is aspiration of gastric contents. This danger is increased in emergencies when fasting may not have occurred before anesthetic induction. There is also an increased risk of neonatal respiratory depression with general anesthesia. To prevent this risk, nursing personnel attempt to complete as much of the preparations as possible before the anesthetic is given. Anesthesia is not administered until the physician is ready to begin the incision. As soon as the nurse anesthetist or anesthesiologist indicates that the woman is sufficiently anesthetized, the physician works very quickly to make the necessary incision and remove the neonate. The remainder of the surgery is completed after the removal of the neonate.

A pediatrician or neonatal nurse usually is present to care for the neonate immediately on delivery. A heated crib, oxygen, and resuscitative equipment are available.

Postoperative Care

Postoperative care after a cesarean birth is similar to that for any abdominal surgery. Additionally, assessments are made similar to those for vaginal deliveries. Frequent assessments are made of vital signs, lochial flow, fundal tone, and urinary output. The infusion of intravenous fluid is maintained until the woman is afebrile, has resumption of bowel sounds, and is tolerating fluids. The fundus is massaged as necessary, and oxytocin is infused. The abdominal incision is observed for bleeding and intactness. Medications are administered as needed for pain and nausea.

The woman who has had a cesarean birth may need a lot of support in the postpartum period. The first day after surgery she may feel weak and have a lot of abdominal pain. Administered analgesias may reduce her ability to bond with her neonate. She may feel too weak to handle her newborn. She needs assistance during this time. Thoughtful, sensitive nursing care helps her to overcome her sense of inadequacy and strengthens her ability to establish a good beginning relationship with her newborn. See the Nursing Care Plan for the Woman Experiencing a Cesarean Birth.

NURSING CARE PLAN
for the Woman Experiencing a Cesarean Birth

ASSESSMENT: Fetal presentation breech
EDD demonstrates 39.5 weeks' gestation
Scheduled for cesarean birth

PREOPERATIVE:

NURSING DIAGNOSIS #1: Anxiety, related to cesarean birth procedures and outcome

EXPECTED OUTCOME: The woman's and her family's levels of anxiety will be decreased with improved understanding of the cesarean birth procedures and expected outcome

Nursing Interventions	*Rationale*
1. Review the cesarean birth procedure with woman and her family. Include in the review the approximate time the newborn will return to the unit, where the woman will recover, approximately how long she will be in the recovery unit.	1. Clearly stated information with guidelines help the woman and her family begin to form a better understanding of the cesarean birth process.
2. Encourage woman and her family to express their fears. Give straightforward answers to alleviate their fears.	2. Unspoken fears increase anxieties. When fears are brought out into the open, acknowledged, and clarified anxiety is decreased.
3. Instruct the support person who will be accompanying the woman to surgery concerning scrub clothes, staff persons accompanying, and specific information about his or her role.	3. The woman's anxiety will be decreased with the knowledge that her support person will be with her.

EVALUATION: The anxiety of the woman and her family are decreased as evidenced by verbal expression and cooperation.

NURSING DIAGNOSIS #2: Knowledge Deficit, postoperative complications related to lack of preoperative preparation.

EXPECTED OUTCOME: The woman learns coughing and deep breathing before surgery, as well as incision splinting methods and comfort measures

Nursing Interventions	*Rationale*
1. Explain to the woman the importance of postoperative deep breathing. Demonstrate use of the incentive spirometer and coughing and deep breathing exercises.	1. The woman will cooperate more readily if she understands the importance of deep respirations. Before surgery the woman is more likely to be able to focus on demonstration of technique.
2. Demonstrate how the woman can use a pillow to support her incision when moving about postoperatively.	2. The woman wishes to be as comfortable as possible postoperatively and is open to suggestions at this time.
3. Stress to the woman the importance of moving about after surgery. Encourage her to use comfort measures and to ask for analgesia when needed.	3. It is necessary for the woman to understand that she is not expected to suffer excessive pain or discomfort, but that moving about is very important to her recovery.

EVALUATION: The woman verbalizes the importance of deep breathing, coughing, and moving about postoperatively. She returns the demonstration of techniques that the nurse has taught her.

Trial of Labor and Vaginal Birth After Cesarean Birth (VBAC)

VBAC is the acronym (letters of words abbreviated to make a new word) for **v**aginal **b**irth **a**fter **c**esarean. It is pronounced "veeback." The old adage "once a cesarean, always a cesarean" does not necessarily hold true in modern obstetric care. In fact, for most patients, vaginal delivery is a safer route than operative delivery. The patient who has a previous low transverse cesarean section may desire an attempt at a trial of labor and vaginal delivery in subsequent pregnancies. Dehiscence of a former low transverse uterine incision occurs less than 1% of the time. A VBAC may be attempted if a prior low transverse or low cervical scar on the uterus is documented, and there is no medical or obstetrical contraindication to labor, and no history of prior uterine rupture.

Intrapartum care of the woman who desires a trial of labor is essentially the same as for any woman in labor. Oxytocin may be used for the usual indications without the need for additional monitoring. Analgesia and anesthesia, including epidural, may be used as desired for labor discomfort. The success rate for women undergoing a trial of labor is reported to be between 65% and 85%. Close observation of fetal status and uterine contractions is maintained throughout the labor. The facility must have the capability to perform an emergency cesarean birth, if necessary. The woman should be cautioned to avoid getting her hopes too high. She may feel greatly disappointed and think of the attempt as a failure if the trial is not successful.

Emergency Delivery by the Nurse

Emergency delivery by the nurse is not a common situation, but can occur. Most frequently, this is the result of a precipitous labor. A precipitous labor is one that lasts less than 3 hours before spontaneous birth of the neonate. The woman may have a history of delivering unexpectedly at home. Factors that contribute to a precipitous labor and birth are multiparity, low resistance of the woman's tissues, large pelvis, small fetus, cocaine abuse, or lack of awareness of contractions. The nurse caring for laboring women must be prepared to handle this unexpected circumstance. A calm, reassuring manner and deliberate actions are necessary to decrease the risk of injury to the mother and infant.

When it is apparent that the woman will deliver without the presence of the birth attendant, the labor nurse makes preparations to ensure a safe environment for delivery. Most birthing units have emergency packs available in the event of precipitous delivery. These packs contain sterile drapes, gloves, and a bulb syringe. This pack is obtained and opened. The woman's hips are elevated, if possible, and her head raised approximately 45 degrees. It is not necessary to provide a totally sterile field, but cleanliness is important. The nurse performs hand washing, puts on gloves, quickly cleanses the woman's perineum, and applies the drapes. The nurse must stay with the woman when precipitous birth becomes apparent. The nurse calls for the additional help of another nurse, if possible. The lower portion of the birthing bed or delivery table should not be removed because a wet, vernix-covered newborn is very slippery and difficult to hold on to.

For the actual delivery, upward pressure is applied on the perineum at the level of the fetal chin, while gentle downward pressure is applied to the occiput. The nurse encourages the woman to pant during delivery of the head. Once the head is through the vaginal opening, mucus is suctioned from the infant's mouth and nose with the bulb syringe. The nurse passes a finger around the neck of the neonate to check for the presence of a nuchal cord. If present, the nurse attempts to remove the cord by sliding it over the head of the neonate. If the cord is wound tightly around the neck, it must be double clamped and cut between the clamps to remove it. To deliver the shoulders, the nurse places a hand on either side of the head of the neonate and applies gentle downward and outward traction while the woman pushes. Once the anterior shoulder is delivered, gentle upward traction is applied to deliver the remainder of the body. The neonate may come so quickly that traction will not be needed. Important points that must be followed are suction the neonate's mouth and nose; hold the neonate close to the vaginal opening to avoid tension on the cord; hold the neonate's head down to promote drainage; and keep the neonate above the level of the vaginal outlet before the cord is cut to prevent transfusion of the neonate by gravity flow. The nurse dries and wraps the neonate in warm, dry blankets. Continuing care follows the procedures of routine care.

Psychosocial Considerations

When a woman has any of the complications of labor, she will experience anxiety and fear. Her labor partner and her family also will be apprehensive and anxious.

The nurse must be sensitive and respond to their anxieties. Acknowledging that the circumstances may be upsetting and reassuring them that their anxiety is accepted can help put them at ease. Clear communication with the woman and her family is essential. Careful, complete explanations are necessary. The woman and the family must be given ample opportunity to ask questions, and the nurse must provide straightforward, simple answers. The nurse must be aware that they may have unspoken questions that they need to be encouraged to vocalize. In some situations, it may be helpful to have an additional staff person assist in providing the support that the family needs during a trying experience. A caring and concerned attitude reflected by the nurse is reassuring to the woman and her family.

REVIEW AND PREVIEW

The number of women who have complicated intrapartum experiences is relatively small. This chapter has presented a description of families at risk. The intrapartum complications covered included preterm labor and its contributing factors, and the induction of labor. Induction by amniotomy, oxytocin induction, and insertion of prostaglandin gel was discussed.

The discussion of dystocia covered the influence of the forces of labor, including power, passenger, passage, and psyche. Other conditions affecting the onset of labor included premature rupture of membranes, hydramnios, and multifetal pregnancies. Complications included cord prolapse, uterine rupture, and uterine inversion. Births assisted by forceps and vacuum extraction were presented. Nursing care for each was addressed. Cesarean birth and VBAC were discussed, including nursing interventions. Finally, also included was the nurse's responsibility in a precipitous labor and birth when the birth attendant is not present. General psychosocial aspects of intrapartum complications also were presented.

The following chapter explores the normal physiologic and psychologic changes associated with the postpartum period. This foundation of information helps the nurse understand the principles of nursing care and nursing interventions. When caring for the postpartum woman, the nurse who has knowledge of the labor and birth process has an appreciation for the adjustments that the woman's body must make in the postpartum period.

◈ KEY POINTS

◆ Preterm labor is the onset of regular uterine contractions resulting in cervical dilatation and effacement between 20 and 37 weeks' gestation. Contributing factors include second trimester abortion, previous preterm delivery, diethylstilbestrol (DES) exposure, late or no prenatal care, poor weight gain, hydramnios, placenta previa, reproductive tract infection, cervical incompetence, multifetal gestation, substance abuse, low socioeconomic status, and poor nutrition.

◆ Induction of labor is the stimulation of uterine contractions before onset of spontaneous labor. Labor can be induced by amniotomy, the administration of oxytocin, or the insertion of prostaglandin gel or suppository.

◆ Dystocia is difficult labor. It is the result of difficulties with one or more of the forces of labor: power, passage, passenger, or psyche.

◆ The position of the fetus can increase the length of labor, causing increased pain, severe backache, and can cause birth to be delayed or difficult.

◆ PROM is premature rupture of membranes. This occurs when the pregnancy is at term but labor has not started. PPROM is preterm premature rupture of membranes occurring between 20 and 37 weeks of gestation.

◆ Hydramnios is an excess accumulation of amniotic fluid, often as much as 2000 mL. Hydramnios can cause abdominal discomfort, difficulty ambulating, edema, dyspnea, and varicosities of the vulva or lower extremities. Prolapsed cord is a greater danger when membranes rupture with hydramnios.

◆ Prolapsed cord can result in compression of the umbilical cord, causing a decreased blood flow to the fetus, which results in fetal distress or fetal death.

◆ When prolapsed cord becomes apparent, the nurse must immediately reposition the woman to relieve the pressure that is pressing against the cord. Pressure can be relieved by placing the woman in Trendelenburg's position, knee-chest position, or by elevating her hips with three pillows.

◆ Cesarean birth is a surgical procedure that results in the birth of the neonate. Cesarean birth may be performed for labor disorders or emergencies, CPD, fetal malpresentations, fetal distress, or previous cesarean birth.

◆ In an emergency delivery, the nurse stays with the woman. The nurse assists the delivery of the neonate, clears the neonate's airway, checks for nuchal cord, keeps the neonate's head down with the body above the vaginal outlet, dries and wraps the neonate, and calls for assistance.

BIBLIOGRAPHY

Creasy, R. K., & Resnik, R. (1994). *Maternal-fetal medicine: Principles and practice* (3rd ed.). Philadelphia: W. B. Saunders.

Cunningham, F. G., MacDonald, P. C., Gant, N. F., Leveno, K. J., and Gilstrap, L. C. (1993). *Williams obstetrics* (19th ed.). Norwalk, CT: Appleton-Lange.

D'Avanzo, C. E. (1992). Bridging the cultural gap with Southeast Asians. *Maternal Child Nursing, 17*(4), 204–208.

Dunn, P. A., York, R., Cheek, T. G., & Yeboah, K. (1994). Maternal hypothermia: implications for obstetric nurses. *Journal of Obstetric, Gynecologic, and Neonatal Nursing, 23*(3), 238–242.

SELF-ASSESSMENT

1. Which of the following patients is *least* likely to experience a uterine rupture?

○ **A.** A woman with a previous classical cesarean delivery
○ **B.** A woman who delivers at 34 weeks' gestation
○ **C.** A woman with a prolonged labor that required oxytocin augmentation
○ **D.** A woman with previous surgery for uterine fibroids

2. The nurse must carefully assess the mother who delivered twins for which of the following conditions?

○ **A.** Endometritis
○ **B.** Deep vein thrombosis
○ **C.** Postpartum hemorrhage
○ **D.** Eclamptic seizure

3. Hydramnios places the woman at higher risk for:

○ **A.** A prolapsed cord
○ **B.** A precipitous delivery
○ **C.** Developing gestational diabetes
○ **D.** Developing preeclampsia

4. Following artificial rupture of the membranes (AROM), the nurse's most important actions should be:

○ **A.** Monitoring maternal vital signs
○ **B.** Monitoring the frequency of contractions
○ **C.** Noting the color of the amniotic fluid
○ **D.** Noting cervical dilation and effacement

5. When the fetus is in a persistent occiput posterior (OP) position, the patient will most likely experience:

○ **A.** A shortened first stage of labor
○ **B.** An uncomplicated delivery
○ **C.** PPROM
○ **D.** Severe back pain

Fawcett, J., Tulman, L., & Spedden, J. P. (1994). Responses to vaginal birth after cesarean section. *Journal of Obstetric, Gynecologic, and Neonatal Nursing, 23*(3), 253–259.

Griese, M. E., & Prickett, S. A. (1992). Nursing management of umbilical cord prolapse. *Journal of Obstetric, Gynecologic, and Neonatal Nursing, 22*(4), 311–315.

Karch, A. M. (1992). *Handbook of drugs and the nursing process* (2nd ed.). Philadelphia: J. B. Lippincott.

Knupple, R. A., & Drukker, J. E. (1986). *High-risk pregnancy: A team approach* (2nd ed.). Philadelphia: W. B. Saunders.

Lynam, L. E., & Miller, M. A. (1992). Mothers' and nurses' perceptions of the needs of women experiencing preterm labor. *Journal of Obstetric, Gynecologic and Neonatal Nursing, 21*(2), 126–136.

Martin, L. L., & Reeder, S. J. (1990). *Essentials of maternity nursing: Family centered care*. Philadelphia: J. B. Lippincott.

May, K. A. (1994). Impact of maternal activity restriction for preterm labor on the expectant father. *Journal of Obstetric, Gynecologic, and Neonatal Nursing, 23*(3), 246–251.

May, K. A., & Mahlmeister, L. R. (1994). *Maternal & neonatal nursing: Family-centered care* (3rd ed.). Philadelphia: J. B. Lippincott.

Pillitteri, A. (1992) *Maternal and child nursing: Care of the childbearing and childrearing family*. Philadelphia: J. B. Lippincott.

Quirk, J. G. (1992). *Perinatal Educational Resource and Learning System— PERLS*. Little Rock: University of Arkansas for Medical Sciences.

Reeder, S. J., Martin, L. L., & Koniak, D. (1992). *Maternity Nursing: Family, Newborn, and Women's Health Care* (17th ed.). Philadelphia: J. B. Lippincott.

Reese, E. A., Hobbins, J. C., Mahoney, M. J., & Petrie, R. H. (1992). *Medicine of the fetus and mother*. Philadelphia: J. B. Lippincott.

Riechert, J. A., Baron, M., & Fawcett, J. (1993). Changes in attitudes toward cesarean childbirth. *Journal of Obstetrics, Gynecologic, and Neonatal Nursing, 22*(2), 159–167.

Scherer, J. C. (1992). *Introductory Clinical Pharmacology* (4th ed.). Philadelphia: J. B. Lippincott.

Scherer, J. C. (1992). *Introductory medical-surgical nursing* (5th ed.). Philadelphia: J. B. Lippincott.

The Family in the Postpartum Period

CHAPTER 14

Normal Postpartum Physical and Psychosocial Changes

Objectives

Terminology

Physical Changes During the Postpartum Period

Psychosocial Changes During the Postpartum Period

Adolescent Considerations

Cultural Considerations

The Role of the Nurse

Review and Preview

Key Points

Self-Assessment

Bibliography

Returning to Non Pregnant state
Puerperium A time of healing
time of change

◆ OBJECTIVES

When the learning goals of this chapter are met, the reader will be able to:

- ◆ Define the postpartum period.
- ◆ Describe the significant physical changes in the reproductive system.
- ◆ List the three types of lochia, including their characteristics.
- ◆ Explain the hormonal changes that take place after childbirth.
- ◆ Describe the physical changes that occur in the cardiovascular system during the postpartum period.
- ◆ List at least three psychosocial events the family typically experiences after childbirth.
- ◆ Discuss the three stages of the maternal response during the postpartum period.
- ◆ Explain parent–newborn attachment and the activities that take place during initial bonding.
- ◆ Discuss the benefits of encouraging siblings and extended family members to visit the couple and newborn after labor and birth.
- ◆ Discuss the significance of cultural considerations for the postpartum family.

TERMINOLOGY

After-pains	Letting-go
Attachment	Lochia alba
Colostrum	Lochia rubra
Ecchymosis	Lochia serosa
Involution	Postpartum depression
Lactation	Taking-in
Let-down reflex	Taking-hold

The family often is very excited after childbirth. The new mother is eager to share the excitement of the birth with her partner, family, and friends. "Is it a girl or boy?" is usually the first question most parents ask. Curious about the health of their newborn, parents often count fingers and toes, looking for any obvious abnormalities. They are encouraged by the reassurance that their newborn is normal and wonderful to behold. Facts such as eye and hair color, and who the baby resembles, are often a part of initial conversations. Most families are relieved that the long period of waiting is over. It is typically a very joyful and emotional time.

The **postpartum period** is the interval between the birth of the newborn until the woman's reproductive system returns to its nonpregnant state. This period lasts approximately 6 weeks. It is a time of enormous physical and psychosocial change for the woman. Each member of the family must adjust to the new roles and responsibilities brought on by the addition of its newest member. This chapter presents the normal physical and psychosocial changes that occur during this period. Chapter 15 builds on this information to present appropriate nursing care during this period.

Physical Changes During the Postpartum Period

Labor and birth place heavy demands on the woman's energy reserves. The nurse encourages the woman to rest and monitors a variety of her responses to labor and childbirth, especially during the immediate postpartum period.

The fourth stage of labor describes the first 2 hours after birth. The woman is closely observed and assessed during this critical time for complications. If she has had general anesthesia and is not completely conscious, the nurse may need to extend the time of close observation. Women who receive regional anesthesia may not regain total feeling in their lower extremities for several hours.

Immediately after childbirth, the woman may state she is feeling chilly and may shake uncontrollably (see Chapter 12). Because the woman expends a tremendous amount of effort during labor and childbirth, she is frequently thirsty and hungry during the early postpartum period. Under usual circumstances, the woman is given fluids and encouraged to drink to replace lost fluids. Ample oral intake often eliminates the need to continue intravenous fluids and helps to return normal kidney function and urinary output. The woman is offered solid food if she tolerates liquids well and wishes to eat.

During the first few hours after childbirth, the woman's blood pressure, pulse, respirations, fundus, lochia, and perineum are assessed every 15 minutes for 1 hour and every half-hour for 1 hour, and every 4 hours at least two times, and then every 8 hours. If the woman had general anesthesia, she is monitored for return of normal levels of consciousness and nausea and vomiting. In many facilities, the woman is kept in the labor and birthing unit for this initial period. Routine assessments are continued when the woman is transferred to the postpartum unit. The Assessment Checklist summarizes the procedure.

Changes in the Reproductive System

After childbirth, the uterus, vagina, perineum, and breasts begin to return to their nonpregnant state in a process called **involution**. This process begins immediately after birth and takes up to 6 weeks to complete. The risk of postpartum hemorrhage is greatest the first few hours after birth but lasts throughout the process of involution.

Uterine Involution

During the first 2 to 3 days postpartum, the woman may experience after-pains. **After-pains** is the common term for the discomfort the woman feels as involution of the uterus occurs. The uterus contracts down to a firm mass. A uterus that has good tone contracts and stays contracted, whereas a uterus with poor tone contracts and then relaxes. Contractions of the enlarged uterus minimize bleeding from the placental site. The capillaries at the placental site are squeezed by the contraction of the muscles, preventing excessive blood loss. Immediately after birth, the uterus is about the size of a grapefruit. Uterine cramping occurs because of contractions of the uterus followed by brief periods of relaxation. The uterus tends to lose some of its tone with each pregnancy. A woman who has had previous pregnancies often experiences stronger contractions as the result of decreased muscle tone. With each successive pregnancy, the uterus has to work harder to return to the prepregnant state. Breast-feeding stimulates the uterus to contract by releasing oxytocin. The woman who is breast-feeding may experience increased discomfort as the neonate nurses.

Fundal Position

For the first 24 hours postpartum, the fundus is normally found at the level of the umbilicus or one finger-

If Systolic goes below 90 then it may indicate danger

School starts at 8

Endometrium Decidua

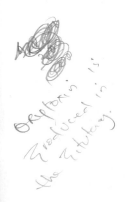

Oxytocin is produced in the pituitary

Physical Changes During the Early Postpartum Period

- Chills and shaking: Common immediately after childbirth, lasts 1–2 hours; provide warm blankets and dry linen
- Fluid and food: Woman is hungry and thirsty; fluids and food help replace fluid loss and supply energy
- Physical assessment (ongoing): Every 15 minutes for first hour; every half hour for second hour; every 4 hours at least twice, then every 8 hours. Blood pressure, pulse, and respiratory rates normally remain stable.
  - Blood pressure: Decrease with rapid, thready pulse may indicate hemorrhage; increase may indicate PIH.
  - Pulse rate: Slow 1 to 2 days (60–70 bpm). Rapid rate (100 bpm or more) may indicate shock, hemorrhage, or infection.
  - Temperature assessed at end of first hour, then every 4 hours for first 24 hours, every 8 hours until discharge. Normal range first 24 hours postpartum: 36.2°C (98°F) to 38°C (100.4°F); dehydration, muscular exertion, and hormonal changes may cause increase. Temperature of 38°C (100.4°F) or higher on 2 consecutive days, after first 24 hours, indicates infection.
- Uterine involution (ongoing): Same schedule as vital signs first 24 hours, then daily. Assess firmness; level in relation to umbilicus; lochial flow: amount, color, odor.
- Bladder function: Empties bladder within 8 hours of delivery; uterine fundus not displaced by full bladder.

breadth above the umbilicus. This is true except when oxytocin is administered after expulsion of the placenta. Fundal height is determined by gently placing the hand slightly above the level of the umbilicus. Forming a small hollow in the hand, the nurse gently palpates the firm, rounded, top of the uterus. The nurse's other hand is placed just above the symphysis pubis to stabilize the position of the uterus (Fig. 14-1). The bladder should be emptied before the height is measured. A full bladder prevents the uterus from contracting. With a full bladder, the uterus may be measured at one or more fingerbreadths higher and may be displaced from the midline (most often to the right).

Fundal height is measured in fingerbreadths in relation to the umbilicus and is used to assess the rate of involution. Conditions that may displace the fundus, causing it to be higher than usual, are a full bladder, overdistension of the uterus by a very large fetus, multifetal pregnancy, or excessive amniotic fluid (polyhydramnios).

If the woman received oxytocin after the expulsion of the placenta, the fundus initially may be one or two fingerbreadths below the uterus. However, within a few hours, it will rise and follow the usual pattern. It re-

mains even with the umbilicus for a day or 2 after birth, and then recedes in height by approximately one fingerbreadth each day postpartum. By the 10th day, the uterus is so low in the pelvis, it cannot be felt during abdominal palpation (Fig. 14-2).

Lochia

The vaginal discharge that follows childbirth is called lochia. As the uterus heals and reduces in size, it cleanses itself by releasing blood, particles of decidua, and mucus. The amount of lochia is described as heavy, moderate, or scant (see Figure 15-1). Lochial discharge is heaviest during the first hour or two after birth. Heavy lochia indicates excessive bleeding and is often accompanied by blood clots. Chapter 16 discusses bleeding complications that occur during the fourth stage of labor.

Lochia is normally odorless or smells similar to menstrual flow. It is characterized by the color, amount, and duration of flow. **Lochia rubra** is bright red to dark red may have small clots, and lasts from day 1 postpartum to day 3. It has a characteristic fleshy odor. The flow changes from red to a pink or pinkish-brown color with no clots, known as **lochia serosa**,

Day 1-3 Moderate to large

3-10 Moderate to scant

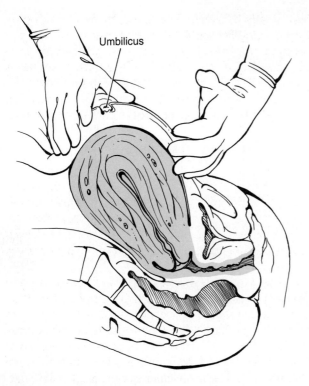

Figure 14-1. *The fundal height is measured in relation to the level of the woman's umbilicus. The nurse gently palpates the fundus and records the accurate number of fingerbreadths above or below "U" (umbilicus). Note the position and shape of both of the nurse's hands.*

and may last until about the 10th day postpartum. There is no odor if the woman practices good hygiene. **Lochia alba** is white or whitish-yellow and lasts about 2 to 6 weeks postpartum.

[handwritten: Moderate to Scant]
[handwritten: It usually stops 15 days when she no longer has lochia the cervix is closed.]

Cervix

Immediately after birth, the cervix is soft and dilated and may be bruised. There is a gradual closing, shortening, and firming of the cervix during the first week postpartum. Closing continues until involution is complete, and the cervix becomes firm. The cervix never closes completely, nor does it return to its prepregnant firmness.

Vagina and Perineum

The perineum may appear swollen and bruised after vaginal childbirth. Discoloration, which appears as a bruise, is called **ecchymosis**. The perineum has been stretched and thinned tremendously to accommodate delivery of the neonate. If an episiotomy was performed, the sutured area should appear intact and

free of bleeding. Lacerations sustained during childbirth are repaired, and the edges of the tear visualized from the perineum should be clean and even. Swelling and discoloration, signs of hematoma formation, are reported.

The vagina resumes its prepregnant appearance in approximately 3 weeks. The prepregnant muscle tone will not be completely regained. Vaginal rugae (ridges) are absent initially but reappear within a couple of weeks. Vaginal lubrication is reduced because of hormonal influences. Lubrication returns to normal once menstruation starts again.

Breasts

The female breasts undergo incredible changes throughout pregnancy in preparation for **lactation** (the secretion of milk by the breasts) and breast-feeding. A thin, yellowish fluid secreted by the breasts called **colostrum** supplies the neonate's first nourishment. Colostrum contains more protein and salts (sodium chloride and zinc) but less fat and carbohydrate than breast milk. Colostrum is secreted by the breasts in the last

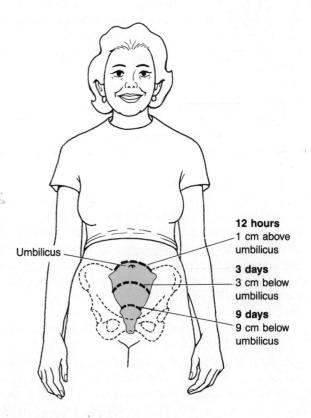

12 hours
1 cm above umbilicus

3 days
3 cm below umbilicus

9 days
9 cm below umbilicus

Umbilicus

Figure 14-2. *Uterine involution is complete between 4 to 6 weeks postpartum. The uterus is no longer palpable from the abdomen by the 10th day following childbirth. Examples are shown here to illustrate usual level in the first 9 days postpartum.*

month before birth until the second or third day postpartum, when mature breast milk appears. It is rich in antibodies. Colostrum acts as a natural laxative, aiding in the passage of meconium. The nurse can reassure the woman that colostrum provides the neonate with all the needed nutrients as well as immunoglobulin A. The neonate does not have immunoglobulin A, an important gastrointestinal antibody.

Lactation and the Let-Down Reflex

Two essential processes are involved in lactation: production of milk and expulsion of milk. Production of breast milk depends on stimulation by the lactogenic hormone (prolactin). Prolactin is released from the woman's pituitary gland. Frequent and complete emptying of the breasts prompts milk production.

Expulsion, or release of milk, is controlled by the let-down reflex. The **let-down reflex** (milk ejection reflex) describes the response of the breasts to stimulation such as sucking or crying of the neonate. Lactogenic hormones result in milk emptying into the lactiferous ducts and forces milk toward the nipple. Oxytocin is another hormone released in the breast-feeding process (see Chapter 2). This contributes to the ejection of milk as the neonate sucks and also produces the uterine contractions felt during the breast-feeding process. Some women describe the let-down reflex as a brief sensation similar to "pins and needles" just before the milk begins to flow. This reflex is influenced favorably by some physical factors such as rest and comfort, and unfavorably by such factors as pain and fatigue. It also is influenced positively by emotional factors such as happiness and contentment, and negatively by worry and tension.

Changes in Other Body Systems

The systems, other than the reproductive system, most significantly impacted by pregnancy, labor, and childbirth include endocrine, circulatory, respiratory, gastrointestinal, urinary, musculoskeletal, integumentary, and the nervous systems.

Endocrine System

In the fourth stage of labor, estrogen, progesterone, and prolactin levels decrease. If the mother is bottle-feeding, estrogen levels begin to increase and serve as a catalyst for the return of menses. The first postpartum menstrual period may occur within weeks of childbirth. During the first menstrual cycle after childbirth, ovulation does not usually occur. In the lactating woman, prolactin levels begin to increase initially as the new-

born nurses. Oxytocin is released by the anterior pituitary, eventually completely taking over as the primary hormone in lactation. An increase in estrogen may occur at any time after childbirth, even if the woman is breast-feeding. Therefore, ovulation can take place. All postpartum women must be warned that conception can take place whether or not they are breast-feeding.

Circulatory System

As described in Chapter 5, circulatory volume increases 50% during pregnancy. This elevation in volume places extra strain on the heart and demands greater work. The cardiac output immediately after birth increases for approximately 48 hours, returning to prepregnancy levels in 4 weeks.

The volume of fluid lost from diaphoresis (profuse perspiration) and diuresis (urinary output) during labor and childbirth is approximately 2.2 kg (5 lbs.). Up to an additional 500 mL of blood loss is normal during childbirth. Amniotic fluid is another source of fluid loss in the birthing process. To avoid severe medical complications, the cardiovascular system must quickly accommodate the incredible changes taking place in the circulatory volume. Decreasing circulatory volume coupled with relaxed muscular tone of the blood vessels results in improvement of varicosities. Because the uterus is no longer placing extra burden on the vena cava, blood flow returns to normal. Women who developed hemorrhoids may find that it takes longer for these to resolve.

Fluids, Electrolytes, and Essential Blood Components

Blood levels return to normal within about 2 weeks after childbirth. Excess fluids in blood and body tissues are excreted by the kidneys. This causes a marked increase in the daily urinary output. Normal postpartum changes in metabolism lead to diaphoresis, particularly at night.

Diuresis and diaphoresis help the body return to the prepregnancy state by helping to remove extra fluid that has accumulated in the tissues. Edema of the hands, feet, and face typically resolve within the first few weeks. Normal fluid and electrolyte balance is restored in about 3 weeks postpartum.

The rapid loss of fluid volume results in some initial changes in hemoglobin, hematocrit, and white blood cell levels. Hemoconcentration increases hemoglobin and hematocrit levels. The white blood cell count is often elevated up to 20,000/mL immediately after childbirth without the presence of infection. Normal laboratory values are indicated in Table 14-1.

Table 14-1. *Blood Values in the Postpartum Period*

Blood Value	Normal Postpartal	Deviation From Expected
Hemoglobin	10.0–11.4 g/dL	< 10.0 g/dL
Hematocrit	32%–36%	< 30%
Leukocytes	14,000–30,000/mm³	> 30,000/mm³

From Reeder, S. J., Martin, L. L., & Koniak, D. (1992). *Maternity nursing* (17th ed.). Philadelphia: J. B. Lippincott; Table 28-3, p. 621.

Respiratory System

After childbirth, many women are able to breathe more easily. This is because of a decrease in the diaphragmatic pressure that had been caused by the enlarged uterus. The chest wall is able to expand more freely without the restrictions of the uterus and growing fetus. If the woman receives general anesthesia for cesarean birth, respirations may be shallow initially because of postsurgical pain. However, respiratory rate and lung capacity should return to normal within the immediate postoperative recovery period. Shortness of breath at any time after childbirth requires further assessment to rule out underlying pathophysiology.

Gastrointestinal System

Some women experience constipation during the early postpartum period. Constipation is attributable in part to relaxation of the abdominal wall and loss of intraabdominal pressure (see Chapter 15). A sluggish bowel may result from overcrowding from the enlarged uterus during pregnancy. In addition, the presence of hemorrhoids or an episiotomy may cause the woman to experience more discomfort when having a bowel movement.

Urinary System

The bladder and urethra often are stressed during labor and childbirth. The woman may have difficulty urinating because the urethra is swollen. The perineum and urethral opening may be sore from the trauma of childbirth. It is not uncommon for the bladder to fill and distend with urine without the woman feeling the urge to urinate. This is usually caused by loss of bladder tone. The reduced sensation and lack of the urge to void may result from trauma during labor. Anesthesia used during labor and childbirth is often associated with bladder distension. Catheterization may be necessary if the woman is unable to void (see Chapter 15). Bladder

tone normally returns within 24 to 48 hours after childbirth.

Musculoskeletal System

The abdominal muscles are stretched and lose much of their tone during pregnancy. There is a flabby appearance of the abdomen in the immediate postpartum period, which normally responds to exercise and involution. Women who give birth to their first child generally gain greater tone than women who have several children. The pelvic muscles and ligaments gradually tighten and return to their prepregnant position within 4 to 6 weeks.

Integumentary System

Striae (stretch marks) on the abdomen, thighs, and breasts gradually become silvery in appearance. Often these marks do not disappear completely because they result from stretching and minute tearing of the skin. The linea nigra, chloasma gravidarum, and darkening of the nipple alveoli typically fade completely (refer to Chapter 5). There may be some sagging of skin from excessive weight gain. Exercise and proper diet are recommended to improve circulation, muscle tone, skin elasticity, and healing.

Nervous System

Central nervous system function may be altered during the postpartum period because of anesthesia or analgesia used during labor and childbirth. Sensory and motor function may be impaired. Headaches from spinal anesthesia are avoided by keeping the woman flat and offering increased fluids. Normally, the woman does not experience a decrease in level of consciousness, severe headaches, or visual disturbances. Sensory and motor function should return to normal as the anesthesia wears off.

The Assessment Checklist highlights essential information about the body system changes that accompany the early postpartum period. The following section addresses the importance of family adaptation and dis-

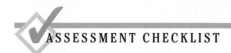

✓ ASSESSMENT CHECKLIST

Changes in Body Systems During the Postpartum Period

- Reproductive:
  - Uterine fundus: firm at midline, one to two fingerbreadths above the umbilicus
  - lochia: lochia rubra, changes to lochia serosa approximately day 3 to day 10, then lochia alba for remainder of involution
  - Cervix: soft and dilated; free of lacerations or hematoma; closes and hardens with involution
  - Vagina and perineum: free of hematomas, lacerations, and edema
  - Breasts: presence of colostrum day 1 to day 2 or 3; lactation begins 48 to 72 hours after childbirth
- Endocrine: Release of oxytocin; estrogen and progesterone levels decrease; prolactin levels increase as newborn suckles; postpartum depression third day postpartum
- Circulatory: Return of prepregnancy blood levels; loss of excessive fluids through loss of amniotic fluid, blood loss, diaphoresis and diuresis; hemoconcentration with elevated Hgb and Hct levels; elevation of white blood cell count (see Table 14-1); increased cardiac output for 24 hours; pulse and blood pressure within normal limits; reduced hand, feet, and facial edema; resolution of varicose veins; hemorrhoids may persist
- Respiratory: Increase chest wall capacity; ability to breath easier; reduction in diaphragmatic pressure; respiratory rate within normal limits
- Gastrointestinal: Desire for fluids and food; experience constipation
- Urinary: Swollen urethra and surrounding tissues; return of bladder tone; urinary output and frequency within normal limits
- Musculoskeletal: Flabby abdominal muscles; gradual tightening of pelvic muscles and ligaments
- Integumentary: Striae gravidarum become lighter and silvery; gradual disappearance of linea nigra, chloasma gravidarum, and nipple hyperpigmentation
- Nervous: Sensory and motor function return postanesthesia; alert level of consciousness

---

cusses the psychosocial changes experienced by the childbearing family.

Psychosocial Changes During the Postpartum Period

In addition to the multitude of physiologic changes that occur during the postpartum period, the mother, her partner, and the family members are often bombarded by an assortment of psychosocial changes. These changes are normal and to be expected. They include reliving the birth experience, parental responses, including maternal and paternal reactions, parent–newborn attachment, sibling response, and grandparenting. Failure of the family to respond adequately to these needs may result in ineffective family coping and adaptation.

Reliving the Birth Experience

Reliving the birth experience is a common event that each parent will communicate many times over. Telling others about labor and the birthing experience helps the parent and support person to integrate the experience into their daily lives. The woman and her support person often compare their actual performance in labor and birth with previous hopes and fantasies. The family may compare this birth with earlier childbirth experiences or with experiences related by other friends and family members.

Parental Response

Maternal and paternal reactions to the labor and birth process vary. The father may be prepared for the birthing experience but may not fully understand and appreciate the physical and psychosocial changes his partner experiences. The mother may be tired and experience pain and discomfort shortly after delivery. Knowledge of normal responses enables the nurse to identify families at risk for poor adaptation and adjustment to parenting responsibilities.

Maternal Responses

In the early 1960s, Reva Rubin, a maternity nurse, observed women during the early postpartum period. She identified certain behaviors that recurred as women assumed their new maternal role. Although maternity care has changed and progressed since the 1960s, the same reactions and behaviors are still identifiable in many women. Rubin described three stages or phases in adaptation after childbirth. These stages include taking-in, taking-hold, and letting-go.

Taking-In Stage
Taking-in is the first maternal stage. Characterized by dependent behavior, it may last from a few hours to 2 days postpartum. There is a strong focus on self during this time. The mother is typically exhausted and desires food and rest. She repeatedly relates her account of the birth experience. Feelings of doubt about her ability to care for the newborn often enter the new mother's mind. She willingly accepts offers to assist in meeting her own physical needs at this time.

Taking-Hold Stage
Taking-hold is the second maternal stage. The woman begins to regain energy and experience greater physical comfort. She is concerned about her bodily functions returning to normal.

Usually, the mother begins to assume greater responsibility for the newborn. She is open to learning about infant care. This is an excellent time for teaching. Chapter 15 discusses this further.

Letting-Go Stage
The third stage, **letting-go**, occurs when the woman adopts more independent behaviors in assuming her new maternal role. This stage usually takes place after discharge, when the woman resumes her position in the home and begins to see the newborn as a separate being. The woman will need to work through her evolving relationship with her partner and other family members. Role upheaval, caused by new responsibilities and added demands, may lead to feelings of mild depression or loss. **Postpartum depression** is the term for the transient, short-lived, emotional reaction experienced by most women during the postpartum period. See the Assessment Checklist for the maternal response and adaptation.

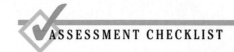

ASSESSMENT CHECKLIST

Maternal Response and Adaptation

The woman typically responds in a predictable pattern and exhibits specific maternal behaviors that are described in three stages:

· Taking-In Stage: The mother is physically exhausted from the birth experience. She looks to the nurse to help her perform her routine daily care. The mother recounts the labor and childbirth experience. She is still in wonderment that pregnancy is over and the newborn is really her baby.

· Taking-Hold Stage: The mother begins to assert her independence in caring for the newborn and herself. She may still feel insecure as a new mother but wishes to actively participate. Independent decision-making is a major behavior observed during this stage.

· Letting-Go Stage: The mother has redefined and accepted her new parenting role. The reality of her baby's appearance, sex, and size is incorporated into her maternal role. This stage may be achieved after the mother is discharged and she is enjoying her new-found motherhood.

Postpartum Depression

Usually, the mother is very happy and excited after the birth of her baby. The long months of waiting are over. However, the mother may experience an almost anticlimatic feeling, and she may even become tearful or irritable as the level of excitement decreases and fatigue builds.

Postpartum blues or **postpartum depression** are terms used to describe the woman's feelings of sadness, which may include crying, unpredictable changes in emotions, and extreme sensitivity. She may sulk or cry openly without being able to explain her mood and emotional outbursts. These feelings are thought to be associated with abrupt hormonal changes, increased fatigue, breast and nipple soreness, and discomfort, all of which are common in the postpartum period. The woman may be upset about her weight and body image or may be anxious and fearful about new parenting responsibilities and reestablishing her relationship with her partner.

These symptoms generally occur around the third day postpartum. They resolve automatically for most women within a week to 10 days. Support, anticipatory guidance, and reassurance that these feelings are normal help the woman cope. The woman may continue to feel depressed or experience intense mood swings. If this occurs, postpartum psychosis should be suspected (see Chapter 16). Professional intervention in the form of counseling or therapy may be necessary.

Paternal (Partner) Response

A new wave of research is underway to gain a better understanding about the father or lesbian partner's reaction to labor, childbirth, and parenting (Fig. 14-3). The father (partner) often experiences reactions to childbirth that are similar to those that the mother feels. Reliving the birthing process and retelling about the ups and downs of labor and childbirth are to be expected. The father (partner) may be unaware of the emotional fluctuations that the mother will experience during the first week or so after childbirth. Parenting responsibilities may shift to the father (partner) initially as the woman regains strength and takes on the maternal role.

Parent–Newborn Attachment

Immediately after birth, the parents and newborn begin to "bond." Bonding is achieved through eye-to-eye contact, touching, and voice and smell recognition. Eye-to-eye contact is an important part of attachment formation. To promote eye contact, the parents are assisted into positions that foster direct eye contact with the

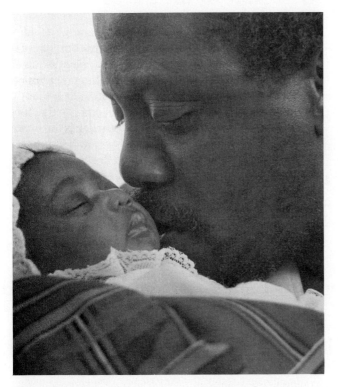

Figure 14-3. *As the father (partner) tenderly embraces the newborn, he experiences a flood of powerful emotions quite similar to the mother's (Photo © Kathy Sloane).*

newborn (see Fig. 14-3). Instinctively, many mothers are able to anticipate when the newborn will open his or her eyes. Both parents usually talk in soft, musical tones to engage the newborn during times of alertness and arousal.

The newborn needs to be held and caressed by the parents to begin attachment to them. Touching of the face, hands, fingers, and stroking of the trunk, legs, and toes are all ways the parents familiarize themselves with the physical features of their newborn. An infant who is separated from parents immediately after birth for long periods may be deprived of the opportunity to form strong attachments. It is nursing's responsibility to promote parent–newborn bonding at the earliest possible opportunity by arranging quiet time together immediately after birth. Within days, a newborn is able to identify the mother by her voice, touch, and smell and respond by turning his or her head toward the mother.

Redefining and Reestablishing the Couple's Relationship

After the parents spend quality time getting to know their newborn and receiving attention from various family members, they need time to get reacquainted and share their experiences. As part of the discharge instructions, the nurse talks about finding time for each other at home. Many couples are grateful for the opportunity to share their feelings and concerns about how they are going to "get it all together" when they arrive home. The couple often wonders how they can find ample time for the newborn and for their relationship. Concerns regarding sexual relations and intimacy are addressed. Maintenance of the couple's relationship is stressed to promote harmony and well-being, enhancing the health of the entire family.

Sibling Responses

Sibling visitation is a creative advance in family-centered maternal-newborn care. These special visits from brothers and sisters contribute to family unity by promoting early acceptance of the newborn by other children in the family (Fig. 14-4).

With advances in epidemiology, the incidence and severity of communicable diseases were reduced, and the public demanded more leniency in hospital visiting regulations. Visits provide children with reassurance that they have not been abandoned. They also help the child recognize childbirth as a normal family event and promote early acceptance of the new family member with a minimum of jealousy and rivalry. Mothers also benefit from sibling visitation. Some mothers have never been separated from their young children.

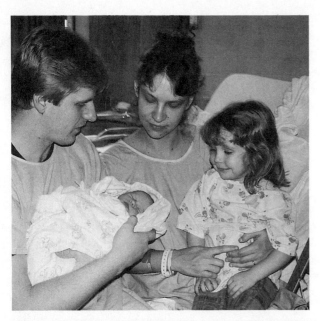

Figure 14-4. The family is strengthened by the involvement of all family members. Children and parents benefit from a visit, and the new member is introduced to the curious sibling.

Adolescent Considerations

The adolescent mother experiences all of the same physical and psychosocial changes as her older counterpart. The postpartum changes may be stressful and create fear, while challenging the adolescent's ability to cope. The body is capable of steady recovery under normal circumstances in adolescence. Excellent health, vitality, and firmer muscle tone all contribute to the rapid progress of the involution process. Substance abuse, poor health habits such as fad diets, and poor living circumstances are examples of factors that may create less favorable postpartum outcomes for the adolescent (see Chapter 16).

Cultural Considerations

Care of the mother and newborn, diet, bathing, and infant feeding often are rooted in cultural, ethnic, and religious customs. Quality nursing care explores these "traditions" and incorporates them into the nursing plan of care as much as possible.

The Mexican American woman is typically supported by another woman during labor and early recovery. This in no way implies that the father is disinterested; it is merely their custom. Women in some cultures believe colostrum is not good for their infants. These women may avoid breast-feeding until their milk supply is established.

Southeast Asian Americans may refrain from direct eye contact and physical contact. These practices should not be misinterpreted as a lack of caring or attachment to the newborn but accepted as cultural practices. Asian Americans and Indian Americans may place higher value on male children. Avoidance of cold water and cold air is a custom practiced by some Chinese American families. They believe warm (hot) is healing, and cold is not. Staying indoors to prevent excess cold from entering the body is a common practice. The woman remains in her home for more than a month to avoid perceived physical ailments associated with cold.

The Role of the Nurse

The nurse supports and guides the new family, provides comfort, promotes parent– and family–newborn attachment, and ensures the family receives essential emotional support. Monitoring the woman's physical response to the enormous changes occurring in her body falls to the nurse. The nurse needs to be equipped to recognize and identify deviations from normal. It is the nurse who generally facilitates the family's smooth transition from labor and childbirth activities to the assumption of new maternal and paternal roles and responsibilities.

REVIEW AND PREVIEW

Among the physical adjustments that the woman experiences during the postpartum period are major adjustments of the reproductive system. Each of the woman's other body systems also undergo changes. The changes that occur in the normal uncomplicated postpartum period were presented in this chapter. This chapter presented the normal psychosocial changes experienced by women and their families. Maternal and paternal responses, parent–newborn attachment, and family adaptation were discussed. Special consideration for adolescent and culturally diverse families were described.

The next chapter presents nursing care after normal labor and childbirth. Based on the nurse's knowledge of normal changes,

nursing care can be planned and implemented using the nursing process. An extremely important aspect of postpartum nursing care is teaching the new family how to care for themselves and their newborn. Health promotion and teaching self-care behaviors will be emphasized within a family-centered context.

◆ KEY POINTS

◆ The postpartum period describes the fourth stage of labor. It begins immediately after the birth of the neonate and ends when the woman's body returns to its nonpregnant state. The process of involution typically takes 6 weeks.

1. Which of the following findings during the first 24 hours post partum should be immediately reported to the physician?

○ **A.** White blood cell count of 15,000
○ **B.** Temperature of 37.5°C
○ **C.** Fundus at the level of the umbilicus
⊗ **D.** Vaginal hematoma

2. Which of the following colors best describes lochia 1 week after delivery?

○ **A.** Dark red
⊗ **B.** Pinkish
○ **C.** Brownish
○ **D.** Whitish-yellow

3. Typical maternal behavior during the taking-in stage includes:

⊗ **A.** Recounting her labor and delivery experience
○ **B.** Depression
○ **C.** Engaging in self-care activities
○ **D.** Asking questions regarding infant care

4. How should the nurse advise a patient who inquires about how long stretch marks last?

○ **A.** They rarely remain after the first pregnancy
○ **B.** They will automatically disappear in 2 to 3 months
⊗ **C.** They may be permanent
○ **D.** Lotion applied daily helps stretch marks disappear

5. Which of the following factors is *least* likely to affect fundal height following delivery?

○ **A.** Fetal size
⊗ **B.** Fetal presentation
○ **C.** Distended bladder
⊗ **D.** Hydramnios

◆ The uterus, cervix, vagina, perineum, and female breasts undergo significant changes to adapt to the woman's and newborn's needs. The uterus contracts and expels debris to resume its prepregnancy size. The cervix, vagina, and perineum regain muscle tone and firmness. The breasts prepare for lactation.

◆ Lochia rubra is the dark red to brownish discharge that typically flows from the uterus for 1 to 3 days. Lochia serosa comes next and is pinkish to pinkish-brown, lasting up to 10 days postpartum. Lochia alba is whitish-yellow and can last up to 4 to 6 weeks after childbirth. Blood clots do not typically occur in normal lochial flow.

◆ Hormonal levels increase and decrease depending on whether the woman breast-feeds or bottle-feeds. The increase in estrogen levels stimulates the return of the menstrual cycle and eventually, the first menstrual period. Ovulation may or may not accompany the first menstrual cycle, depending on the level of hormones that prepare the corpus luteum.

◆ The heart works hard to manage the quick shift in large volumes of fluids after childbirth. Diaphoresis and diuresis result in the postpartum woman losing approximately 2.2 kg (5 lbs.). Cardiac output increases initially, returning to normal within 48 hours.

◆ The family adapts to the newborn and develops positive maternal and paternal roles by going through a variety of stages. Initially the family relives the birthing experience and prepares for new parenting roles by accepting and learning about their responsibilities. Forming strong emotional attachments to the newborn is essential to ongoing psychosocial adaptation.

◆ The postpartum stages of behavioral adjustment include taking-in, taking-hold, and letting-go. The mother initially willingly accepts assistance in caring for herself and the newborn. In taking-hold, the mother becomes more independent in care for herself and her newborn.

◆ Parent–newborn attachment/bonding should be encouraged as soon as possible after birth. Direct eye contact, gentle touching and stroking, and calm reassuring conversation and cooing accompany the family's welcoming of the newborn.

◆ Siblings and extended family members provide comfort and reassurance to the new parents. Younger children benefit from meeting the new baby and visiting with their mother. Sibling visitation often diminishes or eliminates feelings of abandonment, jealousy, and rivalry.

◆ Individuals have unique cultural practices and beliefs. Chinese American women may avoid cold, Southeast Asian women may avoid direct eye or physical contact, Asian Americans and Indian Americans may revere male children more than female. The nurse accepts these beliefs and incorporates them in the plan of care.

BIBLIOGRAPHY

Boyles, J. S., & Andrews, M. M. (1990). *Transcultural concepts in nursing care*. Philadelphia: J. B. Lippincott.

Beck, C., Reynolds, M., & Rutkowski, P. (1992). Maternity blues and postpartum depression. *Journal of Obstetric, Gynecologic, and Neonatal Nursing, 21*(4), 287.

Brazelton, T. B., Tronick, E., & Adamson, L. (1975). Parent-infant interaction. *Ciba Foundation Symposium 33*. Amsterdam: Elsevier Publishing Company.

Jordan, P. (1990). Laboring for relevance: Expectant and new fatherhood. *Nursing Research, 39*, 11.

Karch, A. M. (1992). *Handbook of drugs and the nursing process* (2nd ed.). Philadelphia: J. B. Lippincott.

Klaus, M., & Kennell, J. (1982). *Parent-infant bonding* (2nd ed.). St. Louis: C. V. Mosby.

Martin, L. L., & Reeder, S. J. (1990). *Essentials of maternity nursing: Family centered care* (1st ed.). Philadelphia: J. B. Lippincott.

May, K. A., & Mahlmeister, L. R. (1994). *Maternal & neonatal nursing: Family-centered care* (3rd ed.). Philadelphia: J. B. Lippincott.

Norr, K. F., & Roberts, J. E. (1991). Early maternal attachment behaviors of adolescent and adult mothers. *Journal of Nurse Midwifery, 36*(6), 334–342.

Reeder, S. J., Martin, L. L., & Koniak, D. (1992). *Maternity nursing: Family, newborn, and women's health care* (17th ed.). Philadelphia: J. B. Lippincott.

Rubin, R. (1961). Puerperal change. *Nursing Outlook, 9*, 753–757.

Schuster, C. S., & Ashburn, S. S. (1992). *The process of human development: A holistic life-span approach* (3rd ed.). Philadelphia: J. B. Lippincott.

Thomlinson, P., Rothenberg, M., & Carver, L. (1991). Behavioral interaction of fathers with infants and mothers in the immediate postpartum period. *Journal of Nurse Midwifery, 36*(4), 232.

CHAPTER 15

Nursing Care Following Normal Childbirth

◆ OBJECTIVES

When the learning goals of this chapter are met, the reader will be able to:

- ◆ Describe the nursing actions in postpartum checks and the pertinent observations made with each check.
- ◆ Describe the nursing action taken in the event the fundus feels boggy.
- ◆ Explain how a full bladder affects the involution of the uterus.
- ◆ Describe nursing measures that can be used to encourage a woman to void.
- ◆ Describe perineal care and identify the purpose for it.
- ◆ Discuss postpartum constipation and identify ways it can be relieved.
- ◆ Identify advantages of rooming in postpartum care.
- ◆ Explain mother-baby nursing and state advantages it offers.
- ◆ Identify danger signs the woman is taught to report after discharge.
- ◆ Describe postpartum breast care for the breast-feeding and the non–breast-feeding woman.

TERMINOLOGY

En face	Mother–baby nursing
Boggy	Puerperium
Couplet care	Rooming in
Dorsiflexion	Sitz bath
Engorgement	

Caring for the woman, her newborn, and family after a normal childbirth can be a happy, exciting, and rewarding experience. It also is a time during which nurses are challenged to exercise all of their abilities of observation and sensitivity to provide excellent nursing care. Chapter 14 discussed the normal physical and psychosocial changes that occur in the postpartum period. This chapter uses that foundation of knowledge as a basis for developing a plan of action. In this chapter, nursing care, including nursing assessment, nursing diagnoses, and nursing interventions, are presented.

The postpartum period is divided into three phases: immediate, early, and late. The immediate phase covers the first 24 hours after birth. The early postpartum phase includes the first 2 weeks after birth, and the late phase continues from the end of the second week until the sixth week after childbirth. Another term commonly used for the postpartum period is **puerperium**.

Immediate Postpartum Care

When the woman is received in the postpartum unit, the nurse obtains a complete update on the physical and psychosocial status of the woman. This includes checks for postpartum changes as well as those that indicate complications. The nurse determines what check was last completed, and when the next check is due to be performed.

Physical Care

During the immediate postpartum period, physical care of the woman is directed toward nursing observations and interventions to promote healing and prevent complications. Nursing assessments of the woman's physiologic condition are initiated in the birthing (delivery) unit, at the beginning of the fourth stage of labor. As described in Chapter 14, assessments are performed every 15 minutes for the first hour after birth, every 30 minutes for the next hour, followed by every 4 hours twice and then every 8 hours, depending on the protocol of the facility. These assessments, also called postpartum checks, include the condition of the uterus and level of the fundus, the amount of bleeding, vital signs, the condition of the perineum, and the bladder and voiding. They may be performed in the recovery unit or the post-

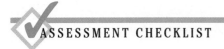

ASSESSMENT CHECKLIST

Procedure for Performing Postpartum Check

1. Explain the procedure to the woman; include what you are going to be doing and the reason.

2. Ask the woman to empty her bladder before beginning the procedure if she has not done so recently.

3. Gather any needed supplies: protective gloves, clean pad, waste container for soiled pad, materials to cleanse perineum; make certain light source is good.

4. Position the woman on her back, knees flexed and feet together.

5. Put on protective gloves.

6. Remove and discard soiled perineal pad in appropriate container; note the time the pad was last changed and amount of saturation (Fig. 15-3).

7. Place outer aspect of one opened hand just above the symphysis pubis to stabilize position of uterus.

8. Place outer aspect of other slightly cupped hand at the umbilicus; press firmly; move hand up or down to feel the top of the fundus, cupping hand around the top of the fundus; measure the distance above or below the umbilicus in fingerbreadths.

9. If fundus is boggy (not firm), gently massage it with a rotating motion until firm. Note any clots that may be expelled.

10. Observe perineal area for bleeding; note trickling, which may indicate unsutured lacerations.

11. Have woman turn on her side to better visualize episiotomy repair and possible hemorrhoids.

12. Note condition of episiotomy, especially ecchymosis (bruising), swelling, tenderness.

13. Cleanse perineum according to facility procedure.

14. Discard any soiled materials, including soiled underpads. Remove and discard gloves. Follow facility's policy for disposing of gloves and soiled items.

15. Assess the woman's vital signs: blood pressure, pulse, and respirations; temperature is checked every 4 hours in the first 24 hours; every 8 hours thereafter.

16. Document level and condition (firm or boggy) of fundus, amount, color, and odor of lochia, clots or excessive bleeding, and condition of episiotomy, perineum, and hemorrhoids, if present. Record vital signs. Report any unusual findings at once.

partum unit, depending on the way in which the facility is set up.

Postpartum Check

When performing a check, the nurse explains the procedure to the woman and positions her on her back with her knees flexed and her feet together. The nurse must glove to prevent contact with the woman's body fluids. The first Assessment Checklist presents the complete procedure for performing a postpartum check.

If at any time the fundus is found to be **boggy** (relaxed, soft to the touch) the nurse massages it until it becomes firm and remains firm. However, vigorous massaging must be avoided because it may cause overstimulation of the fundus. This can result in uterine atony, loss of muscular tone of the uterus that may result in hemorrhage (see Chapter 16).

The woman is taught to assess the height and firmness of her fundus. Early discharge makes this an assessment that the woman must carry on at home. The woman must also be taught to identify danger signs: excessive bleeding, boggy or tender fundus, and foul-smelling lochia.

In addition to the information about the status of the postpartum checks, the nurse gathers information about the birth, intravenous fluids, if the woman has voided, and other relevant information. The nurse also asks for information about the support person and family in attendance.

Urinary Bladder

As mentioned in Chapter 14, a full bladder hinders the uterus from contracting. The bladder lies below and in front of the uterus. When the bladder is full or overdistended, the uterus does not have the space it needs in which to contract (Fig. 15-1). This causes the uterus to feel boggy and usually results in excessive bleeding. The woman may not be aware that her bladder is full. The bladder may have suffered trauma during labor and birth or the capacity of the bladder may have increased after the intraabdominal pressure is lessened with the birth of the baby. Intravenous fluids during labor and physiologic changes in early postpartum contribute to an increased urinary output that causes the bladder to fill more rapidly.

The woman should void within 6 to 8 hours after delivery. Early ambulation encourages bladder function. Because early ambulation has become customary, fewer women have problems with voiding. However, some women continue to have difficulty voiding. The nurse must use nursing techniques to encourage the woman to void, including turning on a faucet to a

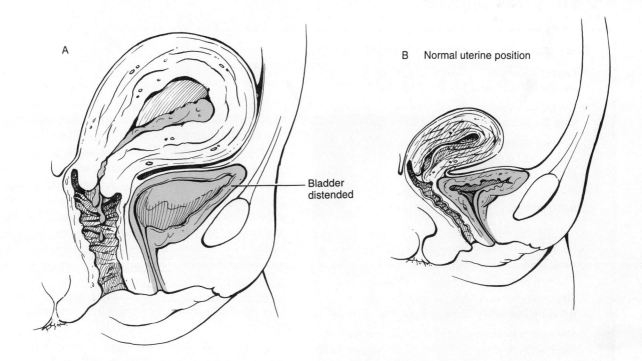

Figure 15-1. *The bladder lies below and in front of the uterus. A full or overdistended bladder pushes the uterus up, often displacing it to the side. The uterus is unable to contract due to crowding and displacement by the bladder. A boggy uterus and excessive bleeding result.*

> ### DISPLAY 15-1
> *Teaching Instructions for Perineal Self-Care*
>
> Taught when woman is able to go to bathroom independently.
>
> 1. Explain the procedure to the woman; assist woman to bathroom.
> 2. Gather supplies and place close at hand in bathroom:
>   Clean perineal pads (1–3, as needed)
>   Clean perineal pad belt or panty, as needed
>   Tissue or other material for drying
>   Container for contaminated waste
>   Container with warm water or cleansing solution
>   Tucks, anesthetic spray, or other medication as directed
> 3. Wash hands and put on protective gloves. Instruct the woman to wash her hands before each pericare.
> 4. Teach the woman to remove the soiled pad from front to back; discard in approved waste container.
> 5. Instruct woman to pour or squeeze the warm water or cleansing solution over vulva and perineum without separating labia.
> 6. Instruct woman to pat dry, from front to back, with tissue or other drying material. Teach woman always to discard tissue after one front-to-back swipe.
> 7. Teach woman to apply any medicated pads, sprays, or ointments as directed.
> 8. Explain to the woman that pad (or pads, as needed) is applied front to back to prevent transferring microorganisms from rectal area to vaginal area. Stress the importance of using a clean belt or panties. Also teach the woman not to touch the part of the pad that will be next to her perineum.
> 9. Wash hands after perineal care.
> 10. Points to stress:
>   Perineal care is performed after each voiding, stool, and at least every 4 hours.
>   Infection is easily transmitted from the rectal area to the vagina.
>   Perineal care is performed until lochial flow ceases.

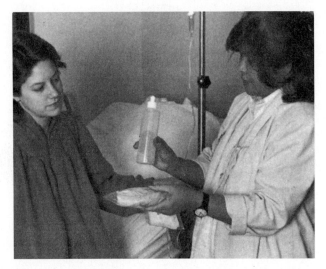

Figure 15-2. *"Peri bottle" used by the woman for self perineal care. The nurse reviews the procedure with the woman before she goes to the bathroom.*

trickle within the woman's hearing; pouring warm water over the woman's perineum; dabbling the woman's fingers in warm water. If the woman is having abdominal or perineal pain, administering analgesia before she attempts to void may be helpful. Some women may simply need privacy. The woman who has had anesthesia or a spinal block may not be able to ambulate. A bedpan and privacy are provided to encourage her to empty her bladder. Urine is measured for the first several times that the woman voids. The amount of urine should be greater than 300 mL. An amount less than 300 mL may mean that she is not emptying her bladder completely. This should be carefully assessed to determine if other measures, such as catheterization, are necessary.

In the event the woman has not voided within 6 to 8 hours after delivery, she must be catheterized. Catheterization is generally considered a last resort because of the risk of infection. Usually a straight catheterization is performed.

Perineal care is performed before catheterization and after voiding. Perineal care may be performed by the nurse or taught to the woman so that she may do it herself if she is ambulatory.

Perineal Care

Regular, properly performed perineal care reduces the risk of infection and helps to promote comfort. The woman is taught to perform her own perineal care as soon as she is able. Display 15-1 presents the procedure for instructing the woman in self-perineal care. The principles of the procedure are reviewed with the woman before she gets out of bed so that she can give full attention to the instructions without worrying about feeling weak or faint (Fig. 15-2). The nurse supervises and assists the woman doing self-perineal care until the woman understands and performs the care satisfactorily.

DISPLAY 15-2
Procedure for Perineal Care Performed by the Nurse

Performed when woman is unable to get out of bed to go to bathroom.

1. Explain procedure to woman including reasons it is performed.
2. Wash hands and gather equipment:
   Protective gloves
   Clean perineal pads (up to 3 pads)
   Bath soap or cleansing solution
   Disposable wipes or gauze to use for cleansing
   Tissues or other disposable drying material
   Basin with warm water
   Container for contaminated waste
   Clean disposable underpads (as needed)
   Clean sanitary belt or panties to secure perineal pads
3. Position woman on her back with knees flexed, feet together, and bed as flat as tolerated.
4. Put on protective gloves.
5. Remove soiled pads, loosen front first, remove in a front-to-back motion and discard in appropriate waste container.
6. Using disposable wipes or gauze, saturate with water and soap or cleansing solution. Use front-to-back motion; start on outer aspect of vulva; make one stroke, front to back, with each wipe and discard in waste container. Continue using one wipe for each stroke, working toward center. Repeat for opposite side.
7. Rinse thoroughly with clear water after completely cleansing with soap or solution. Pat dry with tissues or other drying material.
8. Inspect perineum and vulva for redness, swelling, and ecchymosis.
9. Help woman to turn on her side. Repeat procedure, cleansing well around anus and over buttocks. Continue the front-to-back motion. Inspect for condition of episiotomy and possible hemorrhoids.
10. After completely drying, put clean dry sanitary pad in place, using front-to-back method. Multiple pads may be used, according to the woman's flow. When handling sanitary pad, do not touch inner surface of pad.
11. Change soiled disposable underpads and discard soiled pads in approved waste container.
12. Remove gloves and place in waste container.
13. Dispose of soiled materials in accordance with facility policy.
14. Wash hands. Record procedure and any findings. Report any unusual findings immediately.

The nurse assists the woman when she is getting out of bed for the first time after childbirth, observing for signs of fainting, such as diaphoresis, weakness, or pallor. This may result from hypotension. Providing the woman with fluids to drink and assisting her in getting out of bed slowly helps to avoid a potential fall.

The nurse performs perineal care for the woman who is not able to ambulate because of surgery or anesthesia. Display 15-2 reviews the procedure for perineal care performed by the nurse.

In the immediate postpartum period, cold applications to the perineum may be used to provide comfort and reduce swelling. This therapy is used when the woman has had an extensive episiotomy or perineal repair. Commercially prepared ice packs are readily available. A latex glove filled with ice is inexpensive and may be used effectively. However, regardless of the type used, the ice pack must be covered with a clean, soft, absorbent material to avoid direct contact with the woman's perineal area. Cold therapy is usually discontinued after the first 24 hours. Longer therapy may interfere with healing because of vasoconstriction.

Dyuresis and Dyphorsis are common after childbirth

Psychosocial Care

The length of time the neonate initially stays with the woman depends on the birthing setting and the condition of the neonate. In some settings, the healthy neonate stays in the same room with the mother throughout the entire postpartum stay; in others, the neonate is taken to a central nursery and is with the mother for only part of each day. Many variations between these two opposites are available in various settings.

During the first visit with the newborn, the mother may explore the infant with a finger, gently, almost cautiously. The woman gradually uses her palm in exploring and stroking the neonate, and snuggles the neonate to her. Eye-to-eye contact follows. The woman turns the neonate toward her to look directly at the infant. This is called the *en face* position.

The immediate postpartum period is the time during which the woman undergoes the taking-in response to her experience. She is focused on her own physical and emotional needs. The nurse assists the woman to work through this phase of adjustment by providing supportive nursing care. Providing for opportunities for rest, using comfort measures and administering analgesics to relieve pain, and accepting the woman's retelling of her experience with a nonjudgmental attitude are all methods that assist the woman in this adjustment.

Daily Postpartum Care

After the immediate postpartum phase, the woman enters the early postpartum phase. This includes the first 2 postpartum weeks. Depending on the type of birth setting, the woman is discharged after the first 24 hours or at least by the third day postpartum. During this brief postpartum stay, the nurse must assess the woman's physical condition and psychosocial state. In addition, the nurse must accomplish a great amount of teaching to help the woman adjust to her role as mother.

Physical Care

The nurse must perform postpartum daily checks to determine the woman's physical condition. The woman performs much of her own personal care. The daily checks include assessments of the breasts, fundus, lochia, episiotomy (or incision if woman had a cesarean birth), voiding, stools, hemorrhoids, and lower extremities.

Breasts

Each day the nurse assesses the breast and nipples for tenderness, redness, warmth, firmness, and secretions. The nipples also are observed for cracking if the woman is breast-feeding. The breasts are checked on all women, whether they are breast-feeding or not.

The nurse places one hand on the outer aspect of each of the woman's breasts and gently palpates them to determine their degree of softness or firmness. This is documented as soft, firm, or engorged. The nurse then visually inspects the breasts and nipples. In the first day or two, the breasts are normally soft, and colostrum may leak from the nipples. When, by the second or third day, the breasts are filling with milk, they may feel warm and firm to the touch. By the third or fourth postpartum day, the breast milk may "come in," causing the breasts to become larger, firmer, and tender because of congestion. This is called **engorgement**. Engorgement results from increased blood and lymph in the breast as lactation occurs.

All postpartum women need to wear a good supportive bra to support breast tissue and prevent later sagging. Women are encouraged to wear the bra even when in bed during the period that the breasts are enlarged. The woman who is breast-feeding should only use clear water to cleanse her nipples. Soap or alcohol may dry the nipples and cause further irritation. The non–breast-feeding woman can wash her nipples as part of her daily shower.

Fundus

The involution of the fundus is assessed each day during the daily check. This is performed in the manner described in the Assessment Checklist (see also Fig. 14-1). As discussed in Chapter 14, the rate of involution progresses at about one fingerbreadth per postpartum day.

Evaluation of the fundus after a cesarean birth can be uncomfortable for the woman. With extended fingers, the nurse starts at the side and gently moves toward the midline until the fundus is located. The fundus should be firm and at the midline as in the woman who has had a vaginal birth. This also is the time at which the cesarean birth incision is inspected for redness, drainage, and approximation of the wound edges.

Lochia

The nurse wears protective gloves when checking the sanitary pad (peri pad) for lochia (Fig. 15-3). As described in Chapter 14, lochia initially is bright to dark red and is called lochia rubra. Small clots in the lochia are not unusual, but large clots must be reported at once. The diameter of the clot can be estimated to record the size. When the woman first gets up after resting for a period, she may experience a gush of lochia that has pooled in the vagina. She does not need to be alarmed by this unless the heavy flow continues. A pad that is saturated within 15 minutes is considered hemorrhage (see Chapter 16). As early as the third day, the lochia may change to lochia serosa. This is a pink

to pinkish brown color. The nurse explains to the woman that she will see another change in her lochia around the ninth or tenth day postpartum, when it becomes whitish or whitish-yellow. This is called lochia alba.

The nurse observes the cleanliness of the woman's perineal area when assessing the lochia. Any unpleasant odor is documented and reported because this indicates that further evaluation is needed. Some women do not have good habits of hygiene and need to be urged to clean themselves carefully when doing perineal care. This is an excellent opportunity for the nurse to review and reinforce teaching about perineal care. The woman is reminded to perform perineal care at least every 4 hours to prevent infection and promote healing. She also is encouraged to empty her bladder at least this often.

Episiotomy

The episiotomy or repaired lacerations are inspected during the daily postpartum check. While still wearing protective gloves, the nurse has the woman turn to her side and flex her upper leg toward her chest. Gently the nurse lifts the upper buttocks to inspect the perineum and anal area (Fig. 15-4). The episiotomy or repair is inspected for **r**edness, **e**dema, **e**cchymosis (bruising), **d**ischarge, and **a**pproximation of wound edges (REEDA). In the woman with no episiotomy or repair, the perineum is assessed for ecchymosis, edema,

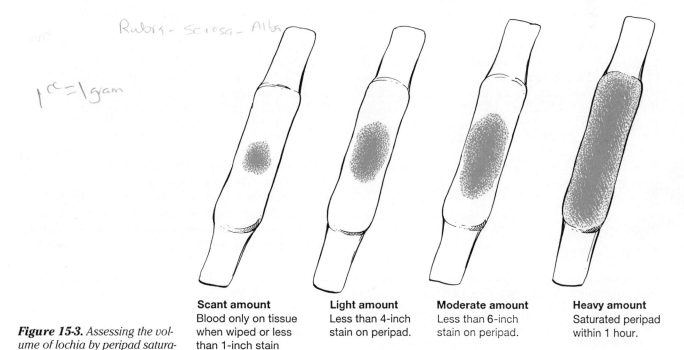

Figure 15-3. *Assessing the volume of lochia by peripad saturation.*

Scant amount
Blood only on tissue when wiped or less than 1-inch stain on peripad.

Light amount
Less than 4-inch stain on peripad.

Moderate amount
Less than 6-inch stain on peripad.

Heavy amount
Saturated peripad within 1 hour.

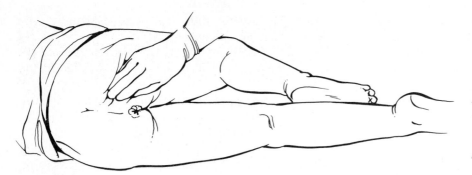

Figure 15-4. *Inspecting the perineal area and anal region with the woman in a lateral position, with her upper leg flexed. The nurse, wearing protective gloves, gently separates the buttocks.*

or discomfort. Any signs of hematoma are reported immediately.

The nurse also inspects the anal area for hemorrhoids. Tucks, a witch hazel–saturated pad, may be used to provide comfort. Other comfort measures are sitz baths or heat lamps, discussed later in this chapter. The nurse can reassure the woman that hemorrhoids gradually reduce in size and eventually resolve.

Bladder and Bowels

The first voiding after childbirth is very important, as discussed earlier. However, the nurse should continue to check daily on the functioning of the woman's bladder. The nurse inquires if the woman is having any dysuria, frequency, or burning on urination. These signs are an indication of a possible bladder infection.

Constipation is a common problem during the early postpartum period. Discomfort from perineal repairs and hemorrhoids are contributing factors in causing the woman to be hesitant to try to have a bowel movement. In addition, the restriction of food and oral fluids and the medications used during labor and childbirth help to compound the difficulty. The nurse questions the woman daily about bowel movements. Often stool softeners such as biscodyl (Dulcolax), docusate sodium (Colace), and milk of magnesia are administered to promote regular bowel habits. The nurse encourages the woman to eat foods high in bulk and fiber and to drink plenty of fluids to aid in reducing problems with constipation. Early ambulation also encourages bowel movements.

Lower Extremities

Venous stasis during the last months of pregnancy contributes to the danger of formation of thrombosis in the lower extremities. This tendency also may be intensified by legs positioned in stirrups during birth or from pressure exerted during pushing efforts in labor. By dorsiflexing the feet (Fig. 7-5), the nurse inspects the woman's legs for redness, swelling, warmth, or pain in the calf. The nurse evaluates each of the woman's legs for a positive Homans' sign, described in Chapter 8.

Psychosocial Care

As the woman moves from the immediate postpartum period to the early postpartum period, she has more energy and is able to focus on caring for her own needs and the needs of her newborn. Although she may still worry about her own body functions, such as bowel and bladder control, she starts to exhibit a desire to care for her infant. This is the taking-hold phase of the woman's adjustment.

During this taking-hold phase, the woman may demonstrate or express a lack of confidence in her ability to adequately care for her newborn. The nurse uses this time to teach the woman. A method that works well is to demonstrate infant care for the woman. The demonstration is followed by the opportunity for the woman to perform the care under the guidance of the nurse. The nurse fills a supportive role, praising and encouraging the woman without criticism. The nurse can support and reassure the woman as she makes decisions about her newborn. Postpartum depression, which may occur around the third postpartum day, is discussed in Chapter 16. As described in Chapter 14, the letting-go phase occurs after the woman is at home.

Family-Centered Care

The family's adjustments to the birth of a newborn begin even before the birth. The actual presence of the new family member makes the need to adjust an immediate reality. Health care facilities have introduced resourceful methods to allow the family to share the birthing experience so that they can form early attachments to the infant.

Rooming In

Rooming in is the term used to indicate a setting in which the neonate is in the mother's room from the time of birth until discharge. Several variations of rooming in are available. In some settings, the newborn is with the mother 24 hours a day. In other settings, there is a central nursery to which the neonate can be returned during visiting hours and at night. If the mother is ill, the neonate can stay in the central nursery.

Much of the nursing care for the newborn can be conducted at the bedside, where the woman can observe and learn. Many incidental questions can be answered by the nurse during these occasions.

Another variable in rooming in settings is the way in which staff members care for the mother and newborn. In some settings, there is a postpartum nurse who cares for the woman's needs and a separate nursery nurse who cares for the needs of the neonate. In some rooming in settings, mother–baby nursing has been established. In **mother–baby nursing** (also called **couplet care**), one nurse cares for both the mother and the baby. The nursing staff is cross-trained to function in both a postpartum and a nursery role. This type of care provides less fragmented care to the family. The mother-baby nurse has a greater opportunity to assess the functioning of the family unit, providing more information to intervene as needed in the family's adjustment.

Grandparent and Sibling Visitation

Grandparents are an important part of any family group. In some cultures, grandmothers play a major role in guiding the new mother in the care of her newborn. However, changes in parenting practices from one generation to another may provide areas of conflict. Many health care facilities offer prenatal classes for grandparents in an effort to inform them about new philosophies and practices in infant care.

Grandparents are encouraged to visit the new family in many facilities (Fig. 15-5). In facilities where they are permitted in the woman's room when the newborn is present, grandparents may be required to scrub and put on a cover gown according to the policy of the facility. However, many facilities do not require scrubbing or gowning. As with any visitor, they must be free of respiratory infections or other communicable illnesses.

Many facilities have prenatal classes for siblings during which the nurse instructor talks about pregnancy, birth, newborns, and the roles of big brothers and sisters. An effort is made to make the sibling feel an important part of the event. Sibling visits are customary in most facilities. The regulation governing sibling scrubbing and covering usually follows those of grandparents in most facilities. If the sibling is required to scrub and cover, the child is supervised by an adult. Siblings who visit must be free of any signs of illness, and an adult, other than the mother, should be responsible

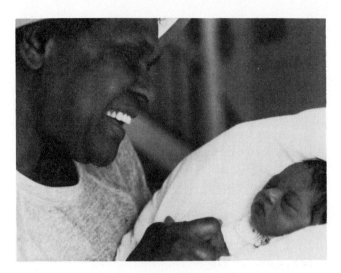

Figure 15-5. *The birth of a child is an important event for grandparents. (Photo by BABES, Inc.)*

for them. Younger siblings may have a greater problem understanding the full impact of the birth of a new family member. Siblings need some time to begin to attempt a relationship with the newborn. Often it is helpful if the mother initially focuses on the sibling and her pleasure at having the sibling visit rather than insisting that the sibling touches or in any way relates to the infant. This gives the sibling an opportunity to "warm up" to the situation.

Postpartum Tasks

The family's immediate tasks of the postpartum period include meeting the daily physical needs of the members of the family while attending to the needs of the newborn; sharing resources of love, affection, time, and money; and deciding how to divide the work that needs to be done in the home. The woman needs a period of restoration after the birth of a child. Whether she is employed outside of the home or not, she will need to have a period during which she can concentrate her efforts on caring for the infant and recovering her own physical well-being. Those with extended family networks (grandparents and other close relatives) available may have fewer problems adjusting to new responsibilities. Other family members, especially siblings or a spouse, need reassurance that they have not been displaced by the newborn in the affections of the mother. The woman will need assistance in carrying out daily household chores until she is physically and emotionally able to assume these tasks. The family that is able to sit down and make an organized plan for division of household tasks, planned rest and recreation time for family members, and allocation of family funds can avoid much of the stress that the postpartum period brings.

Nursing Diagnoses After Normal Childbirth

The nurse uses the nursing process to assess the postpartum woman and determine appropriate nursing diagnoses. Assessing the woman's physiologic condition is the first consideration. Bowel and bladder elimination, pain, fluid volume deficits, nutrition, rest needs, hygiene, and self-care needs are evaluated. The woman's knowledge deficit and level of self-esteem are determined through careful interview and assessment. The results of these assessments are used by the nurse to formulate nursing diagnoses. Some appropriate nursing diagnoses are presented in the Nursing Diagnoses Checklist, Following Normal Childbirth.

Health Promotion

The postpartum woman experiences discomfort for a variety of reasons. Some of these causes of discomfort include uterine cramping; episiotomy or perineal discomfort; and the pain caused by hemorrhoids.

Promoting Comfort

Uterine cramping that results from involution of the uterus (after-pains) can be very stressful for the woman. Administration of analgesia helps to relieve cramping. Explaining to the woman the cause of the cramping can be reassuring in itself. When she understands that her body is going through a natural phase, she may be more accepting of it. The nurse also can explain to her that breast-feeding causes the uterus to contract more, and this causes involution to occur more rapidly. Teaching the woman to ask for analgesia before the pain becomes unbearable helps her to control the pain. Administering analgesia approximately 30 minutes before breast-feeding helps to diminish the pain. The nurse can also tell the woman that ambulation helps to encourage involution and thus decreases the length of time she will have after-pain discomfort.

Another cause of discomfort is an episiotomy or perineal repair. The discomfort from either of these causes can be controlled in several ways. Ice packs may be applied to the perineum in the first hours after birth. These reduce edema and decrease bleeding, which helps to reduce the trauma to the perineum. Heat therapy is frequently used to provide comfort to the perineal area. This can be provided in the form of moist heat or dry heat.

Moist heat is commonly applied by sitz bath. A **sitz bath** is a method of applying warm moist heat to the perineal area by immersion in warm water. A sitz bath can be administered with a small basin that fits on the toilet seat and has an attached bag filled with warm water, which passes into it through plastic tubing (Fig. 15-6). The woman sits on the basin, and warm water flows from the bag into the basin. An overflow opening permits water to flow into the toilet. As the water cools, the woman can unclamp the tubing to allow more warm water to flow into the basin. The sitz bath continues for 20 minutes and is performed three times a day.

Heat lamps have been used in the past to provide dry heat but are currently less commonly used. The heat lamp is administered for 15 to 20 minutes at a time, several times a day. For safety, it should be placed 18 inches away from the perineum. Chemical packs, which provide heat when activated, are sometimes used. However, sitz baths are currently the means by which heat is most commonly provided to the perineal area.

Hemorrhoids cause discomfort for the woman. Witch hazel pads (Tucks), anesthetic sprays (Dermoplast Spray), and topical ointments are frequently used to provide comfort. Sitz baths also help in providing comfort for hemorrhoids.

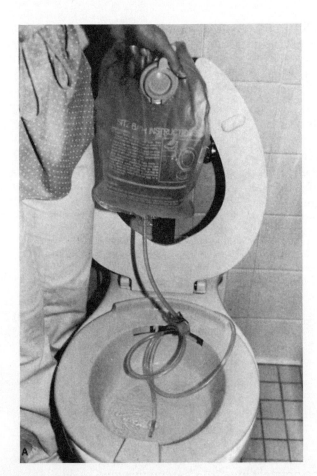

Figure 15-6. *A sitz bath provides perineal comfort. Here the sitz bath is being prepared for use.*

Teaching the woman to tighten her buttocks before sitting helps to reduce some of the discomfort she experiences. The nurse who observes the woman sitting on one buttock, or appearing to be rigid, can help her by teaching her to bring her buttocks together and contracting her pelvic floor muscles before sitting, gradually releasing the contraction after she sits. This helps to relieve tension on the perineal tissues and makes sitting a little easier.

Nutrition Counseling

The dietary intake of the postpartum woman should be well balanced and consist of 2200 to 2300 calories. An intake high in protein along with vitamins and minerals promotes tissue repair. Women who are breast-feeding need a total of 2700 to 2800 calories. The breast-feeding woman also needs to consume at least three milk servings each day to maintain adequate calcium and phosphorus supplies. A high fiber content in the diet aids in reducing constipation.

All postpartum women should have an intake of at least 2000 mL fluids per day. The intake of the breast-feeding woman should be 3000 mL/day. The nurse can tell the woman that she should drink three to four 8-ounce servings of fluids each day. The nurse observes the woman's fluid and food intake to determine if her needs are being fulfilled. Discussing food and fluid needs with the woman helps her to understand their importance in her recovery. This is not the time for the woman to consider dieting.

Breast Care

Every postpartum woman needs to care for her breasts and keep them clean. The breasts should be washed at the beginning of the shower each day. Women who are breast-feeding use no soap on the nipples, to prevent drying and cracking. The non–breast-feeding woman may use soap as she wishes. If leaking of colostrum or milk from the breast becomes a problem, the woman

Figure 15-7. (A) *Normal breast.* **(B)** *Engorged breast. In the engorged breast the alveolus/lobe fill with milk and push forward. Engorgement causes discomfort for the woman until breast-feeding is well established.*

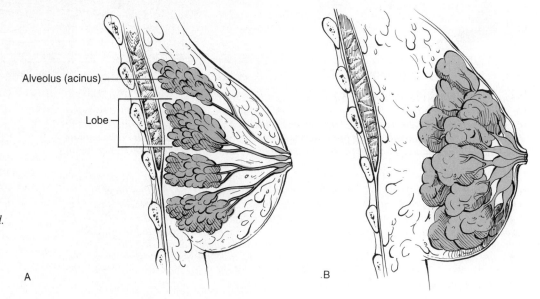

can use disposable pads in her bra to absorb the excess moisture. These should be changed frequently to prevent infection. Plastic liners should not be used, because they keep the nipples moist and will contribute to further soreness and breaking down of the nipple tissue. (See Chapter 7 for breast and nipple care).

The woman's breast may be a source of discomfort to her whether she is breast-feeding or not. Engorgement of the breast occurs on the third or fourth day after delivery in all women (Fig. 15-7). The woman who is breast-feeding will find that the discomfort of engorgement is gone in about 24 hours. Breast-feeding helps to relieve the discomfort. Engorgement and the accompanying pain lasts approximately 2 days for the non–breast-feeding woman. Pumping her breasts, fluid restrictions, or tight breast binders are not helpful. Cold compresses to the breasts several times a day provide comfort for either breast-feeding or non–breast-feeding women. Breast-feeding women may find using ice packs between feedings helpful. Hot compresses or a warm shower just before feedings encourages the flow of milk. Some physicians may prescribe medications to help suppress engorgement in the non–breast-feeding woman.

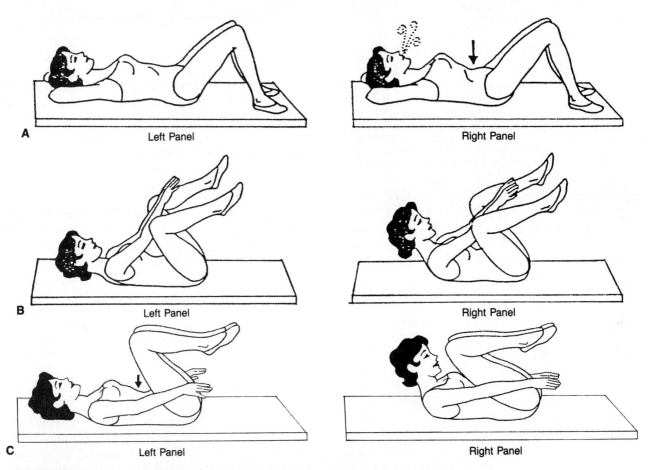

A Left Panel Right Panel

B Left Panel Right Panel

C Left Panel Right Panel

Figure 15-8. Postpartum Exercises. Simple exercises help the postpartum woman strengthen her abdominal muscles and flatten her stomach. They should be done on an exercise mat or a carpeted surface. *(A)* The woman lies on her back with her knees bent. Her feet are flat on the floor and placed the same distance apart as her hips (left panel). The woman breathes out as she pulls in her stomach hard and presses the small of her back firmly to the floor while raising her buttocks slightly. She breathes in and releases 20 times (right panel). *(B)* In a second exercise she lies on her back with her knees bent toward her chest. With her knees in a comfortable open position, she raises her arms between her knees (left panel). She curls her head and shoulder off the floor and holds for 3 seconds. She lowers and repeats these movements. She may gradually increase the number of times she repeats this exercise (right panel). *(C)* In a third exercise, the woman pulls in her stomach hard with her back pressed firmly to the floor. She brings both bent knees toward her chest and raises her arms slightly at her side (left panel). With her chin on her chest, she curls her head and shoulders off the floor, bringing her forehead toward her knees. She rolls back to starting position. Again she starts with a few of these rolls and gradually increases them (right panel).

The woman needs to be taught the signs and symptoms that are important for her to report to her health care provider after discharge. These include redness, swelling, and tenderness of the breasts and cracked nipples accompanied by increasing discomfort during breast-feeding. As part of the postpartum instructions, the nurse should review with the woman breast self-examination and encourage her to examine her breasts each month, preferably a week after the beginning of her menstrual period.

Resumption of Normal Activities

The resumption of normal activities for the woman with a normal childbirth experience occurs gradually over the postpartum period. The woman is given guidance by her health care provider at the time of discharge. Rest needs and exercise limitations are discussed with the woman. She should plan more frequent rest periods and avoid fatigue. Figure 15-8 presents appropriate exercises the woman can perform.

Generally, the woman is instructed to climb only one flight of stairs once a day the first week she is home. This means that she and the newborn should spend the day on the same floor in the home. Supplies to care for the newborn should also be handy so that she does not need to climb stairs to get something she needs. She can increase stair climbing during the second week, if she has no increase in lochia. The woman may be told to avoid lifting anything heavier than her baby for the first postpartum weeks.

Women who work outside the home are encouraged to remain at home for at least 3 weeks after the birth of their child. No heavy work should be done during this time. If the woman's outside job is one that consists of heavy work or lifting, she should avoid returning to work for 6 weeks.

Women who are discharged within 24 hours after birth will benefit from a follow-up visit by a nurse who can assess the home environment and the work that the mother is doing. The nurse may be able to make suggestions that can ease the mother's workload during the postpartum period. The nurse also assesses the physical and psychosocial progress of the woman and her neonate.

Sexual intercourse may be resumed when the woman's lochia is alba and her perineum has healed, if she had an episiotomy or repair. This is approximately 3 weeks after childbirth. The woman should be advised to take precautions to prevent pregnancy when sexual intercourse is resumed. The woman's vaginal tissues may be dry and thin. Use of a lubricating jelly or contraceptive foam will help avoid discomfort during intercourse. The breast-feeding woman may experience leakage of breast milk with sexual arousal. She may find that

---

DISPLAY 15-3
Postpartum Danger Signs to Report

Change in vaginal discharge:

  Increased amount

  Change to earlier character (bright red bleeding)

  Foul smell to discharge

Localized pain, redness, swelling, or warm spot in calf of one leg

Breast has area of pain, redness, tenderness, or swelling

Fever of 38°C (101.4°F)

Pain or tenderness in abdominal or pelvic area

Pain or burning on urination; difficulty urinating

---

breast-feeding just before lovemaking helps to decrease this. She may also want to wear a bra with pads to absorb the leakage during lovemaking. Patience and understanding by both partners is important during the first sexual encounters after childbirth.

Dangers Signs to Report

As part of discharge instructions, the woman needs to learn about the danger signs for which she should be alert. These danger signs should be reported to the health care provider at once if they appear. Display 15-3 presents a list of the danger signs that the woman should report. The availability of a telephone contact reassures the woman that she should seek answers for any concerns that she might have. She is also reassured that she will receive an understanding response to her questions.

Breast-feeding

During pregnancy, the woman has most likely considered whether she wishes to breast-feed her new infant. The nurse must be prepared to support the woman in whatever decision she makes. If the woman has difficulty deciding, the nurse can provide information about the advantages of breast-feeding. Breast- and bottle-feeding is covered in detail in Chapter 18. During the first feedings, the nurse helps the woman with positioning and initiating of feedings.

Rooming in offers the advantage of allowing the woman to breast-feed whenever she or the neonate wishes rather than by the schedule of the facility. This helps to reduce the discomfort of engorgement, because the woman's breast are emptied more frequently. The breast-feeding experience can be rewarding for the woman and very beneficial for the neonate.

NURSING CARE PLAN
Following Normal Childbirth

ASSESSMENT: Marie is a 22-year-old multigravida who delivered a 7 lb 2 oz male 6 hours ago. She has a midline episiotomy and plans to breast-feed.

NURSING DIAGNOSIS #1: Potential for Fluid Volume Deficit, related to excessive blood loss after delivery

EXPECTED OUTCOMES:
1. Marie's uterus will begin the involution process.
2. Marie will void freely without signs of distension or retention.
3. Marie's hemoglobin and hematocrit levels will remain within normal limits.

Nursing Interventions	*Rationale*
1. Monitor patient's lochia according to hospital policy, noting color, amount, and consistency.	1. Excessive lochia may result from lacerations, bladder distention, and/or uterine subinvolution.
2. Monitor the patient's fundus according to hospital policy, noting location and consistency.	2. A distended bladder interferes with involution by preventing the uterus from clamping down.
3. Monitor the patient's hemoglobin and hematocrit (H & H) prior to discharge.	3. Excessive blood loss is reflected in a decreasing H & H.

EVALUATION:
1. Marie's H & H at discharge was 12.6% and 36.1 g.
2. 24 hours after delivery, Marie's fundus is firm, midline, and one finger breadth below the umbilicus.
3. Before discharge, Marie is voiding freely.

NURSING DIAGNOSIS #2: Alteration in Skin Integrity, related to episiotomy

EXPECTED OUTCOMES:
1. Marie's episiotomy will heal without complications.
2. Marie will verbalize an understanding of perineal self-care activities.

Nursing Interventions	*Rationale*
1. Evaluate episiotomy/perineum every shift, noting presence of • redness • edema • ecchymosis • discharge • approximation	1. Frequent assessment ensures prompt recognition and treatment of complications.
2. Explain/demonstrate use of sitz bath and irrigation bottle.	2. Heat from the sitz bath enhances circulation and decreases edema. Irrigation bottles help maintain cleanliness, thus decreasing bacterial concentration.
3. Instruct patient to apply and remove sanitary pad from front to back.	3. Working from front to back decreases the risk of spreading contamination from the rectum to the vagina.

EVALUATION
1. Marie's episiotomy heals without any signs of infection.
2. Marie performs self-care perineal care on a regular basis.

Adolescent Considerations

When doing postpartum teaching with the adolescent, the nurse must plan to give her materials in writing that reinforce what is taught. Materials appropriate for the adolescent should use many drawings that need minimal in-depth reading. Providing the adolescent with reading materials and expecting her to read them is not adequate. The nurse should review all of the materials with her. Many facilities have video programs that they use for teaching purposes. These are effective for the adolescent, but must be followed up with discussion by the nurse to assure that the adolescent actually did watch them and that she got the main messages of the videos. Demonstrating for the adolescent and having her return the demonstration is a helpful technique. The nurse should plan to spend as much time as possible with the adolescent, patiently explaining and supporting her. However, the nurse must not make the adolescent feel that she is inadequate. Strong positive support by the nurse is essential. A referral for a follow-up visit after discharge is appropriate.

Cultural Considerations

The nurse must be sensitive to the differences in cultural practices of the woman and her family. Often older family members are very happy to explain the cultural traditions of the family. Asian and Chinese women may avoid anything cold. This is based on the belief that the body has lost a lot of blood, which is warm; therefore, it must be replenished with warm foods and external warmth.

Bathing practices vary widely among different cultures. Chinese and certain Latin women avoid shampooing their hair. Some cultures believe that the man should not be in the household with the woman while she has lochial flow. At the end of this period, some cultures carry out a ritual cleansing to permit the woman to return to society. Practice and beliefs about the return to sexual activity varies widely. Chinese American couples may avoid sexual activity for 100 days after birth. In those cultures that practice ritual cleansing, the couple abstains from sexual activity until after the cleansing. Few American women adhere to the 6 weeks of abstinence that was once thought to be important in American culture.

The Role of the Nurse

The nurse has an exceptional opportunity to provide the new family with health teaching and information to assist the woman in a successful recovery and a successful family adjustment. Because of early discharge practices, the brief time available requires the nurse to quickly assess, plan, and implement postpartum care. The nurse must make appropriate individualized adjustments to the nursing care plan to meet the needs of the woman and her family. While caring for the woman and her neonate, the nurse serves as a role model for the woman to follow. This is a responsibility and a challenge to the nurse.

REVIEW AND PREVIEW

In this chapter, the immediate postpartum physical and emotional care of the woman was discussed with emphasis on assessments that must be performed during this time. Usual findings were also covered. Daily postpartum care included assessment for the woman's breasts, fundus, lochia, episiotomy, bladder and bowels, and extremities. Each of these were discussed with the usual assessment and presentation of normal findings. Common treatments and procedures were included with explanations for each.

Various types of rooming-in settings were presented. The role of grandparents and the significance of including them in the family visiting was discussed. The adjustment of siblings was briefly presented, including the role of the nurse during sibling visitation. The role the nurse must take in providing postpartum teaching for the adolescent and sensitivity to diverse cultural customs were also discussed.

The following chapter discusses the complications that may occur in the postpartum period. Many of these complications are extensions of the normal physical condition of the postpartum woman.

The nurse must be able to distinguish normal postpartum conditions from complications, which require special intervention. The next chapter presents the nurse's responsibility in addressing complications as part of the complete picture of postpartum nursing care.

◈ KEY POINTS

◆ Nursing care for postpartum checks includes assessment of the level and the firmness of the fundus, the amount and character of the lochia, the condition of the perineum and episiotomy, and presence of hemorrhoids. The fundus should be firm, at the midline, and at or just above the level of the umbilicus during the first 24 hours; the lochia is rubra, with no clots or small clots only; the perineum is free of hematomas and ecchymosis and there is no trickling of blood. Hemorrhoids are described if present.

◆ A boggy fundus is massaged until firm. The nurse must be careful not to use vigorous massage, which may cause overstimulation and uterine atony.

SELF-ASSESSMENT

1. Which of the following statements indicates that a breast-feeding woman requires additional teaching?

- ○ **A.** "I can use absorbent pads in my bra if my breasts leak."
- ⊗ **B.** "I should apply breast cream to my nipples before each feeding."
- ○ **C.** "I should clean my nipples with plain water."
- ○ **D.** "I should change the baby's mouth position each time I feed her."

2. Three days after delivery, a patient complains of severe breast tenderness and a feeling of fullness. Which of the following should be the nurse's initial action?

- ○ **A.** Check the patient's temperature
- ○ **B.** Obtain an order for Parlodel
- ⊗ **C.** Encourage the woman to wear a supportive bra
- ○ **D.** Notify the physician

3. Perineal care includes all of the following EXCEPT:

- ○ **A.** Applying the perineal pad from front to back
- ○ **B.** Performing perineal care at least every 4 hours
- ⊗ **C.** Removing the perineal pad from back to front
- ○ **D.** Drying the perineum from front to back

4. Healing of an episiotomy may be slowed by which of the following?

- ○ **A.** Early ambulation
- ○ **B.** Bladder distension
- ⊗ **C.** Prolonged use of cold applications
- ○ **D.** Sitz baths within the first 24 hours after delivery

5. A breast-feeding woman should change her diet to consume:

- ○ **A.** Less fiber and more vitamins
- ⊗ **B.** More calories and calcium
- ○ **C.** More fiber and less protein
- ○ **D.** Less calories and minerals

◆ A full bladder displaces the uterus and inhibits contraction of the fundus because of lack of space. This may cause excessive bleeding.

◆ The woman can be encouraged to void by providing privacy, pouring water over her perineum, running water in a trickle from a faucet within the woman's hearing, and having her dabble her fingers in warm water. Ambulation also encourages voiding.

◆ Perineal care is the cleansing of the perineum with warm water. A cleansing solution frequently is used in addition to the water. The woman is taught to perform her own perineal care as soon as she is able. It is performed after every voiding or bowel movement, and as needed, at least every 4 hours.

◆ Constipation is a common postpartum problem, which is often made worse by the woman's tender perineum and hemorrhoids. Stool softeners are frequently prescribed. Ambulation, a dietary intake high in bulk and fiber, and ample fluid intake help to alleviate this problem.

◆ Rooming in gives the woman and her partner the opportunity to observe and perform care for the neonate under the guidance and support of the nurse.

◆ In mother–baby nursing, one nurse is cross-trained in postpartum and neonatal nursing to provide care to the mother and the neonate. This affords more flexible care. The nurse who functions as a mother–baby nurse is better able to assess the entire family and provide the guidance and support that benefits all members of the family.

◆ Before discharge from the facility, the woman is taught to report excessive vaginal bleeding, a foul odor to the lochia discharge, or increased discharge; pain in the calf of a leg, which may be accompanied by redness, swelling, or warmth; redness, pain, tenderness, or swelling of a breast in the breast-feeding woman; fever of 38°C (101.4°F); abdominal or pelvic pain or tenderness; and pain, burning or difficulty urinating.

◆ The breast-feeding woman is taught to avoid using soaps or alcohol when washing her breasts. Breasts need only be washed once daily at the time of the shower. Lotions and creams are not generally recommended, but if they are used they are applied after breast-feeding and rubbed in thoroughly to avoid clogging nipple pores. The woman may use clean, absorbent material to absorb leakage from her breasts, but should avoid plastic liners in her bra. All women should wear supportive bras. Changing the feeding position of the neonate may help to prevent sore nipples.

BIBLIOGRAPHY

Ament, L. A. (1990). Maternal tasks of the puerperium reidentified. *Journal Of Obstetric, Gynecologic, and Neonatal Nursing, 19*(4), 330–335.

Bucho, B. L., Pugh, L. C., Bishop, B. A., Cochran, J. F., Smith, L. R., & Lerew, D. J. (1994). Comfort measure in breastfeeding, primiparous women. *Journal Of Obstetric, Gynecologic, and Neonatal Nursing, 23*(1), 46–51.

Evans, C. J. (1991). Description of a home follow-up program for childbearing families. *Journal Of Obstetric, Gynecologic, and Neonatal Nursing, 20*(2), 113–118.

Fritz, P., Galanter, M., Lifshutz, H., & Egelko, S. (1993). Developmental risk factors in postpartum women with urine tests positive for cocaine. *American Journal of Drug and Alcohol Abuse, 19*(2), 187–211.

Gielen, A. C., Faden, R. R., O'Campo, P., Brown, H., & Paige, M. (1991). Maternal employment during the early postpartum period: Effect on initiation and continuation of breast-feeding. *Pediatrics, 87*(3), 298–308.

Gamble, D., & Morse, J. M. (1993). Fathers of breastfed infants: Postponing and types of involvement. *Journal of Obstetric, Gynecologic, and Neonatal Nursing, 22*(4), 358–365.

Gullicks, J. N., & Crase, S. J. (1993). Sibling behavior with a newborn: Parents' expectations and observations. *Journal of Obstetric, Gynecologic, and Neonatal Nursing, 22*(5), 438–444.

Hill, P. D. (1991). The enigma of insufficient milk supply. *Maternal Child Nursing, 16*(6), 312–316.

Knops, G. G. (1993). Postpartum mood disorders: A startling contrast to the joy of birth. *Postgraduate Medicine, 93*(3), 103–107.

Kyena-Isabirye, M. (1992). UNICEF launches the baby-friendly hospital initiative. *MCN, 17*(4), 177–179.

Lim, R. (1993). Postpartum practices throughout the world. *Mothering, 66*(Spring), 86–92

May, K. A., & Mahlmeister, L. R. (1994). *Maternal and neonatal care: Family-centered care*. Philadelphia: J. B. Lippincott.

Pillitteri, A. (1992). *Maternal and child nursing*. Philadelphia: J. B. Lippincott.

Potter, S., Hannum, S., McFarlin, B., & Essex-Sorlie, D. (1991). Does infant feeding method influence maternal postpartum weight loss? *Journal of the American Dietetic Association, 91*(4), 441–446.

Reeder, S. J., Martin, L. L., & Koniak, D. (1992). *Maternity nursing* (17th ed.). Philadelphia: J. B. Lippincott.

Stevens-Simon, C., Beach, R. K. (1992). School-based prenatal and postpartum care: Strategies for meeting the medical and educational need of pregnant and parenting students. *Journal of School Health, 62*(7), 204–206.

Williams, L. R., & Cooper, M. K. (1993). Nurse-managed postpartum home care. *Journal of Obstetric, Gynecologic, and Neonatal Nursing, 22*(1), 25–31.

CHAPTER 16

Nursing Care in the Complicated Postpartum Period

◆ OBJECTIVES

When the learning goals of this chapter are met, the reader will be able to:

- Differentiate between early and late postpartum hemorrhage.
- Identify nursing interventions in the care of the woman with postpartum hemorrhage.
- Describe what happens in disseminated intravascular clotting (DIC).
- List five common sites for puerperal infection.
- Identify nursing actions necessary to prevent puerperal infections.
- State appropriate teaching for the breast-feeding woman to aid in preventing mastitis.
- Describe nursing assessments to identify thrombophlebitis.
- Describe the dangers that deep vein thrombophlebitis presents.
- Differentiate postpartum blues, postpartum depression, and postpartum psychosis.
- Identify nursing assessments and interventions that help a grieving family.

TERMINOLOGY

Atony
Embolectomy
Endometritis
Fibrolytic therapy
Laceration
Mastitis
Parametritis

Placenta accreta
Postpartum hemorrhage
Precipitous birth
Puerperal
Salpingitis
Subinvolution

Nursing care during the postpartum period requires careful assessment of the woman to identify those at risk and to detect early signs and symptoms of postpartum complications. Decisive interventions are necessary to prevent escalation of these complications. Because of the practice of early discharge of mother and baby, it is essential that the woman receive adequate verbal and written instructions regarding danger signs. A contact person and telephone number must be identified for the woman or her family so that they feel comfortable about calling with "silly" questions or concerns.

Physical complications that may arise during the postpartum period are hemorrhage, infection, birth canal injuries, and venous thrombosis. Prenatal complications, such as pregnancy-induced hypertension (PIH) and diabetes (discussed in Chapter 8), may continue to pose a threat to the health of the postpartum woman. Psychosocial postpartum complications include depression, psychosis, and the grief in response to congenital anomalies or fetal or neonatal death. Any of these complications may interfere with the bonding of the mother and her infant.

Postpartum Hemorrhage

Postpartum hemorrhage may occur at any time from immediately after birth up to 4 to 6 weeks postpartum. Thus, it is described as early (first 24 hours) or late (after 24 hours to 6 weeks). Early hemorrhage is most common, occurring in approximately 5% of all deliveries. Late hemorrhage is possibly the more dangerous because it may occur after hospital discharge. Unless the woman experiencing late hemorrhage promptly recognizes the danger and seeks treatment, serious blood loss can result very quickly.

The normal amount of blood lost during delivery is between 300 and 350 mL. Hemorrhage is defined as the loss of more than 500 mL. However, the estimation of blood loss is simply guesswork unless pads and liners are weighed and calculated, with 1 mL of blood equal to 1 g. *Any* suspicion of excessive bleeding should be treated as hemorrhage, with prompt massage of the fundus and notification of the birth attendant.

Causes of Hemorrhage

The major causes of hemorrhage are uterine atony, lacerations of the cervix or birth canal, retained placental fragments, distended bladder, and hematomas. Other causes include subinvolution and inverted uterus. Each of these are briefly described here.

Uterine Atony

After delivery of the placenta, the emptied uterus must contract to shut off the flow of blood from the raw placental attachment site. Contraction of the uterine muscle squeezes the blood vessels of the placental site, effectively stopping the bleeding. If the uterine muscle does not contract, these vessels continue to bleed freely. **Atony** is the lack of normal tone. Uterine atony describes a uterus that is not able to remain contracted, and thus bleeding occurs. This bleeding may consist of a constant trickle to a steady flow of bright red blood and clots from the vagina, or it may be hidden (occult) as the uterus enlarges to hold the blood. On palpation, the uterus feels soft or boggy and may be enlarged. Uterine atony is most likely to occur early when the uterine muscle fibers have been overstretched, exhausted, or relaxed by medications. Thus, the nurse is alert for one or more of the risk factors that are presented in Display 16-1. When uterine atony does not respond to conservative treatment (massage and oxytocics), bleeding can be life threatening, and drastic measures such as hysterectomy may be necessary.

Retained Placenta

Pieces of placenta that remain adherent to the uterus prevent the uterus from contracting effectively and can cause either early or late hemorrhage. Examination of the placenta after its delivery can identify missing pieces, thus indicating the need for additional medical interventions to prevent hemorrhage. Oxytocics are administered to expel retained fragments. If administration of oxytocics is not sufficient to expel the fragments, manual removal of the placenta or dilatation and curettage (D&C) may be necessary. Occasionally the entire placenta remains partially or wholly attached or trapped in the uterus. **Placenta accreta** is the term used for abnormal implantation of the placenta that causes it to adhere to the uterine wall. This rare event becomes evident in the third stage of labor. Profuse hemorrhage may occur. Hysterectomy is often the only solution.

Lacerations

Lacerations are tissue tears caused by trauma during birth. They can result in excessive blood loss during the

uterus remains firm. The woman may be unable to void because of pressure on the urethra, or she may have an urge to defecate because of rectal pressure (Fig. 16-1). Extreme pain is characteristic of hematomas. Hematomas of the broad ligament are difficult to detect, but may be suspected when there is anemia, extreme unilateral pain in the pelvis or abdomen, and abdominal distension. Local incision and drainage or laparotomy may be necessary to drain large or enlarging hematomas. Small perineal hematomas may be treated with ice packs.

Bladder Distention

Bladder distention causes the uterus to be displaced from its center location and prevents it from strongly contracting. After childbirth, the bladder fills quickly as intravenous (IV) fluids are administered and the body begins to rid itself of the extra blood fluid volume acquired during pregnancy. Additionally, after the trauma of labor and childbirth, the woman has diminished sensations of a full bladder. Therefore, she may be unaware of a bladder containing in excess of 500 or even 1000 mL urine. The nurse detects a full bladder when palpa-

early postpartum period. Lacerations may result from forceps use or vacuum extraction, **precipitous birth** (labor less than 3 hours), or a difficult delivery related to the baby's position or size. They may occur on the cervix, vaginal walls, labia, or perineum. The nurse differentiates bleeding caused by lacerations from that resulting from uterine atony or retained placental pieces by fundal palpation and observation of the bleeding. In lacerations, the uterus remains firm and normal in size but bleeding is present as bright red, frank bleeding or continual trickling. In uterine atony and retained placental pieces, the fundus is not firm, and bleeding is free flowing.

Hematomas

Hematomas may result in significant blood loss, but there is no obvious bleeding. Hematomas form when there is injury to a blood vessel without injury to the overlying tissue. They are often visible on the perineum or hidden in the vagina. They can occur elsewhere in the reproductive tract. Perineal pain is a distinguishing characteristic, rather than frank bleeding, and the

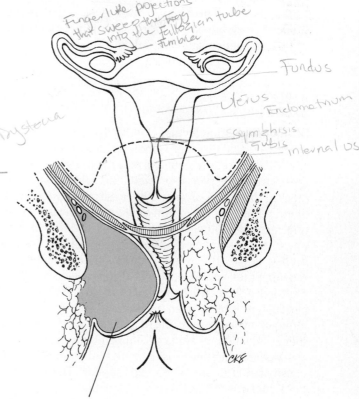

Figure 16-1. *Paravaginal hematoma, showing the large amount of blood that can be contained within a hematoma and the pressure that it can exert on the tissues. The paravaginal hematoma extends over the vulva to the rectal area.*

tion of the uterine fundus shows it to be high (above the umbilicus), displaced, usually to the right, and boggy. The nurse also finds that the lochia is heavy. Catheterization may be necessary to drain the bladder if spontaneous voiding is not possible in 6 to 8 hours. This prevents bladder distention or decompresses a bladder that is already distended.

Subinvolution

Subinvolution is a term used to describe the failure of the uterus to return to its prepregnant size and location, resulting in late hemorrhage. It is most often caused by retained placental fragments, infection, or failure of the placental site to heal. Excessively vigorous massage of the uterus may be a contributing factor. Subinvolution is characterized by a uterus that is large and soft, usually above the umbilicus, prolonged lochia (for 2 or more weeks postpartum), or a return to continuous bright red lochia after the first 3 days, a heavy sensation in the pelvis, and occasionally foul odor when sepsis is present. Conservative treatment consists of administration of oral methylergonovine maleate (Methergine) and antibiotics if infection is present. A D&C may be necessary to remove stray pieces of placental tissue. Sudden heavy bleeding can result in rapid blood loss and shock, necessitating emergency medical or surgical treatment to prevent death.

Disseminated Intravascular Clotting

Problem: Coagulation

Disseminated intravascular clotting (DIC), a serious and potentially fatal disorder, is more common in labor and childbirth as a cause of hemorrhage, but may be seen in the postpartum period as well. DIC results when increased formation of thrombin causes clotting in small blood vessels, which in turn depletes platelets and clotting factors. At the same time, the excessive thrombin stimulates anticlotting mechanisms, and clots are broken down. The result is severe hemorrhage from bleeding sites and vascular occlusion by clots in major organs. DIC is most often associated with abruptio placenta, but is also seen in women with pregnancy-induced hypertension (PIH), retained placental fragments, infection, or amniotic fluid embolism.

Medical treatment is centered on removing the cause of the DIC and physiologic support. This includes fluid, electrolyte, and blood replacement; administering oxygen; insertion of a central venous pressure (CVP) line and urinary bladder catheter. Identification of DIC is difficult in its early stages. The woman with DIC is critically ill and usually is cared for in an intensive care unit.

Nursing Care of the Woman With Postpartum Hemorrhage

Nursing care of the all postpartum women includes assessments to detect postpartum hemorrhage at the earliest possible time. Postpartum discharge instructions to all women include observations to be made and reported to detect late postpartum hemorrhage. In both early and late postpartum hemorrhage, prompt intervention is essential.

Nursing Assessment

Nursing assessments for immediate postpartum care are discussed in Chapter 15. The usual schedule is followed unless there are signs of hemorrhage. More frequent assessments are made when indicated. The Assessment Checklist outlines the nursing assessments appropriate for postpartum hemorrhage.

When assessing the lochia, the nurse assesses lochia not only on the pad, but also under the patient's buttocks or back, as it seeps to the lowest spot. Clots are commonly passed when the woman's position is changed from recumbent to standing and result from blood pooling in the vagina. Clots also can result from blood pooling in a relaxed uterus and may contain pieces of placenta. It is important for the nurse to identify if there is any placental tissue in the clot. Placental tissue appears

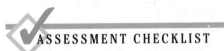

ASSESSMENT CHECKLIST

Postpartum Hemorrhage

· Palpate the fundus for consistency, location, and size

· Check lochia for color, amount, and presence of clots

· Inspect the perineum for hematomas, lacerations, or disrupted episiotomy site

· Monitor urinary output or bladder distention

· Monitor vital signs: blood pressure, pulse, respirations, and level of consciousness, skin color and warmth

· Question regarding perineal pain or excessive after-pains

· Determine presence of risk factors that increase the chance of hemorrhage (see Display 16-1)

· Assess for signs of hemorrhagic disorders (disseminated intravascular clotting [DIC]): bleeding from injection sites, gums, petechiae, purpura

Why would Placenta Previa cause hemorrhage

Fibrous tubours can
cause postpartum bleeding.

fibrous and does not dissolve in cold water. The nurse instructs the woman to save any clots for inspection.

The nurse inspects the perineum and vulva when assessing the lochia. Some swelling of the vulva and perineum is expected. A distinct swelling or ecchymosis of the labia or vulva (Fig. 16-2) or disruption of the episiotomy is usually accompanied by excessive pain in the perineum or rectum. The nurse can differentiate a hematoma from usual swelling by lightly touching the area with a gloved finger. If a hematoma is present, the woman experiences excessive pain. A vaginal examination by the birth attendant is necessary to palpate hematomas of the vagina or identify lacerations of the vagina or cervix.

Vital signs are not reliable as early warning signs of hemorrhage. Because of the increased total blood volume during pregnancy, a woman can lose 30% to 35% of blood volume before a decrease in blood pressure or an increase in pulse occurs. Urinary output and CVP measurements are a measure of circulating blood volume and may more accurately reflect blood loss. Decreasing blood pressure and a rapid thready pulse are indications of major blood loss and impending shock, conditions that must be treated aggressively. Other symptoms include cold, clammy skin; thirst; rapid, shallow respirations; restlessness; and anxiety. Complaints of dizziness, nausea, or ringing in the ears are signs that may precede loss of consciousness.

Assessment of orthostatic changes in blood pressure and review of hemoglobin and hematocrit values are important follow-up assessments once the bleeding

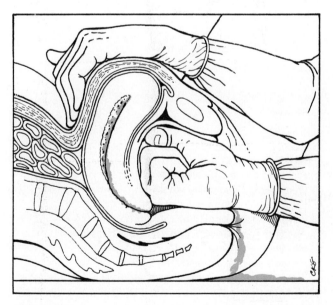

Figure 16-2. *Bimanual compression of the uterus and massage with the abdominal hand usually will control the hemorrhage.*

has stopped. The woman may need to continue iron supplementation after discharge. The nurse must be alert to the increased risk of infection in the woman weakened by postpartum hemorrhage. Assessments of infection are discussed in detail later in this chapter.

Nursing Interventions

Prevention and early detection of hemorrhage are the primary nursing goals in caring for the postpartum patient. The treatment centers on continuing assessment, assisting with operative procedures, administering medications, IV fluids or blood, and providing a supportive calm presence to the woman and her family in a crisis situation. The woman may be transferred to an intensive care unit for more sophisticated monitoring or treatment. Nursing intervention to prevent postpartum hemorrhage include inspecting the placenta thoroughly for missing pieces; administering oxytocic drugs as prescribed to keep the uterus contracted and maintenance of open IV line; applying ice to the perineum to decrease hematoma formation; and inducing voiding with nursing measures or catheterization if bladder is full and patient is unable to void. See the accompanying Nursing Care Plan on the following page for the woman with postpartum hemorrhage.

If excessive bleeding is noted and the fundus is soft or boggy, the first nursing action is to gently but firmly massage the fundus. See Chapter 15 for uterus massage technique. When the uterus is enlarged as well as soft, the presence of clots in the uterus is indicated. These clots must be expressed to allow the uterus to contract effectively. Expression of clots can be accomplished by squeezing and pushing the fundus toward the lower hand. Expression of clots may also be done by the birth attendant, with one hand in the vagina supporting the uterus, while the other hand massages the fundus (Fig. 16-3).

The woman is taught to assess uterine (fundal) firmness and to massage her uterus. This is especially important if she is being discharged early. She also is instructed in the normal involution (shrinking) of the uterus and the expected lochial changes. The mother is given a written list outlining warning signs that require a return visit for additional evaluation. The nurse should review orally the warning signs to be sure she understands. Display 16-2 presents appropriate discharge instructions.

Oxytocics such as Pitocin and Syntocinon are often used in a continuous IV infusion after delivery to prevent atony. The administration rate and concentration of oxytocics may be increased when there is excessive bleeding or the uterus does not stay firm. Pitocin is never given in an IV bolus, because it causes hypotension. It may be given intramuscularly after the placenta

NURSING CARE PLAN
for the Woman With Postpartum Hemorrhage

ASSESSMENT:

Soft or boggy fundus (uterus); larger or higher than normal

Excessive lochia, clots

Severe after-pains

Change in vital signs: decreasing blood pressure, increasing pulse, increased respiration; other symptoms of hypovolemia: thirst, restlessness, anxiety, cool clammy skin, pallor

Full bladder, as identified by absence of voiding, palpable or visible bladder above symphysis, displacement of uterus to side

NURSING DIAGNOSIS #1: Risk for Injury, related to uterine atony

EXPECTED OUTCOME: Prevention of active uterine hemorrhage and injury (hypovolemia or fluid volume deficit) because of recognition of risk factors present and early detection/intervention for uterine atony.

Nursing Interventions	*Rationale*
1. Massage uterus, express clots that may have collected in the uterus; provide for emptying of bladder: nursing measures to promote voiding or catheterization; administer oxytocics as ordered; maintain IV lines.	1. Massage of fundus stimulates contraction of uterine muscle and decreases bleeding; expression of clots permits stronger contraction of the uterus; a full bladder prevents strong contraction of uterus and increases bleeding; emptying the bladder allows for uterine contraction and decreases bleeding. Oxytocics have a stimulating effect on uterine muscle, increasing contraction and decreasing bleeding. Open IV lines are necessary for medication and fluid administration.
2. Notify physician or midwife immediately of changes in fundus, lochia, or vital signs. Document assessments and response to interventions.	2. Prompt early notification of physician or midwife provides for necessary medical assessments and interventions to identify and correct cause of hemorrhage. Documentation is a legal necessity.
3. Monitor vital signs, level of consciousness, skin warmth, and turgor.	3. Early detection of changes in baseline vital signs signals need for continued assessment and treatment to prevent complications of hypovolemia and shock.

EVALUATION: The woman's fundus becomes firm and normal in size, location; lochia is normal in amount, no clots; vital signs are stable, skin warm and dry; woman rests comfortably without severe after-pains, restlessness, or anxiety.

NURSING DIAGNOSIS #2: Fluid Volume Deficit, related to hypovolemia

EXPECTED OUTCOME: Woman will achieve optimal fluid balance.

Nursing Interventions	*Rationale*
1. Prepare for or maintain IV lines for fluid, blood, and medication (oxytocics) administration.	1. Fluids and blood must be administered to replace lost blood and prevent further hypovolemia and shock. Oxytocics are given IV to contract the uterus and to stop further hemorrhage.
2. Monitor and document vital signs, level of consciousness, skin warmth and turgor, color.	2. Continuing evaluation of treatment/response necessary to determine effectiveness of treatment or need for additional measures.
3. Prepare to administer oxygen.	3. Oxygen administration is necessary to prevent hypoxia related to decreased numbers of circulating red blood cells.

EVALUATION: Normal fluid balance is restored as evidenced by stable vital signs, urinary output of at least 30 mL per hour, lochial flow is decreased to normal amount.

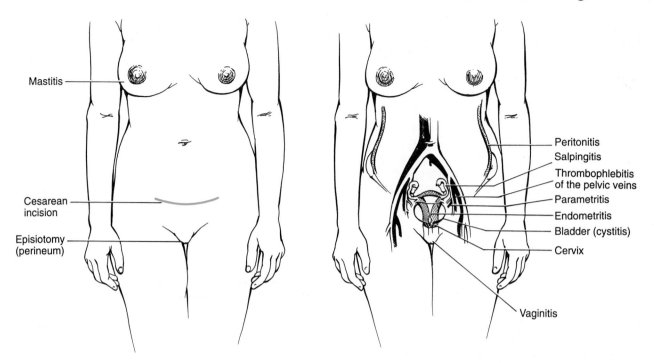

Figure 16-3. *Sites of infection that may occur during the postpartum period.*

is delivered. Ergonovine maleate (Ergotrate) or methyl-ergonovine maleate (Methergine) may be given intra-muscularly, by mouth, or IV to contract the uterus. Transient hypertension may result after IV administration of either of these drugs; therefore, they are contraindicated in patients with PIH or preexisting hypertension.

Intravenous use is usually reserved for true hemorrhagic emergencies.

Most hemorrhages can be controlled with massage and oxytocic drugs. Uncorrected hypovolemia results in loss of consciousness, renal failure, and death. Nursing interventions are presented in the Checklist.

DISPLAY 16-2
Discharge Teaching for Postpartum Complications

Before discharge, the woman is instructed to report the following signs of complications:

· Return of bright red or dark red blood after the 3rd or 4th postpartum day

· Fever over 100.4°F (38°C); pain or tenderness of the uterus (pelvis), breasts, or legs; purulent or foul-smelling discharge from the vagina, incisions, or lacerations

· Burning or pain, urgency, frequency of urination; flank pain

· Flulike symptoms; hot, red, painful lump in one breast

· Recurrent feelings of despair or depression that interfere with ability to sleep, eat, care for infant, or carry out normal activities

---

✔ **NURSING INTERVENTIONS CHECKLIST**

Postpartum Hemorrhage

Continued assessment of blood loss; pad count or weight

Continued gentle but firm fundal massage

Monitor for shock: vital signs every 5 to 15 minutes, assess level of consciousness, urine output (insertion of urinary catheter is indicated), CVP readings, (assist with insertion of central line)

Maintain open IV line with large-gauge needle (#18–#19) and administration of fluids, blood, and drugs ordered by the physician

Assist with preparation for any surgical interventions that may be necessary, such as repair of any lacerations, evacuation of hematoma, dilatation and curettage, hysterectomy

Administer oxygen as prescribed

Document assessment, interventions, and patient response to treatment

Puerperal Infection

Puerperal is a term that means after childbirth. Puerperal infection is infection of the reproductive tract after childbirth. It is characterized by fever higher than 38°C (100.4°F) after the first 24 hours that lasts 2 or more successive days. It generally occurs during the first 10 days, but it is possible for infection to occur before 24 hours. Approximately 6% of women in the United States experience puerperal infection, and its effects range from mild to life threatening.

Sites of Infection

Common sites for puerperal infection include the uterus (endometritis or metritis), vagina, perineum, cervix, and cesarean birth incision. The infection may spread from these sites to produce inflammation of the fallopian tubes (salpingitis) or pelvic cavity (parametritis), and even thrombophlebitis, particularly of the veins of pelvis (Fig. 16-4). The most common causative organisms are the beta-hemolytic streptococcus, staphylococcus, or coliform bacteria.

The highly vascular uterine lining and raw placental implant site are highly susceptible to infection. Prolonged labor, premature rupture of membranes, cesarean birth after labor has started, intrauterine manipulation, and manual extraction of the placenta are all associated with increased incidence of puerperal infection. Anemia, obesity, and diabetes also predispose the woman to infection. There is controversy concerning whether frequent vaginal examinations and invasive fetal monitoring increase the risk of puerperal infection.

Localized Infections

The episiotomy or cesarean birth incision are common sites for local infection. Infection also may occur in the vagina, cervix, or vulva, especially if lacerations are present. The symptoms are the classic signs of inflammation and infection: erythema, warmth, swelling, and tenderness or pain. Purulent discharge also may be present. Warm sitz baths are usually sufficient to promote healing in mild cases; oral analgesics such as acetaminophen (Tylenol), acetaminophen and codeine (Tylenol #3), and topical sprays (benzocaine) may be ordered for pain relief. Antibiotics also may be ordered. In some cases, abscesses may form, and incision and drainage or removal of a suture or clamp may be necessary.

Endometritis

Endometritis, an infection of the uterine lining, is the most common puerperal infection. The symptoms are similar to symptoms of the flu: fever, sometimes chills and tachycardia, fatigue, malaise, headache, backache,

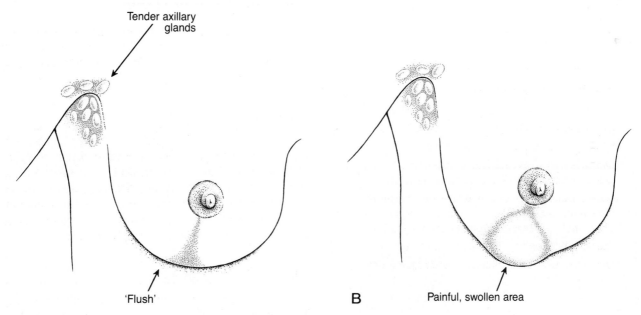

Figure 16-4. Mastitis. **(A)** Early mastitis. Fever is followed by a painful area on the breast and a "flush" that is red and tender but not movable and swollen. **(B)** Overt inflammation in mastitis. A swollen, painful, red-to-brawny area develops. The purulent drainage gradually localizes into an abscess; when movable, it must be incised and drained.

abdominal pain, and foul lochia. Lochia may be scant to profuse, red to brown, and in some cases is normal in odor. A vaginal examination by the physician is performed, and cultures of the lochia are obtained. On palpation, the uterus is very tender and enlarged. A blood culture and complete blood count (CBC) also may be obtained. Antibiotics are initially administered IV, then are followed by oral antibiotics. Antipyretic analgesics for discomfort and fever are prescribed.

Salpingitis, Parametritis, Peritonitis

These infections usually are an extension of endometritis that has traveled through the blood or lymphatics. **Salpingitis** is an inflammation of the fallopian tubes, **parametritis** refers to infection of the pelvic structures, such as the broad ligament, and peritonitis involves the peritoneum. Abscess formation of the uterine ligament, cul-de-sac, or subdiaphragmatic area may complicate the treatment, requiring drainage. Symptoms usually include a high fever, 38.9° to 40°C (102°–104°F), chills, malaise, abdominal pain, and subinvolution of the uterus. With peritonitis, there is severe pain, tachycardia, shallow rapid respirations, abdominal distension, and nausea or vomiting. Broad-spectrum antibiotics are prescribed IV, as well as antipyretics, and analgesics. In severe cases, care in an intensive care unit may be necessary to treat systemic symptoms.

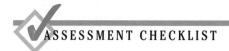

ASSESSMENT CHECKLIST

Puerperal Infections

Identify women at risk for puerperal infection

Assess woman's knowledge deficits concerning hygiene, perineum care

Evaluate vital signs each shift or more often if indicated, with attention to temperature elevation

Inspect perineum or cesarean incision for signs of local infection (each shift): erythema, unusual pain, purulent discharge, separation of wound edges

Assess lochia for odor, abnormal color, amount

Obtain or assist with culture of lochia, exudate, wound

Palpate fundus with attention to size and tenderness; severe after-pains

Attend to complaints of abdominal or pelvic pain, dysuria, malaise, vomiting, diarrhea

DISPLAY 16-3
Risk Factors for Postpartum Infection

Prenatal
- Poor nutrition, anemia
- Poor hygiene
- Preexisting infections
- Diabetes
- Obesity

Intrapartum
- Operative, manipulative procedures, forceps delivery, manual extraction of placenta, catheterization
- Prolonged labor, frequent vaginal examinations
- Intrauterine monitoring
- Premature rupture of membranes
- Cesarean birth after labor is established
- Lacerations or hematoma

Postpartum
- Poor hygiene (especially perineum care)
- Systemic illness
- Hemorrhage
- Retained placental fragments

Nursing Care of the Woman with Puerperal Infection

Prevention of puerperal infection begins with the practice of aseptic technique. Careful, conscientious handwashing by the nurse and the woman is essential in prevention.

Nursing Assessments

The nurse assesses the woman's vital signs, observing for any elevation of temperature. Other assessments include observations for any indication of pain, foul or abnormal lochia, any purulent discharge, abdominal or uterine tenderness and pain, or nausea and vomiting. The Assessment Checklist presents nursing assessments that are appropriate for puerperal infections.

Nursing Interventions

Identification of women at risk for infection (Display 16-3) alerts the nurse to observe for signs of puerperal infection. Early identification helps reduce the incidence and severity of infection by allowing for preventive interventions.

Promoting proper nutrition, hygiene, and the treatment of any preexisting infections during the antepartum period is the most effective means of preventing many postpartum complications. Practicing scrupulous medical and surgical asepsis, teaching handwashing and perineum care, as well reporting signs of infection as identified in the daily assessment, are essential intrapartum and postpartum interventions.

The nurse administers prescribed antibiotics, analgesics, and antipyretics, and maintains the IV site if present. The woman is encouraged to maintain a semi-Fowler's position to localize infection in the lower pelvis (especially with parametritis or peritonitis) and to increase comfort. The nurse promotes comfort and provides rest periods.

Urinary Tract Infections

Bladder infections (cystitis) are common during the postpartum period. They are usually associated with catheterization during labor and birth, trauma to the bladder or urethra during delivery, or failure to completely empty the bladder. In the first 2 days, diuresis increases the urinary output. Voidings of 500 to 1000 mL at a time are not unusual. Perineal pain diminishes bladder sensitivity, and decreased bladder tone results in incomplete emptying of the bladder. Voiding 100 to 200 mL may indicate the woman has retention with overflow. The urine that remains in the bladder provides an excellent medium for bacterial growth. The woman generally has symptoms in 2 to 3 days after delivery. The classic symptoms are frequency, urgency, dysuria, suprapubic pain, fever, and bloody urine. Fever is generally not significant unless the infection travels to the kidneys, producing a pyelonephritis (infection of the kidney pelvis). Untreated or inadequately treated pyelonephritis can progress to the renal cortex, resulting in glomerulonephritis and kidney damage. Treatment consists of antibiotic therapy after the pathogenic organism is identified through urine culture.

Nursing Care of the Woman With Urinary Tract Infection

As with any of the postpartum infections, nursing care is first directed at prevention of a urinary tract infection (UTI) through good basic intrapartum and postpartum care. Once the woman has been identified as having a UTI, nursing care is directed at providing comfort and healing and to teaching measures to prevent recurrence.

Nursing Assessment

Attention to the first voiding after childbirth is essential. This voiding is measured to assess for possible bladder retention. Palpation of the fundus after voiding and inspection for a discernible bladder above the symphysis pubis is performed at each postpartal check. A full bladder of 500 mL or more is visible and palpable as a bulge above the symphysis. The woman who voids frequently, but only 300 mL or less at a time, needs to be evaluated further for urine retention. Symptoms of cystitis, frequency, urgency, dysuria, and suprapubic pain should be assessed each shift as part of each check.

Nursing Interventions

Nursing measures to assist the patient to void are important postpartum interventions. The woman who voids frequent, small amounts is suspected of having urine retention. Catheterization may be necessary to determine residuals and is continued until residuals are less than 60 mL. When catheterizing for residuals, the nurse must perform the catheterization within 5 minutes after the woman has voided for an accurate measurement. The nurse encourages the woman to maintain a fluid intake of at least 1000 mL every 8 hours. The nurse also encourages the woman to ambulate to improve bladder function. Effective patient teaching in regard to perineum care helps to decrease contamination. Once symptoms occur, the nurse must report the symptoms promptly to the physician, obtain a clean-catch urine specimen for culture and sensitivity, and administer the prescribed antibiotics. The nurse instructs the patient concerning the necessity of completing the prescribed antibiotics after discharge, even if the symptoms have disappeared.

Mastitis

Mastitis is a breast infection of the postpartum period largely related to incomplete emptying of the breasts and stasis (pooling) of milk in the ducts of the breast-feeding mother. Milk left in the ducts is easily infected with organisms that gain entrance into the ductwork. The *Staphylococcus aureus* is the most frequently implicated organism. Mastitis usually occurs 2 to 4 weeks after delivery. Local pain, erythema, and heat in the breast are noted by the mother, accompanied by flulike symptoms of fever, chills, malaise, body aches, and headache. It generally affects one side only and is preceded by lumps in the affected breast.

Risk factors for mastitis include sore and cracked nipples (which allow bacteria to enter the ductal sys-

NURSING CARE PLAN
for the Postpartum Woman With Mastitis

ASSESSMENT:

Breast engorgement, painful lumps, redness, warmth
Nipples sore, cracked, bleeding
Fever, malaise, flulike symptoms
Lack of knowledge of breast-feeding techniques
Lack of confidence in ability to successfully breast-feed

NURSING DIAGNOSIS #1: Knowledge Deficit, about breast-feeding techniques

EXPECTED OUTCOME: Mother demonstrates proper breast-feeding techniques

Nursing Interventions	*Rationale*
1. Identify specific areas of knowledge deficit.	1. Nurse individualizes teaching based on identified needs.
2. Discuss techniques of breast and nipple care, feeding, signs and symptoms of mastitis.	2. Nurse provides information to reduce risk factors for mastitis.
3. Provide supportive caring relationship	3. Caring relationship facilitates learning, increases mother's self-esteem, and increases likelihood of compliance with breast-feeding techniques.

EVALUATION: Mother verbalizes and demonstrates techniques of breast-feeding that reduce risk of mastitis.

NURSING DIAGNOSIS #2: Pain, related to infection of breast

EXPECTED OUTCOME: Mother will be pain free, infection free.

Nursing Interventions	*Rationale*
1. Nurse encourages mother to nurse frequently to empty engorged breast. Teach use of breast pump or hand expression of milk if mother is unable to nurse.	1. Frequent nursing (or mechanical expression of milk) empties the breast and promotes healing of mastitis.
2. Administration of analgesics/antipyretic to decrease pain, fever. Use of warm compresses to breast for comfort.	2. Analgesics/antipyretics reduce discomfort, reduce fever.
3. Support and reassurance regarding safety of continued breast-feeding	3. Caring relationship enhances mother's ability to continue breast-feeding.
4. Promotions of careful handwashing before breast-feeding.	4. Handwashing removes transient bacteria that could enter duct work of breast and lead to mastitis.

EVALUATION: Mother indicates that breast-feeding is progressing smoothly, with no complaints of breast tenderness, lumps, or symptoms of mastitis.

tem), poor maternal hygiene, poor positioning of the nipple in the infant's mouth, and excessive or vigorous sucking by the breast-feeding infant. As a result of the sore or cracked nipple, the mother limits nursing time on the breast. This leads to inadequate emptying of the breast. The inhibition of let-down may be caused by maternal discomfort. It too can lead to inadequate emptying of the breast. Milk backs up in the duct, resulting in lumps that can be palpated. Other contributing factors include a decrease in the frequency of breast-feeding related to supplementation with formula, the mother's resumption of outside activities, such as returning to work, and the baby's sleeping through the night (see Fig. 16-4).

Nursing Care of the Woman With Mastitis

Prevention of mastitis includes teaching the woman prenatally to prepare her nipples and breasts for breast-feeding and postpartum teaching in the care of her breasts and proper breast-feeding techniques (see Chapter 18). Because mastitis occurs after the woman has been discharged, the nurse includes complete teaching for the woman in her discharge instructions.

Nursing Assessment

The lactating woman's breasts must be carefully assessed each shift for engorgement, erythema, warmth, and lumps. Bilateral lumpiness is not uncommon in the early postpartal period because engorgement interferes with milk flow. Warmth is also normal with engorgement but is over the entire breast, rather than localized as with mastitis. Nipples are assessed for soreness, pain, or cracks or fissures. Questioning of the mother as to tenderness, which is normal at the beginning of breast-feeding, versus pain that persists throughout the nursing period or is accompanied by bleeding, indicates where especially to look for cracks. In addition, the nurse conducts assessment for the presence of systemic symptoms of mastitis, including fever, chills, malaise, and body aches.

Nursing Interventions

The nurse provides support and patient teaching regarding breast-feeding as the first approach to reduce the incidence of mastitis, especially the importance of handwashing before breast-feeding. When mastitis is mild, warm compresses and frequent feeding on the affected side often are adequate to clear the blockage and any associated infection. The nurse encourages additional rest and fluids and administers analgesics to promote comfort.

Administration of prescribed antibiotics to treat the infection and to prevent abscess formation are nursing interventions for more severe cases. Breast-feeding is rarely discontinued, because emptying of the breast is a primary treatment. The nurse can reassure the woman that she is not exposing her newborn to infection, because the probability is great that the organism initially came from the newborn. The newborn most likely acquired the organism from the woman's skin or from nursery personnel with an upper respiratory infection. The woman needs to be assured of the lack of danger to the baby and the benefit to the woman of continued breast-feeding. This is true even if abscess formation requires drainage. See the accompanying Nursing Care Plan for the woman with mastitis.

◆ Birth Canal Complications

During delivery, there are a number of injuries or complications related to the birth canal that can occur and complicate the postpartum period. Lacerations of the perineum, vagina, cervix, or vulva may involve damage to the rectum or urethra. They also may contribute to the likelihood of early hemorrhage. Even after repair, these lacerations may interfere with normal voiding or defecation. Injury may occur to the levator ani muscle or pelvic joints, resulting in pelvic muscle relaxation, urinary incontinence, uterine prolapse, cystocele, rectocele, or ureteral obstruction leading to hydronephrosis. Fistulas (abnormal connection) between the rectum and vagina or the urinary tract (urethra or bladder) and the vagina may occur as the result of difficult forceps delivery or other trauma during delivery. These fistulas can result in urine or stool being expelled through the vagina.

Nursing Care of the Woman With Birth Canal Complications

The nursing needs of the woman with birth canal complications vary with the particular complication that she has. However, many of the nursing assessments and interventions are the same or similar.

Nursing Assessment

The nurse assesses the woman's labor and birth record for risk factors. These include an abnormally long second stage, fetal malposition, use of forceps or vacuum extractor or other manipulations during delivery, a large infant, an extension of perineotomy through the rectal wall, or the repair of an urethral laceration.

The nurse also assesses the mother's voiding pattern and bowel elimination. Difficulty voiding, incontinence of stool or urine, stress incontinence, or incomplete emptying of the bladder, and dysuria can result from birth canal injuries. Involuntary escape of urine or stool from the vagina is noted with fistulas. The woman who fears disrupting stitches or pain may try to avoid defecation. To prevent this, the nurse assesses the woman's need for and effectiveness of stool softeners such as docusate sodium (Colace), bulk-forming laxatives such as psyllium (Metamucil), or saline-osmotic laxatives such as magnesium hydroxide (milk of magnesia). Mineral oil by mouth also may be ordered by the physician to increase the ease of first bowel movements. However, mineral oil may cause fecal incontinence that is unrelated to the birth canal injury.

The nurse assesses for unusual discomfort or excessive pain of the woman's perineum, vulva, or rectum. She may describe the pain as burning, or a sense of pressure or fullness of the rectum or vagina. The nurse observes for uterine prolapse, which may be visible at the vaginal opening, although it may be detectable only on pelvic examination.

Nursing Interventions

The nurse reports unusual problems such as incontinence, pain, or other symptoms suggestive of birth canal injuries to the physician. The nurse administers medications ordered to prevent constipation and provide pain relief. Sitz baths and local anesthetic medication may also promote healing and increase comfort. The nurse teaches the woman perineal muscle exercise (Kegel), which may improve some pelvic relaxation symptoms.

Usually, rectal treatments such as enemas and suppositories are avoided in the patient with a fourth-degree laceration (through the rectal mucosa) to prevent disruption of the repair. However, if the patient has not had a bowel movement by the third day, the physician may order an oil retention enema or lubricating suppository. The nurse inserts these very gently and carefully to avoid further trauma.

◆ Thrombophlebitis

Thrombophlebitis is the inflammation that occurs in a vein at the site of a blood clot. Blood clots of the veins of the legs or pelvis are a complication whose risk is increased in the postpartum period by immobility, cesarean birth, PIH, and hydramnios. Women who are older than 40 years of age, who are multiparous, or who have preexisting anemia or heart disease also are predisposed to thrombosis. The conditions that lead to formation of thrombi (clots) are venous stasis or diminished flow, injury to the wall of the vein, and clotting factor changes. Clotting factors change in pregnancy because of hormonal changes, and vessels are sometimes injured during birth. However, the change believed to be the strongest contributing factor in the formation of thrombi is the venous stasis that results from the increasing size of the uterus.

Classification of Thrombi and Emboli

Thrombophlebitis is classified by the site of the inflammation. The two types are superficial and deep vein thrombosis (DVT) (Fig. 16-5). The thrombus that moves from the initial site and causes obstruction of circulatory flow is called an embolus. These three types of clots are further discussed next.

Superficial Thrombophlebitis

A clot may occur superficially in a vein of the legs, accompanied by inflammation. This type of clot is firmly attached to the vein and is not so likely to break off and

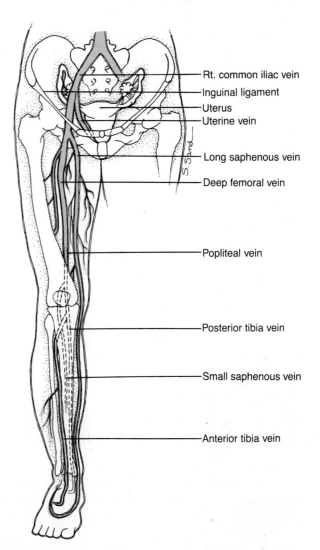

Figure 16-5. *Sites of postpartum thrombophlebitis. Pelvic thrombophlebitis involves the uterine and ovarian veins. Femoral thrombophlebitis involves the femoral, popliteal, and long saphenous veins. When the small saphenous vein is involved, the term is* phlebothrombosis, *because the thrombus is caused more by stasis than infection, although deep calf thrombi do become infected.*

travel. Superficial clots occur most often on the third to fourth day postpartum. Symptoms include a reddened, warm, swollen area over the clot. The vein is palpable and very tender. These superficial clots are termed thrombophlebitis and usually do not require anticoagulation therapy.

Deep Vein Thrombosis

DVT occurs in the larger veins of the central venous system, often without inflammation (phlebothrombosis). The clot is much more likely to break off and travel to the lungs, a potentially fatal complication. The presence of a pulmonary embolus may be the first sign of DVT. It occurs as a result of a venous clot breaking loose and traveling to the lungs, where it obstructs blood flow any further in the lung. DVT can occur in the deep veins of the legs or in the pelvis. Symptoms depend on the location, but generally include complaints of pain in the involved area. Low-grade fever or chills are often noted as well as swelling and paleness of the affected leg. Homans' sign (calf pain elicited on dorsiflexion of the foot; see Chapter 8) is a positive sign for DVT, but the absence of Homans' sign does not rule out thrombosis. Diagnosis of DVT may be made by Doppler ultrasonography, venograms, or computed tomography (CT) scans.

DVT is a serious complication that requires treatment with anticoagulants, bed rest, analgesia, and observant nursing care. Early recognition and treatment can reduce the incidence of emboli. It takes approximately 4 to 6 weeks for thrombophlebitis to resolve.

Embolism

The greatest concern when a DVT occurs is the very serious danger that it may break loose and travel through the right atrium and ventricle of the heart into the pulmonary circulatory system. Pulmonary embolism is a life-threatening condition that requires immediate intervention. Nursing care is geared toward eliminating this danger.

Nursing Care of the Postpartum Woman With a Thrombus

Nursing care for the woman with a thrombus varies somewhat with the location of the thrombus. A superficial thrombophlebitis is not as threatening as a DVT or an embolus. However, the woman with a superficial vein thrombophlebitis needs conscientious nursing care.

Nursing Assessment

Nursing assessment begins with identification of women at risk for thromboembolic disease included in Display 16-4. The nurse identifies the woman's knowledge deficit related to prevention of clots. The nurse also identifies early symptoms and reports promptly any foot, leg, groin, or pelvic pain, erythema, local warmth, swelling, low-grade fever or chills, pallor of one leg, and a positive Homans' sign. The nurse takes a measurement of calf and thigh circumference daily to detect swelling. The woman's bleeding tendencies are assessed, including the amount and type of lochia, especially if anticoagulation is instituted. In addition, the nurse must recognize and promptly report symptoms of

---

DISPLAY 16-4
Risk Factors for Thromboembolic Disease

- History of thrombophlebitis or thrombosis
- Venous stasis: prolonged bedrest, sitting, standing, inactivity
- Women older than 40 years of age, high parity, smokers
- Improperly positioned stirrups, prolonged labor
- Varicosities, trauma to legs
- Obesity
- Postpartum pelvic infection
- Anesthesia and surgery
- Use of estrogen to suppress lactation
- Hypothermia
- Hemorrhage, anemia

---

pulmonary emboli including syncope, arrest, sharp stabbing chest pain, dyspnea, hypotension, tachycardia, diaphoresis, pallor, cyanosis, hemoptysis, and anxiety. The size of the clot and the amount of occlusion that results determine the symptoms and outcome. A small clot may go almost unnoted except for low-grade fever, tachycardia, and chest tightness.

Nursing Interventions

Nursing interventions are aimed at the prevention or early detection of thromboembolic disorders, to prevent the more serious result of pulmonary embolus. Toward this end, recognition of women at risk, and measures to *prevent* clot formation, are instituted. Nursing interventions to prevent clot formation include avoiding prolonged use of stirrups during childbirth, using padding and proper positioning of legs in stirrups to prevent obstruction of circulation, avoiding use of the knee gatch on the bed, teaching the woman to avoid prolonged sitting or standing, and to avoid crossing her legs. The nurse also promotes venous circulation by encouraging early ambulation, leg exercises for the surgical delivery patient, use of support stockings, and adequate fluid intake. The nurse carefully assesses the mother's calves, tests for Homans' sign, and checks for pain in her foot, leg, groin, or pelvis.

If a diagnosis of thrombophlebitis or phlebothrombosis is made, nursing interventions include maintenance of bed rest with legs elevated, support stockings, and application of moist heat to promote venous return and circulation. The nurse also exercises gentle handling of the leg and avoids massage or rubbing to prevent dislodgement of the clot. The nurse administers medications for analgesia and anticoagulation. Anticoagulants may not be ordered for superficial thrombophlebitis. Antibiotics may be indicated with septic thrombophlebitis.

If a diagnosis of pulmonary embolism is made, these additional interventions are indicated, and the woman may be transferred to an intensive care unit. The woman's vital signs and level of consciousness are monitored every 5 to 15 minutes. Cardiopulmonary resuscitation may be necessary. The woman is positioned in high Fowler's to facilitate breathing. The nurse gives the woman and her family simple explanations in a calm, reassuring manner. Oxygen is administered as ordered by the physician. The nurse also assists with insertion of an IV line, electrocardiogram, chest x-rays, arterial blood gas determination, and other blood work. Medications are administered as ordered. These include analgesics such as morphine or meperidine (Demerol) IV for pain relief and to decrease anxiety; heparin IV, and drugs (sodium bicarbonate) to correct pH or electrolyte imbalance. The nurse may assist in preparing the woman for possible fibrolytic therapy (administration of drug to dissolve clot) or embolectomy (surgical removal of clot).

Continuing Prenatal Complications

Some conditions that were diagnosed and treated during the prenatal period continue to present risks during the postpartum period. Two of these common conditions are PIH and diabetes.

Pregnancy-Induced Hypertension (PIH)

Women with PIH are at greater risk for several complications including hemorrhage, DIC, and if a cesarean birth was performed, infection and thromboembolic disease. Additionally, they require continued assessment of blood pressure, reflexes and muscle tone, proteinuria and urine output, and neurologic status. The likelihood of convulsions decreases quickly after delivery, but convulsions may occur up to 48 hours after delivery. Continued provision of a quiet, nonstimulating room, emergency supplies at hand, and maintenance of IV fluids and medication administration are important aspects of the care of this patient (see Chapter 8).

Diabetes

The diabetic woman also has special needs. She often will have delivered by cesarean birth and is more likely to have experienced perinatal loss, anomaly, or prematurity related to complications of diabetes (see Chapter 8). She is at greater risk for wound infection. Her need for insulin must be assessed frequently by blood glucose determination and adjustments made as her body returns to its prepregnant state. Other topics that must be addressed during the postpartum period include family planning and use of barrier methods of birth control if future pregnancies are planned. Safety of oral contraceptives for diabetics is controversial. The nurse also may discuss permanent sterilization options.

Psychosocial Complications

There is a wide variety of mood changes seen in the postpartum period, from the exhilaration after delivery to severe and incapacitating depression or psychosis. Most women (50%–75%), especially first-time mothers, experience a transitory depression approximately 3 to 4 days postpartum. This is most likely related to several factors, including hormonal changes, fatigue, pain, and recognition of lifestyle changes and responsibilities. Symptoms reported by the mother include a feeling of sadness, crying easily and often for no reason, poor concentration, and feelings of anger or irritability toward their husband or partner. These are often referred to as "baby blues," and they resolve without treatment in a day or two.

Classification of Postpartum Psychosocial Conditions

In addition to the postpartum blues that most postpartum women experience, two additional levels of affective disorders are identified. These additional levels are postpartum depression and postpartum psychosis. A brief discussion of each follows.

Depression

Depression may begin as early as the first day postpartum, although it may not appear until 2 to 3 months later and may last as long as a year. It is characterized by a deep persistent sadness, lack of energy, sleep disturbance, loss of appetite, feelings of worthlessness, hypochondriasis (exaggeration of normal physical symptoms), guilt, and anxiety. Infant neglect or abuse can occur, and suicide is a potential threat. Because the onset of postpartum depression is insidious (gradual and subtle), it is often overlooked by health care providers.

Psychosis

Postpartum psychosis usually occurs 2 to 4 weeks after birth and is characterized by loss of contact with reality, hallucinations, delusions, and disorientation. There may be swings between severe depression and mania. The risk of harm to the baby or to the mother is great. Both postpartum depression and psychosis are related to previous history or family history of depression, psychosis, or mood disorders. It is also associated with prenatal stressors such as lack of social support, financial concerns, low socioeconomic status, and low self-esteem. Additional risk factors include ambivalence regarding pregnancy; substance abuse; previous sexual or physical abuse; and primigravida.

Nursing Care of the Woman With a Postpartum Psychosocial Condition

Early identification is essential in the nursing care of the woman with a postpartum psychosocial condition. Because comments by the woman may be misinterpreted, confusion exists in the diagnosis of these conditions. The nurse must be sensitive to the woman's expressions of anxiety, guilt, and other indications of the woman's mood. However, the nurse must be cautious to not overstate the woman's symptoms. An accurate assessment is important.

Nursing Assessment

Risk factors for postpartum depression or psychosis can be identified during the prenatal period. These include ambivalence about continuing the pregnancy, previous history of postpartum mood disorders or bipolar disorder, lack of social support systems, especially lack of supportive partner or parents.

Except for the transient "baby blues," these disorders usually present no symptoms in the hospital setting; thus, assessment of mood disorders occurs in return visit settings or in home visits by public health nurses. Questioning by the nurse in these settings can elicit the woman's feelings of worthlessness, depression, or loss of contact with reality. Assessing the risk of harm either to the baby or the woman is a dominant concern.

Nursing Interventions

Teaching the mother and family members about the symptoms and likelihood of "baby blues" can do a great deal to decrease its impact when it does occur. Counseling should include the identification of symptoms that should be reported to the physician. Referral for a home visit or telephone follow-up at 2 to 3 weeks postpartum may be suggested.

Medical interventions may include medication, psychotherapy, and hospitalization. Electroconvulsive therapy also may be used. Maintaining healthy mother—

infant interaction is a primary goal. The nurse must remember that the woman with postpartum psychosis is at serious risk for committing suicide or infanticide. Identifying family members or neighbors who can assist, referral to community agencies such as the Department of Social Services, or day-care centers that accept infants may be necessary. Family support groups, crisis centers and hotlines, as well as community health centers also may offer assistance to the woman and her family members. The woman who has one episode of postpartum psychosis is highly susceptible to repeat episodes in future pregnancies.

◆ Grieving

The death of a newborn is a complication for which parents as well as staff are usually unprepared. Despite the efforts of the health care team and the parents, failure to produce a healthy baby is often viewed as a personal failure. Along with grief and its predictable stages, there is a sense of having failed to do what other women have done successfully. That sense of failure may be expressed as guilt, anger, inadequacy, helplessness, or anxiety.

Similarly, the loss of the "perfect child" when a child is born with congenital anomalies will result in much the same process of grieving, although the process is never resolved because the child is an ever-present reminder to the parents of the loss of their dream. This process of grieving is also seen in the mother who is giving up her child for adoption.

Stages of the grieving process are identified as shock, denial and disbelief, anger, sadness and guilt, and reorganization and resolution. These are essentially the stages identified in 1969 by Kubler-Ross in *On Death and Dying*. The woman and her family do not move from one stage to another, but rather, will be in one stage, move to another, and then may lapse back to an earlier stage. Finally, they reach the stage of reorganization and resolution when they are able to accept the loss and go on with their lives. This may take many months or even years. In reviewing the stages of grief, the nurse must remember that any person can move to the next stage, then backslide to a previous stage for a period. The grief process is not a smooth transition but has many ups and downs.

Nursing Assessment

Identifying the stage of grief is a primary assessment to permit the nurse to provide the interventions most appropriate for that stage. Active listening, with use of therapeutic communication techniques, encourages the parents to verbalize their feelings. This provides the nurse with direction for future interactions. Assessment of coping skills the family has used in the past, as well as identification of support systems available to the grieving person, are important. Cultural or spiritual aspects that offer solace or direction are also important to identify. The nurse needs to determine if the family wishes to have the baby baptized or if they wish to have clergy notified. When a child born with special needs survives, the nurse must assess parental knowledge of the condition and identify the skills the woman or a family member needs to learn to care for the infant.

Nursing Interventions

Healthy adjustment to the death or anomaly of an infant and maintenance of healthy family relationships are goals of nursing care of a grieving family. See Chapter 20 for a full discussion of nursing interventions.

Cesarean Birth Considerations

The woman who has had a cesarean birth has a longer hospital stay. She may have more opportunity to absorb the teaching available. However, she has additional concerns. The woman and her partner may feel cheated by having missed the vaginal birth experience, particularly if the cesarean birth was unexpected. In addition, the woman may have a long blank period that she cannot recall. She may have difficulty remembering the first time she saw her newborn. These factors can be upsetting to the woman. The nurse can help her verbalize and explore these concerns. The postpartum healing process for the woman who has undergone a cesarean birth may be longer than that for the woman who has had a vaginal birth.

The condition of the neonate also has an impact on the emotional state of the family. If the neonate is in good health, the family may accept the cesarean birth with little disappointment, but if the neonate is in precarious health, the family's main focus will be on the condition of the baby. When the infant's health is in question, the family may have very few emotional resources available to work through their feelings about the birth.

Addicted Mothers

Women who are addicted to alcohol, mood-altering drugs, or cigarettes may present problems in the post-partum period related to their drug dependency. The identification and treatment of the substance-abusing woman in the prenatal period is desirable, but often the problems of addiction are still present after delivery. Additionally, many addicted pregnant women do not seek prenatal care or receive sporadic or late third-trimester care only. Withdrawal symptoms during labor, childbirth, or during the postpartum period may appear if labor is long or the woman is unable to secure the drug after childbirth. The woman's increasing agitation, restlessness, irritability, tremors, increased pulse and blood pressure, and hallucinations may signal alcohol withdrawal symptoms. Medical treatment with tranquilizers or sedatives to prevent convulsions is performed. Close assessment of the woman's vital signs and mental status is necessary because death can result from alcohol withdrawal. Addiction to other drugs such as tranquilizers or barbiturates can also cause serious symptoms similar to alcohol withdrawal, including seizures. Women who are addicted to heroin, crack cocaine, hallucinogens, and amphetamines likely seek the drug soon after delivery to prevent withdrawal symptoms. These women are very prone to simply disappearing. Cigarette smokers often sneak a smoke against hospital rules and may endanger themselves or others, as well as exposing their infants to secondhand smoke.

The nurse's early identification and reporting of the patient exhibiting addictive behaviors or withdrawal symptoms is essential. The woman should be referred to an appropriate smoking cessation program, drug or alcohol detoxification unit, or rehabilitation center. The nurse must provide nonjudgmental care to the woman. Blame and condemnation of the woman for her actions are inappropriate nursing responses. The addicted woman needs support of a multidisciplinary team that is skilled in treating substance abusing women.

Adolescent Considerations

Poor prenatal care, which is common in the adolescent, can contribute to postpartum complications. Adolescents are at greater risk for PIH, which continues as a postpartum problem. In addition, adolescents may have indulged in substance abuse, which adds to postpartum complications. An adolescent who is a smoker is at increased risk for thromboembolic disease.

There is a need for careful assessment of how well the teenage mother is able to assume the parenting role, especially if she has a postpartum complication that affects her feelings of well-being. This is particularly true with the younger teen, who may be quite egocentric and unable to assume responsibility for meeting the newborn's needs before her own. The adolescent mother may need more attention from the nurse before she is able to care for the newborn's needs. Use of videos or one-on-one, "hands-on" practice rather than "classroom" lecture-demonstrations may be more appealing to the teenage mother. Identification of the teenage mother's support system is also important. The baby's father, if present, may need special support and teaching if he is also a teenager learning to care for an infant.

Cultural Considerations

Cultural differences in expectations and behaviors during the postpartum period may be noted. The patient's family configuration varies in different cultures. In some cultures, the "family" includes an extended array of relatives who are available and willing to assist with child care or household duties if complications affect the mother's ability to care for her infant. Cultural influence on behaviors during a crisis also may be seen in a variety of responses to the situation, from dispassionate acceptance to loud wailing or angry confrontation. Practices regarding bathing, nutrition, and activity restrictions can be in conflict with medical or nursing practice. Identification and incorporation of these practices into the nursing care plan when possible will improve the nurse–patient relationship.

Religious beliefs prohibiting blood transfusions for Jehovah Witnesses complicate the treatment of such a woman who hemorrhages. Religious beliefs relating to diet or belief in spiritual healing, to the exclusion of some medical or nursing interventions, also may create difficulties when a woman experiences complications. Conversely, religious faith may facilitate the recovery of the woman. The nurse needs to be aware of and respect the specific beliefs and customs of each woman.

The Role of the Nurse

The nurse must identify risk factors that increase the likelihood of postpartum complications to take measures to prevent or decrease their severity. The Nursing Diagnoses Checklist presents selected nursing diagnoses for the woman with a postpartum complication. In addition to carrying out the specific nursing interventions for the complication, the nurse must present a calm, assured manner of competence and confidence to provide support to the woman. Therapeutic communication that recognizes her fear and anxiety and gives her an opportunity to express her feelings are essential. Simple explanations are needed to keep the woman and her family informed. It is also important for the nurse to give the woman an opportunity to ventilate her feelings of anxiety or fear relating to the experience she has had. Both the woman and her family need to deal with their perceptions of the experience.

Promoting mother–infant interaction is essential. The nurse assists the woman to feed and care for her infant, as permitted by woman's condition. This is a very upsetting time for the mother. The nurse must provide sensitive care, enabling the mother to have contact with her neonate as much as possible. If the woman is not able to care for her newborn, the nurse supports other family members to feed and care for infant.

The nurse provides discharge instructions, which include a list of symptoms to watch for and what to do for them as well as when to contact the doctor or nurse. As in all teaching, the nurse must be certain that the woman understands the teaching and is able to read and recall the instructions.

✔ NURSING DIAGNOSES CHECKLIST

The Complicated Postpartal Period

Activity intolerance, related to anemia

· Impaired Adjustment, related to social or psychological factors

· Alteration in Comfort related to infection, other complications

· Anxiety, related to complication (specify)

· Ineffective or Interrupted, Breastfeeding, related to pain of breast infection

· Altered Family Processes, related to postpartum complication of the woman

· Fluid Volume Deficit, related to hemorrhage

· Anticipatory or dysfunctional Grieving, related to death or anomaly of newborn

· Risk for Injury, related to uterine atony

· Knowledge Deficit, related to complication, medications, or self-care

· Pain, related to birth canal injury

· Altered Parenting, or Risk for Altered Parenting, related to interruption by woman's physical condition

· Altered Tissue Perfusion (specify), related to hypovolemia

SELF-ASSESSMENT

1. Which of the following findings would be *least* helpful in the early diagnosis of shock caused by a postpartum hemorrhage?

- ○ **A.** Vital signs
- ○ **B.** Skin temperature
- ○ **C.** Urine output
- ○ **D.** Level of consciousness

2. A woman with endometritis is likely to exhibit all of the following signs and symptoms EXCEPT:

- ○ **A.** Foul-smelling lochia
- ○ **B.** Fever
- ○ **C.** Uterine tenderness
- ⊗ **D.** Dysuria

3. Methergine may be ordered following delivery to prevent:

- ○ **A.** Endometritis
- ○ **B.** Postpartum hemorrhage
- ○ **C.** DIC
- ○ **D.** Hematoma formation

4. Management of mastitis may include all of the following EXCEPT:

- ○ **A.** The use of antibiotics
- ○ **B.** Administration of analgesics
- ○ **C.** Continuation of breast-feeding
- ⊗ **D.** Application of cold compress

5. Which of the following medications is inappropriate for a patient with a fourth-degree laceration?

- ○ **A.** Milk of magnesia
- ○ **B.** Colace
- ○ **C.** Fleet's enema
- ○ **D.** Mineral oil

REVIEW AND PREVIEW

This chapter presented complications that can occur during the postpartum period. All of the complications interrupt the normal progression of postpartum healing to some extent. In some cases, the complications are serious enough to be life threatening. Hemorrhage, puerperal infections, mastitis, and thromboembolic conditions were presented. PIH and diabetes were discussed as they relate to the postpartum period. Psychosocial conditions ranging from the common postpartum blues to true postpartum psychosis were discussed. Grieving was discussed, both for the infant who died and for the "perfect" infant who was expected. The special problems of adolescent and addicted mothers were explored. In addition, diverse cultural and religious influences were presented. Preventive measures were discussed throughout the chapter.

The next chapter discusses the transition of the neonate from intrauterine to extrauterine life. The neonate has lived a protected life for 9 months and must go through enormous changes to adjust to life in the outside world. These physiologic changes are covered in the following chapter. Each of the body systems are presented with the adaptations that must be made for a successful adjustment to extrauterine life. These presentations lay the foundation for the further study of the neonate and its needs after birth.

◉ KEY POINTS

◆ Early postpartum hemorrhage occurs within the first 24 hours after childbirth. Late postpartum hemorrhage occurs anytime after the first 24 hours until 6 weeks after childbirth.

◆ Nursing interventions appropriate when caring for the woman with postpartum hemorrhage include assessing blood loss, assessing and massaging the fundus, monitoring vital signs, level of consciousness, and urine output, assisting in preparing for surgical interventions, and providing support to the woman and her family.

◆ DIC is a result of decreased platelets and clotting factors as a reaction to clotting in the small vessels. This results from increased formation of thrombin. The excess thrombin causes an overreaction of anticlotting mechanisms and the clots are broken down. Hemorrhage occurs from bleeding sites and major organs are assaulted by clots causing vascular occlusion.

◆ Five common sites for puerperal infection are the uterus, vagina, cervix, perineum, and incisions.

◆ Prevention of puerperal infections is extremely important. Handwashing is the foremost measure to prevent infection. All procedures must be carried out with aseptic technique to prevent puerperal infections.

◆ The nurse assesses the woman's knowledge about the importance of handwashing, care of the breasts and nipples, and proper breast-feeding techniques.

◆ Early symptoms of thrombophlebitis include pain in the foot, leg, groin, or pelvis. Erythema, local warmth or swelling in the calf, low-grade fever or chills, pallor in one leg, or a positive Homans' sign are additional symptoms that are indicative of DVT.

◆ DVT presents the greatest danger for a clot breaking loose and becoming a pulmonary embolism.

◆ Postpartum blues occurs within the first 3 to 4 days postpartum and resolves within a day or 2 with no treatment. Postpartum depression may be first seen on the first day postpartum, but may not be evident until 2 to 3 months later. It may last as long as a year. There is deep sadness, lack of energy, sleep disturbance, loss of appetite, worthless feelings, exaggerating of physical symptoms, guilt, and anxiety. In postpartum psychosis, the symptoms occur within 2 to 4 weeks after childbirth. The woman loses touch with reality, has delusions, and is disoriented.

◆ The nurse must know and understand the stages of grief to assist the grieving family. Active listening and therapeutic communication are essential. Assessing the family's coping skills and support systems is also necessary. Cultural and religious beliefs are important to consider. The woman and her family may benefit from referral to community resources for either reproductive loss or caring for the infant with a congenital anomaly.

BIBLIOGRAPHY

Bastin, N., Tamayo, O. W., Tinkle, M. B., Amaya, M. A., Trejo, L. R., & Herrera, C. (1992). HIV Disease and pregnancy: Part 3. Postpartum care of the HIV-positive woman and her newborn. *Journal of Obstetric, Gynecologic, and Neonatal Nursing, 21*(2), 105–113.

Beck, C. T., Reynolds, M. A., & Rutowski, P. (1992). Maternity blues and postpartum depression. *Journal of Obstetric, Gynecologic, and Neonatal Nursing, 21*(4), 287–293.

Combs, C. A., Murphy, E. L., & Laros, R. K. Jr. (1991). Factors associated with postpartum hemorrhage with vaginal birth. *Obstetrics and Gynecology, 77*(1): 69–78.

Cronin, W. A., Quanash, M. G., & Larson, E. (1993). Obstetric infection control in developing countries. *Journal of Obstetric, Gynecologic, and Neonatal Nursing, 22*(2), 137–144.

Dunn, P. A., York, R., Cheek, T. C., & Yeboah, K. (1994). Maternal hypothermia: Implications for obstetric nurses. *Journal of Obstetric, Gynecologic, and Neonatal Nursing, 23*(3), 238–242.

Freda, M. C., Andersen, H. F., Damus, K., & Merkatz, I. R. (1993). Skin changes and pain in the nipple during the 1st week of lactation. *Journal of Obstetric, Gynecologic, and Neonatal Nursing, 22*(3), 237–243.

Fritz, P., Galanter, M., Lifshutz, H., & Egelko, S. (1993). Developmental risk factors in postpartum women with urine tests positive for cocaine. *American Journal of Drug and Alcohol Abuse, 19*(2), 187–211.

Grevatt, H. (1992). The baby blues club. *Nursing Times, 88*(39), 46–52.

Hudson, P. (1992). Preventing postnatal illness. *Nursing Times, 88*(43), 68–72.

Knops, G. G. (1993). Postpartum mood disorders: A startling contrast to the joy of birth. *Postgraduate Medicine, 93*(3): 103–107.

May, K. A., & Mahlmeister, L. R. (1994), *Maternal and neonatal care: Family-centered care*. Philadelphia: J. B. Lippincott.

Primeau, M. R., & Recht, C. K. (1994). Professional bereavement photographs: One aspect of a perinatal bereavement program. *Journal of Obstetric, Gynecologic, and Neonatal Nursing, 23*(1), 22–25.

Pillitteri, A. (1992). *Maternal and child nursing*. Philadelphia: J. B. Lippincott.

Reeder, S. J., Martin, L. L., & Koniak, D. (1992). *Maternity nursing* (17th ed.). Philadelphia: J. B. Lippincott.

Sullivan, J., Boudreaux, M., & Keller, P. (1993). Can we help the substance abusing mother and infant? *Journal of Maternal Child Nursing, 18*(3), 153–157.

Wolman, W.-L., Chalmers, B., Hofmeyr, G. J., & Nikodem, V. C. (1993). Postpartum depression and companionship in the clinical birth environment: A randomized, controlled study. *American Journal of Obstetrics and Gynecology, 168*(5), 1388–1396.

Family-Centered Care of the Newborn

CHAPTER 17

The Newborn's Transition to Extrauterine Life

◉ OBJECTIVES

When the learning goals of this chapter are met, the reader will be able to:

◆ List the factors that contribute to the onset of extrauterine respirations.

◆ Identify the major physiologic adaptations taking place in the respiratory system during the neonate's transition to extrauterine life.

◆ Describe the major physiologic adaptations of the cardiovascular system, including the closure of the fetal cardiovascular pathways.

◆ List the reasons why the newborn may develop jaundice after birth.

◆ Define neutral thermal environment.

◆ Identify the methods the newborn uses to produce heat.

◆ Define the four mechanisms that cause the newborn to lose heat.

◆ Discuss the nurse's role in preventing heat loss in the newborn.

◆ Explain the effects of cold stress on the newborn.

◆ Discuss the periods of reactivity that occur during the transitional period.

TERMINOLOGY

Atelectasis	Systemic vascular resistance
Cephalocaudal	Thermogenesis
Functional residual capacity	Thermoregulation
Immunoglobulin	Transition
Neutral thermal environment	Viscosity
Pulmonary vascular resistance	

The change from intrauterine to extrauterine life is a period of hazardous instability during which all of the body systems of the neonate undergo many adjustments. (The terms *neonate* and *newborn* are used interchangeably in this discussion.) The greatest challenge that the neonate faces occurs during the **transition** period. This period is usually defined as the first 6 to 8 hours of life.

The initial breath taken by the neonate at birth is an event that marks the newborn's ability to exist independently. The newborn's ability to adjust to the new environment requires a variety of mechanisms working together. Successful transition to extrauterine life is accomplished as the newborn's body systems adjust to the new requirements. The newborn begins to exhibit interest in the surrounding world and is capable of interaction within hours of birth.

The nurse usually is the health care professional responsible for performing the first physical assessment and monitoring the newborn's adjustment to extrauterine life. A thorough knowledge base of how each of the body systems normally adapts enables the nurse to anticipate and identify situations that require immediate evaluation by the medical team.

Body System Adaptations

On emerging into this strange new world, the neonate's body systems must make many adjustments to function as expected. In utero, few of the fetus' systems were functioning as they need to after birth. Each system is discussed here with the adaptations that are necessary for adequate postpartum functioning.

Respiratory System

Breathing movements, which occur as early as 11 weeks' gestation, help prepare the fetal lungs for extrauterine respiration. Fetal lungs are filled with amniotic fluid, rather than air. As a result, these movements simply move the amniotic fluid in and out of the lungs. There is no threat to the condition of the fetus.

There are numerous stimuli during the intrapartum period that trigger respiration in the newborn. These stimuli can be divided into four categories: chemical, sensory, thermal, and mechanical. Each of the factors are necessary to the successful initiation of neonatal breathing. These factors are illustrated in Figure 17-1, along with their relationship to the onset of extrauterine respiration.

Chemical Stimuli

The newborn experiences a temporary asphyxia when the umbilical cord is clamped and placental blood flow stops. Decreased arterial oxygen tension (PaO_2), an increased arterial carbon dioxide tension ($PaCO_2$), and a decreased arterial pH occur. A transient mild acidosis results, which activates the respiratory center in the medulla. Brief periods of asphyxia stimulate the central nervous system. However, prolonged asphyxia acts as a depressant.

Sensory Stimuli

The newborn emerges from warm, quiet, dark security into a cooler atmosphere with bright lights, loud noises, and other sensory stimuli such as movement, touch, and odors. These sensory stimuli are thought to contribute to the initiation of respirations.

Thermal Stimuli

At birth, the newborn is taken from a warm, wet environment and thrust into a much cooler one. This causes an immediate decrease in body temperature as amniotic fluid evaporates from the newborn's body. Thermal receptors located on the newborn's face and chest sense these changes and relay impulses to the medulla, where the respiratory center resides. The medulla prompts the initiation of the first respiration.

Mechanical Stimuli

During vaginal birth, approximately one-third of the lung fluid is squeezed out of the alveoli and airways through the neonate's mouth and nose. The alveoli are the small air sacs, surrounded by capillaries through which gas exchange takes place in the lungs. After the chest is delivered, it recoils by passive motion. This results in a small, passive inspiration of air into partially cleared airways. Newborns born by cesarean do not experience the benefits of the "vaginal squeeze." Therefore, they may experience some respiratory difficulties, such as transient tachypnea, related to retained fetal lung fluid.

Because of the high **pulmonary vascular resistance** (the opposition to blood flow in the blood vessels of the lungs), the lungs receive very little blood supply in utero. When the first breath is taken, the pulmonary vascular resistance decreases because of the effects of oxygen and carbon dioxide on the blood vessels. The blood flow to the pulmonary vascular bed is markedly increased as the pulmonary vascular resistance decreases.

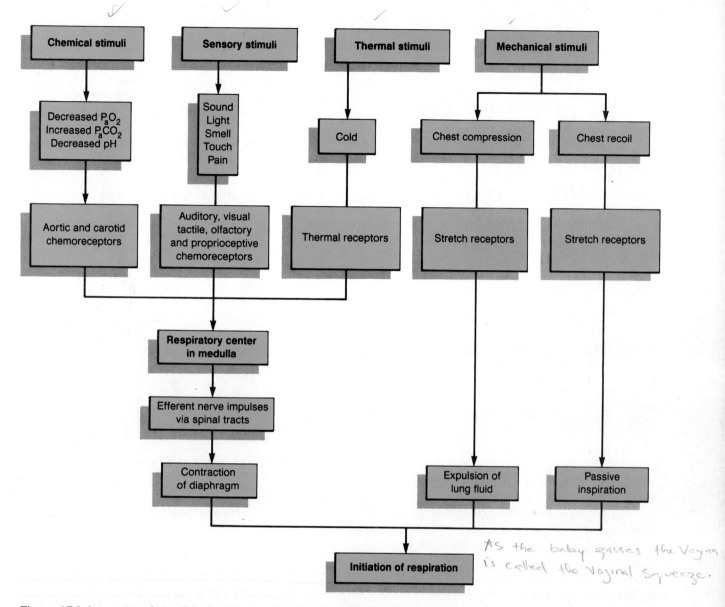

Figure 17-1. Interaction of stimuli in the initiation of neonatal respiration.

Fluid is moved out of the alveoli because of pressure during the "vaginal squeeze." The fluid is moved into the interstitium, where it is absorbed by the lymphatic system. Lung aeration is complete when the alveolar fluid is replaced with an equal volume of air. With the first breath, functional residual capacity (FRC) is begun. Within 24 hours, stable respiratory function is usually complete. **FRC** is that small amount of air that remains in the alveoli and allows them to stay partially open during expiration. The maintenance of a FRC decreases the need for higher pressures during subsequent breaths, making each succeeding breath easier.

Another essential ingredient necessary for successful respiratory adaptation is the presence of surfactant

in the alveoli. **Surfactant** is a phospholipid produced by type II pneumocytes. Surfactant can be compared to soap bubbles. Both help reduce surface tension. Surfactant prevents the sides of the alveoli from sticking together on exhalation, thus decreasing the tendency toward **atelectasis** (failure of the alveoli to expand adequately) and promoting capillary circulation by increasing alveolar size.

There are several factors that oppose the first respirations. These factors include: alveolar surface tension, poor lung compliance, and viscosity of lung fluids. Alveolar surface tension is a force that results in a constant tendency for the alveoli to collapse. As previously discussed, the establishment and maintenance of FRC and surfactant help prevent alveolar collapse. Lung compliance is the lung's ability to fill itself with air easily. If compliance is poor, the lung tissue has difficulty filling with air. Surfactant helps to increase the lung's compliance. **Viscosity** is the property of fluids that affects the way they flow. Fluids with high viscosity are thought of as sticky fluids and flow slowly; fluids with low viscosity are thought of as slippery fluids and flow more rapidly. The high viscosity of lung fluids creates a resistance to the flow of fluids through the lung passages.

The newborn must be able to maintain adequate respirations after the first breath is taken and cardiopulmonary adaptation is begun. The central nervous system must assume the responsibility of respiratory activity. Chemoreceptors in the central nervous system are sensitive to changes in oxygenation. This results in the initiation of a breath.

Circulatory System

The circulatory system undergoes dramatic changes during the transition from intrauterine to extrauterine life (see Chapter 9, refer to Figure 9-6 to review normal fetal circulation). The major changes that occur involve closure of the fetal cardiovascular pathways. The newborn's circulatory system must adapt to the ending of placental function and support. Other factors that play a part in the changes occurring in the circulatory system are the increase in pulmonary blood flow and the beginning of extrauterine respirations.

As previously discussed, pulmonary vascular resistance is very high in utero. Therefore, only a small amount of blood initially circulates in the lung tissue. **Systemic vascular resistance**, the opposition to blood flow in the vessels of the body, is initially low at birth. It increases when the umbilical cord is clamped and the first breath is taken. Because of the effects of oxygen and carbon dioxide on the blood vessels, there is a decrease in pulmonary vascular resistance with the first breath and resulting lung expansion. Blood flow to the pulmonary vascular bed markedly increases as pulmonary vascular resistance falls.

For the fetal circulatory system to successfully adapt to postpartum life, closure of the three fetal cardiovascular pathways—the foramen ovale, ductus arteriosus, and ductus venosus—must occur (Fig. 17-2). Functional closure occurs when blood flow through the structure ceases because of pressure changes. When the structure is obliterated by tissue growth or constriction, anatomic closure results. Functional closure occurs first; therefore, the pathways may open and close intermittently before anatomic closure occurs. Intermittent opening and closing may result in a functional murmur. However, these murmurs do not compromise the newborn clinically; therefore, they are not considered significant.

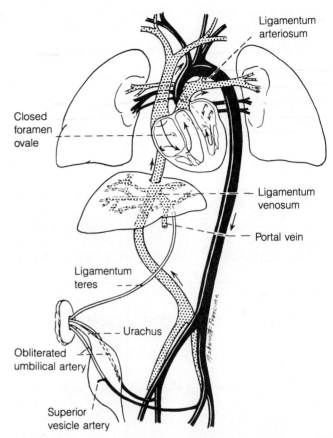

Figure 17-2. *Fetal circulatory accommodations are closed. Indicated are the closed foramen ovale, the ligamentum arteriosus (closed ductus arteriosus), ligamentum venosum (closed ductus venosum), the ligamentum teres (closed umbilical vein), and the obliterated umbilical arteries.*

The foramen ovale is the communication between the right and left atria. The pressure on the right atrium is higher than on the left during fetal life. At birth, when the umbilical cord is clamped and the neonate takes that first breath, pressure changes and becomes greater in the left atrium. The foramen ovale functionally closes when the left atrial pressure is greater than the pressure in the right atrium. Initiation of functional closure normally occurs within several hours after birth. Functional closure is reversible within the first few days of life. The anatomic closure of the foramen ovale takes several months.

The ductus arteriosus, the bypass through which fetal blood flowed from the pulmonary artery into the aorta, usually closes 15 to 24 hours after birth. With the onset of respirations, the arterial oxygen content is increased, and closure of the ductus arteriosus occurs. Anatomic closure occurs by 3 to 4 weeks of age. Continued patency of this fetal pathway can occur if hypoxemia is present. This may result in a flow of blood low in oxygen into the aorta to the general arterial circulation. Failure of the ductus arteriosus to close is termed patent ductus arteriosus and is discussed in Chapter 20.

The ductus venosus functionally closes when the umbilical cord is clamped. This pathway, which by-passed the fetal liver, is no longer necessary as the liver begins to function after birth. The ductus venosus ana-tomically closes in approximately 1 to 2 weeks when it changes into a ligament.

Nervous System

As the fetus reaches term, most of the brain's neurons have been formed and have migrated to their intended destinations. At the time of birth, some cerebellar neu-rons are just completing this process. These neurons are at particular risk for damage related to neonatal as-phyxia and hypoxia.

The normal neonate's cry is lusty and vigorous. Neonates who have weak or high-pitched cries should be evaluated because such cries may result from cen-tral nervous system disorders.

The full-term newborn should exhibit fairly strong muscle tone. Poor muscle tone is abnormal and should be evaluated. The newborn's neurological growth is in a **cephalocaudal** (head-to-toe) and proximal-to-distal (from the center of the body to the outer parts) fashion. The neonate demonstrates many primitive reflexes at birth that disappear as the nervous system matures. It is not unusual to observe fleeting tremors, frequent star-tles, and uncoordinated motor activity in the newborn. Chapter 18 describes the normal reflexes exhibited by the newborn.

First 6-8 hrs

Gastrointestinal System

Despite functional immaturity, the gastrointestinal sys-tem of the neonate is capable of ingesting, digesting, absorbing, and eliminating breast milk and modified cow's milk formulas.

The fetus demonstrates sucking and swallowing movements in utero. These skills become finely coordi-nated during the first few days of extrauterine life. On the first day of life, the gastric capacity of the fetus is ap-proximately 40 to 60 mL (1.5–2 oz.). As feedings are in-troduced, the capacity increases. Gastric emptying time is approximately 2 to 4 hours. Slight regurgitation of milk after feedings is normal in the newborn. This is at-tributable to immaturity of the cardiac sphincter at the entrance to the stomach.

Pepsinogen, which is converted by gastric acid into the enzyme pepsin, is present at birth. It assists with di-gestion, as milk enters the stomach. The enzymes nec-essary for protein synthesis are also present in the new-born. Fats are digested and absorbed less effectively because of inadequate amounts of pancreatic lipase.

Even though breast milk contains fats, it is digested more easily than cow's milk formulas. Breast milk has li-pase, and its composition makes it easier to digest.

The first stool consists of meconium and is passed within the first 24 hours of life in approximately 99% of full-term newborns. Meconium is an odorless, thick, tarry, dark-green substance, composed of bile, vernix caseosa, epithelial cells, lanugo, and amniotic fluid. The passage of meconium is a basic step in the initial functioning and adjustment of the gastrointestinal sys-tem to postpartum life. All newborns should pass their first stool within the first 48 hours of life. The occur-rence of the first stool is important to observe and docu-ment. Newborns who do not pass meconium within the first 48 hours may have an obstruction and require fur-ther evaluation.

Hepatic System

The neonate's liver is immature at birth. The liver plays a significant role in iron storage, carbohydrate metabo-lism, coagulation, and bilirubin conjugation. Iron stores are deposited in the liver of the fetus during the last 3 months of pregnancy. If maternal iron intake was ade-quate during pregnancy, the infant will have enough stores to last for approximately 5 months. The glucose needed to meet the neonate's energy requirements in the first few hours of life are drawn from the glycogen stores accumulated during fetal life.

The neonate experiences a temporary blood coag-ulation deficiency between the second and fifth days of life. This occurs because the maternal coagulation factors cannot cross the placenta. Additionally, the neonate is unable to produce sufficient vitamin K to promote formation of coagulation factors. Vitamin K is administered to the neonate at birth to prevent exces-sive bleeding until the neonate is able to manufacture sufficient vitamin K (see Chapter 18). Vitamin K is pro-duced in the intestines by bacteria. It takes a few days for the vitamin K levels to increase. This is because the gastrointestinal tract is sterile until birth. Normal intesti-nal flora is not established until the newborn ingests milk.

The neonate is born with a high erythrocyte count. When the lungs begin to function adequately, fewer eryth-rocytes are needed. As a result, a large number of eryth-rocytes are destroyed. **Bilirubin** is a by-product of this destruction. The production of bilirubin surpasses the ca-pabilities of the newborn's liver to convert it to conju-gated bilirubin (water soluble) so that it is easily elimi-nated. As this happens, the unconjugated bilirubin (fat soluble) accumulates in the subcutaneous tissue. This is what produces the familiar jaundice appearance seen in newborns between 48 to 72 hours after birth, referred to as physiologic jaundice. For further discussion of physio-

If the baby get Jaundice
After 1st 24hrs Icterus neonatorum

logic jaundice, see Chapter 18. Jaundice that occurs during the first 24 hours of birth is caused by a number of problems and is discussed further in Chapter 20.

Urinary System

The placenta is responsible for fetal excretion of wastes in utero. After birth, the renal system must assume the responsibilities of fluid and electrolyte balance and the excretion of metabolic wastes. The kidneys are immature in their ability to reabsorb electrolytes and concentrate urine.

Among normal newborns, many urinate within the first 24 hours of life. Most all newborns urinate within the first 48 hours of life. The first voiding may be dark amber and cloudy because of mucus and uric acid crystals. As fluid intake increases, the urine becomes clear, straw colored, and less concentrated. The amount initially may be as little as 15 mL (0.5 oz.) with a total output of 30 to 60 mL (1–2 oz.) per day. This amount increases so that by the end of the first week of life the newborn's urine output is approximately 300 mL (5 oz.) per day.

A weight loss of between 5% and 10% of the newborn's birth weight occurs during the first few days of life. Weight loss is due to limited fluid intake, urine and stool losses, an increased metabolic rate, and perhaps the withdrawal of maternal hormones. After this initial expected loss, most infants gain approximately 28 g (1 oz.) per day for the first 6 months of life if they receive adequate daily nutritional intake.

Endocrine System

The transition to extrauterine life is coordinated by the endocrine system. In utero, the placenta acts as the major endocrine organ. It produces precursors for hormones, promotes steroid synthesis, and facilitates the movement of hormones between the fetal and maternal circulations. The neonate's endocrine system, which consists of the hypothalamus, pituitary and pineal glands, thyroid, parathyroid, adrenals, gonads, and pancreatic islet cells, is intact at birth. Several hormones that are essential for the newborn's adaptation to extrauterine life are secreted. These hormones include the growth hormone (GH), thyroid-stimulating hormone (TSH), adrenocorticotropic hormone (ACTH), cortisol, and catecholamines.

Reproductive System

The sex of the fetus is determined at the time of fertilization. External sexual characteristics are not distinguishable until the end of the second month of pregnancy. In the female newborn, pseudomenstruation may occur. This is a condition in which the maternal hormones produce a blood-tinged mucoid vaginal discharge. In both male and female newborns, breast engorgement may be observed. This is a temporary condition caused by stimulation from maternal hormones.

The testes of the male may be palpated in the scrotal sac after 32 to 34 weeks of pregnancy. The communication through which the testes descend into the scrotal sac is not completely closed until several months of age. Male newborns who have one or both testes that are undescended at birth require evaluation to determine the reason and any need for further treatment.

Integumentary System

In the first few hours after birth, the white or Asian newborn has a pink appearance that changes to red in color with activity. The African American newborn has a reddish brown appearance which becomes ruddy on crying or other activity. Newborns whose environment is too cool may exhibit mottling, which appears bluish in the newborn with lighter skin. This quickly disappears if the newborn is provided warmth. The newborn's skin is usually smooth looking and very soft to the touch.

Because of the stresses of the intrapartum period, the nurse may note breaks in the epidermis (skin surface), areas of ecchymosis (bruising), and edematous areas. Breaks in the skin may have been caused by procedures during labor and delivery such as inserting a fetal scalp electrode for internal fetal monitoring, or fetal scalp sampling for acid/base assessment. In addition, areas of edema and ecchymosis may be related to the use of a vacuum extractor, forceps, or pressure from the maternal pelvis on the presenting part.

At birth, the full-term newborn's skin is usually covered with a greasy, yellow-white substance called **vernix caseosa**. Vernix caseosa is composed of sebaceous gland secretions and epidermal cells. It provides the fetus with protection from softening of the outermost layer of the skin by the amniotic fluid in utero. The vernix caseosa that has not been absorbed into the skin is usually lost during the first bath. The removal of this protective layer exposes the newborn's skin to the much drier postpartum environment. Adaptation of the skin to extrauterine life is completed when normal skin flaking is observed. This typically occurs within a week to 10 days after birth.

Musculoskeletal System

Skeletal muscles are used for movement very early in fetal life. This experience helps to promote motor development. In utero, the amniotic fluid reduces the effects of gravity in much the same way that water supports muscle activity when swimming. The uterus provides physical constraints. These physical obstacles are removed after birth, and the newborn must learn to adapt. Fetal movements are usually smooth in comparison to the often erratic, jerky movements of the newborn.

The physical position of the fetus in utero may be apparent on initial inspection of the newborn. For example, it is not unusual to see a newborn exhibiting thigh flexion and knee extension resulting from a breech presentation (Fig. 17-3). Thigh flexion and knee extension from breech presentation generally is self-correcting within several days of birth. It is important to note that breech presentation is a major factor contributing to the development of congenital dislocation of the hip. (See Chapter 20 for further discussion.)

Immune System

The normal newborn produces antibodies in response to an antigen, but not very effectively. Newborns are especially susceptible to infection in the early postpartum period. This is attributable to their delicate skin, limited ability for localization of infection, limited phagocytosis (ingestion of microorganisms by specialized white blood cells), and the large number of portals of entry for organisms, especially the umbilical stump.

Immunoglobulins are antibodies, the major components of the immune response system. There are three major immunoglobulins involved in immunity: IgG, IgA, and IgM. Through the transfer of IgG across the placenta, the newborn acquires passive immunity against bacterial and viral diseases for which the mother has developed antibodies, such as mumps, rubella (German measles), rubeola (measles), and polio. The transfer of IgG occurs primarily during the third trimester of pregnancy. Therefore, neonates born prematurely do not receive adequate amounts of IgG. This is especially true of neonates born before 34 weeks' gestation, causing an even greater susceptibility to infection. Passive IgG decreases over the first few months after birth and is replaced by IgG, which the infant develops through exposure and immunizations.

IgA is not normally produced in utero. Unlike IgG, it does not cross the placental barrier in sufficient amounts to provide immunity to the growing fetus. IgA is secreted in colostrum and breast milk. For this reason, there is some belief that breast-feeding offers some passive immunity to certain gastrointestinal and respiratory infections in breast-fed newborns.

IgM, the largest immunoglobulin, does not cross the placenta. Neonates who have evidence of IgM at birth are believed to have developed them in response to an intrauterine infection such as toxoplasmosis, syphilis, rubella, cytomegalovirus, or herpes. These infections are collectively referred to as the TORCH infections. (See Chapter 20 for further discussion.)

◆ Thermoregulation

Thermoregulation is defined as controlling heat production of an individual. A very important nursing responsibility during transition is the maintenance of a **neutral thermal environment** for the newborn. This is an environment in which the newborn's heat production and heat loss are balanced. In a neutral thermal environment, the newborn's metabolic rate, and therefore oxygen consumption, is maintained with the fewest calories possible being used for temperature maintenance. The normal range of temperature for a newborn is 36.5° to 37.5°C (97.7°–99.0°F).

Heat Production

Heat production occurs as a by-product of the body's metabolic processes. The full-term, healthy newborn attempts to maintain body temperature by assuming a flexed, fetal position. The newborn's peripheral blood vessels constrict by means of a process called nonshivering thermogenesis. The flexed, fetal position provides some protection against cold stress by exposing less surface area to the environment.

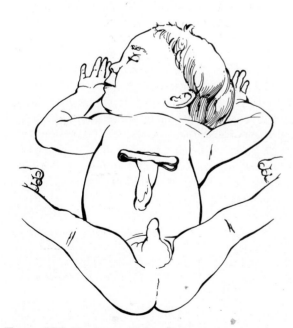

Figure 17-3. *Newborn with breech leg presentation. This neonate has flexed, abducted hips and extended knees as a result of a breech presentation. (Courtesy of David A. Clark, MD, Louisiana State University Medical Center and Wyeth-Ayerst Laboratories, Philadelphia, PA)*

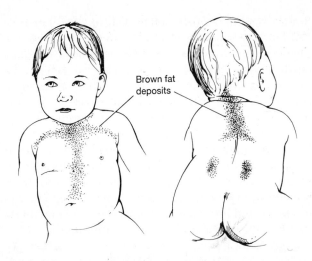

Figure 17-4. *Location of brown fat stores. Deposits of brown fat are found between the scapulae, at the nape of the neck, in the axillae, in the mediastinum, and surrounding the kidneys and adrenals. The skin overlying brown fat deposits feels slightly warmer to the touch. Brown fat reserves usually persist for several weeks after birth unless depleted for heat production required by cold stress.*

Cold stress is the metabolic demands placed on the neonate to maintain adequate body heat. When a newborn is exposed to a cold environment, receptors in different parts of the body, especially the face, relay this impulse to the hypothalamus. The hypothalamus is responsible for coordinating heat production and loss. The sympathetic nervous system activates heat production through the mechanism of nonshivering **thermogenesis** (production of heat). This method of heat production is also known as brown fat metabolism. This process is unique to the newborn.

Brown fat is highly vascular and is specialized for heat production. It is located in the adipose tissue around the axilla, kidneys, adrenal glands, scapulae, behind the sternum, and around the vessels and muscles of the neck. Figure 17-4 illustrates the location of brown fat on the newborn's body. Brown fat starts to be deposited at approximately 28 weeks' gestation and disappears approximately 3 months after birth.

Mechanisms of Heat Loss

The newborn loses heat when body warmth travels toward cooler objects. This can happen through evaporation, convection, conduction, and radiation (Fig. 17-5). These mechanisms can occur alone or in combination.

[handwritten notes: Baby should be in neutral thermal environment in one which the Infants O₂ Consumption are minimal and their body temp stays within normal limits.]

[handwritten note: Normal Resp - 30-60]

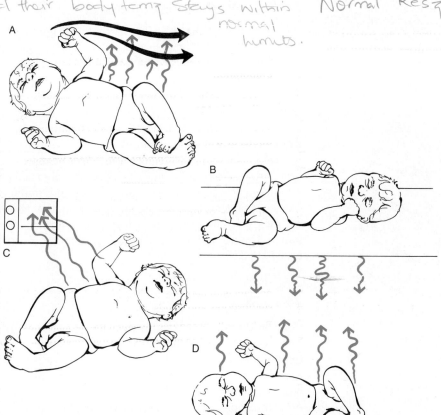

Figure 17-5. *Heat loss mechanisms. Heat loss in the newborn. **(A)** Convection, **(B)** Conduction, **(C)** Radiation, **(D)** Evaporation.*

tachypnea

Evaporation

Heat loss occurs when water evaporates from the skin and respiratory tract. Evaporative heat losses can occur any time the newborn's skin is wet. For example, the skin temperature at birth can drop considerably as the amniotic fluid evaporates from the newborn's skin.

Convection

Heat loss occurs when cool air moves around the newborn. Convection losses occur when the newborn is exposed to cool room temperatures, air conditioning drafts, or when cold oxygen is blown into the newborn's face.

Conduction

The newborn loses heat to objects that come in contact with the body. Conduction occurs when the newborn comes in contact with cold objects. Examples include the provider's cold hands, scales, stethoscopes, or beds.

Radiation

Radiant heat loss occurs when a newborn loses heat from being placed near cold surfaces or objects. Examples include placing the newborn near cold windows, outside walls, or isolette walls. Remember, warmth travels to cooler objects. This heat loss occurs regardless of air temperatures.

Nursing interventions can reduce heat loss from the various mechanisms. The Nursing Interventions Checklist presents nursing interventions to implement in the prevention of heat loss in the newborn.

Cold Stress

Most healthy newborns have the ability to maintain their body temperatures in response to changes in environmental temperatures. However, newborns can only balance their temperature within a fairly narrow range. Normal body temperature does not necessarily indicate the absence of cold stress. It simply means that the newborn is compensating at this time by using calories and oxygen to produce heat.

Other symptoms of cold stress include cool extremities, lethargy, apnea, or poor feeding. If the newborn has other physiologic difficulties such as prematurity or asphyxia, cold stress can cause further complications for the compromised newborn.

The acutely cold-stressed newborn uses more oxygen and glucose and may become hypoxic, acidotic, and show symptoms of respiratory distress. The acidosis that cold stress causes results in a decrease in the production of surfactant. The chronically cold-stressed newborn may lose or fail to gain weight because calories are needed for heat production. If this cycle is not broken, shock, disseminated intravascular coagulopathy (DIC), or death may occur.

The nurse must be alert for symptoms that indicate the neonate is having difficulty adjusting to extrauterine life. Tachypnea, nasal flaring, grunting, and retractions are the cardinal signs of respiratory distress in the newborn. The newborn's nares flare in an attempt to inspire more oxygen. Grunting is the newborn's way of trying to maintain FRC. Retractions symbolize poor lung compliance. During transition, it is not unusual to see one or more of these signs in their mildest form. But if they persist or worsen, medical evaluation is necessary. Display 17-1 serves as a quick reference for respiratory signs and symptoms to report to the provider.

NURSING INTERVENTIONS CHECKLIST

Preventing Neonate Heat Loss

- Dry the neonate thoroughly with warm blankets immediately after birth
- Dry head and cover to prevent heat loss through evaporation
- Remove neonate from wet linens; avoid contact with wet linens
- Protect neonate from drafts from air conditioners, doors, or windows
- Maintain warm environment with radiant warmer
- Warm oxygen before administration
- Place a warm blanket between the neonate's body and scales or any other cool surface
- Encourage skin-to-skin contact with mother after neonate is dried; mother's body heat will warm newborn
- Preheat all materials and equipment that come in contact with neonate, such as blankets, hats, shirts, stethoscope, and hands
- Perform all procedures for which the neonate must be unwrapped as quickly as possible; rewrap immediately
- Remove cribs, isolettes, or radiant warmers from outside walls or windows
- Use double-walled isolettes for very-low-birth-weight neonates

> **DISPLAY 17-1**
> *Observations of Neonate's Respiratory Status*
>
> · Continuously observe neonate's respirations
> · Observe respiratory rate report if greater than 60 breaths per minute
> · Observe mucus membranes for cyanosis
> · Note nasal flaring, grunting, or retractions; report if any of these signs persist
> · Observe for gagging, choking, or other evidence of mucus that needs to be cleared

Neonatal Behavior

The normal newborn is ready to begin to interact with the world soon after birth. A variety of behavioral cues indicate the newborn's readiness for interaction. In the first 6 to 8 hours after birth, the newborn goes through several stages of reactivity.

First Period of Reactivity

The initial period of reactivity lasts approximately 15 to 30 minutes. During this time, the neonate's eyes are open, and the neonate displays random diffuse movements that alternate with periods of immobility (quiet with no activity.) The newborn also demonstrates sucking and rooting reflexes during this time. For this reason, breast-feeding may be initiated if the mother wishes. Heart and respiratory rates are irregular during this time. The neonate's heart rate may reach 180 beats/min, and respirations may be as rapid as 60 breaths/min during this time. Bowel sounds are usually absent.

Period of Inactivity

After the initial period of reactivity, the neonate becomes quiet, gradually falls asleep, and may be difficult to awaken for breast-feeding. This stage may last 2 or more hours. During this time, the newborn's respiratory and heart rates adjust to resting rates, and body temperature may decrease to its lowest point. On auscultation, bowel sounds usually can be heard.

Second Period of Reactivity

Gradually the newborn reawakens, beginning the second period of reactivity. This stage is one in which the neonate goes through many changes. The neonate may have periods of tachypnea, apnea, gagging, regurgitation of mucus, or brief periods of cyanosis. Often the newborn demonstrates interest in feeding again.

Transition from intrauterine to extrauterine life is usually completed in 6 to 8 hours after birth. Dramatic physical and behavioral adaptations prepare the neonate to meet this new world.

Adolescent Considerations

Immediately after the birth, during the newborn's first period of reactivity, the nurse can assist the adolescent mother by helping to position the neonate comfortably on the her chest. The nurse can promote interaction with the newborn by encouraging the adolescent to touch, stroke, talk to, and snuggle the baby. The nurse can explain to the mother the molding of the neonate's head or other "normal" aspects of the newborn's appearance so that the young mother does not become alarmed. If the adolescent plans to breast-feed, the nurse can assist her in proper placement and positioning the baby to her breast. If the adolescent father is present, he also is encouraged to touch, stroke, talk to, and relate to the newborn.

The nurse can explain the stages of reactivity that the newborn will experience in the next few hours of life. This reassures the young mother and father that these are normal phases that their baby is undergoing. Positive statements of support help to reinforce the adolescent's self-confidence.

Cultural Considerations

Cultural and ethnic practices affect the way in which the mother and her family view the birth of a new family member. The nurse must respect these varying attitudes about childbirth. For example, in our Western culture, the role of the father has become very important, but in some cultures, the father is not permitted to be involved in the birth experience in any way. Women from Southeast Asia may view colostrum as "dirty" and refuse to breast-feed the neonate in the early postpartal period. These viewpoints must be respected by the nurse.

Among Mexican Americans and some Southeast Asians, there is a fear of the "evil eye" affecting the newborn if anyone openly praises the baby. The nurse needs to be sensitive to such beliefs to avoid contributing to the mother's apprehensions. Among some Hispanics, there is a belief that the newborn is protected from evil if everyone says "God bless him (or her)" as soon as they first see the neonate. The nurse can put this mother at ease by making this comment immediately on the birth of the neonate. In other cultures, the mother may wish to put an amulet (a special charm) on the newborn's clothing to provide protection from evil spirits. The nurse assists with this or any other cultural custom desired by the family in a nonjudgmental way.

The Role of the Nurse

During the transitional time, the nurse bears the primary responsibility for assessing the neonate. Immediate recognition of signs that the neonate is not adjusting successfully is essential. Respiratory, thermoregulation, or circulatory problems of the neonate must be met with quick action.

In addition to responding to the physiologic needs of the newborn, the nurse also must know about the neonate's periods of reactivity. With this information in hand, the nurse can provide guidance to the woman and family in early responses to the neonate. Nursing diagnoses that may be useful in planning the care of the neonate are included in the Checklist.

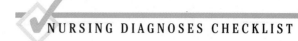

NURSING DIAGNOSES CHECKLIST

Neonatal Transition to Extrauterine Life

· Ineffective Airway Clearance, related to secretions in the oropharynx

· Ineffective Breathing Pattern, related to alteration in response to extrauterine life

· Ineffective Thermoregulation, related to extrauterine transition

· Risk for Infection, related to immature immune system

· Risk for Impaired Tissue Integrity, related to lack of normal skin flora

· Risk for Fluid Volume Deficit: Bleeding, related to immaturity of blood coagulation mechanism

· Sensory/Perceptual Alterations, Visual, related to excessive lighting

· Risk for Altered Parenting, related to addition of new family member

---

REVIEW AND PREVIEW

The fetus prepares in utero for entry into the extrauterine world. This chapter highlighted the key changes that occur in each of the newborn's body systems after birth, including implications for the neonate's adjustment to postpartum life. Changes in fetal circulation necessary to successfully adapt to postpartum life were described in detail. The basic principles of thermoregulation were described, emphasizing actions that prevent heat loss in the early postpartum period. Changes in the respiratory system were detailed, and nursing interventions were described to assure adequate air exchange for the neonate.

The periods of reactivity in the first few hours of life were described, with guidelines for reinforcing parent–infant bonding during this time. The nurse's role during this critical time in the life to the neonate presented nursing concerns, observations, and interventions.

The next chapter will discuss physical and behavioral assessment of the newborn. Nursing assessments and appropriate interventions will be presented. Routine procedures, health promotion, and home care instructions will be explored. Each family's learning needs will need to be considered as the individualized plan of care is developed. Smooth transition includes successful adaptation of each family to its newest member.

⬦ KEY POINTS

◆ The onset of respirations is one of the biggest challenges the newborn faces. Factors that contribute to the onset of respirations include chemical, sensory, thermal, and mechanical stimuli.

◆ The success of the newborn's respiratory adaptation to extrauterine life is dependent on the effectiveness of the first few respirations. Surfactant, a phospholipid, decreases surface tension in the lung tissues and promotes circulation by increasing alveolar size.

◆ The closure of the fetal cardiovascular pathways (foramen ovale, ductus venosus, and ductus arteriosus) must take place for successfully adaptation from fetal to neonatal circulation. Factors that contribute to the closure of the fetal pathways include the onset of extrauterine respirations, an increase in pulmonary blood flow, a decrease in pulmonary vascular resistance, an increase in arterial oxygenation, and closure of the umbilical arteries and vein occur at the time of clamping of the cord.

◆ At birth, the neonate has a high erythrocyte count. Extra erythrocytes are destroyed because they are no longer needed, resulting in increased bilirubin. The neonate's immature liver is not able to adequately conjugate the bilirubin. Thus, unconjugated bilirubin (fat soluble) collects in the subcutaneous tissues of the newborn, causing a jaundiced appearance, which occurs between 48 and 72 hours of birth.

◆ A neutral thermal environment occurs when heat production and heat loss are balanced. In a neutral thermal environment, the newborn does not have to consume more oxygen or burn more glucose to produce heat or to maintain body temperature.

SELF-ASSESSMENT

1. Vitamin K is administered to newborns to prevent:

- ○ **A.** Hyperbilirubinemia
- ◉ **B.** Excessive bleeding
- ○ **C.** Nutritional deficits
- ○ **D.** Jaundice

2. The presence of IgM in the neonate may be indicative of:

- ○ **A.** Immunity to certain viral diseases
- ○ **B.** Protection against respiratory infections
- ◉ **C.** Intrauterine infection
- ○ **D.** A congenital anomaly

3. Oxygen administered to the neonate must be warmed to prevent heat loss via:

- ○ **A.** Evaporation
- ◉ **B.** Radiation
- ○ **C.** Conduction
- ◉ **D.** Convection

4. Acute cold stress in the neonate can lead to:

- ◉ **A.** Hypoglycemia
- ○ **B.** Metabolic alkalosis
- ○ **C.** Decreased oxygen consumption
- ○ **D.** Increased surfactant production

5. After the umbilical cord is cut, respiratory centers in the brain are activated in response to:

- ○ **A.** Increased arterial pH
- ○ **B.** Decreased arterial carbon dioxide tension
- ◉ **C.** Decreased arterial oxygen tension
- ○ **D.** Prolonged asphyxia

◆ Newborns produce heat by a process called nonshivering thermogenesis or brown fat metabolism, which is exclusive to the newborn. Starting at approximately 28 weeks' gestation, the fetus begins to collect brown fat stores. These stores are specialized for heat production.

◆ There are four mechanisms that cause newborns to lose heat. The first, evaporation, occurs when water or fluids evaporate from the newborn's skin. In conductive heat loss, the newborn loses heat to a cooler object in direct contact with the body. Heat loss attributable to drafts is called convective heat loss. Radiative heat loss occurs when the newborn loses heat to a nearby cooler object that is not touching the body.

◆ Heat loss can be prevented by prewarming items that come in contact with the newborn, avoiding drafts and cool environments, thoroughly drying the newborn, using a hat, and moving cribs and isolettes away from cold walls. The first bath should be delayed until the newborn's temperature has stabilized.

◆ In the acute stage of cold stress, newborns consume more oxygen, use more glucose, become acidotic, and have decreased surfactant production. Severely cold-stressed newborns may exhibit disseminated intravascular coagulopathy (DIC), shock, and eventually death, if appropriate intervention is delayed.

◆ Patterns of activity observed in the newborn after birth include three distinct periods. During the first period of reactivity, the newborn is awake, alert, and visually exploring the environment. Next, there is a stage of inactivity, as the newborn sleeps. Finally, there is the second period of reactivity, during which the newborn is awake and alert again.

BIBLIOGRAPHY

American Academy of Pediatrics and American College of Obstetricians and Gynecologists. (1992). *Guidelines for perinatal care* (3rd ed.). Elk Grove Village/Washington, DC: Author.

Blackburn, S. T., & Loper, D. L. (1992). Maternal, fetal, and neonatal physiology: A clinical perspective. Philadelphia: W. B. Saunders.

Carpenito, L. J. (1993). *Nursing diagnosis: Application to clinical practice* (5th ed.). Philadelphia: J. B. Lippincott.

Corrine, L., Bailey, V., & Valentin, M. (1992). The unheard voices of women: Spiritual interventions in maternal-child health. *MCN, 17*(3), 141– 145.

D'Avanza, C. E. (1992). Bridging the cultural gap with Southeast Asians. *MCN, 17*(4), 204–208.

Fanaroff, A. A., & Martin, R. J. (1992). *Neonatal perinatal medicine: Diseases of the fetus and infant* (5th ed.). St. Louis: C. V. Mosby.

Kenner, C., Brueggemeyer, A., & Gunderson, L. P. (1993). *Comprehensive neonatal nursing: A physiologic perspective*. Philadelphia: W. B. Saunders.

Marks, M. G. (1994). *Broadribb's introductory pediatric nursing*. Philadelphia: J. B. Lippincott.

May, K. A., & Mahlmeister, L. R. (1994). *Maternal & neonatal nursing: Family-centered care* (3rd ed.). Philadelphia: J. B. Lippincott.

Moore, K. L. (1989). *Before we are born: Basic embryology and birth defects* (3rd ed.). Philadelphia: W. B. Saunders.

NAACOG OGN Nursing Practice Resource. (1990). *Thermoregulation*. Washington, DC: Author.

Nugent, J. (1991). *Acute respiratory care of the neonate*. Petaluma: Neonatal Network.

Pillitteri, A. (1992). *Maternal and child health nursing* (1st ed.). Philadelphia: J. B. Lippincott.

Reeder, S. J., Martin, L. L., & Koniak, D. (1992). *Maternity nursing: Family, newborn, and women's health care* (17th ed.). Philadelphia: J. B. Lippincott.

Tappero, E. P., & Honeyfield, M. E. (1993). Physical assessment of the newborn. Petaluma: NICU Inc.

CHAPTER 18

Nursing Care of the Normal Newborn

◆ OBJECTIVES

When the learning goals of this chapter are met, the reader will be able to:

- ◆ Discuss the major aspects of the newborn health history.
- ◆ Identify and explain the components of the newborn physical assessment.
- ◆ List the features of a newborn behavioral assessment.
- ◆ Explain routine procedures performed in the first few hours of the neonate's life.
- ◆ Discuss the nurse's role in prevention of infection in the newborn nursery.
- ◆ Discuss safety issues related to the care of the newborn.
- ◆ List advantages and disadvantages of breast-feeding and bottle-feeding.
- ◆ Define parent–newborn interaction.
- ◆ Describe six areas of discharge teaching that help prepare family members to care for their newborn.
- ◆ Identify the function of the nurse when teaching the adolescent mother.

TERMINOLOGY

Acrocyanosis	Jaundice
Bradycardia	Milia
Caput succedaneum	Molding
Cephalhematoma	Mongolian spots
Crepitation	Phimosis
Erythema toxicum	Pseudomenstruation
Fontanelle	Tachycardia
Icterus neonatorum	

In the short time the newborn is in the health care facility, the nurse has a great responsibility to assess the neonate's physical and behavioral condition, conduct routine procedures, and teach the new family important aspects of infant care. Throughout this time, the nurse looks for deviations from the norm or other concerns that may need further evaluation or intervention. Nursing care of the newborn emphasizes neonatal assessments, procedures, infection prevention, and the teaching of infant care to the mother and family.

Newborn Assessment

At the birth of the neonate, the nurse makes initial assessments to establish Apgar scores. A general examination of the neonate's physical appearance is also performed. Later, in the nursery setting, the nurse conducts a complete assessment. Before beginning the complete assessment of the newborn, the nurse gathers information about the health history of the neonate. The nurse uses the findings of the health history and assessment to make an individualized plan of care for the newborn. The Assessment Checklist serves as a quick reference for normal findings in the newborn.

Health History

The health history is usually available from the mother's records. A copy of this information is included as part of the newborn's record. (See Chapter 5 for information gathered in the mother's prenatal history.) The nurse reviews this information to determine the presence of any medical or genetic disorders in the family. Information concerning the current pregnancy, labor, and childbirth, as well as the neonate's Apgar scores and assessments in the transition period, are also obtained. Once the records are reviewed, the nurse interviews the mother to gain any omitted in-depth data.

Physical Assessment

Complete assessment is usually postponed until the neonate's temperature is stable. The nurse must be certain that the newborn is kept warm throughout the examination. Cold hands startle the neonate. The nurse can prevent cold hands by washing with warm water immediately before the examination. During the assessment, the nurse uses slow, gentle movements while talking softly to the newborn. The nurse may find that a pacifier will help quiet a neonate who is upset and crying.

A complete physical assessment is divided into three areas: general appearance, vital signs and measurements, and head-to-toe assessment. Generally, the nurse begins by performing assessment techniques that require the newborn to be in a quiet state. Examples include observation of general appearance, measurement of vital signs, observation of respiratory effort, and auscultation of the heart, lungs, and bowel sounds. Bowel sounds are assessed, followed by palpation of the abdomen, while the newborn is relaxed. The nurse completes inspection and palpation of the rest of the neonate's body. The physical examination ends with measurements of the length, head and chest circumferences, and weight.

General Appearance

The nurse begins the physical assessment by observing the newborn at rest. Posture is observed before touching the newborn. The full-term neonate posture is flexed. A normal variation in posture occurs after breech presentation in utero (see Fig. 17-3). After a breech birth, the neonate may either assume a "frogleg" position or lay with legs fully extended. Findings that require further investigation include hypotonia (poor muscle tone, flaccid; a "floppy baby") or hypertonia (high muscle tone), lethargy, jitteriness, or irritability. Observe the newborn during movement and note any restricted or asymmetrical (not the same for both sides) movement. Deviations from normal are reported to the neonate's physician and documented.

Skin

The skin is inspected throughout the physical examination. There may be areas of dryness or peeling, especially on the hands and feet. The skin turgor, assessed by lightly pinching the skin over the abdomen, is elastic, that is, it returns quickly to its original state. Remnants of vernix caseosa may still be noticed, especially in the folds of the skin. Lanugo, fine downy hair, may be seen on the face, brow, and shoulders, especially in preterm neonates.

It is important to look closely for any discolorations, markings, or variations in the skin. A common rash, called **erythema toxicum,** may be observed on the trunk of the newborn. It is characterized by small isolated areas of redness with a yellowish-white wheal in the center. The lesions range from a few millimeters to 1 or 2 cm and are commonly seen on the trunk. The appearance of the lesions are short term, usually seen in the first 24 hours up to 10 days. The rash is temporary. No treatment is indicated. Figure 18-1 shows a newborn with erythema toxicum.

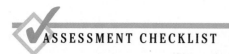

ASSESSMENT CHECKLIST

Normal Newborn

Assessment	Normal Findings
Posture	Flexed, good muscle tone
Skin	Soft, smooth, good turgor, possible peeling and dryness of hands and feet, pink to ruddy color; lanugo may be present on face, brow, and shoulders; vernix in folds; acrocyanosis, erythema toxicum, mongolian spots, and harlequin sign normal variations
Respiratory rate	30 to 60 breaths per minute, may have passing tachypnea, short periods of apnea; breath sounds clear
Heart rate	120 to 160 beats per minute; may increase to 180 when crying or decrease to 100 during sleep
Blood pressure	70/45 during first 36 hours in quiet alert state
Temperature	36.5°C to 37.5°C (97.5°F–99.3°F)
Weight	2500 to 4000 g (5 lbs 8 oz to 8 lbs 13 oz); weight loss of 5% to 10% normal in first few days
Length	45 to 55 cm (17.75–21.5 in)
Head circumference	31 to 38 cm (12.2–15 in)
Chest circumference	31 to 36 cm (12.2–14.2 in)
Head	Vaginal birth: molding evident; cesarean birth: well rounded unless prolonged labor preceded surgical intervention; anterior and posterior fontanelles palpable, flat and soft; no bruising, abrasions, or swelling
Face	Face symmetrical; milia over nose and chin; nares patent; mouth midline, symmetrical, mucous membranes pink; eyes symmetric, slate blue, dark gray, or brown; sclera white to bluish white; strabismus and nystagmus may be present; ear pinna recoils rapidly, placement in line with eyes
Neck	Short, symmetrical, supple, no masses
Chest	Round, symmetrical, and slightly smaller than head; areola stippled and raised; no crepitation or evidence of fractured clavicle
Abdomen	Protrudes, no distention; umbilical cord has 2 arteries, 1 vein; bowel sounds present; no masses palpable
Genitals	Female: labia majora covers clitoris and labia minora; vaginal opening patent, may have discharge; Male: penis straight, testes palpable in scrotum
Extremities	Symmetrical, flexed; nail beds pink; 3 creases in palm, no creases on plantar surface
Anus	Present and patent
Spine	Straight, at midline; no visible defects
Reflexes	Rooting, sucking, palmar and plantar grasp, Moro's, startle, Babinski's, step, and tonic neck reflexes present

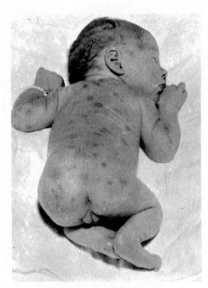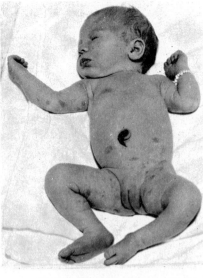

Figure 18-1. *Newborn with erythema toxicum. This "newborn rash" develops more frequently on the back, the shoulders, and the buttocks. (Courtesy of MacDonald House, The University Hospitals of Cleveland, Cleveland, OH)*

The newborn may have vascular or pigmented lesions present on the skin. These birthmarks are measured and documented. Some of the common birthmarks are described in Table 18-1. Parents should be reassured that many birthmarks are not associated with health problems.

As the newborn is resting quietly, the skin is observed for color variations. A normal variation in skin color is **acrocyanosis**. This is a bluish discoloration of the newborn's hands and feet. The hands and feet may have almost a charcoal-like appearance. It results from poor peripheral circulation and may occur in the first hours to a few days. The harlequin sign is a normal variation found only during the newborn period. It occurs when one side of the body is red and the other side remains pale. It is a result of vasomotor instability.

Generalized cyanosis (cyanosis of large portions of the body) is abnormal and may indicate respiratory or cardiac problems. Other abnormal findings in the skin

Table 18-1. *Common Birthmarks*

Type	Characteristic
Vascular nevi	
Telangiectatic nevi (stork bites)	Tiny pink to red spots found commonly on nape of the neck, eyelids, and bridge of the nose; blanch on pressure; usually disappear spontaneously during infancy; may persist to adulthood
Nevus vasculosus (strawberry marks)	Dark red, rough textured sharply demarcated elevations usually found on head and face; continue to grow for several months, then shrink spontaneously and usually disappear by 7 to 10 years of age.
Pigmented nevi (mongolian spots)	Gray-blue pigmented areas seen most often on lumbosacral region and buttocks of dark-skinned and Asian infants; usually spontaneously disappear during late infancy or early childhood; have no relationship to Down syndrome
Café au lait spots	Patch, flat brown areas that are lighter in color than surrounding skin; single small lesions are common and of no significance (see Chapter 20 for further discussion)

Adapted from Reeder, S. J., Martin, L. L., & Koniak, D. (1992). *Maternity nursing* (17th ed.). Philadelphia: J. B. Lippincott, Table 29-3, p. 659.

that require further investigation include pallor, ruddiness, or grayness. **Jaundice** in the first 24 hours or significant jaundice after day 1 of life can be abnormal. Jaundice is assessed by applying pressure to the newborn's nose. The skin will appear yellow when the pressure is released. The mucous membranes are the best indicators of systemic color in babies of all races. The mucous membranes in a healthy newborn are pink and moist. Variations of mucous membrane color may indicate need for further evaluation. Chapter 20 highlights the common cardiovascular and hematologic problems associated with the neonatal period.

Vital Signs and Measurements

The nurse assesses the vital signs before the newborn is stimulated during the head-to-toe physical examination. Temperature, pulse, respirations, and blood pressure are recorded. The newborn's weight, length, and vital circumferences are measured and recorded. These baseline values serve as useful indicators of deviations from normal. Temperature, pulse, and respirations are assessed and recorded frequently during the transition period. The schedule is established by the policy of the facility, but these measurements are taken at least every half hour for the first 2 hours or until stable.

Respiratory Rate

The nurse counts respirations by visually watching the rise and fall of the neonate's chest. Respirations are counted for a full minute. In a quiet newborn, the normal range is 30 to 60 breaths per minute. Chest movement is normally unlabored and symmetrical. There may be some passing tachypnea (rapid respirations) in the first few hours after birth. This should not persist. Another normal finding is periodic breathing. This describes an intermittent cessation of respirations for up to 10 seconds.

An apneic episode refers to cessation of respirations for more than 20 seconds in the newborn. Cyanosis or duskiness may accompany apnea. Signs of respiratory distress include tachypnea, retractions of the sternum, clavicle area, and costal margins, nasal flaring, or respiratory grunting (see Chapter 20). Abnormal findings are reported immediately to the physician.

Breath sounds are auscultated bilaterally. Breath sounds are normally clear and equal both anteriorly and posteriorly. Abnormal findings include rales (crackles), wheezing, grunting on expiration, decreased breath sounds, and unequal breath sounds. Occasionally a newborn may have fine rales for a few hours after birth because of some remaining, uncleared alveolar fluid. This finding is considered normal if the neonate remains asymptomatic.

Heart Rate

The heart rate is auscultated with a warmed stethoscope. The best place to hear the apical pulse rate is normally at the fourth or fifth intercostal space. The heart rate is counted for 1 full minute. Normal range is 120 to 160 beats/min. The apical rate may increase up to 180 during crying episodes and decrease to 100 during sleep and still be considered within the normal range. Murmurs are common in newborns, but need to be evaluated further because they may indicate congenital heart defects. **Bradycardia** refers to a heart rate less than 100 beats/min. **Tachycardia** is a heart rate above 160 beats/min.

Blood Pressure

Blood pressure is obtained while the newborn is still relatively quiet. Obtaining an accurate blood pressure is much easier since Doppler ultrasound equipment has become available. The nurse uses an appropriately sized cuff and measures the blood pressure in all four extremities. The measurement should be approximately equal. Significant differences of blood pressure, especially between the upper and lower extremities, are abnormal. In this case, the neonate is evaluated for congenital heart disease.

Blood pressure values are dependent on birth weight, gestational age, and state of alertness. In the full-term newborn, the average systolic value is 70 mm Hg, and the average diastolic value is 45 mm Hg. These values relate to the newborn in the quiet alert state during the first 36 hours of life. During the first week of life, the systolic blood pressure increases by an average of 1 mm Hg per day. During the next 3 weeks, an increase of 2 mm Hg per week normally occurs in the systolic pressure. During the sleep state, blood pressure values are generally 5 to 10 mm Hg lower. When the newborn is crying, sucking, or faces stressful situations, the blood pressure values are 10 to 20 mm Hg higher than quiet alert state values.

Temperature

In some facilities, an initial rectal temperature is taken to determine rectal patency. Taking a rectal temperature may pose a risk of perforating the rectum. Therefore, after the initial measurement, the temperature is taken in the axilla (Fig. 18-2). Care is taken to place the end of the thermometer into the armpit. The nurse must make certain that skin-to-skin contact is made and no clothing is in the way. Normal values for

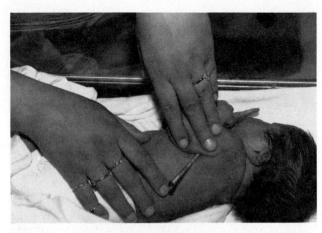

Figure 18-2. *Measuring the axillary temperature in the newborn. The infant's arm is held gently but firmly against his side while the thermometer is in place to ensure a more accurate temperature reading.*

axillary temperature range between 36.5°C and 37.5°C (97.5°F–99.3°F).

An increasing number of facilities have begun to use tympanic membrane sensors. A disposable speculum is used for each infant. The manufacturer's directions are followed in the use of the tympanic sensor. The temperature registers in approximately 2 seconds, with very little disturbance to the neonate.

Weight and Length

Every newborn is weighed on admission to the nursery. The newborn is weighed at the same time each day while in the facility. All weights are performed with the newborn naked or wearing a diaper but no other clothing. A protective cloth or paper liner is placed on the scale. The scale is balanced, and the newborn is placed on the scale and weighed. The nurse holds a hand within an inch of the neonate's body to be ready to quickly grasp the neonate if necessary. A full-term newborn's average weight is between 2500 and 4000 g (5 lbs. 8 oz. to 8 lbs. 13 oz.). The newborn typically loses weight in the first few days. A weight loss of 5% to 10% is considered normal. The birth weight in the healthy neonate is gained back in approximately 2 weeks or sooner. The weight loss is partially a result of limited intake and loss of excess fluids.

The newborn's length is measured from crown to heel. The nurse places the newborn flat on the back with the legs extended as much as possible. The normal length for the newborn is between 45 and 55 cm (17.75–21.5 in.).

Head and Chest Circumference

The head is measured over the most prominent part of the occiput and around to the frontal prominence, just above the eyebrows. It is best to use a measuring tape that does not stretch. The normal range of the head circumference for a full-term newborn is between 31 and 38 cm (12.2–15 in.). It is important to remember that if molding or caput succedaneum (edema of the scalp) is present, the head circumference may not be accurate. Molding and caput succedaneum are discussed later in this chapter.

In many facilities, chest circumference is not routinely measured. However, to measure the chest, the tape measure is placed around the chest at the nipple line and measured during expiration. Chest circumference is normally 31 to 36 cm (12.2–14.2 in.) in full-term newborns. Typically the chest measures approximately 2 to 3 cm (0.8–1.2 in.) smaller than the head circumference.

Head-to-Toe Assessment

The nurse continues the physical assessment with a detailed examination of the newborn from head-to-toe. This systematic approach helps organize the assessment process.

Head and Face

The large head normally makes up approximately one fourth of the newborn's body length. The birth may effect the shape of the newborn's head. Most newborns born by cesarean birth have a well-rounded head. Vaginal birth newborns may have an asymmetrical (lopsided) head. The skull bones override each other during labor and vaginal birth for the head to fit through the vaginal canal. This causes an elongated appearance called **molding** (Fig. 18-3). It usually diminishes

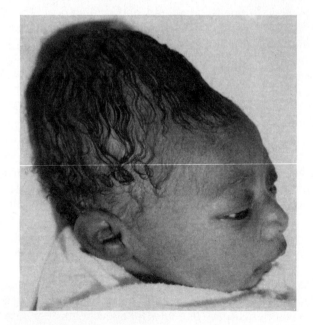

Figure 18-3. *Molding of the head.*

within the first few days but may last as long as a few weeks.

The nurse inspects and gently palpates the newborn's head. The suture lines where the bones of the skull meet may be open or overlapping. A **fontanelle** is often called the *soft spot*. The anterior fontanelle is diamond shaped, 3 to 4 cm long (1.2–1.6 in.) by 1 to 3 cm (0.4–1.2 in.) wide. It usually closes by 12 to 18 months of age. This is the fontanelle that is most commonly thought of as the soft spot. The posterior fontanelle is triangle shaped, 1 to 2 cm wide (0.4–0.8 in.). This fontanelle generally closes by 2 months of age. Fontanelles may bulge when the newborn cries; thus, they should be assessed during a quiet time. The fontanelles are normally soft and flat. A bulging fontanelle when the newborn is at rest is a sign of increased intracranial pressure. A sunken fontanelle is a sign of dehydration.

The head is inspected for bruising or bleeding. Small abrasions may have been caused by an internal fetal monitor electrode. Common variations that are caused by pressure or trauma during labor and birth include caput succedaneum and cephalhematoma. **Caput succedaneum** is subcutaneous edema (soft tissue swelling) of the head caused by pressure during labor. It crosses the suture lines, is present at birth, and is reabsorbed within the first few days of life. **Cephalhe-matoma** is the accumulation of blood between a bone of the skull and the periosteum that covers it. It is not always obvious at birth. In the first 48 hours of life, cephalhematoma becomes larger. It is gradually reabsorbed, taking up to 3 weeks or longer. A cephalhematoma does not cross suture lines (Fig. 18-4).

Next, the nurse observes the face and nose. The infant's face appears symmetrical both when crying and at rest. The nurse observes the face for forceps marks on the cheeks or jaw areas. The nurse may observe whitish pinhead-sized spots on and around the nose or on the chin. These tiny white papules, formed by plugged sebaceous glands, are called **milia**. They usually disappear within a few weeks. The nose appears midline and symmetrical in the normal newborn. Patency of the nostrils is assessed because newborns are obligatory nose breathers. Nasal patency can be determined by holding one naris shut at a time. A wisp from a cotton ball can be held up to the open nostril to detect air movement. A mirror also can be held under the open nostril to detect fogging from expired air. Nasal flaring is abnormal and a sign of respiratory distress (see Chapter 20).

Observation of the eyes includes noting placement, shape, and symmetry. The distance between the inner canthus of each eye is equal to the width of the eye itself. The eyes are normally clear and without red-

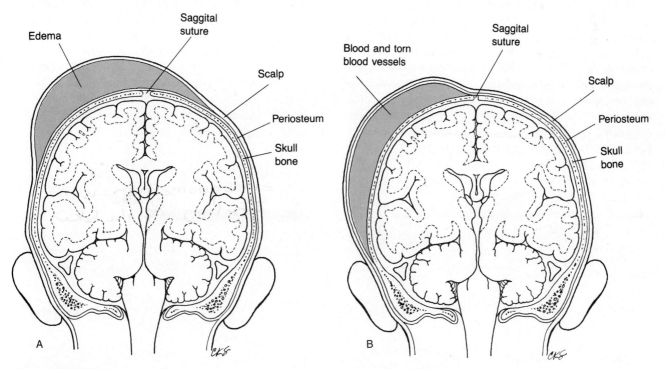

Figure 18-4. (A) *Caput succedaneum is swelling of the soft tissue of the scalp. Note that it crosses the suture line.* **(B)** *Cephalhematoma is bleeding that collects between the periosteum and the bone; it is confined by the periosteum and does not cross the suture line.*

ness or drainage. The eyelids may be slightly swollen from pressure during birth or after administration of eye drops.

The sclera are white to bluish white. Blue sclera are abnormal and associated with osteogenesis imperfecta, a rare inherited condition commonly called brittle bone disease. Scleral hemorrhages, or ruptured capillaries, occur from pressure during birth. These hemorrhages resolve within 2 to 3 weeks. The iris is initially slate blue, dark gray, or brown. Eye color is not final until approximately 6 months of age.

Other normal variants in the eye are strabismus and nystagmus. Strabismus is the appearance of crossed eyes. It is caused by muscular incoordination and improves as the muscle coordination matures. When the eyeball has rapid, involuntary, cyclical movements, it is called **nystagmus.** This can occur occasionally up to 3 to 4 months of age and is of no significance unless it continues beyond this time.

Ear formation is an indication of maturity. In the full-term newborn, the ear cartilage is firm. The pinna (external part of ear) is curved with ready recoil after folding. The auricular area (directly in front of the ear lobe) is observed for skin tags and sinus tracts. Ear position is assessed as shown in Figure 18-5.

Ear malformations may be associated with chromosomal abnormalities, kidney anomalies, or hearing loss. The nurse assesses hearing by observing how the neonate responds to noises. Early detection of hearing loss is important so early intervention can be initiated.

The newborn's mouth is midline and symmetrical. The lips, mucous membranes, and gums are pink and moist. The tongue is pink and midline. It should be proportional in size to the mouth. The hard and soft palates are visualized and palpated with a gloved finger. The palate is normally intact. There may be small white cysts present on the gums or hard palate. These are called Epstein's pearls and are normal. Occasionally, a tooth may be present. These are usually re-moved, especially if they are loose, since they pose a risk for aspiration.

Neck and Chest

After the head and face are carefully assessed, the physical examination continues with observation of the neck and chest. The neck is symmetrical, with full range of motion. Masses or enlarged lymph nodes are not normally present. The clavicles are gently palpated. They should appear symmetrical and smooth both to the touch and sight. If there is **crepitation** (crackling sound or sensation of fractured bone ends moving across one another) or asymmetry, the clavicle may be fractured from birth trauma.

The chest is normally round, symmetrical, and slightly smaller than the head. As described earlier, respirations are symmetrical, relaxed, and diaphragmatic (coming from the diaphragm) in nature. During normal respirations, the lower thorax pulls in, and the abdomen bulges out. The newborn is assessed for retractions. Retractions are the drawing in of the chest and can be substernal (below the sternum) or intercostal (between the ribs). Retractions normally may be seen immediately after birth. If they persist, they indicate respiratory distress (see Chapter 20).

The breasts are inspected. In the full-term newborn, the areolae are stippled (have small elevations) and raised. The breast tissue can be palpated and is approximately 1 cm in diameter. The breasts of both female and male newborns may be enlarged. They may have milky white discharge called "witch's milk." This is normal and results from the influence of maternal estrogen.

The nurse observes for the presence of accessory or supernumerary (more in number) nipples. These appear as small raised or pigmented areas that lie in vertical alignment below or above the true nipple. Accessory nipples may be associated with congenital anomalies.

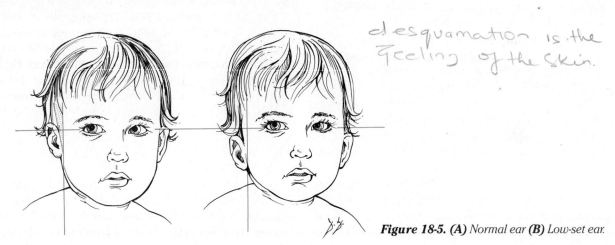

Figure 18-5. **(A)** *Normal ear* **(B)** *Low-set ear.*

Abdomen

Moving downward, the normal full-term newborn's abdomen appears slightly protuberant and symmetrical. It should not be distended or show signs of visible peristaltic waves or herniation. In some normal neonates, there may be visible bulging at the midline of the abdomen. As long as there is no hernia present, this is a normal finding. It is a gap between the rectus muscles called diastasis recti.

The umbilical cord is assessed during examination of the abdomen. Initially, the umbilical cord is white and gelatinous, with two arteries and one vein. The cord is normally free of oozing, redness, or foul odor. As the umbilical cord dries, it darkens and shrivels. Generally, it falls off within 10 to 14 days.

After observing the abdomen, the nurse auscultates for bowel sounds in all four quadrants. A good time to listen for bowel sounds is after the heart and lungs have been auscultated. Normal bowel sounds may be heard within 15 minutes after birth. They may not be present until up to 2 hours of age.

The nurse palpates all four quadrants of the abdomen after auscultation. Using the fingertips, the nurse moves through all four quadrants with shallow, gentle pressure. These movements then are repeated, using deeper palpation. The abdomen should be free of masses. The liver may be palpated in the right upper quadrant. It is normally approximately 1 to 2 cm below the right costal margin at the midclavicular line. The liver is firm and smooth to the touch and has a sharp, well-defined edge. The spleen is not normally palpable. The kidneys are difficult to palpate, especially the right kidney, which is covered by the liver.

Genitals

After the abdominal assessment, the nurse examines the genitals to determine the newborn's sex. The newborn should be further evaluated for ambiguous genitalia if the nurse has difficulty determining the sex. In the full-term female newborn, the labia majora (which may be edematous) completely cover the labia minora and clitoris. The vagina is open. There may be a small amount of whitish or bloody discharge present. **Pseudomenstruation** (false menstruation) is a normal finding and results from the influence of maternal estrogen. The female newborn's urethral meatus is located above the vaginal opening. Hymenal tags are commonly seen. These are small tags of tissue protruding from the vaginal opening.

The full-term male neonate's penis is straight. Average length is 2.8 to 4.3 cm (1–1.7 inches). The foreskin generally covers the entire glans. The urethral meatus is normally located at the tip of the glans and midline. The testes should be descended and can be palpated bilaterally in the scrotum. The scrotum is full with numerous rugae (ridges).

Most neonates void within the first 24 hours of life, often at or immediately after birth. The nurse must be alert for the first voiding and document and report it. If the newborn has not voided by 24 to 36 hours of age, the physician is notified. The first voidings may be scanty and infrequent. The frequency ranges from two to six times a day initially up to 20 times a day as intake increases, until bladder control is developed. The first voiding may be dark amber and cloudy, changing to straw colored, pale, and less concentrated as intake increases. The neonate total daily urine amount ranges from 15 to 60 mL/day.

Extremities

The nurse observes the neonate's arms and legs. Both arms and legs should appear symmetrical and in proportion to each other and to body size. There is full range of motion and symmetrical bilateral movement in the normal newborn. The radial, brachial, and femoral pulses are palpated bilaterally. They are strong and equal in the healthy newborn. If the femoral pulses are decreased or not equal to the upper extremity pulses, the physician is notified. The newborn needs to be evaluated further for congenital heart disease.

The hands and feet are normal in size. Each hand and foot normally has five fingers or toes. The fingers and toes have full range of motion. They are inspected for syndactyly (webbing of digits) and polydactyly (extra digits). Nails are present and extend to the tips of the digits. The nail beds are pink and have a capillary refill time equal to less than 3 seconds. Three creases running at an angle across the palm are normal. A single crease running across the palm is called a simian crease and is common in Down syndrome (see Chapter 20). The feet do not have creases on the soles and are flat at birth, until approximately 3 years of age. The leg and buttock creases are normally symmetrical. Asymmetrical leg length and buttock creases are associated with dislocation of the hip. The hips should be examined for dislocation using Ortolani's maneuver. Figure 18-6 shows how to perform this maneuver. The feet are inspected for club foot (talipes equinovarus), which is a common congenital deformity (see Chapter 20; Fig. 20-13).

Anus

The nurse turns the neonate to a prone position. The perianal area is visually inspected to confirm that the anus is present. Documentation of the first stool is very important. Meconium is passed from the anus

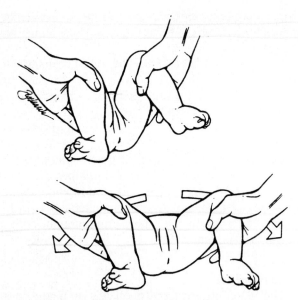

Figure 18-6. *Ortolani's maneuver. The neonate's legs are flexed and abducted laterally toward the bed. The examiner may feel a "click," which is called Ortolani's sign. This is a positive sign of congenital dislocation of the hip.*

by 24 hours of age in all but a small percentage of neonates. If the newborn has not passed meconium by 48 hours of age, the physician is notified. Some facilities may require that the physician is notified of the lack of a meconium stool after 24 hours so that further evaluation can be initiated.

Spine

The spinal column is normally straight and midline. There are no visible defects. Any dimples or hair tufts are documented. The entire length of the spine is palpated. The vertebrae in the normal newborn are intact without bulging. The newborn is free of pain during the palpation of the spine.

Behavioral Assessment

The behavioral assessment helps the nurse determine when the neonate is most accepting of outside stimulation and interaction with the family. The nurse shares this information with the newborn's family. The nurse observes the neonate's sleep and awake states, reflexes, sensory capabilities, and gestational age to understand the individual newborn.

General Behavior

There are six states of consciousness, ranging from deep sleep to vigorous crying. The full-term newborn makes frequent transitions from one state of consciousness to another. The transition from state to state should be smooth. Abrupt changes between sleep and awake states in a full-term newborn are abnormal. The newborn's cry is evaluated. It is normally vigorous and lusty, not high pitched or weak. Display 18-1 highlights the characteristics of the six states of consciousness in the newborn.

DISPLAY 18-1
Characteristics of States of Consciousness in the Newborn

Deep sleep:	Eyes closed; regular respirations; no eye movements; no spontaneous activity; external stimuli elicits a delayed startle response; state changes are unlikely
Light sleep:	Eyes closed; irregular respirations, rapid eye movements; random movements; sucking off and on; brief fussing or crying noises; external stimuli elicits a startle response and may elicit a state change
Drowsiness:	Eyes open and close and appear dull; eyelids flutter and appear heavy; variable activity; delayed response to external stimuli; will move back to sleep state or to a more alert state
Quiet alert:	Eyes open and bright; attention alert and focused, minimal movement; best state for interaction
Active alert:	Eyes open, less bright; less attentive; increased movement; fussy but consolable
Crying:	Intense crying with increased motor activity; color changes; often stimulation makes agitation worsen; infant may be able to console self, but likely to need assistance from others

Reflexes

The newborn's central nervous system is normally immature at birth. There are several newborn reflexes that are assessed, indicating neurological well-being. However, certain reflexes appear in all neonates. For example, all newborns smile, even if they are blind, and all infants tightly grasp objects placed in their palms. Most of the reflexes disappear during the first year of life. The most commonly discussed reflexes are rooting, sucking, grasp (palmar and plantar), Moro, startle, Babinski, step or dance, and tonic neck reflex.

Rooting Reflex

The rooting reflex is seen when the cheek is stroked and the newborn responds with a turn of the head toward the side that was touched. For example, when the mother places a hand on the neonate's cheek to turn the head toward the breast, the neonate turns instead toward her hand.

Sucking Reflex

The sucking reflex is so well developed at birth that health care personnel attending the birth may be startled by the loud sucking noises coming from the newborn. Newborns suck on almost anything that comes near their mouth in the first months of life.

Grasp Reflex (Palmar and Plantar)

Pressure on the palms of the hands or soles of the feet near the base of the digits causes flexion of hands and toes. The palmar grasp is so strong in a healthy newborn that the neonate can be lifted off the examining table (Fig. 18-7). The palmar grasp diminishes after 3 months; the plantar grasp persists until 9 to 12 months of age.

Moro's Reflex

Any sudden jarring or abrupt change in equilibrium elicits Moro's reflex in the normal newborn. It consists primarily of abduction and extension of arms. All digits extend except finger and thumb, which are flexed to form a C-shape (Fig. 18-8). If the response is not immediate, bilateral, and symmetric, possible injury to the brachial plexus, the humerus, or the clavicle may be present. Persistence of this reflex beyond 6 months of age may indicate brain damage.

Startle Reflex

Similar to Moro's reflex, the startle reflex follows any loud noise and consists of abduction of the arms and flexion of the elbows. Unlike in Moro's reflex, hands remain clenched. Absence of this reflex may indicate hearing impairment.

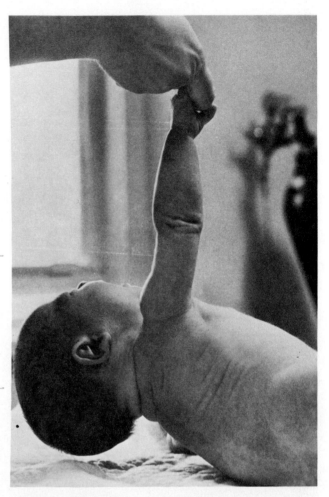

Figure 18-7. *Grasp reflex present in all normal newborns is sufficiently strong to lift them from the examining table. (Courtesy of Mead Johnson Laboratories, Evansville, IN.)*

Babinski's (Plantar) Reflex

When the lateral plantar surface of the neonate's foot is stroked, the toes flare open (Fig. 18-9). This usually disappears by the end of the first year. If it is found later in life, it is an indication of neurologic damage.

Step, or Dance, Reflex

Until 6 weeks of age, most normal infants when held in an upright position will make stepping movements (Fig. 18-10).

Tonic Neck Reflex

The tonic neck reflex, also called the fencing reflex, can be observed when the newborn lies on the back, with the head turned to one side, the arm and leg on the same side extended, and the opposite arm flexed as if in a fencing position (Fig. 18-11). Normally this reflex disappears between 3 to 4 months of age.

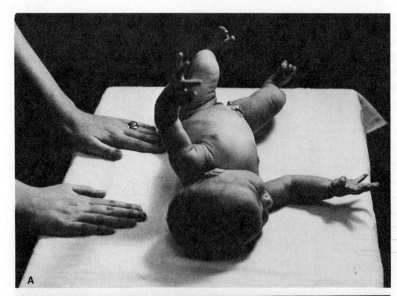

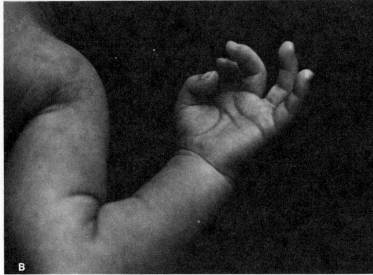

Figure 18-8. *Moro's reflex. Moro's reflex is elicited by sudden jarring or change in equilibrium. (**A**) Arms abduct at the shoulder and extend at the elbow. (**B**) All digits extend except the index finger and the thumb, which curve into a C-shape. (Courtesy of Mead Johnson Laboratories, Evansville, IN.)*

Sensory Behaviors

The newborn experiences the world by seeing, hearing, tasting, smelling, and touching. The family is eager to learn about ways to stimulate the newborn's senses as they interact with their baby. Although sensory stimulation may not increase intellectual performance of the newborn, it does promote the development of a well-rounded, well-balanced infant.

Vision

The normal full-term newborn sees objects without blurriness as long as the object is within the newborn's visual field. The newborn can see up to 9 to 12 inches away from the eyes and 30 degrees in either direction from the midline.

Faces, geometric figures, and moving objects are favorite sights for newborns. They like objects that have sharp contrast, such as big black dots on a white background or a black and white checkerboard.

Hearing

When the newborn hears a sound, heart rate increases, followed by a mild startle reflex. Newborns turn toward the sound. Within the first few days of life, the newborn discriminates the parents' voices from others. Preference for the mother's voice is observed.

Taste

The ability to taste is developed during pregnancy by the time the fetus is 20 weeks of age. Studies have shown that newborns prefer sweet fluids over salty solutions.

Palate should close 6 to 8 wks

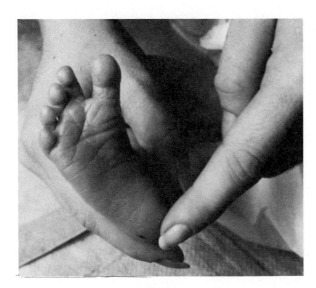

Figure 18-9. *Babinski's reflex.*

Smell

The neonate's sense of smell is highly sensitive. Studies have shown that newborns exhibit physiologic changes when exposed to strong odors. Changes in breathing patterns and activity levels have been documented. By 1 week of age, the neonate can recognize the mother's breast pad by her individual scent.

Touch

The newborn is very sensitive to touch. Tactile stimulation is important in the growth and development of the newborn. Gentle massage and stroking are soothing to the newborn. Skin-to-skin contact is a wonderful way to relax the newborn during feedings. The neonate also responds to painful stimuli.

Gestational Age

Tools have been designed to assess the newborn's physical and neurologic development to make an educated calculation of the neonate's gestational age. This can be important to determine if the newborn is preterm (born before 37 weeks' gestation), term (38 to 42 weeks' gestation), or postterm (greater than 42 weeks' gestation). This calculation also determines, then, if the neonate is small, average, or large for gestational age. Neonates who are preterm or postterm have special nursing needs.

There are two common tools that have been designed to assess gestational age. These are the Dubowitz and the Ballard scoring systems. The Ballard scoring system is a simplification of the Dubowitz system and is commonly used by nurses. Each facility determines the scoring system of choice. Gestational scoring is per-

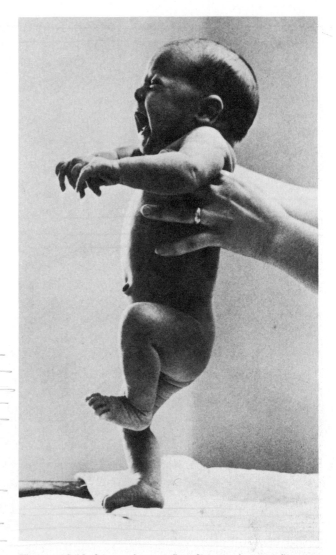

Figure 18-10. *Step or dance reflex. Step, or dance, reflex simulates walking when infant is held so that the sole of the foot touches examining table. (Courtesy of Mead Johnson Laboratories, Evansville, IN.)*

formed within the first few hours of birth and is repeated again at 24 hours after the neonate has neurologically settled somewhat. The Ballard scale is shown in Figure 18-12.

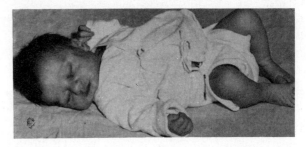

Figure 18-11. *Tonic neck reflex.*

Assessment Tool

Estimation of Gestational Age by Maturity Rating

NEUROMUSCULAR MATURITY

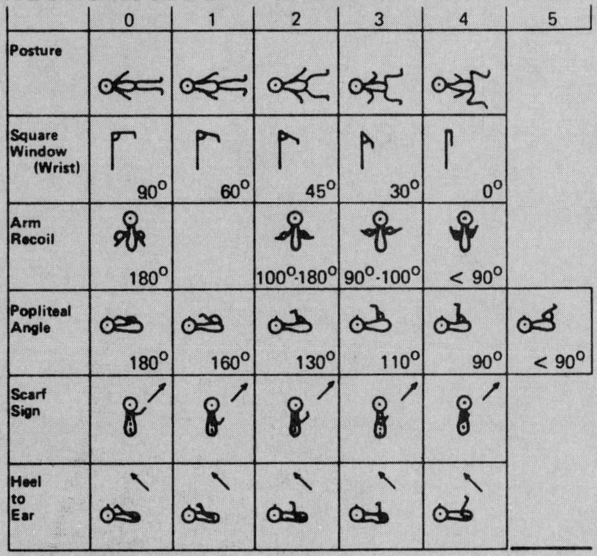

	0	1	2	3	4	5
Posture						
Square Window (Wrist)	90°	60°	45°	30°	0°	
Arm Recoil	180°		100°-180°	90°-100°	< 90°	
Popliteal Angle	180°	160°	130°	110°	90°	< 90°
Scarf Sign						
Heel to Ear						

PHYSICAL MATURITY

	0	1	2	3	4	5
SKIN	gelatinous red, trans-parent	smooth pink, visible veins	superficial peeling &/or rash, few veins	cracking pale area, rare veins	parchment, deep cracking, no vessels	leathery, cracked, wrinkled
LANUGO	none	abundant	thinning	bald areas	mostly bald	
PLANTAR CREASES	no crease	faint red marks	anterior transverse crease only	creases ant. 2/3	creases cover entire sole	
BREAST	barely percept.	flat areola, no bud	stippled areola, 1–2 mm bud	raised areola, 3–4 mm bud	full areola, 5–10 mm bud	
EAR	pinna flat, stays folded	sl. curved pinna, soft with slow recoil	well-curv. pinna, soft but ready recoil	formed & firm with instant recoil	thick cartilage, ear stiff	
GENITALS Male	scrotum empty, no rugae		testes descend-ing, few rugae	testes down, good rugae	testes pendulous, deep rugae	
GENITALS Female	prominent clitoris & labia minora		majora & minora equally prominent	majora large, minora small	clitoris & minora completely covered	

Gestation by Dates _____ wks

Birth Date _____ Hour _____ am/pm

APGAR _____ 1 min _____ 5 min

MATURITY RATING

Score	Wks
5	26
10	28
15	30
20	32
25	34
30	36
35	38
40	40
45	42
50	44

SCORING SECTION

	1st Exam=X	2nd Exam=O
Estimating Gest Age by Maturity Rating	_____ Weeks	_____ Weeks
Time of Exam	Date _____ Hour _____ am/pm	Date _____ Hour _____ am/pm
Age at Exam	_____ Hours	_____ Hours
Signature of Examiner	_____ M.D.	_____ M.D.

Scoring system from Ballard, J. L., et al. (1977). A simplified assessment of gestational age. Pediatric Research, 11, 374. Figures adapted from Sweet, A. Y. (1977). Classification of the low-birth-weight infant. In M. H. Klaus & A. A. Fanaroff (Eds.), Care of the high-risk infant. Philadelphia: WB Saunders.

Figure 18-12. *Ballard gestational age assessment tool. Scoring system from Ballard, J. L., et al. (1977). A simplified assessment of gestational age.* Pediatric Research, 11, 374. Figures *adapted from Sweet, A. Y. (1977). Classification of the low-birth-weight infant. In M. H. Klaus & A. A. Fanaroff (Eds.),* Care of the high-risk infant. *Philadelphia: WB Saunders.*

Dubrowitz and ballard are tools that assesses the gestational age of the baby.

Port Wine Nevi will not disappear
white spot on top of Nose
Muller

Routine Procedures

The nurse performs routine procedures on all neonates after birth. Some of the procedures are performed very soon after birth before the newborn leaves the birthing area. One of the primary concerns is keeping the newborn warm and dry. Identification of the neonate is completed before the newborn and mother are separated. Vitamin K administration and eye prophylaxis are also performed during this immediate time. Other laboratory tests, immunization, and general care are performed after the neonate is under the care of the nursery personnel. These procedures are covered in the following discussion.

Thermoregulation

The nurse keeps the neonate warm in one of several ways, depending on the practices of the facility. Chapter 17 explains the principles of heat loss and highlights measures to maintain thermoregulation in the neonate. In some facilities, the newborn may be placed in a pre-warmed, radiant warmer set on the servocontrol mode. In other facilities, the newborn is wrapped in several warmed blankets and placed in the bassinet under warming lights. The newborn is dry and usually is wearing a diaper and often a hat on arrival in the nursery. The temperature is taken in the axilla or by tympanic sensor every 30 minutes until it has stabilized for 2 hours. Once the temperature is stable, the newborn may be dressed and wrapped in blankets and placed in an open crib without an external heat source. The temperature is taken again 1 hour later and then every 2 to 4 hours per protocol. If the temperature falls below 36.4°C (97.5°F), the newborn should be placed under warming lights or in a radiant warmer and rewarmed gradually. Either hyperthermia or hypothermia can cause the newborn to experience increased metabolic requirements, which may lead to metabolic acidosis.

Identification

Identical identification bracelets are put on the mother and the neonate before they are separated in the birthing room. The identification bands and birth records are checked by the labor and birth nurse and the nursery nurse when the neonate is admitted to the nursery. This is a safety measure to verify that the numbers match. The identification bands (usually one on the arm and one on the leg) remain on the newborn during the entire stay. The baby's identification bands are matched with the mother's band each time the newborn is taken to her. This is practiced even in rooming-in settings. Some facilities place an identification band on the father or one other person of the mother's choosing. This allows another person to pick up the newborn from the nursery. It also serves as a safety measure against abduction. The neonate's footprints and the mother's thumb or finger prints are also taken before they are separated for identification purposes. The identical serial number of the mother's and newborn's bracelets is documented on the same record as the neonate's footprint and mother's fingerprints.

Before discharge, the mother is assisted in completing the birth certificate by someone authorized by the facility. It records the name of the mother, the father, and other statistical information used by the individual state's health department.

Administration of Vitamin K

Every newborn receives a single dose of vitamin K within 1 hour of birth. This injection prevents vitamin K–dependent hemorrhagic disease and coagulation disorders. The normal dose is 0.5 to 1.0 mg natural vitamin K (phytonadione). It is administered intramuscularly in the middle third of the vastus lateralis muscle.

Eye Prophylaxis

Crede prophylaxis is given at birth.

Prophylaxis against gonococcal ophthalmia neonatorum is required for all neonates. Infection in the newborn can result in blindness. Silver nitrate 1% (two drops in each eye) or ophthalmic ointment with 1% tetracycline or 0.05% erythromycin (1–2-cm ribbon in each eye) is recommended. Ophthalmic ointment may be preferred because it is less caustic to the eyes. Silver nitrate is the least expensive and appears to be the best agent for the penicillinase-producing *Neisseria gonorrhoeae*, although it causes more chemical conjunctivitis. Silver nitrate is not effective against *Chlamydia trachomatis*, another common cause of ophthalmic conjunctivitis. Erythromycin ointment is less expensive than tetracycline and is effective in the prevention of chlamydial conjunctivitis. The physician or nurse midwife prescribes the medication of choice.

The ophthalmic preparations are available in single-use containers. The nurse ensures the agent reaches all areas of the conjunctival sac. After instillation, the eyes are not irrigated. Excess medication may be wiped away with sterile cotton after 1 minute. Instillation of either agent is often delayed up to 1 hour after delivery to allow time for parent–newborn interaction.

Hepatitis B Vaccination

Recommendations by the Centers for Disease Control and Prevention and the American Academy of Pediatrics state that all infants need to receive the hepatitis B vaccination, regardless of the mother's HBsAg (hepatitis B surface antigen) status. The first vaccine is given within the first 12 hours of life. Subsequent doses are given at 1 to 2 months of age and again at 6 months of age. The recommended dosages are 0.5 mL (10 mg) for newborns of HBsAg-positive mothers and mothers with an unknown status, and 0.25 mL (5 mg) for HBsAg-negative mothers. If the mother is HBsAg positive, the newborn also receives HBIG (Hepatitis B immune globulin) 0.5 mL within the first 12 hours of life. Both Hepatitis B vaccine and HBIG are given intramuscularly, using the same procedure described for administering vitamin K.

Laboratory Tests and Newborn Screening

Laboratory tests are performed on umbilical cord blood to determine blood type and Rh, complete blood count, serology, and total bilirubin. The results of these tests are reported to the nursery nurse. The nursery nurse must be familiar with expected normal values and alert to abnormal results so that they are quickly brought to the attention of the physician. Tables 18-2 and 18-3 present the range of normal values. These laboratory tests are not repeated on the normal newborn but are evaluated and repeated if any fall outside of the normal range.

State laws mandate screening of neonates for inborn errors of metabolism. Each state has a protocol for screening and reporting the results. As a minimum, newborns are screened for phenylketonuria (PKU) and congenital hypothyroidism. Additionally, some states screen for hemoglobinopathies, including sickle cell disease, and metabolic disorders, including galactosemia and maple syrup urine disease. See Chapter 20 for further discussion.

A heel stick blood sample is obtained from the newborn before discharge (Fig. 18-13). Screening is repeated for PKU no later than 3 weeks of age if there is question about the validity of the results of the first test. It is important to obtain the blood sample for PKU after the newborn has fed for 24 hours. The level of phenyl-

Table 18-3. Normal Neonatal Values: Total Bilirubin

Age	Preterm (mg/dL)	Full Term (mg/dL)
Cord	<2	<2
0–1 day	<8	<6
1–2 day	<12	<8
2–5 day	<16	<12

Adapted from May, K. A. & Mahlmeister, L. R. (1994). *Maternal & neonatal care: Family-centered care* (3rd ed.). Philadelphia: J. B. Lippincott, Table B-2, p. 1110.

alanine begins to increase after feedings have been started. Most affected newborns are detected 24 hours after adequate protein intake.

Daily Care

The nurse performs a detailed physical assessment at least once a shift. Vital signs may be taken more than once a shift, depending on the neonate's status and facility protocol. The assessment includes general appearance, skin color, and behavior. Abnormal findings may indicate the need for a more detailed assessment. At this time, the nurse also assesses the umbilical cord and circumcision for signs of infection or hemorrhage.

The nurse carefully monitors the neonate's fluid intake, including the type and amount of feeding. Breastfeeding is recorded according to how long and how vigorously the newborn suckles on each breast. Recording of formula feedings includes the amount in milliliters or ounces. The nurse assesses the newborn's sucking ability and tolerance of feedings.

All output, urine, stools, and emesis is accurately documented. The amount and character of the emesis is recorded. It is not unusual for neonates to regurgitate after a feeding because of an immature cardiac sphincter. The nurse must be able to differentiate between vomiting and regurgitation. Regurgitation usually is simply relieving an overflow of the stomach. Conversely,

Table 18-2. Normal Neonate Values: Complete Blood Count

Age	Hemoglobin (g/dL)	Hematocrit (%)	MCV (fl)	WBC ($10^3/mm^3$)	Neutrophils (%)	Lymphocytes (%)	Platelets ($10^3/mm^3$)
Birth	13.5–21	42–65	100–140	9–30	60	30	100–300
1 week	13.5–21	42–65	95–125	5–21	40	50	100–300
1 month	10–16	30–48	85–125	5–21	35	50	100–300

Adapted from May, K. A. & Mahlmeister, L. R. (1994). *Maternal & neonatal care: Family-centered care* (3rd ed.). Philadelphia: J. B. Lippincott, Table B-1, p. 1110.

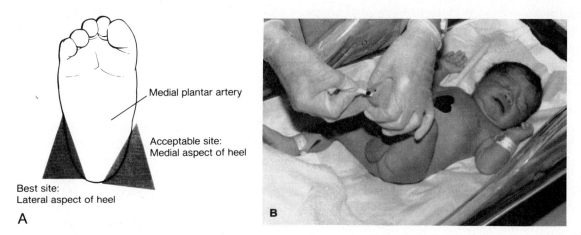

Medial plantar artery

Acceptable site:
Medial aspect of heel

Best site:
Lateral aspect of heel

A

B

Figure 18-13. *Heelstick procedure. The heelstick procedure is used to perform several blood tests. (A) Appropriate sites for the heelstick are illustrated. (B) A microlancet is used to puncture the heel. After elimination of the first drop of blood, the nurse collects the specimen.*

vomiting can occur at any time, can be projectile in nature, and may deplete the neonate's body fluids and electrolytes.

The stools are described according to their consistency. During the first day of life, the stools are meconium. The stools change from greenish-brown to yellowish-brown. They become less sticky and may contain some milk curds. These are called transitional stools and occur usually during days 2 to 3. After the transitional stools, the stools change according to whether the newborn is breast or bottle fed. A breast-fed baby's stools are golden-yellow, loose to mushy, and have a sweet-type odor. The formula-fed baby's stools are pale yellow to light brown, firmer, and may have a slightly foul odor.

The nurse is responsible for assessing the family's knowledge of infant care, their coping behaviors when caring for their newborn, and the interactions between the family and their baby. After the assessment, the nurse implements an individualized teaching plan for the family. (See Family Teaching Checklist.)

Physiologic Jaundice Screening

When observing skin color of the neonate, the nurse carefully assesses the neonate for signs of jaundice. Physiologic jaundice, which occurs in approximately half of all full-term neonates, is also called **icterus neonatorum**. Physiologic jaundice occurs after the first 24 hours of life. It usually is the result of inadequate fluids to flush the direct water-soluble bilirubin from the neonate's body. Increased fluid intake helps to ease this condition. The nurse observes the color of the neonate's sclera to determine if there seems to be an increase of jaundice. If the neonate's sclera appears

more yellow than previously, a microbilirubin may be performed. It is performed by a heel stick, described earlier. Normal values are found in Table 18-3. If the microbilirubin is elevated, the infant may undergo phototherapy (see Chapter 20).

Infection Prevention

Infection prevention is an area of prime concern for nurses. Universal precautions are essential in caring for all childbearing women and their babies. Display 18-2 describes when protective gloves are worn by the nurse. It is best to remember, when in doubt, glove.

Most nursery nurses change into scrub suits or dresses when they come to work. The scrub clothes are short sleeved to allow handwashing up to the elbows. In some nurseries, all personnel and visitors who have contact with neonates are expected to put on cover gowns and follow handwashing protocols. This is especially true for any individuals planning to touch the newborn. When the nurse leaves the nursery or maternal-newborn area, it is important to cover the scrub clothes with a lab coat or cover gown. This protects the scrub clothes from microorganisms in other areas of the health care facility. The cover is removed before reentering the nursery and handwashing is performed.

Handwashing

Handwashing is the single most important method of infection prevention in the newborn nursery. At the beginning of a shift, all personnel should wash their hands and arms up to the elbows with antiseptic preparation according to the protocol of the facility. Rings and watches are removed before handwashing. A 15-second handwash, using an antiseptic preparation and vigorous friction, takes place before and after contact with each newborn. Bacterial organisms can be transmitted from one newborn to another by the caregiver. Handwashing is necessary before performing an invasive procedure and after touching an object or surface that may be contaminated. This includes hair, face, clothing, diapers, equipment, and the telephone. In addition, the nurse washes before feedings, after diaper changes, and between handling babies.

Newborn Skin Integrity

After the neonate's temperature has stabilized, the nurse administers the first bath. It is best to obtain single-use containers of any agent that comes in direct contact with the neonate's skin. If single-use containers are not available, each neonate should have private supplies. Sterile cotton sponges or soft, disposable wipes are ideal when caring for the newborn's skin. Gauze can tear and break the neonate's fragile skin. Plain warm water or warm water with mild nonmedicated soap may be used. After the initial bath, the buttocks and perianal areas are cleaned during each diaper change (refer to Bathing and Diapering sections).

Cord Care

The umbilicus is an open site that is highly susceptible to infection. It should be assessed daily for signs of infection. Foul odor, oozing, or redness at the cord's base may indicate infection. The umbilicus is also assessed for signs of bleeding. The cord is kept clean and dry. The diaper is folded down below and the shirt up above the umbilicus to provide air circulation.

Current methods, determined by provider preference or facility protocol, include the local application of triple dye, an antimicrobial agent such as bacitracin, or alcohol. These agents promote drying or provide an antimicrobial effect. To facilitate drying, the cord may be cleansed with a cotton ball and alcohol after each diaper change and bathing. The cord clamp is removed when the neonate is 24 hours old. Before the clamp is removed, the cord stump is inspected to make certain that it is dry. Cord clamp cutters are used to remove the plastic cord clamp. After the clamp is removed, the cord stump is treated with an application of the preferred agent of the facility.

Circumcision Care

At one time, circumcisions were done almost routinely on all male neonates. However, circumcision has become controversial in more recent years.

Parents should be thoroughly informed by the physician about both the risks and the benefits of the procedure (Table 18-4). Circumcision of the newborn male is performed frequently for religious reasons, most notably by those of Jewish faith. Circumcision does prevent the accumulation of the secretions collectively called *smegma*. If the foreskin of the newborn male is so tight (**phimosis**) that it obstructs the urinary system, circumcision is performed at once.

Circumcision is performed by the Gomco (Yellen) clamp method or the Plastibell method. The choice of the physician determines the method used. A surgical consent is required before the procedure is performed. The neonate is not fed for several hours before the procedure to eliminate the danger of aspiration. The neonate is placed on a molded plastic restraining board with his arms and legs restrained by Velcro straps. A heat source should be available to protect the neonate from cold stress. The neonate may wear a shirt, but the diaper is removed. The nurse assists the physician as needed. Some physicians use a local anesthetic to de-

Table 18-4. *Advantages and Disadvantages of Neonatal Circumcision*

Advantages	Disadvantages
Prevention of	Complications of
Penile cancer	Hemorrhage
Inflammation of glans and prepuce	Infection
Complications of later circumcision	Dehiscence
Possible decrease of	Meatitis from loss of protective foreskin
Urinary tract infections in males	Adhesions
Sexually transmitted disease	Concealed penis
Preserves male body image	Urethral fistula
To be same as circumcised father or peers	Meatal stenosis
when older	Pain at time of procedure

Marks, M. G. (1994). *Broadribb's introductory pediatric nursing* (4th ed.). Philadelphia: J. B. Lippincott, Table 5-3, p. 90.

crease the pain of the surgery. After the procedure is completed, the nurse comforts the neonate and observes the surgical site for bleeding. When the clamp has been used, sterile petroleum jelly gauze or an antibiotic ointment is applied to the glans according to the physician's preference. If the Plastibell is used, nothing is applied. The Plastibell ring falls off in 7 to 10 days. The nurse observes the site for bleeding every 15 minutes for the first hour, then every 30 minutes for the next several hours. The first voiding after circumcision is documented. When used, the sterile petroleum jelly gauze or ointment is reapplied with each diaper change. After the first 24 hours, plain petroleum jelly may be substituted for the sterile petroleum jelly gauze. The nurse continues to observe the site for bleeding and signs of infection. The nurse teaches the family circumcision care (discussed later in this chapter).

◆ *Health Promotion*

According to the American Academy of Pediatrics, injuries caused by accidents result in one million children needing medical care each year. Of those children, 40,000 to 50,000 suffer permanent damage, and 4000 die. These statistics are sobering. Nurses are in a key position to advocate for health promotion and accident prevention. Nurses also must advocate immunizations for the infant. A pediatric nursing text, such as Broadribb's *Introductory Pediatric Nursing*, Fourth Edition, by Margaret G. Marks, includes a complete discussion of immunization requirements.

Safety

The nurse teaches the family about safety. Simple instructions that the family can understand may save a life. Preventing accidental injuries can be accomplished with little effort. Families need to learn about measures such as safe positioning, use of an infant car seat, abuse prevention, aspirations, scaldings and burns, falls, electric shock, suffocation, poisoning, and cardiopulmonary resuscitation (CPR).

Positioning

Over the years, families have been taught to avoid placing their infants in a supine position to sleep. However, new evidence from studies about sudden infant death syndrome (SIDS) indicates that many infants with SIDS have been found in a prone sleeping position. Therefore, a high relationship between a prone position and SIDS appears to exist. As a result, current recommendations are to maintain the infant in a side-lying position for sleeping until they are 6 months old. The nurse can teach the family to prop the back and abdomen of the infant to help maintain the side-lying position. These must be placed so that there is no danger that the infant's nose and mouth are blocked by the supports.

Infant Car Seat

The newborn or infant must be secured in a federally approved car seat in most states. The newborn leaves the hospital in the car seat. The infant car seat is placed on the seat, preferably the back seat, facing the rear of the car. The seat belt should be in the correct place to secure the car seat. The infant needs to be snugly buckled into the car seat with the harness and straps provided. The nurse teaches the family the importance of never traveling in a vehicle without placing the infant securely in the car seat.

Accident Prevention

The nurse reviews safety practices with the family. Common sense and sound judgment are key to protecting the newborn. The newborn or infant should never be left alone on a bed, changing table, or sofa. It is easy for the infant to scoot, wiggle, roll, or fall. The infant should never be left alone in the house or car. The infant is unable to move from a dangerous environment or situation. An adult must always be responsible for the newborn. The tub can pose a major hazard for drowning or burns. The infant is never left alone in a tub or without an adult present. Many families fall into the habit of giving their infant a bedtime bottle. The nurse teaches the family the danger of aspiration when bottles are propped. In addition, a bedtime bottle can cause otitis media (middle ear infections) or bottle mouth caries in an older infant.

Abuse Prevention

Child abuse is a social problem that may occur in any family regardless of race, income, or education. Physical abuse is one of the more common forms of child abuse. Being a parent can be difficult and stressful. Families need to learn techniques for dealing with their frustration and anger. The nurse teaches families to recognize their anger and to remove themselves from the situation. There are many support groups in the community. There are 24-hour hotlines to call if a family member needs support. Sexual abuse frequently is committed by a family member or close acquaintance. Careful observations and immediate action in the case of any suspicion are the best methods to prevent sexual abuse of the infant. The family member who becomes suspicious of possible sexual abuse of the infant must immediately take the infant to the infant's primary health care provider to discuss these concerns.

Cigarette smoking in the presence of an infant is a form of abuse. Secondhand smoke is harmful. It doubles the risk for respiratory illnesses. Smoking around an infant must be avoided.

CPR Classes

It is highly recommended that all families learn basic CPR. Courses are provided by the American Red Cross or the American Heart Association. It is important for the nurse to stress to the family that CPR can save their child's life if an accident occurs. The family may want to post the instructions for CPR and choking techniques in a visible place in the home. Child care providers and babysitters need to be prepared to handle an emergency in the absence of the family members.

Feeding and Nutrition

Most women decide whether to breast-feed or bottle-feed their newborn before childbirth. For those who are undecided, it is important to provide facts to allow them to make sound decisions. Display 18-3 highlights the advantages and disadvantages of breast- and bottle-feeding. Some supplements may be needed in either type of feeding. Supplements recommended for breast-fed infants are vitamin D, vitamin K, iron, and fluoride. The infant has iron stores at birth, but by approximately 4 months of age the infant has used all those iron stores. Iron must be provided by supplements or iron-enriched infant cereals. Vitamins D and K are also essential for the infant's healthy development and are not available in adequate amounts in breast milk. Fluoride, needed for development of tooth enamel, is available in most public drinking water. Fluoride is present in breast milk if the mother drinks fluoridated water. However, many families use bottled water or have well water as their source of drinking water. Therefore, a supplement of fluoride is desirable. Most formulas provide the vitamins needed for healthy infant development. Iron-enriched formulas are available, which the infant needs by the age of 4 months. Many neonates are started on the iron-enriched formulas at birth. As for fluoride, if the formula is being prepared with fluoride-enriched public drinking water, the infant's needs are being met. However, if ready-to-use formula is used or the formula is prepared with bottled water, the infant needs supplements of fluoride. Fluoride preparations are available and are administered in drop form twice a day.

The Women Infants Children (WIC) food program is a special supplemental food program for pregnant, breast-feeding, or postpartum women, infants, and children up to 5 years of age. There is no cost to any who are determined eligible, and the family's food stamp benefits or schoolchildren's breakfast and lunch program benefits are not affected. Many hospital nurseries currently give WIC information to eligible mothers at prenatal visits or at the time of childbirth to encourage the use of WIC services.

Breast-feeding

Colostrum is the first milk that is produced from early pregnancy to several days after birth. It is a thick, yellow, creamy fluid. Colostrum contains higher levels of antibodies, protein, minerals, and fat-soluble vitamins. After 2 to 4 days, colostrum is replaced by transitional milk. This milk is produced until approximately 2 weeks postpartum. The transitional milk provides more calories than colostrum. It is also higher in fat, lactose, and water-soluble vitamins.

DISPLAY 18-3
Advantages and Disadvantages of Breast- and Bottle-Feeding

Breast-Feeding

Advantages

Provides all nutrients plus valuable antibodies easily digested

Cost-effective, no preparation

Always available and at the proper temperature

Emotionally satisfying

Increases maternal confidence in nurturing abilities

Promotes development of facial muscles, jaw, and teeth

Aids in uterine involution

Reduces incidence of allergies

Disadvantages

No one can nurse the newborn but the mother; other family members may feel left out

For working mothers, pumping is time consuming

Mother must be careful about her diet and medications

Bottle-Feeding

Advantages

All family members can participate in feeding

Frees mother from being on call 24 hours a day

Know exactly how much the newborn is eating

No worry about mother's diet and medication

Takes longer to digest so infants eat less often

Disadvantages

Does not supply antibodies found in human milk

Costly

Takes time to prepare bottles and formula

Requires cleanliness of hands, water, and equipment

Requires adequate refrigeration and storage

Mature milk is generally produced by 2 weeks postpartum. It has a high water content, causing the breast milk to look thin. The mature milk typically appears bluish in color. The mother must be alert for signs of dehydration in the infant, such as poor skin turgor, sunken fontanelles, and a decrease in voidings. She must consult with the health care provider immediately if the infant shows any signs of dehydration.

Initiating Feeding

The best time to initiate breast-feeding is during the first period of reactivity when the newborn is awake and alert. The mother is taught to wash her hands before touching the breast. Contact with breast milk requires the nurse to wear gloves.

Initially, the newborn is limited to 5 to 10 minutes on the first breast, increasing to a maximum of 15 minutes. The mother does not need to limit the time the newborn nurses on the second breast. Feedings are "on demand"; the newborn sets the frequency of feedings. To prevent sore nipples, the mother is instructed to vary positions during breast-feeding sessions. This changes the area of the areola and nipple in the newborn's mouth. The mother is taught to use her fingertip in the corner of the mouth to release the suction before ending each feeding. The breast-feeding mother may appreciate a referral to the La Leche League. The La Leche League is an international organization support group for breast-feeding women. Many communities have local 24-hour hotlines through which a mother can contact a member for support with breast-feeding problems. Some facilities employ a lactation educator or consultant who can consult with the mother to assist her in adjusting to and solving breast-feeding problems.

Positioning

The mother and newborn can try several positions as they practice breast-feeding. The mother may prefer to lie on her side with the newborn beside her. This position is especially helpful for the mother who is nursing immediately after childbirth. The mother may prefer to sit up. In the sitting position, the newborn is cradled at breast level. After cesarean birth, the mother may wish to use the "football hold." The newborn lies facing the mother, tucked into her side. The newborn's head is supported with the mother's hand and the body with her arm. Figure 18-14 shows pictures of the common breast-feeding positions.

Once the newborn is properly positioned, the mother holds her breast using the C-hold (see Fig. 18-14C). This is done by supporting the breast from below with the fingers and placing the thumb on top of the breast above the areola. Next, the mother slightly compresses the breast and strokes the newborn's cheek or tickles the mouth with her nipple. This stimulates the rooting reflex. The newborn opens the mouth widely and turns toward the breast. The mother guides the nipple into the newborn's mouth, pulling the baby close to her. This encourages the newborn to place part of the areola into the mouth, resulting in proper "latching on" and complete emptying of the breast. The nurse reminds the mother to gently compress the breast away from the newborn's nares. Newborns are obligatory nose breathers, and they will stop sucking if the nose is not free to provide an open airway. The infant is burped every 5 minutes or so during the feeding.

The infant can be held on the shoulder, laid in a prone position over the lap, or sitting in the lap with one hand supporting and rubbing the back while the other hand supports the infant's chest and the chin is held between the caregiver's thumb and forefinger. Both breasts are used at each feeding. The mother should alternate the starting breast each time. A safety pin can be placed on the bra strap to keep track of which breast to use. When breasts are emptied at a feeding, they refill for the next feeding. If the breast is only half emptied, it only needs to half fill for the next feeding. As this occurs, the breast produces less and less milk.

Chapter 15 discusses nutritional needs of the breast-feeding woman. Many medications taken by the mother during breast-feeding are secreted in breast milk. This occurs in varying amounts and is sometimes accumulative. Research needs to be continued in this area of information. The mother is best advised to avoid taking any medication, including over-the-counter drugs, unless specifically approved by her health care provider.

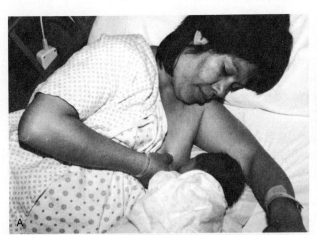

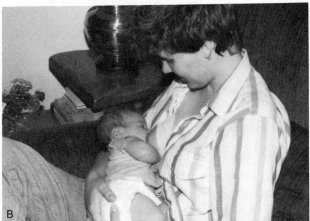

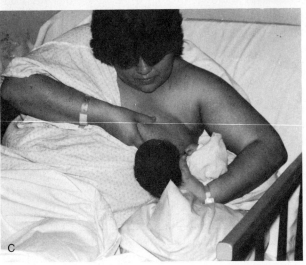

Figure 18-14. *Breastfeeding positions. **(A)** Side lying. The mother who breast-feeds her newborn while lying down turns her baby toward her and curves her arm around the baby. **(B)** Sitting. The mother may prefer to assume a sitting position while nursing. She should prop her feet or legs so she is comfortable and can comfortably hold the baby. **(C)** Football hold. The mother may position the newborn in a football hold. The baby is supported by a pillow. The side rail is up for added security.*

Bottle-feeding

Parents need to be assured that both breast milk and commercially prepared formula provide adequate nutrition for the growing infant. The health care provider selects the formula based on the individual needs of the newborn. Preparing the formula is a skill easily taught by the nurse. The nurse teaches the family to wash their hands before preparing formula and feeding the newborn. This reduces the risk of contamination and infection.

Types of Formulas

There are three major types of formula: cow's milk–based formula, soy-based formula, and predigested formula. Most newborns tolerate cow's milk–based formulas fortified with iron. These formulas contain lactose as the added carbohydrate. Some newborns are allergic to cow's milk or have difficulty digesting lactose. These infants are typically changed to a soy-based formula. It contains soy protein instead of cow's milk protein. The soy formula has glucose polymers or sucrose added instead of lactose. Predigested formulas are reserved for infants who do not tolerate either cow's milk or soy-based formulas. The infant's health care provider supervises the use of predigested formulas.

Formula and Bottle Preparation

Formula is available in different forms: ready-to-feed liquid, liquid concentrate, or powder. Powder is the least expensive preparation, and ready-to-feed liquid is the most expensive. The family is instructed that it is important to follow the manufacturer's preparation instructions. If the formula is incorrectly mixed, the infant faces risks. When the formula is too concentrated (too little water), diarrhea and electrolyte imbalance may occur. When the formula is too weak, the infant receives inadequate calories and nutrients. This results in dehydration and inadequate growth.

Formula prepared in advance may be refrigerated for up to 48 hours. It should not remain at room temperature for longer than 4 hours before it is discarded. Each bottle should be prepared with the amount the infant is expected to take at a feeding. The feeding should be completed within 30 minutes. The prepared bottle should not be unrefrigerated for more than an hour. It should be discarded if it is not used by the end of the hour. Formula can be given at room temperature or it may be warmed. The nurse warns the family that bottles must never be warmed in the microwave. There is great danger of the bottle exploding, causing burns. In addition, the internal temperature of the formula may be too hot and burn the newborn's mouth and gastrointestinal tract.

Bottles are available in glass, plastic, and plastic with disposable liners. Several types of nipples are also available. Some nipples even come color coded to be used with milk, water, or juice. The family can determine which type they wish to use. Often cost is the guiding factor. Regardless of the type used, the pieces that are reused should be thoroughly cleaned after each use. If the family's water is chlorinated, the bottles and nipples may be placed in the dishwasher. They may also be washed with dishwashing detergent and hot water. If the family has nonchlorinated or well water, the bottles and nipples should be washed with dishwashing detergent and water. Bottles are then placed in boiling water for 5 to 10 minutes.

Positioning

The bottle-fed newborn needs to be held closely during feeding in the same way that the breast-feeding newborn is. The neonate is cradled in a semi-upright position, supporting the neck and head. The nurse instructs the family to avoid feeding the infant who is lying down. This increases the risk of aspiration. It also allows the milk to flow into the middle ear, which may cause an ear infection. The nurse teaches the family to hold the bottle at an angle that fills the nipple and prevents air from being swallowed. The caregiver strokes the nipple on the newborn's cheek to stimulate the rooting reflex. Similar to breast-feeding, the newborn naturally turns and opens the mouth. The nipple is placed completely in the mouth. The newborn eats 2 to 3 ounces of formula every 3 to 4 hours. The nurse teaches the family that burping for the bottle-fed infant is done every 5 minutes or every 15 mL (0.5 oz.), following the same methods that are described earlier for the breast-fed infant.

After the feeding, the breast-fed or bottle-fed infant is positioned on the right side, with the back supported. This decreases the probability of regurgitation, because gravity places the milk or formula toward the distal end of the stomach away from the cardiac sphincter. The side-lying position is also the best for drainage of any regurgitated material.

Parent–Newborn Interaction

Parent–newborn interaction and attachment is the tie or bond that forms between the newborn and each parent. The nurse plays an important role in facilitating the attachment process, which influences the future relationship between parents and their children. The process is affected by many factors, among them the mother's physical and emotional condition after labor, the infant's condition and behavior, and the comparison of the real infant with the "fantasy" infant that the mother has imagined throughout her pregnancy. This imaginary baby is likely quite different from the real infant the family meets soon after birth.

At first sight, the newborn does not present the chubby, well-formed baby pictured by the world in general. The head is large in proportion to the body and may be misshapen by the birth process. Blood and vernix still cling to the body, and the neonate probably is crying. The newborn may appear completely self-centered and displeased over this abrupt introduction to the world. It is important that the family understands that each infant is unique, with individual characteristics and developmental potential. Studies have shown that pointing out to the family their infant's unique characteristics can help develop a more positive attitude, reduce feeding and sleeping problems, and bring about greater activity and alertness in the infant. The nurse encourages family members to hold, cuddle, inspect, and feed the newborn as early and often as possible. By pointing out normal newborn reflexes, such as the grasp, the nurse plays a significant role in parent–newborn bonding. The psychosocial task of the infant is to develop trust. A secure loving environment helps the newborn to begin to develop that sense of trust.

Family Teaching

Nurses are instrumental in teaching the family how to care for their newborn. One-on-one teaching and small group settings are ideal for instruction in infant care. Many videos and pamphlets are available to assist with the teaching. Teaching needs to consider includes the learners' needs, the learners' level of comprehension, and any language barriers. The nurse also must evaluate the learner's understanding of the material that is presented to clarify and amplify information as needed. The Family Teaching Checklist provides a quick reference for topics and skills discussed with the family before discharge.

Providing a Safe Environment

The family needs to understand that it is important to support the newborn's head at all times. The head is large in comparison with the rest of the body. Neck muscles are unable to hold the head up at this age. Therefore, the newborn depends on the caregivers to protect the head.

The nurse stresses to the family that they must never leave the newborn unattended on elevated surfaces such as a bed, couch, or changing table. The infant can easily roll or fall off surfaces. If the infant is placed in a

---

✔ FAMILY TEACHING CHECKLIST

Care of the Normal Newborn

The nurse includes the following topics in family teaching to promote health and well-being:

Car-seat use

Safe environment

Feeding and nutrition

Clothing

Activity and rest

Behavioral characteristics

General hygiene and bathing

Elimination and diapering

Cord and circumcision care

Nasal and oral suctioning

Temperature assessment

Medication administration

Signs and symptoms of illness

Follow-up visits

---

carrier or swing, the seat belt should always be securely fastened, and the carrier must not be left on an elevated surface. Families with other young children must be advised that the infant should never be left alone in the company of young siblings. In addition, families with pets must be alerted to the possibility of aggressive behavior by the pet toward the infant. The animal may see this new being as a challenge to the pet's position in the family's affections. Pet's have been known to be attracted to an infant by the smell of milk. These are dangers which can be easily avoided. The family must become aware of the infant's changing abilities and expand their safety practices to meet the child's development.

Clothing

Clothing for the newborn should be appropriate for the weather. A good rule of thumb is to dress the infant in about the same amount of clothing that the caregiver finds comfortable. In hot weather, a shirt and diaper may be sufficient. The nurse should advise the family to avoid exposing the infant to direct sunlight for any length of time. The infant's skin must be protected from the strong, direct sun. A hat is needed in sunlight. In cold weather, the infant's head should be covered with a cap or close-fitting hood. Dressing the infant in layers allows the caregiver to add or remove clothing based on the infant's needs.

Clothing, diapers, and blankets for the infant must be laundered regularly in moderately warm water and mild nondetergent soap. The clothing must be thoroughly rinsed to remove any soap residue. Two rinsings are recommended, especially for diapers. The nurse advises the family to avoid detergents and laundry softeners because they may cause skin irritation in the infant.

During the first few weeks of life, the newborn may prefer to be swaddled. Being snug in a blanket provides a sense of security. Figure 18-15 presents the technique and directions for swaddling an infant.

Activity and Rest

Most newborns sleep for much of the time. The total amount of sleep time can vary from 15 to 20 hours a day during the first 3 months of life. The infant will settle into a routine of quiet, alert, and fussy periods during the day. Nighttime sleeping usually is interrupted every 2 to 4 hours for hunger pains in the early months. The infant may cry for a total of up to 2 hours a day and be within normal limits. The nurse advises the family that the infant has no other means of communication at this stage of development. The infant whose cries are met with comfort develops a feeling of trust.

Behavioral Characteristics

Each newborn has its own individual personality. The family needs to learn to interact with the newborn during times of alert behavior. They also need to be able to identify the behaviors that indicate overstimulation so that they let the infant rest. Some behaviors that indicate overstimulation are stiffening or arching of the body, averting gaze, sudden color change, hiccups, facial grimace, and fussing. When these behaviors occur, the infant is usually sending the message that enough is enough.

The nurse can teach the family that talking, singing, cooing to, and cuddling the infant are important means of stimulation. The infant does not need expensive toys and equipment for stimulation. Newborns react positively to human faces. They also respond to black geometric figures on a white background. Skin-to-skin contact is especially appreciated by the newborn. Stroking and resting bare skin to bare skin against a parent are excellent ways to promote touch. Infants also respond to rocking. Rocking an infant while talking or singing softly is a rewarding experience for both baby and parent.

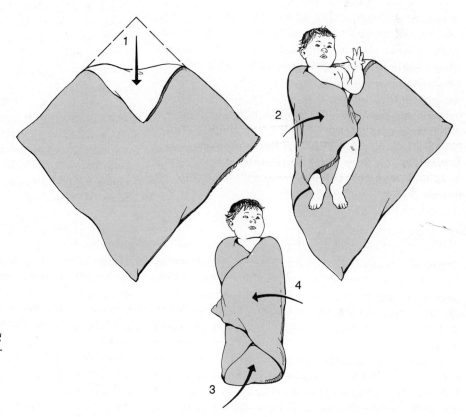

Figure 18-15. Technique for swaddling the newborn. Swaddling an infant. 1. Fold down top corner of blanket and place infant on blanket with neck near fold; 2. Bring corner of blanket around from infant's right side and tuck under left side; 3. Bring bottom corner up to chest 4. Bring remaining corner around and tuck under right side. Wrap securely, but not too tightly—leave some room for infant to move.

General Hygiene

The general hygiene needs of the newborn are an important aspect of family teaching. The nurse has a responsibility to carefully teach the family, making certain that they understand the principles involved, and that all questions and apprehensions are addressed.

Bathing

Newborns do not need complete baths every day. A sponge bath every other day is sufficient until the umbilical cord falls off. Once the umbilicus has healed, the newborn may be given a tub bath. However, the face and neck are cleaned daily, and the diaper area must be well cleansed after every diaper change. The newborn is dressed in clean clothes every day.

The nurse teaches the bath procedure. Family members are instructed to gather necessary supplies before starting the bath. The infant should never be left unattended in the tub. The bath water should be warm, not hot. Water temperature is assessed on the inside of the caregiver's wrist. It should be comfortable to the wrist, neither hot or cool. A mild nonperfumed, nondeodorant soap is recommended for bathing. When giving a sponge bath, the eyes and ears are cleansed first. This can be done with a clean cotton ball or the corner of a clean washcloth and plain water, no soap. Each eye is wiped with clear water from the inner canthus to the outer canthus (the nose side to the ear side of the eye). A new cotton ball or area of the cloth is used for the other eye or if the eye needs to be wiped again. The external part of the ears are wiped next, again with a clean cotton ball of clean area of the cloth. Care is taken to remove any crusting of milk or formula which may have dribbled into the ear. Nothing is put into the infant's ear. Next wash the face while the washcloth is still free of soap. A clean corner of the cloth is used to gently clean the nares. Continue by washing one area at a time, keeping the rest of the body covered as much as possible. Dry each area after it is washed. Cleanse the diaper area to complete the bath.

Skin, Hair, and Nail Care

Most pediatricians and nurse practitioners recommend mild soap and water for skin care. Baby lotions, powders, and baby oils are not recommended. Lotions are frequently perfumed and may have other toxic chemicals in their ingredients that may cause a reaction in the infant. In addition, many of the skin rashes seen in infants can be caused or aggravated by use of lotions. Baby oils clog the pores of the neonate's skin, so their use is discouraged. Inhalation of baby powder has been responsible for causing pneumonia and infant deaths; therefore, the nurse teaches the family that the use of baby powder is avoided.

The infant's hair is washed with mild soap or baby shampoo at bath time. The hair is washed no more than every other day. Rinse and dry the hair thoroughly. The hair is brushed with a soft bristled brush to prevent formation of cradle cap (seborrheic dermatitis). Cradle cap is a yellowish crust that is a collection of oil, sebum, and dirt that forms on the scalp. The newborn may be wrapped in a towel and held in a football hold to wash the hair. A wet baby is slippery, and a towel makes the infant easier to hold.

The nails are best cut while the newborn is sleeping. The nurse teaches the family to cut the nails straight across very carefully with scissors. The infant's arm is held securely to avoid sudden movements that might cause the scissors to slip and cause injury to the infant. The nurse cautions the family not to cut the nails too close to avoid cutting the tender fingers.

Cord Care

The nurse teaches the family to cleanse the base of the umbilical cord with alcohol. This is performed at least three times a day and can be done with the bath or diaper changes. The diaper is folded down below the level of the umbilicus to facilitate drying of the cord. The undershirt is turned up to expose the cord. The family can expect the cord to fall off in 10 to 14 days. Tub baths are not given until the cord falls off. The nurse teaches the family to notify the infant's health care provider if the cord appears moist, has a foul smell, redness, or if there is bleeding or a discharge from the cord. An infection of the cord, called omphalitis, can be very serious and needs immediate attention.

Elimination

The nurse tells the family to expect 6 to 10 wet diapers each day. Every newborn's stool pattern varies. Stools that are hard, as well as loose, runny stools, need to be reported to the health care provider. In the absence of stools for 48 hours, the physician or nurse practitioner should be notified.

Diapering and Diaper Rash

The nurse teaches the family to change the infant's diaper whenever it is wet or soiled with stool. As mentioned, the diaper is folded down to allow air to circulate to the umbilicus until the cord falls off. If cloth diapers are used, care must be taken to carefully rinse the diapers with double rinsing to remove any trace of ammonia that results from the breakdown of urine. The nurse teaches the family that clear water and a clean cloth are satisfactory for cleansing the infant's diaper area.

The best prevention for diaper rash is frequent diaper changes. Diaper rash occurs as a result of ammonia irritation. Some infants may develop a diaper rash in re-

NURSING CARE PLAN
Circumcision in the Newborn

ASSESSMENT: Jamal was born 24 hours ago to a 17-year-old primigravida. He was circumcised a few hours ago and is scheduled for discharge later today.

NURSING DIAGNOSIS #1: Potential for Injury, related to removal of foreskin

EXPECTED OUTCOMES:
1. Jamal's circumcision will heal without any complications.
2. Jamal will urinate within 6 to 8 hours of the circumcision.

Nursing Interventions	*Rationale*
1. Document first void following procedure.	1. Tissue edema may interfere with voiding.
2. Check circumcision site for excessive bleeding every 15 minutes for the first hour and then every 30 minutes for the next several hours.	2. Signs of excessive bleeding must be promptly identified and treated in order to minimize complications.

EVALUATION:
1. Jamal urinates 3 hours after circumcision
2. Bleeding from the circumcision site is minimal

NURSING DIAGNOSIS #2: Knowledge Deficit, related to care of circumcision site

EXPECTED OUTCOMES:
1. Jamal's mother will perform circumcision care with each diaper change until the site is healed.
2. Jamal's circumcision will heal without complications.

Nursing Interventions	*Rationale*
1. Demonstrate the application of petroleum jelly or antibiotic ointment to the circumcision site.	1. A jelly/ointment helps prevent the introduction of bacteria to the site and prevents the diaper from adhering to the tip of the penis.
2. Instruct mother regarding signs of infection versus signs of normal healing.	2. Removal of the foreskin alters skin defenses, thus allowing possible introduction of bacteria. Purulent, foul-smelling discharge may be indicative of an infection. A yellow exudate is a normal sign of healing as long as it is neither foul-smelling, nor bloody.

EVALUATION:
1. Jamal's mother demonstrates circumcision care to the nurse.
2. Jamal's circumcision was completely healed at his first well-baby check-up.

---

action to the plastic in disposable diapers. If this occurs, the family is advised to change to cloth diapers. For most diaper rashes, the area should be kept clean and dry. The nurse can instruct the family that the infant's buttocks may be exposed to air for 30 minutes or so several times a day to help heal diaper rash. Application of A and D ointment may help protect the area. The nurse teaches the family to notify the provider if the infant develops diaper rash after receiving antibiotics or if the rash is persistent. A special ointment may be indicated.

Care of the Female Genitals
The genitalia are cleansed at bath time and during each diaper change. The female should always be cleansed from front to back. A clean area of the cloth or a new wipe is used for each front to back sweep. This prevents the spread of microorganisms from the anal area to the urethra and vagina. Urinary tract and vaginal infections are avoided with proper hygiene.

Care of the Male Genitals
The penis is cleansed at bath time and with each diaper change. It is important to cleanse the folds underneath the scrotum. In the uncircumcised male, the foreskin should not be forcibly retracted. Gentle retraction to clean the glans is acceptable.

The nurse teaches the family with a circumcised male to use petroleum jelly on the surgical site until it is well healed unless the Plastibell method was used. The circumcision is observed for bleeding and a purulent, foul-smelling discharge, which need to be reported to the health care provider. A yellow exudate over the surgical site is normal if it is not bloody or does not have a foul odor. (See Nursing Care Plan: Care of the Neonate With a Circumcision.)

Nasal and Oral Suctioning

Many facilities provide a bulb syringe and teach the family how to use it (Fig. 18-16). The nurse teaches the family to use the bulb syringe when the airway is blocked by regurgitated milk or mucus. The nurse instructs the family on the use of the bulb syringe and observes the mother demonstrate its use. The nurse makes certain that the family is very clear that the air must be expelled from the bulb syringe before it is inserted into the infant's nose or mouth. The family is also instructed to discard a bulb syringe and buy a new one after the infant has an upper respiratory infection.

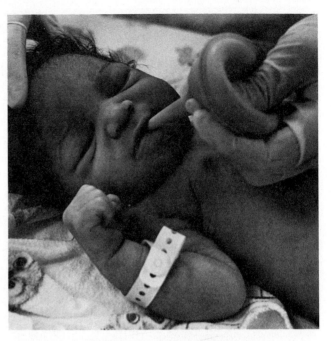

Figure 18-16. Bulb syringe. A bulb syringe is used to suction mucus from the neonate's nose and mouth. The bulb is compressed before insertion into the nares or mouth and then slowly released to create suction. (Photo © Kathy Sloane.)

✔ FAMILY TEACHING CHECKLIST

Signs and Symptoms of Infant Illness

The nurse includes the following information in family teaching to promote health and well-being:

- Call the health care provider if you observe remarkable changes in skin color; if infant looks dusky to you, has a blueness around the mouth, or if the infant's sclera (whites of the eyes) look yellow.
- Watch the infant's breathing. If there is absence of breathing for longer than 15 seconds or if the infant is having difficulty in breathing, call your health care provider immediately.
- Take axillary temperature and report if greater than 37.8°C (100°F) if infant looks or acts sick.
- Call the health care provider if projectile vomiting occurs 2 or more times. Projectile vomiting is emesis which is expelled with great force.
- Report to your health care provider if infant refuses to take 2 consecutive feedings.
- Report excessive crying, fussiness, lethargy (listlessness), or difficulty waking the infant.
- Notify health care provider if infant has 2 or more green, watery, stools, if the infant's stools are hard, or if infant urinates fewer than 6 times in 24 hours.
- Observe for local signs of infection and report to your health care provider: redness, swelling, or drainage from the eyes; redness, swelling, drainage, or bleeding from umbilicus or circumcision site; frequent rubbing ear or shaking head.

Temperature Assessment

The family should be instructed on the proper technique for axillary temperature assessment (see Fig. 18-2). The temperature is not routinely monitored unless the parent believes the infant may be sick. The nurse teaches the family that the normal range of axillary temperature is 36°C to 37.2°C (96.8°F–99°F). An axillary temperature over 37.8°C (100°F) is reported to the health care provider. However, the healthcare provider is notified if the infant looks and acts ill even though the temperature is not elevated.

✳ Medication Administration ✳

Vitamin supplements may be prescribed for the normal newborn. Medicine droppers or syringes are the easiest methods for administering medication and supplements. Careful cleansing after each use reduces the risk of contamination. The nurse teaches the family to place vitamin or acetaminophen (Tylenol) drops in the side of the infant's mouth toward the back. Drops are administered slowly, allowing the infant to swallow between small amounts. As a last resort, the family may mix medication with a small amount of formula or breast milk. However, this is not an accurate means of providing medications to the infant.

Signs and Symptoms of Illness

Parents often have a hard time recognizing when the infant is sick. Unlike older children, the newborn is unable to communicate with words when something is wrong. The Family Teaching Checklist provides essential information for parents to report to the pediatrician or provider.

◆ Discharge and Follow-up

The usual routine for the newborn is to be seen by the health care provider 2 weeks to 4 weeks after discharge, unless otherwise specified at the time of release. Often the provider sees the breast-fed neonate at 2 weeks to evaluate the newborn's weight and determine that breast-feeding is meeting the neonate's nutritional needs. In addition, the newborn discharged in 24 hours after birth may be seen in 2 weeks. Home visit follow-ups may be planned for neonates who are discharged within 24 hours. Neonates who are discharged early may need to be seen by the health care provider for additional screening, particularly for PKU. In addition, the family may be notified to return with the neonate to the facility or to the health care provider's office for additional testing if initial screening results are questionable. The family is provided with a telephone contact number and encouraged to call if they have questions and concerns.

◆ Adolescent Considerations

The adolescent with no prenatal parenting instruction and weak or nonexistent support has enormous teaching needs. The nurse functions as a role model, teacher, and support person for that adolescent while providing parenting information to the young mother. Teaching for adolescents must be presented in a simple and interesting manner. Videos, comic books, and easily read well-illustrated instructions are helpful. Demonstrations that include return demonstrations are an essential aspect of teaching the adolescent. Active listening is a tool the nurse must use in assessing the attitudes, fears, and anxieties of the adolescent to plan appropriate interventions.

The nurse must take care to be nonjudgmental throughout contacts with the adolescent. A helpful, friendly, warm approach is much more effective than a competitive or hostile approach. A referral to community health or social services may be in order to assist the adolescent in housing, financial, educational, and child care needs. Most adolescents are referred to WIC for food and nutrition support.

◆ Cultural Considerations

Cultural practices influence the family's view of the care of the newborn. One of the practices that varies from culture to culture is the care of the umbilical cord in the newborn. African American, Filipino, and Hispanic families frequently use a "belly band," an abdominal binder, to cover the umbilical cord. Often coins, or stones are placed over the cord stump and wrapped under these bands. Women who practice this must be advised to keep the cord stump clean and dry. The practice of male circumcision varies from culture to culture and is common in the United States. In families of Jewish faith, circumcision is performed by a special rabbi, called a mohel, on the eighth day of life. This is a sacred ritual and usually is accompanied by a celebration with friends, relatives, food, and drink. Female circumcision is practiced by some Middle East and African families. Although this procedure is not performed anywhere in the United States, some families may choose to take their infant daughter back to their native country to have it done. This practice is dangerous and has extreme risks. Health professionals must try to educate these families about the disadvantages of this procedure.

◆ The Role of the Nurse

Ongoing assessment is a vital aspect of neonatal nursing care. The nurse continuously observes and assesses

✓ NURSING DIAGNOSES CHECKLIST

Care of the Normal Newborn

- Ineffective Thermoregulation, related to inadequate fat stores and improper environmental control
- Risk for Infection, related to immature immune system and portals of entry for microorganisms through the umbilicus, breaks in the skin, and if applicable, the circumcision site
- Risk for Injury, related to immaturity
- Altered Nutrition: Less than body requirements, related to uncoordinated suck
- Risk for Altered Parenting, related to impaired parent–newborn attachment, initial separation from the newborn after cesarean birth
- Risk for Fluid Volume Deficit, related to decreased fluid intake.
- Ineffective Airway Clearance, related to remaining alveolar fluid and decreased ability to mobilize secretions
- Health Seeking Behaviors, related to the family's desire to learn about care of the neonate
- Ineffective Breastfeeding, related to mother's knowledge deficit
- Altered Parenting, related to the changed dynamics in the family constellation

the neonate as care is given, in addition to the specific assessments that are necessary. The nurse is the health care person who is with the neonate during these first hours and days. Because the time is brief, the nurse must be constantly alert to any signals from the neonate that may indicate a need for further evaluation. Selected nursing diagnoses are presented in the Checklist for Care of the Normal Newborn.

Another essential part of the nurse's role is teaching the new family. In assessing the family's knowledge deficits, teaching the family, and determining that they understand, the nurse is helping them get started in a new, healthy, and rewarding life together.

The family often comes to the birth experience with many anxieties. The nurse identifies these anxieties, acknowledges them, and helps the family resolve them. The nurse functions as a calm, reassuring, supportive person ready to assist the family as they begin life together with their newborn. Each newborn is distinctive, and the nurse has the gratifying task of introducing the family to the special qualities of their newborn.

REVIEW AND PREVIEW

The newborn is a miracle to behold. Appearing delicate and fragile, the newborn is surprisingly well equipped to survive in our world. Caring families provide the basic needs for their newborn. Nurses spend a great deal of time teaching family members how to meet the newborn's needs for safety, rest and activity, food, hygiene, and love.

All aspects of normal newborn care have been presented in this chapter. The chapter emphasized health promotion and family teaching. Suggestions were presented for a nursing care plan that the nurse adjusts to meet the individual needs of each newborn and their family. Assessing the childbearing family's learning needs helps the nurse identify knowledge deficits that must be considered when planning. The plan of care includes health teaching geared to the level of understanding of the family. The newborn's health and well-being depends on the family's ability to properly love and care for their baby.

Recognizing deviations from normal helps identify newborns at risk. The next two chapters focus on the special needs of high-risk neonates. The preterm neonate is defined as any neonate of 37 weeks' or less gestation. Nursing care is highly specialized for preterm neonates and is described in Chapter 19. The book concludes with a chapter devoted to the care of other high-risk neonates, such as those with birth injuries, respiratory dysfunction, congenital and developmental problems, hematologic problems, and infections.

◈ KEY POINTS

- ◆ The neonatal health history includes family, pregnancy, and labor and birth history.
- ◆ Physical assessment is a vital part of nursing care. To identify abnormal deviations, the nurse must be capable of as-

SELF-ASSESSMENT

1. During a newborn assessment, the nurse notes the infant's hands and feet are cyanotic What should be the nurse's initial action?

- ○ **A.** Monitor the infant's glucose level
- ○ **B.** Check the infant's temperature
- ⊙ **C.** Document the finding
- ○ **D.** Immediately notify the physician

2. When there is a significant difference between the blood pressure in an infant's upper and lower extremities, the nurse should anticipate further evaluation of which body system?

- ○ **A.** Renal
- ⊙ **B.** Cardiac
- ○ **C.** Neurological
- ○ **D.** Gastrointestinal

3. Which reflex may be abnormal when there has been an injury to the clavicle during delivery?

- ○ **A.** Grasp
- ○ **B.** Tonic neck
- ○ **C.** Babinski's
- ⊙ **D.** Moro's

4. The nurse recognizes a sunken fontanel to be a possible sign of:

- ⊙ **A.** Dehydration
- ○ **B.** Infection
- ○ **C.** Increased intracranial pressure
- ○ **D.** A normal deviation

5. Estrogen from the mother is responsible for:

- ○ **A.** Epstein's pearls
- ○ **B.** Crepitation
- ⊙ **C.** Witch's milk
- ○ **D.** Milia

sessing normal findings. The physical assessment is divided into the general appearance, assessment of vital signs and body measurements, and a head-to-toe assessment of the neonate.

◆ Behavioral assessment includes general behavior, the reflex responses of the neonate, and sensory assessment, and may include determining gestational age.

◆ There are several routine procedures performed on the newborn within the first hours of birth. These include administration of vitamin K, eye prophylaxis, laboratory testing, and cord care. Newborn screening, hepatitis B vaccination, and circumcision (if desired) are procedures that are carried out during the neonate's stay.

◆ Handwashing is the single most important method of infection prevention in the newborn nursery. The nurse has the responsibility to teach the family and other visitors and to monitor the handwashing practices of everyone who comes in contact with the neonate.

◆ It is critical to teach the family ways to prevent injury to the infant at home. The nurse teaches the family safe practices regarding car seat use, positioning the neonate, potential for falls, burns, scalds, and drownings. In addition, the nurse alerts the family to potential aggressive behavior by siblings or pets that would endanger the neonate.

◆ Breast-feeding advantages include cost-effectiveness, no preparation required, correct temperature, essential antibodies provided, facial muscle, jaw, and teeth development, and that it aids in mother's uterine involution. Disadvantages of breast-feeding include its availability from only the mother, and the fact that the mother must be careful about her dietary and medication intake.

Advantages of bottle-feeding include the fact that any family member can bottle-feed the newborn, the newborn's intake can be measured, mother's diet is not affected, the mother is not on call all the time, and the infant eats less often because it takes longer to digest. Disadvantages of bottle-feeding are that it does not supply antibodies, formula and bottle preparation takes time and is expensive, aseptic methods are necessary, and refrigeration and storage are required.

◆ Parent–newborn interaction refers to the tie or bond that forms between the newborn and parents. While facilitating this process, the nurse teaches the family the importance of helping the neonate to develop trust. The nurse provides support and guidance to enhance the interaction between the family and the neonate.

◆ There are several key areas in discharge teaching. These include providing a safe environment for the newborn, nutrition, clothing, general hygiene and bathing, elimination and diapering, and when to call the health care provider.

◆ The nurse functions as a role model, teacher, and support person for that adolescent while providing parenting information to the young mother. Teaching is presented in a simple interesting way.

BIBLIOGRAPHY

Auerbach, K. G. (1990). The effect of nipple shields on maternal milk volume. *Journal of Obstetric, Gynecologic, and Neonatal Nursing, 19*(5), 419–427.

Baird, S. C., White, N. E., & Basinger, M. (1992). Can you rely on tympanic thermometers? *RN, 55*(8), 48–51.

Bottorf, J. L., & Morse, J. M. (1990). Mothers' perception of breast milk. *Journal of Obstetric, Gynecologic, and Neonatal Nursing, 19*(6), 518–527.

Briggs, G. G. (1994). *Drugs in pregnancy and lactation* (4th ed.). Baltimore: Williams & Wilkins.

Crawford, N. G., & Pruss, A. M. (1993). Preventing hepatitis b infection during the perinatal period. *Journal of Obstetric, Gynecologic, and Neonatal Nursing, 22*(6), 491–497.

Donaher-Wagner, B. M., & Braun, D. H. (1992). Infant cardiopulmonary resuscitation for expectant and new parents. *Maternal Child Nursing, 17*(1), 27–29.

Fleming, B. W., Munton, M. T., Clarke, B. A., & Strauss, S. S. (1993). Assessing and promoting positive parenting in adolescent mothers. *Maternal Child Nursing, 18*(1), 32–37.

Freeman, C. K., & Lowe, N. K. (1993). Breastfeeding care in Ohio hospitals: A gap between research and practice. *Journal of Obstetric, Gynecologic, and Neonatal Nursing, 22*(5), 447–454.

Gamble, D., & Morse, J. M. (1993). Fathers of breastfed infants: Postponing and types of involvement. *Journal of Obstetric, Gynecologic, and Neonatal Nursing, 22*(4), 358–365.

Guidelines For Perinatal Care (3rd ed.). (1992). Elk Grove Village, IL: American Academy of Pediatrics and American College of Obstetricians and Gynecologists.

Gullicks, J. N., & Crase, S. J. (1993). Sibling behavior with a newborn: Parents' expectations and observations. *Journal of Obstetric, Gynecologic and Neonatal Nursing 22*(5), 438–443.

Hill, P. D. (1991). The enigma of insufficient milk supply. *Maternal Child Nursing, 16*(6), 313–316.

Kyenka-Isabirye, M. K. (1992). UNICEF launches the baby-friendly hospital initiative. *Maternal Child Nursing, 17*(4), 177–179.

Lerner, H. (1993). Sleep position of infants: Applying research to practice. *Maternal Child Nursing, 18*(5), 275–277.

Long, C. A. (1992). Teaching parents infant CPR: Lecture or audiovisual tape? *Maternal Child Nursing, 17*(1), 30–32.

Marks, M. G. (1994). *Broadribb's Introductory pediatric nursing* (4th ed.). Philadelphia: J. B. Lippincott.

Matthews, M. K. (1991). Mothers' satisfaction with their neonates' breast-feeding behaviors. *Journal of Obstetric, Gynecologic, and Neonatal Nursing, 20*(1), 49–55.

May, K. A., & Mahlmeister, L. R. (1994). *Comprehensive maternity nursing: Nursing process and the childbearing family* (3rd ed.). Philadelphia: J. B. Lippincott.

Reeder, S. J., Martin, L. L., & Koniak, D. (1992). *Maternity nursing: Family, newborn, and women's health care*. Philadelphia: J. B. Lippincott.

Robbins, M. J. (1992). Breast-feeding in the face of adversity. *Maternal Child Nursing, 17*(5): 243–245.

Roller, C. G. (1992). Drawing out young mothers. *Maternal Child Nursing, 17*(5), 254–155.

Tappero, E. P., & Honeyfield, M. E. (1993). *Physical assessment of the newborn: A comprehensive approach to the art of physical examination*. Petaluma, CA: NICU Ink Book Publishers.

Williams L. S., & Cooper, M. K. (1992). Nurse-managed postpartum home care. *Journal of Obstetric, Gynecologic, and Neonatal Nursing, 22*(1): 25–31.

CHAPTER 19

Nursing Care of the Preterm Neonate

◆ OBJECTIVES

When the learning goals of this chapter are met, the reader will be able to:

- ◆ Define criteria for the preterm, small for gestational age (SMA), large for gestational age (LGA), and appropriate for gestational age (AGA) neonate.
- ◆ Identify families at risk for premature birth.
- ◆ Describe the physical appearance of the preterm neonate.
- ◆ Compare at least seven physical developmental characteristics of the full-term and preterm neonate.
- ◆ Discuss the nursing assessment of the preterm neonate.
- ◆ Identify potential complications of the preterm infant.
- ◆ Identify factors relating to the caregiver role strain.
- ◆ Identify nursing considerations and special needs of the pregnant adolescent.
- ◆ Discuss cultural influences of the mother at risk for preterm labor.
- ◆ Identify appropriate nursing diagnoses related to nursing care of the preterm infant.

TERMINOLOGY

Appropriate for gestational age (AGA)	Neonatology
	Phototherapy
Hyperbilirubinemia	Postterm
Hypoglycemia	Preterm
Large for gestational age (LGA)	Respiratory distress syndrome (RDS)
Kernicterus	
Micronate	Small for gestational age (SGA)
Necrotizing enterocolitis (NEC)	

For most families, the birth of a baby is a joyous occasion filled with anticipation and expectation. However, for some families who face the unexpected premature birth of their infant, the occasion can be filled with worry and fear. The nurse plays a vital role, not only in identifying, assessing, and meeting the physiologic needs of the preterm infant, but also in meeting the emotional needs of the family.

Identification of the "at risk" neonate and predicting the ability of the neonate to survive is based on gestational age as well as birth weight. The neonate's gestational age is an indicator of the maturity of the physiologic functioning of the neonate's body systems.

Classification of Neonates by Gestational Age and Birth Weight

The weight of the average full-term infant is 3500 g (7½ pounds). Historically, an infant weighing less than 2500 g (5½ pounds) was considered premature. However, with the advent of **neonatology**, the study of the newborn, came the realization that a neonate weighing more than 2500 g could also be premature. In other words, weight was not the factor used to determine whether the neonate's body systems were mature. Rather, gestational age is the primary indicator of the maturity of the neonate's body systems and ability to adapt to the environment outside the uterus.

As discussed, the **preterm** neonate is one who has completed 37 weeks or less of gestation; the full term neonate is one who completed 38 to 41 weeks of gestation; and the **postterm** neonate is one who completed 42 weeks or more of gestation. This definition of the classification of the gestational age of a neonate is accepted internationally.

Neonates of more than 37 weeks' gestation are classified by weight for gestational age and compared with the norms for that age. The **small for gestational age** (SGA) neonate is one who weighs less than 90% of other neonates of the same gestational age. The **large for gestational age** (LGA) neonate weighs more than 90% of other neonates of the same gestational age. **Appropriate for gestational age** (AGA) neonates weigh less than the heaviest 10% and more than the lightest 10% of neonates of the same gestational age (Fig. 19-1).

The low-birthweight (LBW) infant, who weighs less than 2500 g, is also small for gestational age and therefore at risk.

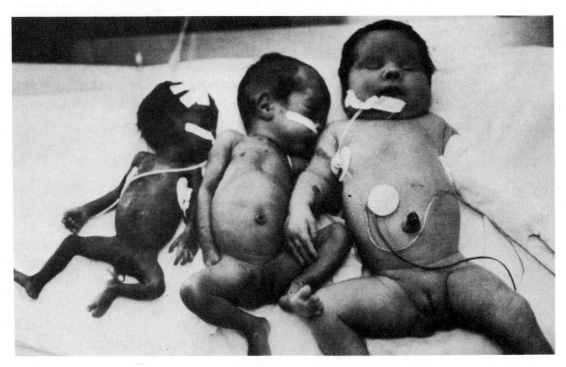

Figure 19-1. Variations in Infants of Identical Gestational Ages. These three infants are the same gestational age but weigh 600, 1400, and 2750 g, respectively, from left to right. The smallest infant is malnourished, probably because of impaired placental function, the middle infant is premature, and the largest infant is characteristic of an infant from a diabetic mother. (From Korones S. & Lancaster J: High-risk newborn infant. St. Louis, C. V. Mosby, 1981.)

The knowledge gained through the study of neonatology, the advanced technology of diagnostic equipment, and highly trained medical professionals have all contributed to decreased mortality rates associated with the preterm infant. However, premature births still account for approximately two-thirds of infant mortality in the United States.

The degree of immaturity of the systems of the body is determined by the number of completed weeks of gestation and therefore is also an indication of the neonate's survival risk. Those preterm infants born before 26 weeks' gestation or who weigh less than 500 g (1 pound) have a very poor survival rate. These very early preterm infants have been termed **micronates**.

Families at Risk

Factors that predispose the pregnant woman to premature delivery have been presented in earlier chapters. Display 19-1 presents a list of risk factors.

Effects on the Neonate

At first glance, the preterm neonate often looks like a perfectly formed little doll. The uninformed onlooker may see only the outer appearance of a small, fragile being. However, unfortunately for the preterm neonate, the immaturity of the neonate's systems creates the gravest problem that must be solved in the fight to maintain life. A discussion of the problems created by immaturity of each of the systems follows.

General Appearance

The typical preterm infant has the appearance of a "wrinkled old man" because of the lack of subcutaneous adipose tissue. The chest is small, and the ab-

domen and head are large in relation to the chest. The bones of the skull are soft, particularly near the suture lines and the fontanelles. Because of the small size, there is very little molding of the preterm infant skull during the birthing process. The hair is very fine and is matted against the head easily. Unlike the well-developed cartilage in the ear of the term infant, the cartilage of the preterm infant is poorly developed. As a result, the ears lie flat against the head. The soles of the feet of the preterm neonate are smooth with very few creases, in contrast to the well-creased soles of the full-term infant. The skin is very thin and fragile with a transparent appearance, resulting in easy visualization of the underlying blood vessels. The body is covered with lanugo and vernix caseosa. The clitoris is exposed by the labia majora of the female preterm genitalia until after 32 weeks' gestational age. In the male, the testes are found high in the scrotal sac at 37 weeks. The rugae do not appear on the scrotal sac until after the 36th week of gestation (Fig. 19-2).

The immaturity of all body systems causes the preterm neonate to experience difficulty adapting to extrauterine life. The extent of the difficulty in adaptation depends on the gestational age of the neonate and the development of each system.

Thermoregulation

The immature temperature-regulating system of the preterm neonate presents special challenges to maintaining a stable body temperature. Chapter 17 presented a complete discussion of thermoregulation.

Several factors increase the problems of thermoregulation in the preterm neonate. These factors include decreased brown fat and glycogen stores, large body surface area in relation to weight, lack of body flexion, decreased subcutaneous tissue, and location of blood vessels close to the body surface because of lack of subcutaneous adipose tissue. The decrease in brown fat and glycogen stores limits the preterm neonate's ability to produce heat. The greater body surface area provides more surface through which heat can be lost. Lack of body flexion exposes a greater amount of body surface, contributing to greater heat loss. Decreased subcutaneous tissue permits body heat to be lost to the outer surface. Each of these factors must be considered when caring for the preterm neonate (Fig. 19-3).

Body Systems

The immaturity of each of the preterm neonate's body systems plays a role in the degree of risk the neonate

Premature Infant

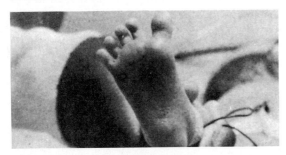

Full-term Infant

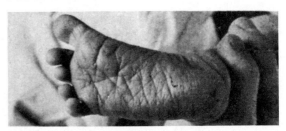

SOLE CREASES *The sole of the premature infant has very few or no creases. With th increasing gesta-tion age, the number and depth of sole creases multiply, so that the full-term baby has creases involving the heel. (Wrinkles that occur after 24 hours of age can sometimes be confused with true creases.)*

A

Premature Infant, 34–36 Weeks

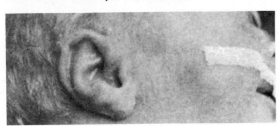

Full-term Infant

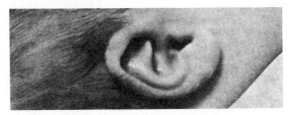

EARS *At fewer than 34 weeks' gestation infants have very flat, relatively shapeless ears. Shape devel-ops over time so that an infant between 34 and 36 weeks has a slight incurving of the superior part of the ear; the term infant is characterized by incurving of two thirds of the pinna; and in an infant older than 39 weeks the incurving continues to the lobe. If the extremely premature infant's ear is folded over, it will stay folded. Cartilage begins to appear at approximately 32 weeks so that the ear returns slowly to its original position. In an infant of more than 40 weeks' gestation, there is enough ear cartilage so that the ear stands erect away from the head and returns quickly when folded. (When folding the ear over during examination be certain that the surrounding area is wiped clean or the ear may adhere to the vernix.)*

B

Figure 19-2. (A) *Sole creases. The sole of the premature infant has very few or no creases. With the increasing gestation age, the number and depth of sole creases multiply, so that the full-term baby has creases involving the heel. (Wrinkles that occur after 24 hours of age can sometimes be confused with true creases.)* **(B)** *Ears. At fewer than 34 weeks' gestation infants have very flat, relatively shapeless ears. Shape develops over time so that an infant between 34 and 36 weeks has a slight incurving of the superior part of the ear; the term infant is characterized by incurving of two thirds of the pinna; and in an infant older than 39 weeks the incurving contin-ues to the lobe. If the extremely premature infant's ear is folded over, it will stay folded. Cartilage begins to appear at approximately 32 weeks so that the ear returns slowly to its original posi-tion. In an infant of more than 40 weeks' gestation, there is enough ear cartilage so that the ear stands erect away from the head and returns quickly when folded. (When folding the ear over during examination be certain that the surrounding area is wiped clean or the ear may adhere to the vernix.)*

Full-term Male

Premature Male

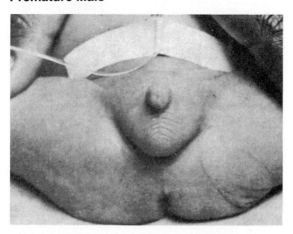

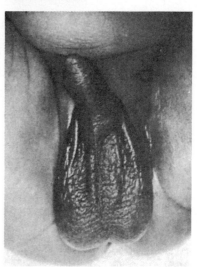

MALE GENITALIA *In the premature male the testes are very high in the inguinal canal and there are very few rugae on the scrotum. The full-term infant's testes are lower in the scrotum and many rugae have developed.*

C

Full-term Female

Premature Female

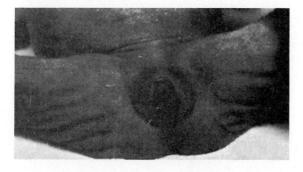

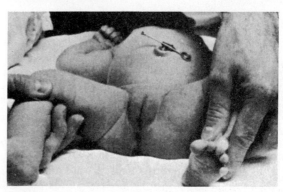

FEMALE GENITALIA *When the premature female is positioned on her back with hips abducted, the clitoris is very prominent and the labia majora are very small and widely separated. The labia minora and the clitoris are covered by the labia majora in the full-term infant.*

D

Figure 19-2 (Continued) *(C)* Male genitalia. In the premature male the testes are very high in the inguinal canal and there are very few rugae on the scrotum. The full-term infant's testes are lower in the scrotum and many rugae have developed. *(D)* Female genitalia. When the premature female is positioned on her back with hips abducted, the clitoris is very prominent and the labia majora are very small and widely separated. The labia minora and the clitoris are covered by the labia majora in the full-term infant.

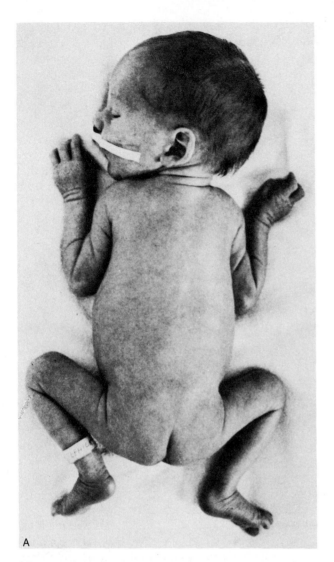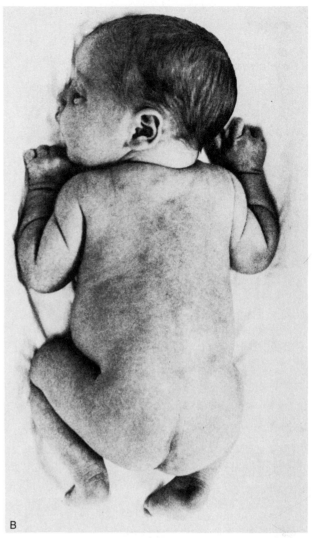

Figure 19-3. *It is easy to distinguish the premature newborn from the term infant when both are in the prone position. (A) The premature infant lies with pelvis flat and legs spread in a froglike position. (B) Term infant lies with limbs flexed, pelvis raised, and knees drawn up under abdomen. (Courtesy of Mead Johnson Laboratories, Evansville, IN.)*

faces. The nurse needs a good basic knowledge of the prenatal development of each system to understand the effect that preterm birth has on the neonate.

The Respiratory System

Although the lungs begin developing during the third week of gestation, they are not fully mature until after the 35th week of gestation.

The most important consideration is the preterm's ability to produce an adequate amount of surfactant. Insufficient surfactant results in collapse of the alveoli when the neonate exhales (see Chapter 17). Collapse of alveoli results in hypoxia, reduced blood flow to the lungs, and depletion of the neonate's energy. In addition, when sur-

factant supply is decreased, the pressure required to fill the lungs with air increases. This places increased energy demands on the already stressed preterm neonate.

The respirations of the preterm neonate may be irregular, with periods of apnea. Apnea is a common problem in the preterm infant of less than 36 weeks' gestation. For this reason, they must be monitored continuously by an apnea monitor. Respiratory distress syndrome, a common serious problem of the preterm neonate, is discussed later in this chapter.

Circulatory System

The muscular coating of the pulmonary arterioles (small arteries in the pulmonary system) does not develop completely until late in the gestational period and therefore is not completely developed in the preterm infant. The exact amount of development depends on the gestational age of the neonate. Because of the decreased development of the muscular coating in the pulmonary arterioles, the preterm neonate has a lower pulmonary vascular resistance than the full-term neonate (see Chapter 17). This leads to the shunting of blood through the ductus arteriosus and increased blood flow back into the lungs.

In the full-term neonate, the ductus arteriosus usually closes by means of vasoconstriction in response to increased oxygen concentration. However, in the preterm infant, the ductus may remain patent because of the presence of hypoxia. With the increased volume of blood returned to the lungs, there is subsequent pulmonary congestion and edema. This requires an increased pulmonary effort and the need for additional oxygenation.

Nervous System

The third trimester of pregnancy marks a period of rapid brain growth and development. The maturity of the neonate's nervous system therefore is directly dependent on gestational age. At birth, the nervous system is immature in both the full-term and preterm neonate. The nurse assesses central nervous system (CNS) function by checking the neonatal reflexes, including the infant's ability to suck and swallow. The suck, gag, and swallow reflexes are uncoordinated or not present before 34 to 35 weeks' gestation. The Moro and tonic neck reflexes are present in the preterm neonate, but vary with gestational age (see Chapter 18).

Gastrointestinal System

The premature infant is able to take in some nourishment because of the early gestational formation of the gastrointestinal (GI) tract. However, the GI tract is not completely functional until after the 36th week of gestation, when the digestive and absorptive processes mature. As a result, the neonate is unable to adequately digest and absorb some nutrients such as saturated fats and protein high in casein. Providing adequate nutrition and fluids to meet the caloric needs of the preterm neonate is of major concern to the nurse. The immaturity of other body systems also can affect the nutritional status of the preterm infant. For instance, difficulties in feeding may occur because of weak or absent sucking and swallowing reflexes. This may result in the necessity for gastric gavage (tube feeding) or intravenous feedings given by way of an umbilical catheter. The danger

of aspiration is also a concern directly related to immaturity of the nervous system as exhibited by a poor gag reflex.

Most preterm infants tire easily during feeding. They have to expend a great amount of energy to take in an adequate amount at a feeding. Most are placed on a 2- or 3-hour feeding schedule to meet their nutritional needs. Once the infant's tolerance for water and glucose is documented, oral feedings generally progress to a formula or breast milk. The mother may pump her breasts and freeze the milk so that breast milk is available when needed for the preterm neonate. The preterm's stomach has a limited capacity. Abdominal distention may occur, resulting in vomiting and subsequent aspiration of formula. For this reason, the preterm neonate is offered only very small amounts of nourishment, usually 1 to 5 mL, at frequent intervals. The amount, of course, depends on the gestational age and maturity of body systems.

Urinary System

The immature kidneys of the preterm infant cause problems with the management of fluid and electrolyte balance. Preterm infants have a limited ability to concentrate urine or to handle large amounts of fluid. For these reasons, the preterm infant is at risk for fluid retention and overhydration. Metabolic acidosis is a danger because excessive bicarbonate losses may occur.

The decreased kidney filtration rate of the preterm neonate results in delayed excretion of medications. Therefore, the intervals between administration of medications may need to be increased to avoid toxic drug levels. The urinary output of the preterm infant receiving medication also should be monitored to ensure excretion of the drug to avoid toxic side effects of excessive accumulation of the medication.

Integumentary System

The skin of the preterm infant varies in color from red to dark pink. It is smooth in texture and very thin and fragile because of the lack of subcutaneous tissue. The veins are distinct and quite visible. Depending on gestational age, the skin is covered with lanugo in varying amounts. Lanugo diminishes with increasing gestational age. Vernix caseosa is abundant.

Particular care must be taken to maintain the integrity of the skin and preserve its function as a barrier against infection. In addition, the preterm neonate under 30 weeks' gestational age has a large insensible (not detectable by the senses) water loss through the immature skin.

The preterm neonate's skin absorbs chemicals readily. The nurse must take care to protect the neonate's skin when using ointments and other solutions. Reactions and systemic absorption of the materials can occur easily in the preterm neonate.

Musculoskeletal System

The preterm infant lacks muscle tone because of the immaturity of the musculoskeletal system. Movements of the preterm neonate are jerky and uncoordinated. As muscle tone increases, movement of the extremities becomes less jerky and more coordinated. Flexion of the extremities gradually takes place as the infant assumes the posture of the full-term neonate (see Chapter 18).

Immune System

The preterm infant is at high risk for infection. The integrity of the fragile, thin skin of the neonate is compromised by invasive procedures such as intravenous infusions. Each invasive procedure places the neonate at risk for nosocomial infection (infection acquired in the hospital). The nurse must practice good handwashing techniques while delivering nursing care to the neonate. The nurse also must monitor others caring for the neonate to ensure that they are practicing aseptic technique and good handwashing practices. The nurse must be certain that adhesive used with monitoring equipment does not cause tears or breaks in the skin to create a prime site for invasion of microorganisms.

Passive immunity received from the mother protects the full-term infant from various infections. The preterm infant is deprived of much of this passive immunity because it primarily is acquired during the last trimester of pregnancy. The shorter gestational time results in fewer antibodies for the preterm infant. Therefore, the preterm neonate is at greater risk for infection.

The Endocrine System

One of the most common endocrine disorders affecting the preterm neonate is hypoglycemia. The shortened gestational period results in inadequate amounts of brown fat and glycogen stores. The preterm infant has an increased need for glucose to supply the energy needs for continued growth and the needs of vital tissues such as the heart and brain. Stress on the infant, such as chilling, creates an increased need for energy in the form of glucose. This additional need causes a rapid depletion of the infant's glycogen stores.

The blood glucose levels of the preterm infant are closely monitored for hypoglycemia. **Hypoglycemia** in the neonate weighing less than 2500 g is defined as a blood glucose level less than 20 to 25 mg/dL during the first 72 hours after birth and less than 40 mg/dL after that time. The nurses assesses for hypoglycemia with a Destrostix. A heelstick is performed to obtain the blood specimen (see Fig. 18-13).

Nursing Assessment and Care of the Preterm Neonate

To anticipate the special needs and problems of the premature infant, an accurate, detailed physical assessment of the infant is performed. This assessment discloses important information regarding the preterm's level of physiologic maturity by estimating the gestational age.

The Ballard scale, which is a modern, simplified version of the Dubowitz scale, offers an easy-to-use tool for the estimation of gestational age. The Ballard scale (see Chapter 18) incorporates a scoring system that indicates the neuromuscular maturity and physical maturity of the infant. Using the information obtained, the nurse may then prepare an appropriate plan of care for the preterm infant.

Nursing care for the preterm infant is often provided in an intensive care setting. It is delivered by a nurse highly skilled in the special needs of the preterm infant.

The nurse performs the initial assessment of the neonate, full-term or preterm, at the time of birth, using the Apgar scoring system (see Chapter 12). The nurse further evaluates the neonate's respiratory effort, noting any difficulty the neonate is experiencing. The infant is assessed for signs of retraction or grunting during the respiratory effort. A clear airway must be maintained. The neonate's body temperature must be maintained at or slightly above 36.5°C (96.8°F). An Apgar score of less than 8, respirations less than 30 or more than 60 breaths/min, with associated respiratory grunting or retractions, an apical pulse rate less than 120 or more than 160 beats/min, or a body skin temperature less than 36.5°C (98.6°F), pale blue skin color, or the presence of circumoral pallor, requires immediate efforts to stabilize the neonate. Appropriate treatment is instituted as quickly as possible.

Common Complications of the Preterm Neonate

When caring for the preterm neonate, the nurse continuously assesses for possible complications. Commonly seen complications of the preterm neonate include thermoregulation instability, retinopathy of prematurity (retrolental fibroplasia), respiratory distress syndrome (hyaline membrane disease), patent ductus arteriosus, intraventricular hemorrhage, hyperbilirubinemia, and infection. Each of these complications carries a serious threat to the preterm neonate's state of health. These complications and their nursing care are further discussed in the following section. Throughout the care, the nurse also must be continuously aware of the anxiety and stress the family is experiencing.

Thermoregulation

Low-birthweight and premature infants are susceptible to heat loss through evaporation, conduction, radiation, and convection (see Chapter 17). The neonate's body temperature must be maintained with the least expenditure of energy.

When the preterm neonate is cared for in a warmer or isolette, the temperature of the skin is monitored constantly by a sensor electrode attached directly to the neonate's skin. The nurse periodically compares the electronically monitored temperature readings with those obtained with a clinical thermometer to assure proper functioning of the electronic sensor.

Isolettes may be used to maintain a constant temperature-controlled environment for the neonate. However, the open radiant warmer bed is more frequently used and permits easy handling of the infant by nursing personnel and parents.

Airway and Irregular Breathing Pattern

The immaturity of the preterm neonate's neurologic and respiratory systems contribute to an irregular breathing pattern and frequent periods of apnea that result in decreased oxygenation. Apnea may occur at any time in the preterm neonate. For this reason, the nurse must be alert to intervene promptly. An apnea monitor, which attaches externally to the infant's chest, continuously monitors respirations. An alarm sounds should respirations fall below preset limits. The nurse checks the apnea monitor each shift to assure that it is functioning properly and the settings are correct. Should apnea occur, the nurse first briefly observes the neonate to assess whether spontaneous respirations return. The nurse may be able to stimulate the neonate to breathe by gentle tactile stimulation such as rubbing the back or extremities. The nurse responds with more intense interventions if the infant does not respond, becomes cyanotic or dusky, or develops bradycardia.

The preterm neonate is at risk for respiratory obstruction caused by accumulation of mucous from the bronchi and trachea. Aspiration is also a threat because of a weakened or absent gag reflex. Frequent suctioning may be necessary. In addition, the infant should be positioned with the head slightly elevated to ensure a patent airway. Electronic cardiac and respiratory monitors aid in early identification and intervention of respiratory and cardiac difficulties (Fig. 19-4).

Retinopathy of Prematurity (ROP)

Retinopathy of prematurity (ROP), commonly known as retrolental fibroplasia (loss of vision or blindness) is associated with prolonged high concentrations of oxygen administration. In ROP, the immature retinal blood vessels of the eyes rupture and partially or completely detach from the posterior surface of the eyes. For this reason, it is extremely important to monitor oxygen concentrations and arterial blood gases to evaluate the general condition of the neonate and maintain the appropriate blood oxygen concentration. An umbilical artery catheter may be inserted to allow easy access for frequent sampling of blood for arterial blood gas determination. To reduce the frequency of the invasive blood gas sampling, transcutaneous oxygen/carbon dioxide ($TcPCO_2$) monitoring is used. This is carried out by using a heated electrode that gives a constant measurement of the partial pressure of oxygen (PaO_2) and partial pressure of carbon dioxide ($PaCO_2$). Another noninvasive means of monitoring the neonate's blood oxygenation is with the pulse oximeter. This can be attached to the neonate's hand, toe, or foot (Fig. 19-5). However, the pulse oximeter provides the best monitoring in the neonate who is not receiving oxygen administration because it is not as accurate at high oxygen concentrations.

Respiratory Distress Syndrome (RDS)

Hyaline membrane disease, also known as respiratory distress syndrome (RDS), is a common complication of premature neonates, especially those of less than 36 weeks' gestation and neonates of diabetic mothers. RDS is thought to be caused by the lack of an adequate amount of surfactant in the lung. The lack of surfactant causes the alveoli to collapse each time the infant exhales. This leads to increasing atelectasis and hypoxia. The neonate's attempt to maintain adequate oxygenation results in increasing respiratory effort and expenditure of energy. Symptoms may first be reflected by a low Apgar score at birth. However, they may develop within a few hours of birth. The neonate

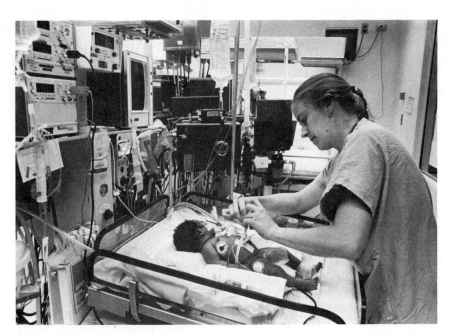

Figure 19-4. *Sophisticated equipment and highly skilled nursing and medical care are the hallmark of the NICU. (Courtesy of The Children's Hospital of Philadelphia)*

may exhibit respiratory difficulty in the form of expiratory grunting and nasal flaring. If an early termination of the pregnancy by cesarean birth is planned, an amniocentesis may be performed. Assessment of the amniotic fluid indicates lung maturity. Immature lungs are indicated by a low L/S ratio. The L/S ratio is a comparison of two lipoproteins, lecithin and sphingomyelin (see Chapter 10).

The use of synthetic surfactant, made from animal sources or extracted from human amniotic fluid, has recently been successful in treating neonate's with RDS. Neonates at risk receive surfactant at birth, or shortly thereafter, through an endotracheal tube. Surfactant replacement supplies the neonate's needs until production of surfactant occurs at approximately 5 days of age.

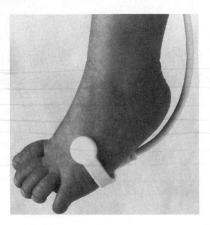

Figure 19-5. *Pulse oximeter probe applied to neonate's foot. (Used with permission, Ohmeda, Boulder, CO.)*

Treatment of RDS is directed toward oxygenation and ventilation as supportive measures until the neonate's lungs are mature enough to produce adequate amounts of surfactant. The type of assistance depends on the severity of the symptoms and can range from oxygen delivered by an oxyhood to continuous positive airway pressure (CPAP) applied through an endotracheal tube. Adequate hydration, maintenance of body temperature, and proper acid–base balance are of vital importance. The nurse must remember that increased handling of the neonate causes tiring and consumes the neonate's energy. The infant should be handled gently, as little as possible, and allowed to rest.

Patent Ductus Arteriosus (PDA)

In prenatal life, the ductus arteriosus allows most of the circulating fetal blood to bypass the lungs (see Chapter 9). In the full-term neonate, the ductus closes shortly after birth (see Chapter 17). However, in the preterm infant, the undeveloped muscular coating of the ductus arteriosus causes incomplete closure of the ductus. When the ductus arteriosus remains open, an increased load is placed on the left ventricle, resulting in a left-to-right shunting of blood. This causes an increased amount of blood to be shunted from the aorta into the pulmonary artery, resulting in pulmonary congestion and hypoxia. As a result, the infant experiences increased respiratory distress.

Treatment includes fluid restriction and diuretic therapy to decrease the effect of the volume overload on the cardiovascular system. Indomethacin, a prostaglandin inhibitor, may be used to constrict the ductus arteriosus. Side effects include GI bleeding and possible renal shutdown. The ductus can be closed surgically, but this poses a major risk for the already compromised preterm neonate. If the patent ductus is not treated, the infant is at even greater risk for complications arising from decreased oxygenation to the mucosal lining of the bowel, resulting in necrosis, perforation, and sepsis (necrotizing enterocolitis).

Necrotizing Enterocolitis (NEC)

Necrotizing enterocolitis (NEC) is an acute inflammatory process of the bowel characterized by necrosis. Although it can occur in full-term neonates, it is seen much more frequently in preterm infants of 33 weeks' gestation weighing less than 1500 g. The cause of NEC is not clear, but there is reason to believe that episodes of asphyxia may shut down circulation to all but the vital organs, causing areas of necrosis in the mucosa of the bowel. These weakened, necrotic areas form gas as a result of bacterial action. They may perforate, spilling intestinal contents into the abdominal cavity, resulting in peritonitis. Signs of NEC are distension of the abdomen with an increased amount of residual feeding (feeding remaining in the stomach). Aspiration of the residual may be 2 mL or more of undigested formula. With increased abdominal distention, bowel loops may be visible, bowel sounds diminished or absent, diarrhea present, and occult blood detected in the stools.

All oral feedings for the neonate are discontinued to provide bowel rest. Intravenous fluids are administered, and nasogastric suction may be implemented to clear the stomach contents. Surgery may be necessary to remove necrotic portions of the bowel. A temporary colostomy may be performed. The nurse caring for the neonate at risk for NEC must be constantly alert to the initial signs, especially how the neonate tolerates feedings. The neonate with NEC is critically ill. NEC can cause death in the preterm neonate.

Intraventricular Hemorrhage (IVH)

The most common type of intracranial hemorrhage in the preterm infant is intraventricular hemorrhage (IVH). Increased cerebral blood flow and venous congestion dilate cerebral blood vessels, causing them to rupture easily. Any condition that causes hypoxia, such as respiratory distress, trauma, or asphyxia during the birthing process, can lead to intraventricular hemorrhage.

Nursing care includes careful monitoring of vital signs and blood pressure for evidence of increasing intracranial hemorrhage as well as observation for changes in muscle tone and seizure activity. The nurse assesses the fontanelles for bulging or tenseness, which indicates increased intracranial pressure caused by hemorrhage.

Hyperbilirubinemia

The liver of the preterm infant is immature and therefore is not able to adequately modify and excrete bilirubin through the bile duct into the intestine. This results in increased levels of serum bilirubin in the neonate. **Hyperbilirubinemia** is characterized by serum bilirubin levels in excess of 12 mg/100 mL or the appearance of jaundice within the first 24 hours after birth. When the serum bilirubin level reaches 20 mg/mL, it is termed **kernicterus**. Kernicterus can result in permanent brain damage. However, with the success of phototherapy, kernicterus rarely occurs.

Phototherapy is the treatment of choice for increased serum bilirubin, both for the preterm and the full-term neonate. The neonate's skin is exposed to high-intensity light. The nurse protects the neonate's eyes with an eye shield during the phototherapy (Fig. 19-6). The neonate is turned on a regular schedule to expose all parts of the body. The nurse observes the neonate's skin for rashes or "sunburn" or tanning; the stools for green, loose stools ("bili stools"); signs of hyperthermia; or dehydration. The nurse increases the neonate's fluid intake during phototherapy.

Because phototherapy is usually successful, exchange transfusions are rarely necessary. Exchange transfusion is discussed further in Chapter 20.

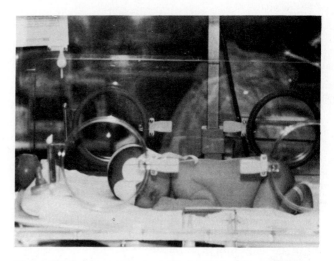

Figure 19-6. *A neonate's eyes are shielded while receiving phototherapy. (Photo by BABES, Inc.)*

Nutrition

The type and method of feeding the preterm infant depends on the neonate's general health status, fatigability, and ability to suck and swallow. Even though the preterm is offered only small amounts of feeding at frequent intervals, the infant may tire easily because of the energy demands of sucking and swallowing. To save the neonate's energy resources, gavage or tube feeding may be required. This type of feeding is completely passive, requiring no energy expenditure on the part of the infant.

Before feeding, the abdomen should be palpated and observed for signs of distention. The abdomen then is auscultated for bowel sounds. If the infant is being fed by gavage, the nurse assesses for gastric residual by aspirating gastric contents. Should there be formula remaining in the stomach, it may indicate intolerance to the formula being fed or it may indicate the amount of the feeding is excessive. When the stomach is assessed by aspiration of contents, the residual is readministered. This is important because the contents contain digestive juices. During feeding, the nurse should assess the tolerance of the infant, paying particular attention to fatigue, signs of respiratory distress, sucking effort, and ability to swallow. The length of the feeding is limited to avoid overtiring the neonate.

The nurse places the neonate on the right side after feeding to facilitate the emptying of gastric contents. This position also decreases the possibility of aspiration because gastroesophageal reflux is common in the preterm neonate as a result of an immature cardiac sphincter. Adequate back support is necessary to ensure that the infant remains in position. The nurse weighs the neonate daily to monitor weight gain or loss.

The nurse provides emotional support to the caregiver and involves the caregiver in the feedings to increase parental attachment and decrease fear of caring for the preterm infant.

Fluid Volume

The premature infant is susceptible to water loss through increased respirations and evaporation caused by use of open radiant warmer beds and phototherapy. It is important for the nurse to monitor the infant's state of hydration and fluid therapy management. This is done by monitoring and accurately documenting daily weight, intake and output, and urine specific gravity. Hourly monitoring of intravenous fluid delivery is critical because the preterm neonate is especially prone to alterations in hydration.

DISPLAY 19-2
Signs of Infection

Nonspecific, sometimes obscure
Temperature instability
Lethargy
Feeding difficulties
Skin color changes
Vomiting
Diarrhea
CNS signs
Respiratory signs

Infection

The immaturity of the immune system, the fragile skin, and the many invasive procedures, such as blood gas sampling, contribute to the preterm neonate's susceptibility to a variety of infections. It is the nurse's responsibility to protect the preterm infant from nosocomial infection. For this reason, it is imperative that the nurse maintain strict medical aseptic technique in every aspect of care. A 2- to 3-minute scrub is necessary at the beginning of the shift, followed by frequent handwashing during the course of delivering care. Visitors also must be instructed in and adhere to handwashing protocols.

The nurse may be the first to observe infection in the preterm neonate. The nurse reports findings indicative of infection immediately. Clinical signs of infection or sepsis in the preterm infant are nonspecific and often obscure. They can include temperature instability, lethargy, feeding difficulties, vomiting, color changes such as cyanosis, and diarrhea. CNS signs of infection include jitteriness, muscle tremors, and seizure activity, whereas respiratory infection and cold stress may be manifested by respiratory symptoms. Signs of infection are summarized in Display 19-2.

Caregiver Role Strain

The early, unscheduled birth of a preterm newborn is upsetting and frightening for the entire family. They have planned for months for their newborn, and now they face the unexpected birth of a neonate whose life is in jeopardy. Many emotions swirl in each of them. They may be faced with the rapid transport of their neonate to a distant tertiary care facility. Even if the birth occurred in a facility that can provide adequate care for the newborn, they are separated by a transfer to the neonatal intensive care unit (NICU).

Family caregivers frequently experience grieving for the loss of their idealized child. The mother may have feelings of guilt. She may blame herself for something that she believes brought about the premature birth of her child. Mothers of full-term infants progress through a process of preparation and anticipation for the birth of their infant. The mother of the preterm infant is deprived of the completion of this process and therefore may not be prepared emotionally to "let go" of the pregnancy.

Family caregivers should be allowed time to grieve the loss of their "perfect" infant. They need to do this to work through their emotional crisis. After they let go, they can begin the process of parental attachment and bonding with their infant. The nurse must understand that this emotional crisis is a grieving process and offer empathy and emotional support to the caregivers.

The special needs of the preterm infant may require prolonged separation of the infant from the caregiver. The nurse must realize that it is essential for the mother to be reunited with her infant as quickly as possible. Only then can the mother begin the process of successful attachment with the infant.

Until the time the mother and infant are reunited, it is vital for the nurse to implement measures to promote the parental bonding process. The nurse acts as an intermediary, relaying information and explaining procedures. The nurse also explains the purpose of medical equipment used in the care of the infant. All of this seems strange and overwhelming to the family members. The nurse can do much to decrease their feelings of being overwhelmed.

The nurse offers constant emotional support to the family of the preterm infant. In many NICUs, one neonatal nurse is the primary nurse caring for the infant. The nurse keeps in contact with the family. The family gains the feeling that someone special is the advocate for their infant and reassures them that they can check on their neonate at any time.

The sight of sophisticated medical equipment and intravenous (IV) tubing may be frightening to the family caregivers of the preterm infant and may initially delay their bonding process. The nurse must prepare the family caregivers by describing the environment of the specialized neonatal intensive care unit and acquainting them with some of the equipment before they visit the infant. The family caregivers also may become alarmed at the physical appearance of their infant. The nurse explains the physical development of the preterm infant and describes what they will see. The nurse reminds the family that their neonate still has developmental time to complete to attain the expected appearance of the full-term neonate.

It is advisable for the nurse to stay close at hand for the family caregivers during their initial visit, while at the same time providing privacy for this special time between parent and child. The nurse can encourage the family to bring clothing the neonate can wear, place photos of family members on the neonate's isolette or unit, and provide small soft stuffed animals for the neonate. These practices often help the family feel closer to their neonate. The family is encouraged to visit the neonate and assist with the care as much as possible.

Adolescent Considerations

Adolescents are at a greater than average risk for having preterm births. The adolescent may have avoided prenatal care because she was trying to deny the pregnancy. This is another contributing factor to the increased incidence of preterm births. In addition, the adolescent's prenatal nutrition may have been poor. Any list of families at risk includes age younger than 17 years, poor nutrition, and general health as factors. The adolescent often falls within these groups. The adolescent who has good prenatal care improves her chances of having a full-term newborn.

The adolescent often has poor family support and may or may not be in touch with the neonate's father. In addition, the adolescent is still experiencing psychosocial and physical growth and development herself. The additional emotional stress that being the parent of a preterm neonate places on the adolescent may be very difficult for her to handle. The nurse must be especially sensitive to the needs of the adolescent. Some of the adolescent's needs may be as simple as needing transportation to the facility where her infant is receiving care.

Cultural Consideration

Although most Western cultures seek prenatal care early in the pregnancy and anticipate and plan extensively for the birth of the infant, some cultures, such as that of the Middle East, do not plan ahead for the coming of the baby. This cultural influence may keep the Middle Eastern woman from seeking early prenatal care and may place her at greater risk for preterm birth. This orientation to the present may be a cultural consideration related to the high infant mortality rate experienced in the past by the Middle Easterners.

The Hispanic culture views pregnancy as a normal, natural, healthy process. The extended family is valued and traditionally relied on for advice. For this reason, the Hispanic woman may not seek early prenatal care or may ignore the guidance of the health care provider when a problem arises. Many African American and Asian families also share the Hispanics' value of the extended family and therefore do not seek prenatal care.

The Role of the Nurse

The nurse who cares for the preterm neonate must be highly skilled. The neonatal nurse fulfills this role. The nurse is skilled in the physical and psychosocial care of the neonate. Although to the casual onlooker, the neonatal nurse's role may seem to be that of meeting many physical needs, the neonatal nurse has a major concern for the psychosocial needs of the neonate. The neonatal nurse realizes that the preterm neonate is only able to accept small amounts of sensory stimulation at a time. The nurse also must help the family to understand this. Protecting the neonate from sensory overload is an essential nursing role.

Nursing diagnoses that address the special needs of the preterm infant are presented in the Nursing Diagnoses Checklist. Once the appropriate nursing diagnoses are selected, the nurse can then plan the required intervention for nursing care of the preterm neonate. The nursing care plan for the preterm neonate presents several common nursing interventions.

✓ NURSING DIAGNOSES CHECKLIST

Nursing Diagnoses for Care of the Preterm Infant

Impaired Gas Exchange, related to decreased functional lung tissue secondary to atelectasis and lack of surfactant

Ineffective Breathing Pattern, related to prematurity of CNS

Altered Nutrition: Less than body requirements, related to inadequate sucking and swallowing reflexes

Fluid Volume Deficit, related to insensible water loss and dehydration

Risk for Altered Body Temperature, related to immaturity of the temperature-regulating system

Decreased Cardiac Output, related to increased ventricular load

Risk for Infection, related to inadequate immune system and invasive procedures

Activity Intolerance, related to poor oxygenation and weakness

Risk for Impaired Skin Integrity, related to urinary excretion of bilirubin and exposure to phototherapy light

Altered Family Processes, related to prolonged hospitalization and separation from family

NURSING CARE PLAN
for the Preterm Neonate

ASSESSMENT: Male neonate 72 hours old. 33 weeks gestation. Birth weight 1800 grams (3 lb. 15 ½ oz.). Apgar scores 6 and 8 at 1 and 5 minutes. Surfactant rescue treatment at birth. Minimal respiratory problems. Jaundice requires phototherapy. Receiving intravenous fluids. Oral feedings initiated. Mother is pumping breast milk for neonate.

NURSING DIAGNOSIS #1: Altered Nutrition: Less than body requirements, related to inadequate sucking, gag, and swallowing reflexes

EXPECTED OUTCOME: The neonate will take oral feedings without tiring and will gain 10 to 15 grams per day.

Nursing Interventions	*Rationale*
1. Offer sterile water for first feeding.	1. To determine neonate's swallowing ability. Sterile water is less irritating if aspirated.
2. Observe sucking and swallowing efforts. Check gag reflex.	2. Neonate must be able to suck and swallow adequately to take oral fluids. Gag reflex helps protect neonate from aspirating.
3. Limit amount of feeding to a maximum of 5 mL initially.	3. The neonate's stomach is small. 1 to 5 mL may be all that can be tolerated.
4. Use special preemie nipple.	4. Eases the effort that the preterm neonate must make to obtain nutrition.
5. Check stomach residual before next feeding.	5. To determine that previous feeding has been digested.
6. Position neonate on right side after feeding. Prop securely.	6. Through gravity this position removes feeding away from cardiac sphincter, decreasing possibility of regurgitation.
7. Feed neonate every 2 hours.	7. Frequent feeding provides more nutrition without over tiring neonate.
8. Weight neonate daily at the same time, on the same scales, and in the same amount of covering.	8. To determine by the weight gain that neonate is receiving adequate nutrition.

EVALUATION: Neonate takes breast milk well; no residual in stomach at time for next feeding; no regurgitation; gains 10 to 15 grams per day.

NURSING DIAGNOSIS #2: Altered Family Processes, related to prolonged hospitalization and separation from family

EXPECTED OUTCOME: The mother and other family members visit neonate and become involved in neonate's care.

Nursing Interventions	*Rationale*
1. Instruct mother in procedure of pumping and care of her breast milk.	1. Mother feels she is contributing to vital nutrition of neonate.
2. Encourage family to visit neonate.	2. Helps family begin to establish relationship with neonate.
3. Provide family with a contact person who will keep them informed about their infant.	3. Reassures family that the neonate has an advocate and helps them remain in touch.
4. Encourage and assist mother and other family members to hold neonate when possible.	4. Helps to relieve the family's fear and anxieties about the neonate.
5. Post family photos on neonate's unit.	5. Establishes neonate as part of the whole family.
6. Refer to neonate by given name.	6. Identifies the neonate as an individual person and member of the family.

EVALUATION: The mother successfully pumps breast milk and provides it for neonate. The family visits neonate and becomes involved with care. Family members speak of neonate in terms that indicate integration into family constellation.

SELF-ASSESSMENT

1. Preterm infants have problems with thermoregulation primarily due to:

- ⊙ **A.** Altered metabolism of brown fat
- ○ **B.** Lack of body flexion
- ○ **C.** Increased glycogen stores
- ○ **D.** Well-developed sweating responses

2. Indomethacin may be given to a premature infant for the management of:

- ○ **A.** Hypoglycemia
- ○ **B.** Patent ductus arteriosus
- ○ **C.** Necrotizing enterocolitis
- ○ **D.** Intraventricular hemorrhage

3. Bilirubin levels must be carefully monitored to prevent:

- ○ **A.** Hypoxia
- ○ **B.** Necrotizing enterocolitis
- ○ **C.** Brain damage
- ○ **D.** Intracranial hemorrhage

4. Nosocomial infections in the newborn can be best prevented via:

- ○ **A.** Liberal administration of antibiotics
- ○ **B.** Changing of IV sites every 3 to 4 days
- ○ **C.** Monitoring of vital signs every 2 hours
- ⊙ **D.** Good handwashing techniques

5. Which physical characteristics would you expect in an infant born at 28 weeks' gestation?

- ⊙ **A.** Abundant lanugo and vernix
- ○ **B.** Well-creased soles and soft ears
- ○ **C.** Descended testes and wrinkled skin
- ○ **D.** Thin skin and clitoris hidden by labia majora

REVIEW AND PREVIEW

In this chapter, those families at risk for preterm delivery are identified, and guidelines for prevention of preterm labor are discussed. The physical appearance and immature functioning of the body systems of the preterm infant are compared with those of the full-term neonate, and defining criteria for gestational age is identified. Common complications and nursing care of the preterm infant are described as well as the special needs of the family caregivers of the preterm infant.

Although the greatest number of neonates are healthy and have no major physical problems, there are a number of serious congenital anomalies and conditions that are apparent in the first days after birth. Often these conditions are best handled with early intervention. The following chapter addresses the assessment and nursing care of the newborn with these special needs.

◆ KEY POINTS

◆ The preterm infant is defined as having 37 weeks or less completed gestation; full-term is 38 to 41 weeks' completed gestation; postterm is 42 or more completed weeks gestation. The SGA neonate weighs less than 90%, the LGA neonate weighs more than 90%, and the AGA neonate weighs more than the lightest 10% and less than the heaviest 10% of neonates of the same gestational age.

◆ Conditions or risk factors that may predispose the pregnant woman to premature delivery include socioeconomic background, nutritional status, general health status, health history, maternal age younger than 17 or older than 40, history of previous preterm births, frequency and number of previous pregnancies, and pelvic size.

◆ The typical preterm infant has the appearance of a "wrinkled old man" because of the lack of subcutaneous adipose tissue. There is very little molding of the preterm's skull because of the softness of the bones; the hair is fine and easily matted. The skin of the preterm is thin and transparent and covered with lanugo and vernix caseosa. The ears lack cartilage formation.

◆ The initial assessment of the preterm neonate begins at the time of birth with the Apgar scoring system to assess the functioning of the heart, respiratory effort, muscle tone, reflex irritability, and skin color. The completion of a thorough physical assessment enables the nurse to identify potential and actual problems that require nursing intervention.

◆ Potential complications include instability of thermoregulation, retinopathy of prematurity, respiratory distress syndrome, patent ductus arteriosus, intraventricular hemorrhage, hyperbilirubinemia, and infection.

◆ Family caregivers should be allowed time to grieve the loss of their idealized child so they may work through their emotional crisis and begin the process of attachment and bonding with the infant.

◆ Prenatal care is not seen as a priority in many non-Western cultures. As a result, the pregnant women may be at an increased risk. Problems are not identified at an early stage when they may be more readily treated.

◆ Adolescent have an increased incidence of pregnancy-induced hypertension, which may be related to poor nutritional habits. Low birth weights are also associated with adolescent pregnancies.

◆ Nursing diagnoses that address the special needs of the preterm infant include gas exchange, impaired, related to decreased functional lung tissue secondary to atelectasis and lack of surfactant; breathing pattern, ineffective, related to prematurity of the CNS; nutrition, altered, related to inadequate sucking and swallowing reflexes; fluid volume deficit related to insensible water loss and dehydration; body temperature, altered, related to the immaturity of the neonate's temperature regulating system; cardiac output, decreased, related to increased ventricular load; infection, high risk for, related to inadequate immune system and invasive procedures and finally; and caregiver role strain related to premature birth.

	Preterm Neonate	*Full-term Neonate*
Skin	Thin, fragile	Soft, smooth
Blood vessels	Easily seen	Not easily seen
Head	Small, little molding	Large, may be molded
Ears	Little cartilage	Well formed
Feet	Smooth, few creases	Well creased
Testes	High in scrotal sac	Descended in sac
Scrotum	No rugae	Rugae present
Labia	Labia minora exposed	Labia majora closed
Clitoris	Exposed	Not exposed

BIBLIOGRAPHY

Affonson, D. D., Hurst, I., Mayberry, L. J., Haller, L., Yost, K., & Lynch, M. E. (1992). Neonatal network. *Journal of Neonatal Nursing, 11*(6), 63–70

Carlson, G.-E. (1991). Retinopathy of prematurity: Nursing interventions. *Pediatric Nursing, 17*(4), 348–351.

Church, J. L. (1991). Neonatal implications of adolescent pregnancy. *NAACOG's Clinical Issues in Perinatal and Women's Nursing. 2*(2), 245–253.

Cusson, R. M., & Lee, A. L. (1994). Parental interventions and the development of the preterm infant. *Journal of Obstetric, Gynecologic, and Neonatal Nursing, 23*(1), 60–67.

Dorsten-Brooks, F. (1993) Kangaroo care: Skin-to-skin contact in the NICU. *Maternal Child Nursing, 18*(5), 250–253.

Freda, M. C., McDamus, K., & Merkatz, I. (1991). What do pregnant women know about preventing preterm birth? *Journal of Obstetric, Gynecologic, and Neonatal Nursing, 20*(2), 245–253

Gennaro, S., Brooten, D., & Bakewell-Sachs, S. (1991). Postdischarge services for low-birth-weight infants. *Journal of Obstetric, Gynecologic, and Neonatal Nursing, 20*(1), 29–36.

Green, A. (1991). Intravenous immunoglobulin for neonates. *Maternal Child Nursing, 16*(4), 208–211.

Kinneer, M. D., & Beachy, P. (1994). Nipple feeding premature infants in the neonatal intensive-care unit: Factors and decisions. *Journal of Obstetric, Gynecologic, and Neonatal Nursing, 23*(2), 105–112.

Marks, M. G. (1994). *Broadribb's introductory pediatric nursing* (4th ed.). Philadelphia: J. B. Lippincott.

May, K. A., & Mahlmeister, L. R. (1994). *Maternal and neonatal nursing: Family centered care* (3rd ed.). Philadelphia: J. B. Lippincott.

Oehler, J. M., Goldstein, R. F., Catlett, A., Boshkoff, M., & Brazy, J. E. (1993). How to target infants at highest risk for developmental delay. *Maternal Child Nursing, 18*(1), 20–28.

Papke, K. R. (1993). Management of preterm labor and prevention of premature delivery. *Nursing Clinics of North America, 28*(2), 279–288.

Pickler R. H., Higgins, K. E., & Crummette, B. D. (1993). The effect of nonnutritive sucking on bottle-feeding stress in preterm infants. *Journal of Obstetric, Gynecologic, and Neonatal Nursing, 22*(3), 230–235.

Pillitteri, A. (1992). *Maternal and child health nursing*. Philadelphia: J. B. Lippincott.

Pridham, K. F., Sondel, S., Chang, A., & Green, C. (1993). Nipple feeding for preterm infants with bronchopulmonary dysplasia. *Journal of Obstetric, Gynecologic, and Neonatal Nursing, 22*(2), 147–155.

Schwab, S. V., & O'Dowd, S. (1994). Partnerships in neonatal care: a model in reverse neonatal transport. *Journal of Obstetric, Gynecologic, and Neonatal Nursing, 22*(3), 210–213.

Reeder, S. J., Martin, L. L., and Koniak, D. (1992). *Maternity nursing: Family, newborn, and women's health care* (17th ed.). Philadelphia: J. B. Lippincott.

Smith, P. B., Weinman, M., Reeves, G. C., Wait, R. B., & Hinkley, C. M. (1993). Educational efforts in preventing preterm delivery among inner city adolescents. *Patient Education and Counseling, 21*(1/2): 71–75.

Stevens, B. J., Johnston, C. C., & Horton, L. (1993). Multidimensional pain assessment in premature neonates: A pilot study. *Journal of Obstetric, Gynecologic, and Neonatal Nursing, 22*(6): 531–541.

Thurman, S. K., & Gonsalves, S. V. (1993). Adolescent mothers and their premature infants: Responding to double risks. *Infants and Young Children, 5*(4), 44–51.

Urrita, N. L. (1991). Sorting the complexities of respiratory distress syndrome. *Maternal Child Nursing, 16*(6), 308–311.

CHAPTER 20

Nursing Care of the Newborn With Special Needs

◉ OBJECTIVES

When the learning goals of this chapter are met, the reader will be able to:

- ◆ Identify risk factors in the antepartum, intrapartum, and transition periods that predict the birth of a special-needs newborn.
- ◆ Discuss the family's psychological reaction to the birth of their newborn with special needs.
- ◆ Explain the immediate care of a special-needs newborn in the birthing area and the nursery.
- ◆ Identify signs seen at birth and during the transition period that indicate the neonate has special needs.
- ◆ Describe how the nurse can assist the family during the early period when congenital anomalies are first obvious.
- ◆ Identify ways in which the nurse can ease the family's concerns when the neonate is transferred to a neonatal intensive care unit (NICU).
- ◆ Name the most common fracture that occurs as a birth injury.
- ◆ Describe the process that occurs in meconium aspiration syndrome.
- ◆ Differentiate the three types of spina bifida.
- ◆ Explain parental grief as it relates to perinatal loss.

TERMINOLOGY

Asphyxia neonatorum

Congenital

Cryptorchidism

Extracorporeal membrane oxygenation (ECMO)

Hemangioma

Hemolysis

Macrosomia

Meconium aspiration syndrome (MAS)

Myelomeningocele

Omphalocele

Phenylketonuria

Pigmented nevus

Tachypnea

Transient tachypnea of the newborn (TTN)

The role of the nurse in the newborn nursery is exciting, challenging, and rewarding. However, when the newborn is identified as having special needs, the role of the nurse expands to a new level. Care of the newborn is modified when special problems present during the postpartum period. Often, the newborn who requires additional monitoring and nursing care is transferred to a specialized neonatal nursery, a neonatal intensive care unit (NICU). Nurses in the NICU must possess excellent assessment skills to provide comprehensive nursing care. The nurse caring for the neonate with special needs also must be exceptionally skilled in caring for, relating to, and teaching the family of the neonate. The new parents need to learn about physical care as they are struggling to accept the special needs of their newborn. Family members experience a wide range of emotions and require sensitive support and guidance from the nurse.

Factors Placing Families at Risk

The prenatal history or record may indicate factors that hint at the possible birth of a newborn with special needs (see Table 8-1). Symptoms of hydramnios and oligohydramnios may be warning signs. Maternal conditions such as malnutrition, diabetes, and premature rupture of the membranes serve as warnings signs for possible placental insufficiency or congenital infection. **Congenital** is a term meaning that a condition is present at or before birth. This applies not only to inherited conditions, but any other condition present at birth. The newborn at risk may be identified during the antepartum period through diagnostic testing. Chapter 10 provides information about prenatal testing.

In some pregnancies, the diagnosis of a special-needs newborn is not made until the congenital anomaly is apparent at or soon after birth. Injuries that occur during childbirth and infections can necessitate specialized care for the newborn. Early identification and management of high-risk conditions are essential. Neonatal outcomes often are improved with early diagnosis and intervention. Open communication with the parents and family promotes healthy adaptation.

Birth of a Newborn With Special Needs

At a time when most new families are delighting over their newborn's individuality and learning basic newborn care, the family of a special-needs newborn are faced with a world they may never have anticipated. Friends and other family members may be at a loss about how to acknowledge the birth event. The family often turns to the nurse for support and guidance. The nurse helps them adjust as they begin to accept their special-needs newborn.

Identification of the Newborn At Risk

Some newborns are easily recognized as newborns with special needs (Fig. 20-1). Low Apgar scores, grunting respirations, bradycardia, obvious anomalies, and injuries are often diagnosed in the birthing area. Other newborns may appear normal at birth but demonstrate difficulties during their stay in the nursery. Although the physician is responsible for diagnosing a newborn's condition, nurses are often the first to identify a problem. It is the nurse's responsibility to notify the physician of any abnormal findings. It may be necessary to

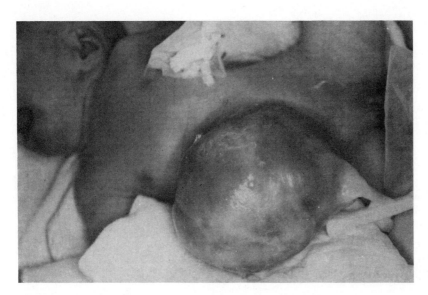

Figure 20-1. The newborn with special needs. The neonate with a large omphalocele. The anomaly is easily observed at birth, creating an immediate crisis situation in the birthing area.

intervene to stabilize the newborn until the physician can arrive to oversee and direct care.

Emergency Procedures at Birth

During the initial emergency and rush to stabilize the newborn, it is imperative that identification bracelets be placed on the newborn according to facility protocol before leaving the birthing area. Early nursing care of the special-needs newborn focuses on stabilization of the newborn. The airway is always the first priority in the care of the newborn.

Special resuscitation intervention may be necessary for the newborn with respiratory difficulties. Nurses in the birthing area and nursery must be knowledgeable regarding resuscitation procedures, including cardiopulmonary resuscitation, suctioning, and oxygen administration. During resuscitation, the nurse stabilizes the newborn's body temperature between 36.5° to 37.5°C (97.7°–99.0°F) axillary as quickly as possible. It is more difficult to resuscitate the newborn once the body temperature drops. Whenever possible, resuscitation should be performed under an overbed radiant warmer.

Parental Perception and Care

The physician informs the parents about their baby's condition and discusses diagnostic tests and immediate medical care required by the newborn. If the diagnosis is certain, the family is informed about the diagnosis, the treatments, and possible outcomes. During this time of crisis, the family may be overwhelmed and feel that information is being given at a pace they are unable to control or understand. Conversely, when the diagnosis is not conclusive and further tests are pending, the family may interpret the lack of information as willful withholding of information by the health care staff.

The nurse must answer the family's questions with easy-to-understand explanations. Information shared with the family focuses on reinforcing what the physician has already told them. Providing the family with opportunities for open expression of fears and concerns helps them cope with their situation.

In the birthing area, the appearance of a newborn with congenital anomalies may silence the normal noise and increase the activities of the team members. The nursing staff may suddenly become very busy with emergency procedures and resuscitative activities. It is important to maintain a calm, controlled situation during emergency procedures to avoid alarming the family. The family's questions may be difficult to answer or may cause the nurse to feel uncomfortable. Responses should be honest but limited until the physician has talked with the family. It is often a good idea to have a

specified nurse address the family's concerns while others tend to the immediate needs of the compromised newborn. The nurse must exercise caution and good judgment when answering the questions of other family members.

Transfer to the Neonatal Intensive Care Unit

The usual nursery is generally not equipped to handle all newborns with special needs. Some high-risk neonates need to be transferred to specialized nurseries equipped to handle their acute needs (see Fig. 19-6). Transferring the neonate to a special care unit should be accomplished in a systematic and orderly fashion.

Before transport, a complete record is prepared to accompany the newborn. The transfer record includes prenatal data and information about childbirth. Any additional reports related to nursery stay, including diagnostic tests and procedures, are also sent. The transferring nurse is responsible for acquiring and completing all records needed for transfer.

The newborn is monitored and supported by portable equipment during the transfer. Most newborns are moved in a transport isolette that maintains a consistent temperature and enables close observation of the entire body. To maintain appropriate blood gases in an unstable newborn, the transport isolette may be accompanied by oxygen.

It is critical to prepare the family for transfer of the newborn. The nurse describes to the family what they may see when they visit their neonate in a NICU. The family needs frequent updates about the condition of their newborn. This is accomplished through the cooperation of the staffs in the sending and receiving facilities. Many NICU units encourage the family to contact them at any time for updates on the neonate's condition.

Special Assessment Needs

Observation and initial assessment of the newborn is completed immediately after birth. A thorough assessment is conducted on admission to the nursery. Ongoing evaluation and continuous monitoring of the newborn is essential during transition from intrauterine to extrauterine life (see Chapters 17, 18). Recorded data may become the basis for recognizing changes in the newborn's condition. Documentation needs to be completed in a timely fashion. The nurse is responsible for maintaining an accurate and complete record of nursing assessment and care. Documentation of normal findings can be as significant as abnormal findings in determining a diagnosis.

Health Promotion

Because the neonate's condition can deteriorate rapidly, resuscitation equipment and emergency medications must be available at all times. A radiant warmer provides external heat to stabilize the newborn's temperature (see Fig. 19-5). The warmer's design facilitates observation of the newborn.

Neonates have small airways, placing them at risk for problems that interfere with gas exchange such as a blocked airway. Deep suctioning may be required to clear the airway. Special care is taken to avoid stimulating laryngeal spasm. Deep suctioning is performed by a highly skilled nurse or physician, depending on the state's nurse practice act and the protocol of the facility.

Positioning is an excellent method of facilitating respirations in the newborn with special needs. Elevating the head of the bassinet places the newborn in semi-Fowler's position (Fig. 20-2A). In this position, gravity pulls the intestines away from the diaphragm promoting respiratory expansion. Placing a roll under the newborn's shoulders in the supine position, puts the head in the neutral "sniffing" position (Fig. 20-2B). This position helps open the airway. Caution is necessary to avoid hyperextending the neck, resulting in interference with respirations. The use of a bulb syringe is discussed in Chapter 18 (see Fig. 18-16).

The special-needs neonate may be especially susceptible to infection. Therefore, it is important that all personnel who come into contact with the newborn practice strict aseptic technique.

The umbilical cord is not painted if the newborn may require umbilical catheterization as an intravenous site. This may be the case with preterm neonates or those with gastrointestinal abnormalities. Neonates requiring

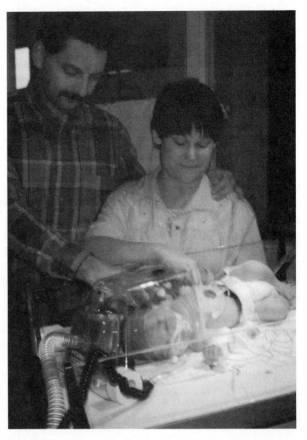

Figure 20-3. *The parents visit their newborn with special needs.*

parenteral fluids and medications need to have the umbilical stump preserved.

If the newborn is unable to leave the nursery, the parents should be encouraged to visit their newborn (Fig. 20-3). Before the first visit, the nurse prepares the

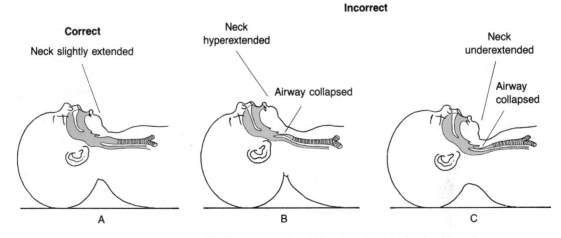

Figure 20-2. *Neonatal resuscitation.* **(A)** *The neonate should be placed on the back with neck slightly extended. This is known as the "sniffing" position.* **(B)** *Hyperextension of the neck will cause decrease in air entry.* **(C)** *Underextension of the neck also will decrease air entry.*

Handwritten margin notes: *History — Pregnancy Test / Urinalysis Pelvic Exam / CBC / Pap Smear*

Table 20-1. *Birth Injuries*

Injury*	Assessments	Nursing Interventions
Intercranial hemorrhage	Frequently seen in preterm neonate Bulging tense fontanelles Increasing head circumference High pitched, shrill cry Poor feeding Cyanosis, apnea Seizures	Measure head circumference daily Report symptoms Observe, describe, document, and report seizures Keep oxygen and suction on hand
Facial paralysis (Figure 20-4)	History of forcep delivery Asymmetrical facial appearance when crying Eye on affected side may remain open Feeding difficulties	Assist and support mother with feeding; preemie nipple may help Position nipple on side that is not paralyzed If eye remains open, protect from excessive drying with artificial tears and eye patch
Brachial plexus palsy (also called Erb's palsy) (Figure 20-5)	Poor or absent Moro's reflex on affected side Arm limp, elbow extended	Position affected arm in natural position, pin shirt sleeve to hold arm in place Instruct family on gentle passive range-of-motion exercises; exercises to start when neonate is a week old Limit movement of affected arm or body part
Fractures and dislocations	Clavicle most common site of fracture Moro reflex asymmetrical Cries in pain when affected body part moved Crepitus (crackling sound or sensation of bone fragments rubbing together) may be felt or heard with movement or palpation	Observe for hyperbilirubinemia secondary to local bleeding Monitor circulation to affected part In fracture of clavicle, affected arm stabilized by pinning sleeve to shirt Splints and casts rarely used

Handwritten margin notes: *Moro's*; *↑ Edema / Proteinuria / Hypertension TB/P*; *Rise from the Pelvis 3rd month / End 1st trimester*

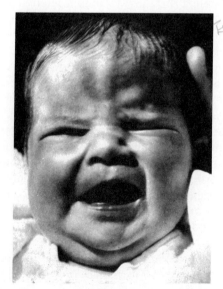

Figure 20-4. *Facial nerve paralysis. The infant's face is markedly assymetric when the infant cries.*

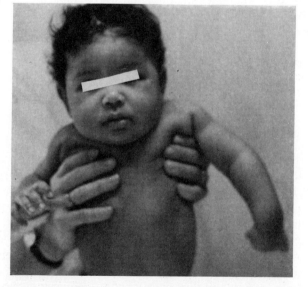

Figure 20-5. *Brachial palsy. This 2-month-old infant has Erb's palsy of the left arm. Note that the elbow is extended, the wrist pronated, and the arm rotated internally.*

*Note: Cephalhematoma and caput succedaneum are discussed in Chapter 18.

Hemotocrit — Blood Volume — Erythrocyte

Hemoglobin — O₂ in the blood (Amount).

family for the experience so they know what to expect. The nurse describes how the neonate will look. Any equipment and treatments are described in terms the family understands. Pointing out the positive features of the neonate helps to soften the negatives the family sees.

If the newborn has to be transferred to another facility, the family needs to spend time with the newborn before the transfer takes place. The nurse should stay with the family during this visit. Before the transfer, nurses in many facilities offer to take pictures of the baby for the family. If this is not common practice, the family may wish to photograph the neonate. The nurse encourages the family to verbalize their feelings about the transfer. The health team at the birth facility stays in close contact with the transfer facility. Most transfer facilities encourage the family to keep in close touch to get an ongoing report of how their infant is progressing, especially when the facility is some distance away.

◆ Birth Injuries

Neonates born after a difficult labor or birth may receive birth injuries. Examples include the use of forceps or vacuum extraction during childbirth. Premature and macrosomic (large body size) newborns are more likely to experience injuries at birth. The nurse assesses each newborn for injuries after birth. If injury is suspected, the nurse supervisor and physician provider are notified. Table 20-1 summarizes the common injuries observed in the newborn.

◆ Respiratory Dysfunction

The respiratory system makes significant modifications during transition as the newborn adjusts from intrauterine to extrauterine existence. As soon as the umbilical cord is clamped, the newborn absorbs amniotic fluid in the lungs. The lungs inflate and fill with oxygen for transfer to the blood. When the newborn is separated from the placental blood supply, oxygen and carbon dioxide transport between the alveoli, and pulmonary blood flow must meet the requirements of the body.

A variety of respiratory conditions can occur in the newborn. Some pose greater threats than others. The more commonly occurring respiratory conditions include asphyxia neonatorum, meconium aspiration, and respiratory distress.

Asphyxia Neonatorum

Asphyxia neonatorum refers to the newborn whose respirations are depressed by elevated levels of carbon dioxide at the time of birth. The increasing CO_2 level causes the newborn to take the first breath. When oxygen does not enter the lungs, the CO_2 level continues to increase. High levels of CO_2 result in depression of the respiratory center in the brain. This is known as asphyxia neonatorum. Maternal analgesia or anesthesia, maternal hemorrhage, and other conditions that decrease maternal blood pressure are the most common causes. The earliest observable symptom of asphyxia is **tachypnea** (rapid respirations). Apnea results if treatment is unsuccessful.

Meconium Aspiration Syndrome (MAS)

Meconium aspiration syndrome is common in newborns who suffer stress in utero. **Meconium aspiration syndrome** (MAS) is the inhalation at birth by the neonate of amniotic fluid contaminated with meconium. The only time meconium passage in utero is considered normal is in the breech presentation of the fetus during labor. Other newborns that pass meconium before birth have experienced hypoxia at some time in utero.

Whenever meconium-stained amniotic fluid is evident during labor or birth, the nurse should prepare for the possibility of MAS. Meconium interferes with oxygen exchange in the neonate's alveoli. It prevents CO_2 exhalation even though it does not interrupt oxygen inhalation, because it acts as a valve, allowing air in but inhibiting its exit. As air gets trapped, the newborn's alveoli become overdistended and the newborn develops pneumonia and pneumothorax. The neonate with MAS is very ill.

One of the newest methods of treatment for MAS and other problems causing respiratory failure is **extracorporeal membrane oxygenation (ECMO)**, a long-term cardiopulmonary bypass system for neonates. Basically, the ECMO setup is a modified heart–lung machine for neonates that allows the neonate's pulmonary or cardiovascular system to rest and heal while the work of oxygenation is conducted outside the neonate's body. This provides time for the treatment of the underlying problem. It must, however, be a problem that is reversible within a short period. Five days is the average amount of time that ECMO is used.

Respiratory Distress

Respiratory distress syndrome (RDS) is a common problem for the premature newborn. This syndrome was discussed in Chapter 19. However, other respiratory problems may present symptoms of respiratory distress at birth or may arise during the transition period or later in the nursery. The nurse monitors the newborn continuously for signs and symptoms that signify the development of respiratory problems.

A type of respiratory distress commonly seen in infants who had a cesarean birth or large neonates of diabetic mothers is transient tachypnea. **Transient tachypnea of the newborn (TTN)** is the temporary elevation of the rate of respirations in an effort to get rid of amniotic fluid in the neonatal lungs. TTN occurs within the first few hours after birth, before the neonate is 6 hours old. The first indications are nasal flaring, expiratory grunting, and mild cyanosis in neonates breathing room air. Respirations increase and may reach a rate between 100 to 140 breaths/min.

TTN is treated with oxygen administration and respiratory support. TTN may last for 4 days, but improvement is usually seen within 48 hours. There is some belief that TTN occurs more frequently in cesarean births because the neonate does not experience the squeezing of the chest that occurs during the vaginal birth process.

The nurse evaluates the newborn's respirations on a continuing basis. Figure 20-6 illustrates the Silverman-Andersen index to determine respiratory status in the newborn. Respiratory distress is evident in the presence of a rapid respiratory rate, nasal flaring, grunting, seesaw respirations, cyanosis, or apnea. Any of the signs are an indication that the neonate requires close observation and respiratory support.

The nurse is responsible for identifying and reporting early signs and symptoms of respiratory distress.

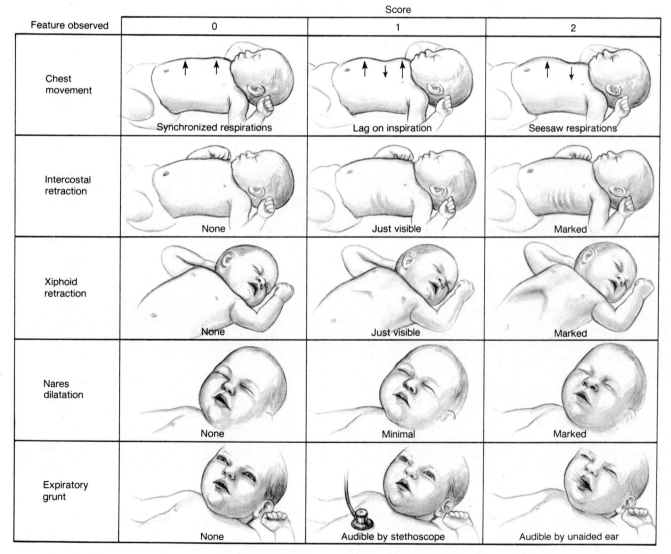

Feature observed	Score		
	0	1	2
Chest movement	Synchronized respirations	Lag on inspiration	Seesaw respirations
Intercostal retraction	None	Just visible	Marked
Xiphoid retraction	None	Just visible	Marked
Nares dilatation	None	Minimal	Marked
Expiratory grunt	None	Audible by stethoscope	Audible by unaided ear

Figure 20-6. *Grading of neonatal respiratory distress using the Silverman-Andersen index.*

Hypoxia, as a result of respiratory distress, can lead to hypoglycemia, brain injury, seizures, mental retardation, learning disabilities, and eventually death. Newborns experiencing respiratory distress develop acidosis as a result of cellular metabolism under anaerobic conditions. Because of immature lungs and kidneys, the newborn is generally unable to effectively modify blood pH.

Congenital Problems

Congenital problems are those that are present at birth. They may be genetic (inherited), the result of an antepartum condition in the mother, the result of the birth process itself, or may not have any clear cause. The family of the neonate may have been aware through prenatal testing that a problem was expected. Conversely, they may be completely surprised by the birth of neonate with a congenital problem. Even when the problem is predicted in prenatal testing, the family experiences great emotional turmoil when faced with the actual presence of the newborn. Nursing care for the individual neonate varies with the condition. However, all families need special care and sensitivity from health care personnel as they work through acceptance of their neonate's condition. The Family Teaching Checklist demonstrates a family teaching plan for a specific congenital anomaly, the neonate with a cleft lip/palate, discussed later in this section. Birthmarks, gastrointestinal, neural tube, genitourinary, or orthopedic problems, and congenital heart defects are the common congenital conditions that may occur. They are briefly presented here. The reader is urged to do further research in a pediatric nursing text for additional information.

Birthmarks

Babies may be born with a variety of birthmarks, including pigmented nevi and hemangiomas (see Table 18-1). A common type of **pigmented nevus** is a mole. They may vary in size and appearance. Mongolian and café au lait spots are pigmented nevi. **Hemangiomas** con-

---

✔ FAMILY TEACHING CHECKLIST

For the Neonate with Cleft Lip/Cleft Palate

The nurse includes the following information when teaching the family who has a neonate with cleft lip/cleft palate:

Hold neonate upright when feeding to prevent choking.

Stop at once if neonate shows signs of aspiration.

Use soft nipple, lamb's nipple, specialized nipple, or other method that works to ease flow of milk or formula.

Take care to avoid flow too rapid for neonate to swallow.

Burp neonate frequently, because a large quantity of air is swallowed while feeding.

Limit feeding times to avoid tiring neonate; may need to build up from 10 or 15 minutes per feeding.

Feed neonate more frequently if necessary to attain adequate daily intake.

Milk or formula may seep out through nose by way of the cleft; this is common and is no cause for alarm.

Talk to the infant when caring for infant, but avoid baby talk; encourage infant's babbling and cooing.

Be alert for ear infections when infant has upper respiratory infection; have infant's ears checked.

Elbow restraints may be required to be worn before cleft lip repair to accustom infant to them.

Cleanse passages by giving water after feeding.

Good oral hygiene is essential, especially after lip or palate repair.

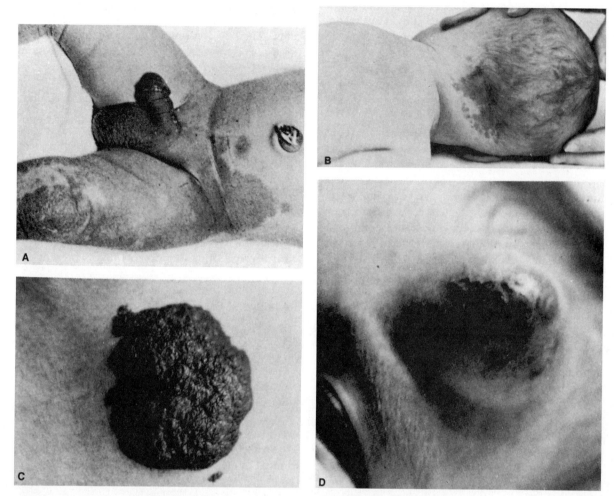

Figure 20-7. *Types of hemangiomas found on the newborn.* **(A)** *Nevus flammeus (port-wine stain) formed of a plexus of newly formed capillaries in the papillary layer of the corium. It is deep red to purple, does not blanch on pressure, and does not fade with age.* **(B)** *Stork's beak mark, commonly occurring on nape of neck. It blanches on pressure; although it does not fade, it is not noticeable as it becomes covered by hair.* **(C)** *Strawberry hemangiomas consist of dilated capillaries in entire dermal and subdermal layers. They continue to enlarge after birth but usually disappear by age 10 years.* **(D)** *Cavernous hemangiomas consist of a communicating network of venules in subcutaneous tissue and do not fade with age. (Courtesy of Mead Johnson & Company, Evansville, IN.)*

sist of blood vessels clustered together to form a red, blue, or purple lesion. Capillary hemangiomas consist of small superficial vessels. Among these are the common stork bite, strawberry marks, and port wine stains. Cavernous hemangiomas are soft and spongy and may consist of a large amount of blood. They may grow and may cause additional problems. Most birthmarks only affect appearance (Fig. 20-7). Occasionally, a birthmark can indicate other problems. For example, a port-wine stain on the face may be associated with the severe mental retardation of Sturge-Weber syndrome. Even minor birthmarks take on significant importance to the family when the marks appear on the face. The nurse must be sensi-

tive to the family's questions and concerns about the long-term effect. This is especially true if the neonate's face has an unsightly birthmark. Many birthmarks fade as the child matures. Others may grow or become more distinctive. Cosmetics and surgery may be required at a later date. All birthmarks are recorded on the newborn's record, and the physician is notified.

Gastrointestinal Problems

Some gastrointestinal anomalies such as cleft lip, omphalocele, and gastroschisis are apparent at birth. Other problems may not be apparent on observation. These

Universal weight loss of Newborn.

Table 20-2. *Congenital Gastrointestinal Problems Commonly Observed in the Newborn*

Defect	Knowledge Base	Nursing Interventions
Cleft lip (Figure 20-8)	Failure of fusion of upper lip May be unilateral or bilateral Often associated with cleft palate Interferes with sucking; baby swallows air, increased vomiting Visible defect may interfere with parental bonding Surgical correction within weeks of birth aids parental acceptance	Support bonding Encourage parental verbalization of feelings and concerns Promote nutrition, determine most effective nipple—preemie, lamb's, cleft palate nipple, rubber-tipped asepto. Feed in high Fowler's position. Burp after every ½ to 1 ounce Follow feeding with sips of water to clear nasal passages (See Family Teaching Checklist for the Neonate with Cleft Lip/Cleft Palate)
Cleft palate	Failure of fusion of hard and soft palate May be unilateral or bilateral Interferes with sucking; baby swallows air, increasing vomiting Often associated with cleft lip Associated with dental deformities when teeth erupt Associated speech defects and upper respiratory infections as infant grows Surgically corrected at 12 to 18 months of age to allow palate growth. May require additional surgery to correct speech problems.	Nutrition as with cleft lip Infant is weaned from breast or bottle prior to surgical correction. Postop infant is fed liquid diet from a cup Speech therapy as needed in early years
Tracheoesophageal anomalies	Involves esophageal and tracheal anomalies including combinations of esophageal atresia and tracheoesophageal fistulas Associated with maternal hydramnios Postnatally newborn has excessive mucous secretions	Use sterile water for first feeding to check for choking Notify physician of feeding difficulties immediately Withhold further feedings until newborn has been evaluated

Condition	Assessment/Description	Nursing Care
Diaphragmatic hernia (Figure 20-9)	With feedings, infant chokes; may become cyanotic, may vomit	Maintain in semi-Fowler's position to prevent gastric contents from entering lungs
	Prone to aspiration pneumonia	Keep suction equipment close at hand
	Newborn maintained NPO with IV fluids until surgical intervention	Notify physician immediately of findings; neonates deteriorate quickly
	Anomaly of diaphragm, usually on left	Keep NPO
	Abdominal contents located in thoracic cavity	Position in high semi-Fowler's position to shift abdominal organs away from chest cavity
	Absent breath sounds heard in chest	Position *on affected side* to allow unaffected lung to expand
	Appears barrel chested; abdomen appears small	
	Cyanosis may be present	
	Surgical correction required	
Omphalocele (Figure 20-1)	Herniation of abdominal contents into the base of the umbilicus. Intestines are covered by a thin transparent membrane.	Maintain membrane covering defect
	Abdomen is small	Reduce infection and loss of fluids through evaporation by covering with sterile gauze moistened with warm sterile saline; plastic wrap or plastic bag may be used to cover
	Complete surgical correction may not be possible until skin of abdomen can be stretched to cover intestinal contents	Position newborn in lateral position and support bowel to prevent injury
Gastroschisis	Similar to omphalocele except defect is not an umbilicus	Similar to omphalocele
	Intestines are not covered by a membrane, resulting in irritation of the tissues	
	Treatment similar to omphalocele	
Imperforate anus	Congenital malformation of the anorectal area resulting in intestinal obstruction	Report findings to physician
	Failure to pass meconium	Keep accurate records of intake and output
	Rectal thermometer usually cannot be inserted	Evaluate all newborns who do not pass meconium within 24 hours of birth
		Observe for abdominal distention

conditions are typically manifested as obstructions such as a tracheoesophageal fistula. A neonate born to a mother who was diagnosed as having hydramnios prenatally is suspect for a gastrointestinal obstruction. The support for this is the theory that amniotic fluid is increased when there is an imbalance between fetal swallowing and micturition (urination). Another early indication of a gastrointestinal anomaly is the presence of only two vessels (one vein and one artery) in the umbilical cord.

If the newborn appears normal at birth, routine nursery care is implemented. The nurse monitors all neonates' intake and output to assess gastrointestinal function. Emesis is noted on the neonate's chart. Notes should include the frequency, amount, and the appearance of the vomitus. Bile-stained emesis indicates that food has progressed in the gastrointestinal tract past the stomach. Failure of the newborn to pass meconium within 24 to 48 hours of birth is reported to the physician for evaluation.

Abdominal circumferences can be measured over time, although this is not necessarily routine. Measurement of the abdominal circumference helps determine

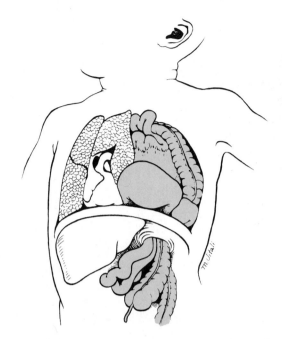

Figure 20-9. *Diaphragmatic hernia showing abdominal contents within the thoracic cavity. This is considered a true pediatric emergency. (Mayer B. W.:* Pediatric anesthesia: A guide to its administration. *Philadelphia, J. B. Lippincott, 1981)*

if abdominal distention is occurring. When the nurse suspects an obstruction, feedings are withheld until evaluation by the physician takes place. Table 20-2 summarizes the gastrointestinal problems (see also Figs. 20-8 and 20-9 and the Family Teaching Checklist on page 362).

Genitourinary Problems

Congenital anomalies of the genitourinary tract may not be immediately evident on visual inspection. The nurse must observe closely during care of the neonate to be alert for a genitourinary anomaly. Recording and reporting the neonate's voidings are part of this observation. Genitourinary tract problems often are not life threatening, but they may have long-lasting effects on the social adjustment of the child. Genitourinary defects may range from a slightly deviated ureter and urinary meatus in the male to exstrophy of the bladder or ambiguous genitalia. The families of neonates born with ambiguous genitalia (gender difficult to determine by observation only) undergo tremendous emotional reactions. Chromosomal studies may be needed to determine the biologic sex of the neonate. Reconstructive surgery may be performed early to prevent problems with sexual identity. Internal reproductive anomalies also may be present in these neonates. Exstrophy of the bladder (the absence of the anterior bladder wall exposing the open bladder on the surface of the abdomen) is an emergency situation at birth. Surgical re-

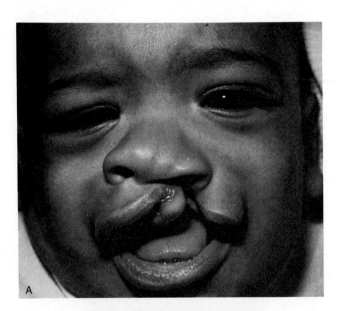

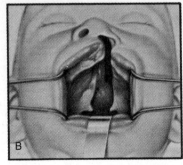

Figure 20-8. (A) *Infant with unilateral cleft lip and cleft palate.* **(B)** *Illustration of internal view of unilateral cleft lip and cleft palate.*

pair is necessary as soon as possible. Prognosis may be poor because of additional anomalies of the urinary tract that may accompany the defect. Table 20-3 presents the most common of the genitourinary abnormalities and appropriate nursing care (Fig. 20-10).

Neural Tube Problems

Neural tube anomalies refer to defects occurring during the development of the nervous system. Many of the defects of the neural tube have associated anomalies in other systems. For instance, one of the major neural tube anomalies is myelomeningocele (Table 20-4), which often has the additional complication of clubfoot (see discussion of orthopedic problems). The meningoceles refer to a defect in the development of the spinal column where the meninges are displaced outside the vertebral body. If the spinal cord and its nerves are involved, it is termed **myelomeningocele**. For the neural tube defect to occur, a defect in the vertebral body is present. Anomalies affecting the nervous system frequently leave the newborn with neurologic deficits. Figures 20-11 and 20-12 illustrate various spinal cord anomalies.

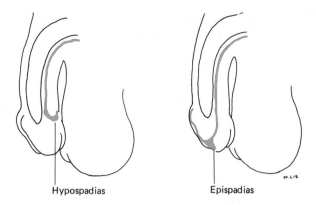

Hypospadias   Epispadias

Figure 20-10. *Hypospadius and epispadius. Drawing on left is an example of the more common hypospadias; drawing on the right is an example of epispadias.*

Orthopedic Problems

Two common orthopedic problems seen in the newborn nursery are talipes equinovarus (clubfoot) and congenital hip dysplasia (Figs. 20-13, 20-14, 20-15). Treatment for both anomalies is usually begun before the newborn is discharged from the newborn nursery. Therefore, the nurse needs to be aware of the diagnoses

Table 20-3. *Congenital Genitourinary Problems Commonly Observed in the Newborn*

Defect	Knowledge Base	Nursing Interventions
Hypospadias (Figure 20-10)	Occurs more commonly in males	Observe urinary output
	Opening to urinary meatus is posterior to normal site on ventral side (underside) of the glans or shaft of the penis	Circumcision is not performed (foreskin may be used in reconstruction)
	May be located anywhere along the shaft or at base of penis	
	Interferes with reproduction if sperm cannot be introduced into woman's vagina	
	Surgical correction performed between 6 months and 18 months through microsurgery; definitely before school age	
	In females the urinary meatus opens into the vagina	
Epispadias	Opening to urinary meatus is on dorsal surface (top side) of penis	Similar to hypospadias
	Rarer than hypospadias	
	Often associated with other anomalies of the genitourinary system	
	As above	
Cryptorchidism	Failure of testes to descend into scrotum, which usually occurs in late fetal life or shortly after birth	Evaluate during daily bath
	May be unilateral or bilateral	Observe for lump in inguinal area that may be testis
	Body heat damages undescended testicles, leading to sterility	No special nursing care required
	Surgical correction is delayed but is performed before school age	

Table 20-4. Congenital Neurologic Problems Commonly Observed in the Newborn

Defect	Knowledge Base	Nursing Interventions
Spina bifida occulta	Defect in one or more vertebral arches May have tuft of hair or dimple at base of spine No neurologic symptoms; no repair needed	No special nursing care required
Spina bifida meningocele	Sac apparent along spine, covered by skin or thin, transparent membrane Meninges and cerebrospinal fluid in sac High risk for rupture with loss of cerebrospinal fluid and infection Weakness of lower extremities may be evident	Pre op care: Protect membrane; cover with sterile nonadhesive dressing or antiseptic impregnated dressing if ordered Position on abdomen No clothing or diaper Observe sac for signs of leaking cerebrospinal fluid Prevent feces from contaminating sac Maintain neonate's temperature by placing in isolette or radiant warmer
Spina bifida meningomyelocele (Figure 20-11)	Similar to meningocele in appearance Spinal cord or nerves present in sac Paralysis from site of defect to lower extremities Lack of sphincter control of bladder and bowel, resulting in urinary and bowel incontinence Surgical correction does not restore neurologic function; long-term follow-up required	Similar to meningocele Catheterization at regular intervals may be needed Meticulous skin care to avoid breakdown Observe for signs of infection Passive exercises to lower extremities Change position frequently; keep off of back Observe for signs of increased intracranial pressure indicating possible hydrocephalus (see below)
Hydrocephalus (Figure 20-12)	Excessive accumulation of CSF in ventricles of brain Head enlarges, fontanelles bulging and tense; scalp thin and transparent May have "setting sun eyes" and high-pitched cry from increased pressure Brain damage and mental retardation as a result of pressure inhibiting brain cell growth Surgical treatment places shunt with pump device. Shunt usually directed from ventricle to peritoneal cavity.	Measure head circumference daily Reposition head often to prevent pressure sores; neonate unable to more heavy head Observe for signs of increased intracranial pressure (ICP) including irritability, high-pitched cry, projectile vomiting

and common treatment. Table 20-5 presents these two common orthopedic problems and appropriate nursing care.

Early treatment of orthopedic problems results in quicker correction of the defect and reduces the severity of the treatment. Clubfoot and congenital hip dysplasia defects interfere with walking if they go undiagnosed or if treatment is delayed until late infancy. Surgery is usually required for either anomaly if treatment is not begun until late infancy.

In some instances, a neonate's foot may appear to be turned as in clubfoot as a result of fetal "position of comfort." The positional problem is easily manipulated and can be corrected with passive exercises.

The nurse should be aware of this differentiation to provide reassurance to the family. The family of the neonate with congenital orthopedic problems faces long-term, perhaps costly, treatment. The nurse must be supportive, encouraging the family to express their fears and anxieties. The nurse reviews with the family teaching that will enable them to care for their neonate. See the Family Teaching Checklist for appropriate family teaching.

Congenital Heart Defects

The neonate born with a congenital heart defect may be identified in the newborn nursery. Conversely, the

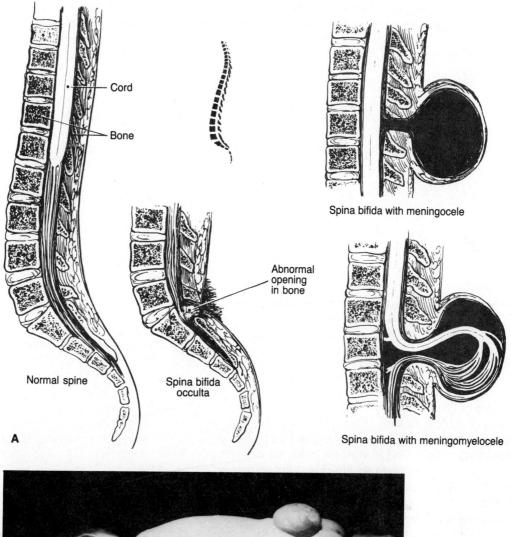

Cord

Bone

Spina bifida with meningocele

Abnormal opening in bone

Normal spine

Spina bifida occulta

Spina bifida with meningomyelocele

A

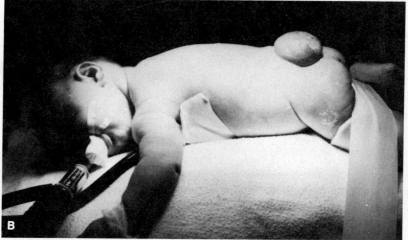

B

Figure 20-11. *(A) Spina bifida. (Spina Bifida: Hope Through Research. PHS Publication No. 1023, Health Information Series No. 103, 1970) (B) Meningomyelocele in the lumbosacral area. The patient is in a prone position with supporting blanket rolls beneath a heating blanket. (The heating blanket is not shown.) (Mayer B. W.:* Pediatric anesthesia: A guide to its administration. *Philadelphia, J. B. Lippincott, 1981)*

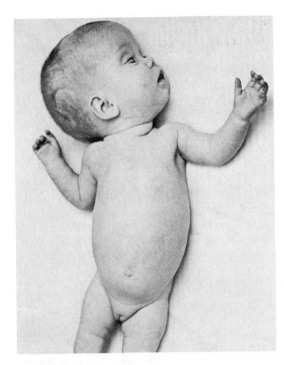

Figure 20-12. *Infant with hydrocephalus. Note site of incision for shunt; also note "setting sun" appearance of eyes.*

defect may go unrecognized until some period after discharge from the nursery. Prenatal information often warns of the possibility of congenital heart disease. Rubella and other viral infections, maternal diabetes, and malnutrition during pregnancy can result in congenital heart disease. The use of alcohol and selected medications during the antepartum period increases the risk of heart disease in the newborn. The nurse assesses all neonates for murmurs, apneic spells, abnormal heart rate or rhythm, and cyanosis. The newborn with a congenital heart defect may exhibit breathlessness and fatigue while feeding. Any abnormal findings should be reported to the physician immediately. Early

diagnosis helps to indicate appropriate treatment and nursing care for the neonate.

In the past, congenital heart defects were classified as acyanotic and cyanotic. However, this classification is no longer used because children with those conditions formerly classified as acyanotic defects may have periodic episodes of cyanosis, and those with conditions classified as cyanotic may be free of cyanosis at times. Table 20-6 describes some of the more common congenital heart defects.

The newborn suspected of having congenital heart disease should be closely monitored. The nurse observes for respiratory difficulty, increasing cyanosis, and symptoms of congestive heart failure (CHF). Tachycardia, tachypnea, diaphoresis, or enlargement of the liver and heart may indicate CHF. Respirations may need to be supported with warmed, humidified oxygen. Mist may be added to thin respiratory secretions. Activities are limited. During oral feedings, a special nipple for premature infants with a large opening reduces sucking and minimizes the newborn's fatigue. Gavage feedings may be initiated to reduce the stress of feedings. Nursing care is planned to decrease the number of times the neonate is disturbed and therefore to reduce the work load of the neonate's heart. Elevating the neonate's head and shoulders may improve respirations and reduce the workload of the heart. The nurse monitors the environment to make it more restful, to reduce excessive noise and light, and to prevent the threat of infection.

Cardiac catheterization and chest x-rays help determine the diagnosis of heart conditions. Digoxin (Lanoxin) and furosemide (Lasix) may be ordered to promote cardiac functioning. Surgical correction may be warranted but may need to be postponed until the infant is older. In some conditions, initial repair can be performed immediately, with additional repair needed when the infant is larger.

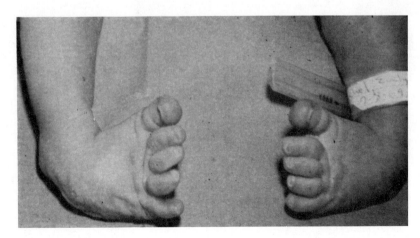

Figure 20-13. *Bilateral talipes equinovarus (clubfoot).*

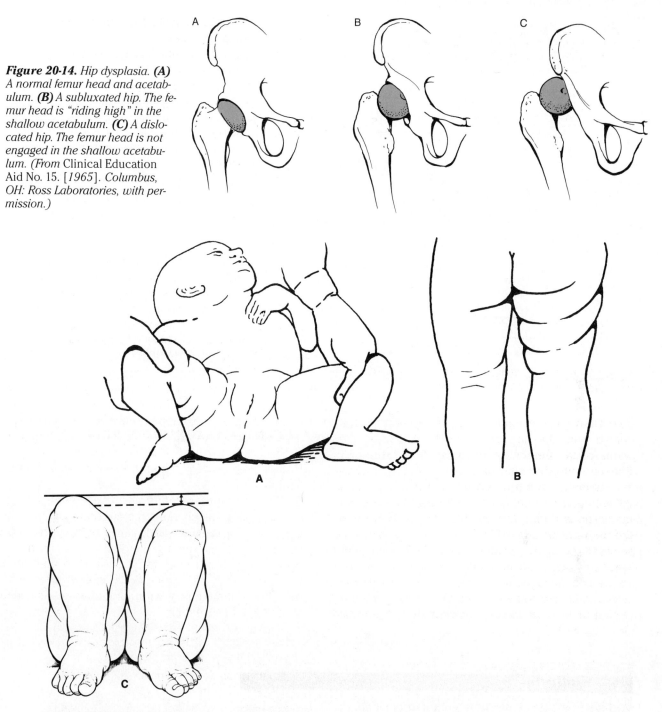

Figure 20-14. *Hip dysplasia.* **(A)** *A normal femur head and acetabulum.* **(B)** *A subluxated hip. The femur head is "riding high" in the shallow acetabulum.* **(C)** *A dislocated hip. The femur head is not engaged in the shallow acetabulum.* (*From* Clinical Education Aid No. 15. [1965]. Columbus, OH: Ross Laboratories, with permission.)

Figure 20-15. *Observations made to identify congenital hip dysplasia.* **(A)** *Limitation of abduction in the affected leg.* **(B)** *Asymmetry of the gluteal folds of the thighs.* **(C)** *Apparent shortening of the femur.*

Table 20-5. Congenital Orthopedic Problems Commonly Observed in the Newborn

Defect	Knowledge Base	Nursing Interventions
Clubfoot (talipes equino-varus) (Figure 20-13)	Most common form is talipes equinovarus; foot and ankle deviate toward midline with plantar flexion of foot. May be unilateral (one foot) or bilateral (both feet). Occurs twice as often in females Treatment starts early with long-term follow-up Casts applied in progressive correction Braces as child gets older	After casting, allow cast to dry, avoid finger pressure when handling Protect cast edges with tape and padding Protect cast from soiling by urine and feces Observe for circulation and pressure sores Teach family home care, including cast care and observations for needed change due to growth—tightness, circulatory signs, pressure areas.
Congenital hip dysplasia (Figure 20-14)	First identified during examination through Ortolani's maneuver (Chapter 18) Head of femur rides out of (subluxation) or dislocates (luxation) from acetabulum Treated by positioning and maintaining head of femur in acetabulum until muscle and cartilage form to make stable joint Triple diapers, Frejka pillow splint, or Pavlik harness may be used to maintain abduction and external rotation of femur Hip spica followed by braces used if splint or harness not effective	Observe carefully during physical assessment for apparent shortening of femur; limited abduction of affected leg; asymmetry of gluteal folds (Figure 20-15) Meticulous skin care to protect skin around appliance Protect appliance from soiling by urine and feces Encourage and assist family in holding and caring for neonate Teach home care of appliance or cast Pavlik harness can dig into shoulders, protect with extra padding and massaging Avoid powders and lotions to prevent skin irritation around cast resulting from "pilling" and "caking"

Chromosomal Abnormalities

Chromosomal abnormalities range from abnormal numbers of chromosomes to translocation of chromosomes. There are normally two chromosomes in a pair, but in abnormal numbers one chromosome may be missing (monosomy) or there may be an extra chromosome present (trisomy). Either of these anomalies in numbers may be incompatible with life. Translocation of chromosomes are structural abnormalities. This occurs when chromosomal material breaks away from one pair and attaches to or becomes part of another pair. One of the most common chromosomal abnormalities is Down syndrome.

Down Syndrome

Down syndrome is the result of a chromosomal abnormality. It results from an extra chromosome in the 21st pair or a translocation, usually from the 15th to the 21st pair, hence the name *trisomy 21*. Down syndrome may tend to recur in some families. It occurs more frequently in newborns born to older women. In other situations, Down syndrome may be pure chance. Genetic counseling can help parents determine why Down syndrome occurred, including the risk of recurrence in future pregnancies. Chorionic villi sampling and amniocentesis are tests that can detect chromosomal abnormalities, including Down syndrome (see Chapters 9 and 10).

✓ FAMILY TEACHING CHECKLIST

For the Neonate with a Casted Congenital Orthopedic Problem

The nurse includes the following information while teaching the family care of the infant in a cast:

Protect perineal area of cast with plastic covering.

Replace plastic covering when soiled with fresh, clean covering.

Covering can be washed, dried well, and reused.

Observe skin around edges of cast for signs of redness, swelling, or irritation; report to health care provider if these signs are present.

Avoid using powders or lotions that will cause pilling and caking under the cast.

Keep small food items or toys away from infant's cast; watch that an older sibling does not put anything down the cast.

Provide for growth and development activities within the restrictions of the cast. Plan activities that use the infant's hands.

Engage in activities with infant that provide stimulation of sensations of feeling (touch), seeing, and hearing.

Hold, cuddle, stroke, and croon or talk to infant to provide feelings of warmth, love, and safety.

Table 20-6. *Congenital Cardiovascular Problems Commonly Observed in the Newborn*

Defect	Symptoms	Comments
Patent ductus arteriosus	Murmur Feeding difficulties Upper respiratory infections	Seen commonly in preterm neonates Open ductus arteriosus allows left-to-right shunting of blood from the aorta to the pulmonary artery
Atrial septal defect (ASD)	Murmur Growth failure Upper respiratory infections	Shunts blood from left atrium to right atrium, recirculating blood through pulmonary system Tends to be small, causes fewer problems than ventricular septal defect Surgically corrected to prevent subacute bacterial endocarditis later in life
Ventricular septal defect (VSD)	Murmur Feeding difficulties Upper respiratory infections Growth failure Congestive heart failure	Most frequent cardiac anomaly Left-to-right shunting in ventricles Tends to be more significant than ASD Symptoms vary with size of defect; may be asymptomatic or severe enough to cause pulmonary edema and congestive heart failure Surgical prognosis good if no other anomalies
Coarctation of the aorta	Murmur Blood pressure differences between extremities (high in upper extremities; low in lower extremities) Early congestive failure	Narrowing of the aorta (stenosis) causing increased pressure on left ventricle and upper extremities Can occur before or after ductus arteriosus If stenosis minimal, may show no symptoms
Tetralogy of Fallot	Neonate may be cyanotic within hours of birth; may not have severe cyanotic episodes until 4 to 6 months of age Cyanosis and respiratory distress increased by stress, such as crying or feeding	Consists of four defects: VSD, pulmonary stenosis, right ventricular hypertrophy, and overriding aorta Combination of defects cause right-to-left shunting of blood Surgical correction usually performed later in childhood
Transposition of the great vessels	Inconsistent with life unless a congenital opening between left and right side provides a passageway from one side of the system to the other Cyanosis	Aorta arises out of right ventricle, pulmonary artery out of left ventricle Surgery performed as soon as possible Surgical prognosis poor

Newborns with Down syndrome can be identified by observing certain hallmark appearances (Fig. 20-16). The newborn with Down syndrome has an upward slant to the eyes because of an epicanthal fold. Speckles, known as Brushfield's spots, are seen on the iris. The nose is small with a wide flat bridge. The ears are low set. The tongue appears to be too large for the mouth. The body muscles tend to be hypotonic. A *simian crease* may be noted; this refers to a single transverse crease in the palm of the hand. Neonates with Down syndrome frequently have associated congenital heart defects or gastrointestinal obstruction. Mental retardation is associated with Down syndrome.

In the newborn nursery, feeding difficulties may be observed because of the hypotonicity of the muscles. Newborns with Down syndrome are prone to respiratory infections. Parents need support and guidance to learn to accept their newborn's condition. Family teaching needs to include information on feeding, prevention of infections, and early developmental stimulation. Referral to a Down syndrome support group is often beneficial for family members.

Inborn Errors of Metabolism

Inborn errors of metabolism often do not cause symptoms that are readily detected at birth. Therefore, nurses must be knowledgeable about these conditions, because newborn screening is performed to detect them. Some of the screening tests are required by law in most states. Other tests are performed when there is evidence to suggest that the infant may have such a condition.

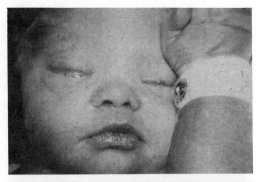

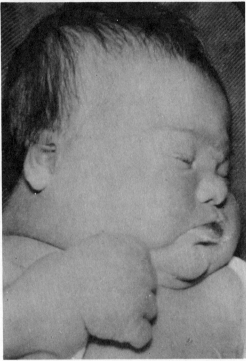

Figure 20-16. *Infant with Down syndrome. (Avery G. B.: Neonatology: Pathophysiology and management of the newborn, 3rd ed. Philadelphia, J. B. Lippincott, 1987)*

For example, if there is a history of a particular condition in the family, screening is performed so treatment can be started as early as possible.

Phenylketonuria

Phenylketonuria (PKU) is inherited as an autosomal recessive disease. In other words, both parents must be carriers for the disease. In PKU, the newborn is unable to convert the essential amino acid phenylalanine to tyrosine because of the missing liver enzyme, phenylalanine hydroxylase. Phenylalanine is found in all protein foods. When the newborn ingests protein, phenylketones, the breakdown products of phenylalanine, build up in the bloodstream. These phenylketones accumulate in the brain, causing mental retardation. Phenylketones are excreted through the skin and in the urine. The newborn typically has eczema and musty-smelling skin and urine. Tyrosine, an amino acid needed to produce melanin, the coloring agent of the body, is not present in neonates with PKU. As a result, the skin color of the neonate, normal at birth, becomes increasingly lighter until treatment is instituted.

Babies born with PKU are normal at birth. They develop progressive mental retardation as phenylketones accumulate in the blood and are deposited in the brain. Phenylketonuria can be diagnosed by a blood test after the newborn has ingested protein foods for 24 hours or longer. The time of the first formula or breast-feeding is recorded, and the blood test is scheduled for 24 hours later. With early discharge, this has caused some problems. However, the test is performed on all neonates. The neonate who is discharged in 24 hours is required to return to the health care provider for a retest in the third week of life. The nurse must stress to the early-discharge family the importance of the return visit for testing. Early detection is essential in preventing harmful effects to the newborn from phenylketones.

The newborn diagnosed with PKU is placed on a special diet with limited phenylalanine intake. An example of a low-phenylalanine formula is Lofenalac. A special diet prevents the development of mental retardation. For maximum benefit, the phenylalanine-restricted diet should be started before the newborn is 3 weeks old. Close monitoring of phenylalanine levels is essential as the infant grows. Normal development depends on appropriate diagnosis and treatment of PKU.

Congenital Hypothyroidism

Congenital hypothyroidism is a result of an inborn error of metabolism, a maternal iodine deficiency, or prenatal use of antithyroid drugs by the mother. At birth, the neonate may appear normal but soon shows evidence of lack of thyroid, with poor weight gain, poor feeding, lethargy, constipation, hypothermia, and neonatal jaundice. If congenital hypothyroidism is not diagnosed and treated with thyroid replacement early, mental retardation and arrested growth occur. Neonatal screening for congenital hypothyroidism is required in most states and includes thyroxine (T_4) and thyroid-stimulating hormone (TSH). These tests are usually performed as part of the heel stick for PKU screening.

Handwritten margin notes (top): Kernicterus / Baby→♀Mother / RH pos & RH neg—starts building up resistance / Destroys baby's RBC / Antibodies

Maple Syrup Urine Disease

Maple Syrup Urine Disease (MSUD) is so named because of the distinctive odor of the untreated neonate's urine. It can be detected by a neonatal screening test. MSUD is branched-chained ketoaciduria, an enzyme defect in which the branch-chained amino acids, leucine, isoleucine, and valine are not metabolized. MSUD is a rapidly progressive disease resulting in central nervous system (CNS) depression and death. If treated very early with a special formula (MSUD formula) that is low in the branch-chained amino acids, normal CNS development appears likely.

Galactosemia

Galactosemia is an inborn error of carbohydrate metabolism. The neonate is unable to metabolize galactose and lactose into glucose. CNS symptoms of seizures, poor feeding, and lethargy result from rising levels of galactosemia. Prosobee and Nutramagen are lactose-free formulas used in the treatment of galactosemia. Galactosemia is detectable through neonatal screening. Early diagnosis and dietary elimination of galactose and lactose result in an excellent prognosis.

Handwritten margin notes: Pathological – hyperbilirubinemia 24hrs / 1st / TX RHGam / begins or 72hrs after birth / Physiological – Icterus neonatorum – after 24hr

Hemolytic Disease of the Newborn

The term *hemolytic disease of the newborn* is currently used instead of erythroblastosis fetalis, because it more accurately describes the disease process. Hemolytic disease occurs when the blood types of the woman and her fetus are not compatible. The primary incompatibilities are Rh incompatibility and ABO incompatibility. In either incompatibility, antibodies cross the placenta, enter the bloodstream of the fetus, and attack the fetal red cells, which results in hemolysis. The by-product of hemolysis is bilirubin. Bilirubin, hyperbilirubinemia, and kernicterus is discussed in Chapter 19.

Rh Incompatibility

Rh incompatibility occurs when the mother is Rh negative (Rh–) and the fetus is Rh positive (Rh+). Rh+ is dominant; therefore, if the father is Rh+ and the mother is Rh–, the fetus usually will be Rh+. The father may be heterozygous, meaning that he is carrying genes for both Rh– and Rh+. This explains why it is possible that an infant of an Rh+ father and an Rh– mother may be Rh–. A fact that must be understood when discussing Rh incompatibility is that Rh+ means that the Rh factor is present, and Rh– means simply that the Rh factor is not present. When blood cells that are Rh+ enter the bloodstream of the woman who is Rh– through the placental site, the woman's system immediately musters its forces to defend against the invader and manufactures antibodies. Thus, the woman becomes sensitized (see Fig. 8-2). Sensitization usually occurs at the time of the birth of the first Rh+ fetus. The first Rh+ fetus generally is born healthy. With the second and succeeding pregnancies of Rh+ fetuses, the maternal antibodies, formed at the time of the first pregnancy, cross the placental barrier. These antibodies attack the red cells of the fetus, destroying them. The response of the fetus' system is to produce large numbers of immature red blood cells to replace those that were destroyed. This leads to anemia and CHF in the fetus, resulting in a condition known as hydrops fetalis. If the condition does not become serious until after birth, hyperbilirubinemia develops, and kernicterus may occur if the newborn is not treated.

Handwritten margin note: check bilirubine frequently / Brain damage

Sensitization of the woman is prevented if she receives RhoGAM before developing antibodies. RhoGAM coats, neutralizes, and destroys the Rh red blood cells from the fetus. This prevents the maternal development of natural antibodies. The nonsensitized Rh– woman must receive RhoGAM within 72 hours of every abortion, amniocentesis, or birth involving an Rh+ fetus or fetus of unknown blood type. RhoGAM is also administered prophylactically at 28 weeks of pregnancy to all nonsensitized Rh– women to reduce the probability of sensitivity occurring before birth. For example, sensitization can occur before birth if the placenta pulls away from the uterine wall as in abruptio placenta. Once the woman is sensitized, RhoGAM is ineffective in preventing Rh incompatibilities. *(handwritten: Coombs test is done)*

In the sensitized woman with an Rh-incompatible pregnancy, the newborn's condition is monitored by amniocentesis to determine the bilirubin level of the amniotic fluid. If the fetus displays symptoms of increasing anemia (increased bilirubin level), the fetal condition may be improved by an intrauterine transfusion with O-negative blood. As soon as the fetus is mature enough to survive, childbirth is induced or the newborn is delivered by cesarean. After birth, the newborn with Rh incompatibility is treated with phototherapy. The newborn also may need to receive an exchange transfusion. Exchange transfusion may be necessary if hyperbilirubinemia does not decrease adequately with phototherapy. The negative form of the newborn's blood type is administered during exchange transfusion. For example, if the newborn is A-positive, the exchange transfusion uses A-negative blood. This provides the neonate with sufficient blood that will not be destroyed

Handwritten notes (bottom): Liver & spleen will be enlarged. / does not affect the 1st Pregnancy but the others that follow / Coombs test is done č the Mother's blood or the baby's blood / RH+ is more common / RHGam / RHGam – is given Im

Phototherapy

PURPOSE: To convert bilirubin to an excretable form by means of exposure to high intensity lights.

EQUIPMENT: Bili lite, isolette or radiant warmer, protective eye cover, and diaper or shield to protect the genitalia, especially the testes of the male neonate.

PROCEDURE:

Nursing Intervention	*Rationale*
1. Explain the procedure to the family.	1. To prepare family for the procedure.
2. Remove neonate's clothing.	2. To expose the largest amount of skin surface.
3. Place face mask (eye shield) over eyes, making certain the nasal passages are clear.	3. To protect eyes from damage to vision. To facilitate breathing since neonate is obligatory nose breather.
4. Place the shield to protect the genitalia.	4. To protect genitalia from damage from lights.
5. Place neonate in neutral thermal environment. Monitor temperature every 2 hours, or according to policy of the facility.	5. To promote thermoregulation. Lights can overheat neonate; air can cool neonate.
6. Change position every 2 hours. Do not use lotions or oils on the neonate's skin.	6. To provide maximum skin area coverage; to prevent skin breakdown from pressure areas. Lotions or oils may cause burns.
7. Keep skin clean and dry.	7. To prevent skin irritation or breakdown from loose stools and urine.
8. Monitor number, type, and color of stools.	8. Phototherapy may cause loose green stools.
9. Offer water between feedings. Monitor intake and output.	9. To prevent dehydration from phototherapy through insensible losses and output.
10. Inspect carefully during feedings and bathing to determine skin, mucous membrane, and sclera color. Check skin turgor.	10. To observe the progress and effectiveness of phototherapy between microbilirubin tests.
11. Check skin turgor.	11. To determine if neonate is becoming dehydrated.
12. Talk to neonate during care. Hold during feedings.	12. To provide sensory stimulation to the neonate when possible.
13. Answer family's questions and encourage them to express their anxieties.	13. To help the family understand the process and reassure them.
14. Document all skin, sclera, mucous membrane, urine and stool observations, turnings, and all procedures.	14. To have a complete record of the procedure and the neonate's response.

Leave Light 15-20mins at atime

by hemolysis until the bilirubin level is brought under control.

Nursing care for the neonate includes careful assessment and monitoring. Signs of hyperbilirubinemia are reported immediately. Treatment should be started as soon as possible. Jaundice is discussed in Chapter 18. The umbilical cord stump is preserved in case it is needed for exchange transfusions.

To reduce bruising, the nurse must exercise special care in handling newborns with hematologic diseases. Bruising increases red blood cell breakdown. The release of bilirubin results, requiring conversion by the immature liver. The newborn's liver is able to convert bilirubin more effectively when a stable body temperature is maintained. Good fluid intake also helps the neonate's system rid itself of bilirubin because it is excreted through the urine.

ABO Incompatibility

The most common of the blood incompatibilities is called an ABO incompatibility. Blood types A, B, and AB carry a natural antigen, but type O carries no antigen. Thus, type O blood is the universal donor, because there is no antigen to cause the recipient to produce antibodies. Type AB is the universal recipient, because it carries antigens for both A and B. The most frequent type of ABO incompatibility is when the mother is O and the fetus is A or B. If red blood cells cross into the mother's system during the prenatal period, the mother's system sees this as an invasion and manufactures antibodies that cross the placenta into the fetus. Little fetal red cell destruction occurs during fetal life, but in the neonatal period hemolytic disease may be seen. Generally, the reaction is mild, with hyperbilirubinemia seen in the first 24 hours of life. Phototherapy is usually adequate treatment. See Appendix E for a quick reference for information regarding blood incompatibilities. Refer to Nursing Procedure Display, Phototherapy, for information about nursing care during treatment.

Infections

Newborns may acquire infections in utero, or during the intrapartum or postpartum period. Infections acquired in utero are termed congenital infections because they are present at birth. These are typically viral in nature. Fetal infection is preceded by maternal infections. The maternal infection may be so mild that it is not recognized in the woman. The earlier in pregnancy the fetus is exposed, the more significant the effects. Among the congenital infections a neonate may have are those that are called TORCH (toxoplasmosis, rubella, cytomegalovirus, and herpes simplex) infections and human immunodeficiency virus (HIV) and acquired immunodeficiency syndrome (AIDS) (see Chapters 8, 9). Table 20-7 provides information about a variety of neonatal infections, including sexually transmitted diseases.

Nursery care of newborns with an infection is aimed primarily at early recognition of symptoms and prevention of its spread within the nursery. The infected newborn demonstrates nonspecific symptoms. Behavioral changes such as poor feeding, vomiting, diarrhea, and lethargy may be symptoms of early infection. The newborn may manifest skin color changes. Cyanosis or jaundice may occur as the newborn's body becomes overwhelmed by the infection. Hypothermia (low body temperature) is a common initial symptom of infection. This results from the immaturity of the thermoregulation center in the brain. It is important to note that some newborns may demonstrate hyperthermia (fever). As the infective process continues, apnea and shock may follow.

Isolation of infected newborns is of primary importance. If bacterial infection is suspected, antibiotics are administered until cultures are negative for bacterial infection. Antibiotics are most often administered intravenously, often through a heparin or saline lock. Common drugs used in treatment for the specific condition are included in Table 20-7. Isolation of the newborn is accomplished in an isolette in an area separate from the regular nursery. The design of the isolette enables close observation of the newborn. A cover gown, used only for the specific infected neonate, is worn over scrubs by the nurse when caring for an infected neonate. This protects the nurse's scrubs from carrying organisms to another neonate. Proper handwashing technique by all nursery personnel is essential. Universal precautions are carefully followed. Each neonate must have a private linen and equipment supply to prevent the spread of organisms to other newborns.

Acquired Immunodeficiency Syndrome

Acquired immunodeficiency syndrome is caused by the human immunodeficiency virus (HIV) (see Chapter 4). The newborn may acquire HIV across the placenta, through amniotic fluid, through contact with maternal blood during the birth process, and through breast milk. Not all newborns born to HIV-positive women develop congenital AIDS. The enzyme-linked immunosorbent assay (ELISA) serologic test does not accurately identify the HIV-positive neonate, because of the pres-

Text continues on p. 381

Table 20-7. *Neonatal Infections*

Infections	Infective Agent	Maternal Effects	Fetal/Neonatal Effects	Treatment
Toxoplasmosis	*Toxoplasma gondii* (protozoan)	Maternal contact through poorly cooked meat or infected cats. Infection may not be noticed in pregnant woman	Transferred through placenta. May lead to abortions, hydrocephalus, blindness, deafness, or mental retardation	Prenatal damage not reversible. Drug therapy includes pyrimethamine and sulfadiazine. Folinic acid given to prevent anemia
Rubella (German measles)	Rubella virus	A nonimmune woman exposed to virus during pregnancy. Woman may show no symptoms	Acquired in utero, neonate may have cataracts, congenital heart disease, deafness, and intrauterine growth retardation. Infant continues to shed rubella virus up to a year after birth	Only effective measure is prevention by rubella vaccination. No effective drug therapy for disease.
Cytomegalovirus (CMV)	Cytomegalovirus	Most common perinatal infection. No symptoms in woman.	May result in fetal death. Neonate may have hydrocephalus, microcephaly mental retardation, learning disabilities, hearing loss	No effective prevention or treatment. Nursing care supportive.
Herpesvirus, Type 2 (HSV)	Herpesvirus	Most commonly spread to neonate during birth process. Cesarean birth is performed when woman has genital tract lesions at time of birth.	If acquired in first trimester, fetus may be spontaneously aborted or stillborn. When acquired during intrapartum period, neonate has seizures, jaundice, and skin lesions may occur.	Neonate is highly contagious and is isolated. Vidarabrine and acyclovir are antiviral drugs that have been used with limited success

Condition	Organism			
Group B streptococcus	Group B ß-hemolytic streptococcus	Woman may be silent carrier. Can be found in maternal cervix or vagina	May be acquired during prenatal, intrapartum, or postpartum periods. May be stillborn, or develop respiratory distress, apnea, or shock. Onset of symptoms within hours of birth or up to 3 months later (late onset)	Newborn treated with antibiotics such as gentamicin, penicillin, or ampicillin administered intravenously
Syphilis	*Treponema pallidum*	Results in second trimester abortions, stillbirths, and preterm births	Neonate of untreated woman is born with congenital syphilis. Neonate's symptoms are snuffles, mouth fissures, cataracts, and hepatomegaly	Pregnant woman and newborn treated with penicillin
Gonorrhea	*Neisseria gonococcus*	Woman with gonorrhea transmits it to the neonate during the birth process	Untreated neonate develops ophthalmia neonatorum. All neonates are treated prophylactically within 2 hours of birth with silver nitrate solution or erythromycin ophthalmic ointment.	Neonatal infection prevented with appropriate eye prophylaxis. Woman is treated with penicillin.
Thrush Monilia	*Candida albicans*	Woman has candida vaginitis, which is acquired by neonate during birth.	Neonate has small white patches that adhere to the mucus membranes of the tongue and mouth. May also cause candida diaper rash. Highly contagious in nursery setting. May spread by direct contact with infected person.	Treated with nystatin (Mycostatin)

NURSING CARE PLAN
Neonate Whose Mother is HIV Positive

ASSESSMENT: Jason is a 2-day-old infant whose mother has been HIV positive for 3 years. It is too early to make a definite diagnosis regarding Jason's HIV/AIDS status.

NURSING DIAGNOSIS #1: Risk for Infection, related to uncertain status of immune system

EXPECTED OUTCOMES:
1. Mother will recognize and minimize potential sources of infection.
2. Signs/symptoms of infection are quickly identified and treatment initiated.

Nursing Interventions	*Rationale*
1. Observe infant for possible signs of infection, noting Color Lethargy Temperature instability Change in feeding patterns	1. Prompt recognition and management of infections helps minimize complications.
2. Practice universal precautions at all times by wearing gown, gloves and/or masks as indicated when in contact with body fluids.	2. Universal precautions help prevent transmission of disease between the patient and health care workers.
3. Instruct parents regarding signs/symptoms and prevention of infection.	3. An infant with a possibly compromised immune system is at risk of developing potentially fatal infections

EVALUATION:
1. Jason's mother verbalized signs/symptoms and potential sources of infection.
2. Jason's mother identified health care resources to contact for future care and follow-up.

NURSING DIAGNOSIS #2: Anticipatory Grieving, related to infant's uncertain diagnosis and future health

EXPECTED OUTCOMES:
1. Jason's mother will verbalize fears/concerns regarding Jason's future
2. Jason's parents will understand the need for ongoing medical evaluation and management.

Nursing Interventions	*Rationale*
1. Encourage the mother to verbalize feeling/emotions regarding the infant's condition.	1. Mother may have misconceptions that need to be cleared up to decrease tension and anxieties
2. Encourage mother to actively participate in the planning and performing of the infant's care.	2. Participation in the infant's care helps enhance parental/infant bonding, increases parental self-esteem and enhances a sense of control.
3. Encourage mother to seek emotional support from family, friends, and/or outside support groups	3. Use of support systems helps increase coping abilities, thus decreasing anxiety.

EVALUATION:
1. Jason's mother's verbal and nonverbal behavior indicates initiation of bonding.
2. Jason's mother openly discusses her fears/anxieties with staff.
3. Jason's mother is referred to a community support group.
4. Arrangements were made for medical follow-up for Jason following discharge.

Pyloric stenosis — vomiting and choking
Narrowing of pyloric sphincter

ence of the maternal antibodies in the exposed newborn. The ELISA test is repeated at 6 months of age because of the early inaccuracy. New test procedures are currently being developed to assess newborns for congenital AIDS.

Nursing care includes normal newborn care. Methods to prevent the spread of infection, universal precautions, are the same used by nursery personnel when caring for any newborn. The HIV organism is spread through contact with blood or body fluids of the infected neonate. Gloves are worn whenever contact with blood or body fluids is anticipated. These procedures include the initial bath, diaper changes, cord care, and circumcision care. Any time blood samples are being obtained, gloves are worn. Goggles and other coverings are worn as needed. One of the most common symptoms of the HIV-positive newborn is failure to thrive (see Table 20-7 for explanation and appropriate nursing interventions). Diarrhea and susceptibility to infections pose challenges in providing quality nursing care for the HIV-infected newborn.

In the HIV-infected newborn, attention to sound nutrition and maintenance of skin integrity are important in reducing the incidence of infection. The nurse should be observant to changes in the newborn's behavior and skin condition. Color, appetite, stools, and temperature may serve as early indicators of arising problems. The nurse assesses, documents, and reports any changes to the health care provider. See the Nursing Care Plan, Neonate Whose Mother is HIV Positive for several nursing interventions.

The Newborn of a Diabetic Mother

Diabetes is a disease of carbohydrate metabolism. It is caused by insufficient insulin production by the pancreas. Diabetes carries a risk for the fetus of the pregnant woman. Women with long-standing diabetes may have vascular disease that can interfere with nutrients reaching the fetus in utero. This may result in fetal death or intrauterine growth retardation.

Uncontrolled or poorly controlled diabetes in the pregnant woman may result in an elevated maternal blood glucose level. Under the influence of the high blood glucose, the fetus can develop **macrosomia** (large body size for gestational age) and congenital anomalies. Difficult birth and birth injuries may result from the macrosomia. Congenital anomalies seen in the newborn of a diabetic mother include congenital heart defects, CNS anomalies, and tracheoesophageal fistula. After birth, the most common problem for the newborn is hypoglycemia. This occurs especially in the infant of the mother whose diabetes is not well controlled. During fetal life, the fetus receives excessive amounts of glucose, which stimulates the fetus' pancreas to produce increased amounts of insulin. After birth, the maternal glucose supply is no longer available. The neonate's pancreas is not able to slow insulin production quickly enough, and hypoglycemia results. For this reason, early and frequent heel sticks are performed to assess the neonate's blood glucose level. Early oral feedings or intravenous glucose is administered to maintain the neonate's blood glucose levels. A Dextrostix (Miles) determination of less than 40 mg/dL is considered hypoglycemia in the full-term neonate. Laboratory blood glucose determinations should be performed periodically to confirm the accuracy of the Dextrostix results. Left untreated, hypoglycemia can lead to seizures, brain damage, and death.

When the prenatal history indicates diabetes, when the newborn is small for gestational age, large for gestational age, or weighs more than nine pounds, the nurse monitors the newborn for hypoglycemia. Blood glucose levels can diagnose the condition before the onset of symptoms. Symptoms of hypoglycemia include jitteriness, seizures, and apnea. Early oral feedings of breast milk or formula within the first 30 minutes after birth help maintain blood glucose levels within the normal range. The normal range for laboratory-determined blood glucose for the full-term neonate at birth is 30 to 60 mg/dL. At 1 day of age, the normal range is 40 to 60 mg/dL.

Newborns of diabetic mothers are prone to respiratory distress syndrome. The cause of this is uncertain, but it is thought to be a result of the inability of the fetus to use phospholipids because of hyperinsulinism. This interferes with the establishment of an adequate L/S ratio (see Chapter 19). The nurse should carefully monitor respiratory adaptation of the newborn, providing nursing care that supports respirations. Transient tachypnea of the newborn (TTN) is the most common respiratory distress seen in the neonate of a diabetic mother (see earlier discussion in this chapter). The newborn of a diabetic mother responds to the environment in an immature manner, regardless of size. Liver functioning is delayed, and the newborn is prone to hyperbilirubinemia, possibly because of polycythemia (increased number of red blood cells).

The Newborn of a Substance-Abusing Mother

Newborns born to women who abuse alcohol or drugs may be born physiologically dependent on the abused substance or substances. These newborns may suffer

[handwritten: hyperbilirubinemia — 24hrs after birth]

[handwritten: 1 portion goes to a blind pouch then the other one goes to the trachea]

congenital anomalies. The substances most commonly abused are alcohol, cocaine, and opiates, including methadone, a synthetic drug with properties similar to those of heroin and morphine. These neonates may suffer from neonatal abstinence syndrome, formerly referred to as narcotic withdrawal. Display 20-1 lists some of the characteristic symptoms seen in neonates of substance-abusing mothers.

Neonatal Abstinence Syndrome

Nursing care of newborns born to substance-abusing mothers focuses on monitoring the condition of the newborn. The nurse caring for a newborn with neonatal abstinence syndrome must have advanced skill and lots of patience. Crying for no apparent reason is common in these neonates. They are very difficult to console. Providing adequate rest and nutrition are nursing priorities. Stimulation of the newborn is reduced. These babies tend to rest more comfortably while swaddled tightly. Special "rocker beds," which rhythmically rock the neonate and transmit uterinelike sounds, seem to provide comfort. The neonate is snugly swaddled and placed in this type of bed. Avoiding brightly lit and noisy environments reduces irritability. Attention to nutrition and prevention of vomiting are important aspects of care of the neonate born to substance-abusing mothers. Although these neonates may display almost frantic non-nutritive sucking, they seem unable to coordinate the suck–swallow reflex to feed adequately. Gastrointestinal hypermotility is common. Paregoric may be administered to quiet gastric motility that causes regurgitation, weight loss, diarrhea, and results in excoriated buttocks. Maintenance of skin integrity and body temperature promote newborn health. Respirations are monitored and supported as needed. Medications, such as phenytoin (Dilantin) and phenobarbital, may be given to reduce seizures and promote rest. Frantic activity results in the knees, elbows, and nose of these neonates becoming red, raw, and tender from rubbing against bedding. Conscientious skin care and protection of bony prominences are essential.

The nurse may have a difficult time caring for the substance-abusing woman without being judgmental. However, the nurse must support and accept the woman. The woman may need encouragement and guidance to enter a treatment program. She may have overwhelming guilt and remorse. Conversely, she may not be able to focus on the fact that her substance-abusing behavior caused the problems of her newborn. Social service and public health referrals are necessary to provide the care the family needs. Long-term follow-up care is necessary to assess the developing infant and child for learning and behavioral disabilities. Foster

---

DISPLAY 20-1
Some Symptoms Seen in Fetal Alcohol and Neonatal Abstinence Syndromes

Alcohol Abuse

Characteristic facial anomalies

Microcephaly

Developmental delay; mental retardation

Fine motor dysfunction

Hypotonia

Failure to thrive

Cardiac septal defects

Malformations of limbs, joints, phalanges

Cocaine Abuse

Intrauterine growth retardation (IUGR)

Prematurity

Cardiac defects

Irritability

Inconsolable crying

High-pitched cry

Gaze aversion

Increased incidence of SIDS

Poor feeders

Hypersensitivity

Tremors and seizures

Hyperactive nonnutritive sucking

Opiate Abuse

Hyperthermia

Irritability

Hypertonicity

High-pitched cry

Easily startled

Short sleep cycles

Tachypnea

Tachycardia

Hyperactive nonnutritive sucking

Poor feeder

Regurgitates feedings

Stuffy nose

Seizure activity

---

care may be a necessary step while the family is attempting to solve its problems.

Fetal Alcohol Syndrome

There is no known safe level of alcohol ingestion during pregnancy. Newborns born to women who abuse alcohol are born with fetal alcohol syndrome (FAS). Neonates with this syndrome have characteristic facies. This includes a thin upper lip, short, upturned nose, small lower jaw, short opening between eyes, and a flat philtrum (vertical groove in upper lip). They usually suffer learning disabilities or mental retardation. Newborns born with FAS demonstrate a growth lag at birth. This lag may continue into the postpartum period. Display 20-1 lists common symptoms. Nursing care is directed toward reducing symptoms and improving nutrition using many of the techniques that are used in caring for neonates with abstinence syndrome.

NURSING CARE PLAN
The Family Experiencing Loss

ASSESSMENT:
- Stillborn neonate at 40 weeks' gestation
- Family afraid to look at infant
- Family appears stunned by loss

NURSING DIAGNOSIS #1: Ineffective Family Coping, related to death of neonate

EXPECTED OUTCOMES:
1. Family members identify coping mechanisms that have helped them in the past.
2. Family members identify resources to help with grief resolution.

Nursing Interventions	*Rationale*
1. Same staff nurses assigned on each shift.	1. Continuity of care promotes improved nurse–family relationships.
2. Encourage family to talk openly through use of communication techniques.	2. Talking allows family to begin to work through their feelings.
3. Provide physical care to woman in an unhurried manner.	3. Encourages woman to express feelings and an opportunity to discuss loss.
4. Offer woman and her partner the chance to see and hold the infant.	4. Allows them to bond with infant; promotes grief resolution.
5. Provide family with written information about neonatal losses and the grieving process.	5. Allows family to refer to the information when they are ready.
6. Provide family with information about bereavement groups.	6. Facilitates continued work towards grief resolution.

EVALUATION: The family begins to identify their coping strengths, makes necessary decisions, and expresses feelings openly.

ASSESSMENT:
- Mother states, "How will we ever tell the other children?"
- Grandmother weeping loudly; grandfather stony silent, looking grim

EXPECTED OUTCOMES: Mother identifies age-appropriate ways to discuss the death with the other children in the family.
Grandparents are assisted in expressing their grief and identifying ways to support the parents.

Nursing Interventions	*Rationale*
1. Inquire about ages of siblings at home and their previous experience with death, if any.	1. Children's perception of death is affected by their developmental stage and past experiences with death, including death of pets.
2. Provide family with story or reading material dealing with death that is age-appropriate for children.	2. There are many excellent age-appropriate resources to help children deal with death. Knowledge of age-appropriate understandings of the child assists the adult family members to interact with the children.
3. Encourage family to name the neonate.	3. Naming the neonate provides an identity and makes it more real.
4. Spend time with grandparents in an unhurried atmosphere; talk about their past experiences with death, especially in the family.	4. Grandparents can be a resource for the parents. Recognizing them, encouraging them to express their feelings, and acknowledging their life experiences helps to mobilize them to support the rest of the family.
5. Make contacts with religious counselors, as desired by family members	5. Religious counselors can provide support to the family and help them make the immediate decisions they must make.

EVALUATION: The mother is able to talk with her other children about the death of the neonate. She encourages them to express their feelings in an age-appropriate manner. The grandparents provide strength to the family by assisting with the children and openly talking about their feelings with the parents. The family is comforted by the support of the family religious counselor.

Fetal Loss and Grief

Just as the birth of a healthy, robust newborn is a highly charged emotional event, so is the experience of fetal loss or death. Parents of a stillborn newborn and those who suffer a perinatal loss endure intense emotional trauma. The newborn may die before, during, or after birth. To incorporate the loss and accept this traumatic event, the family needs to work through the grieving process. The stages of the grieving process have been identified as denial and isolation, anger, bargaining, depression and acute grief, and finally acceptance. The family members must work through each of these stages at their own pace. The process is not one that flows easily from one stage to another. An individual family member may be in one stage while another is in a different stage. A person can complete one stage only to regress back to an earlier stage. The nurse caring for the grieving family must be very sensitive, kind, and patient when providing support to the family. The family who experiences a reproductive loss or neonatal death must release the dreams that they had for the infant they lost. This may be a long and traumatic process.

Parents work through their grief more effectively if they bond with their newborn. The body of the newborn should be treated with respect. Parents may want to see and hold their newborn. This activity helps parents accept the reality of their loss while beginning the resolution of grief. The baby should be dressed and wrapped in a receiving blanket. The nurse prepares the parents for their baby's appearance.

The nurse spends time with the grieving family to offer support and to encourage open expressions of sorrow. The family needs as much time as they want to say goodbye to their newborn. They may want to take pictures to remember what their newborn looks like. Many facilities have a camera and film available for this purpose. If the family refuses the pictures, inform them the pictures will be retained by the facility, in case they wish to see them at a later date. The family may request the identification band, receiving blanket, a lock of hair, or other "memory" objects. Some facilities prepare a memory booklet for this purpose. Burial arrangements and baptism may be desired by the family. Efforts to assist the parents with these arrangements may be helpful to the grieving family.

Although the family may wish to have privacy, the family should not be avoided. All health team members caring for the grieving family need to be informed of the loss. Inappropriate comments are avoided, such as "You're young, you can have another baby," "Another baby will help you forget this one," or "You have to think of the rest of your family." Opportunities for the family to express feelings about their loss are encouraged. Some families may not wish to openly express their feelings at this time. It is important to view the family's response to the loss in a nonjudgmental manner. A sensitive, caring approach is appropriate. Referral of the family to a support group for bereavement counseling allows family members to continue work on grief resolution. Organizations such as SHARE and Compassionate Friends have chapters throughout the United States and Canada. The members of these organizations have experienced the death of an infant or child and can provide needed support. Just knowing that they are not alone in their grief may be helpful to the family.

There is no correct time or way to grieve. The nurse should help the family recognize that they will progress through the grief stages at different rates. Families with other children also may need support and guidance in explaining the death to the neonate's siblings. The accompanying Nursing Care Plan provides sample nursing diagnoses and interventions for families experiencing loss. The nurse needs to be aware of dysfunctional grieving behaviors such as psychosomatic illnesses, inappropriate hostility, hyperactive behavior patterns, and unhealthy changes in family relationships.

Discharge Planning

Plans for discharge are begun on admission. Each newborn needs to be discharged to family who are physically and emotionally prepared to care for their newborn. In addition to normal newborn care, families of special-needs newborns often have to be familiar with specialized treatments and equipment. Allowing family members to handle equipment and care for their newborn, under the supervision of the skilled nurses, allows the family to build self-confidence. Opportunities for positive feedback and reinforcement are important in helping the family develop a sense of competence. Special equipment necessary for care of the newborn must be determined before discharge. This allows the family to obtain necessary equipment and gain skills before their infant comes home. Specific instructions on types of equipment to purchase or rent are helpful. The family needs ample opportunity to practice their skills and demonstrate the techniques they are learning before the infant is discharged.

Community resources should be identified for the family. A variety of support groups allow families to continue to grow and cope with the challenges of caring for a special-needs infant. With the support of the nursing staff, families of special-needs newborns can acquire the skills necessary to provide physical care. With appropriate emotional support, the family learns to accept their newborn's condition. Healthy parent–newborn bonding is promoted. The nurse must identify the family's coping strengths and support systems to determine the their needs.

Successful discharge of a newborn with special needs to a loving, attentive, and capable family is very rewarding. The health care team can view the beneficial results of their care. Nurses can feel a sense of shared pride and accomplishment in supporting a positive family-centered childbearing experience.

Adolescent Considerations

Adjusting to and caring for a special-needs infant requires a caregiver with maturity. The adolescent may not be sufficiently mature to handle these responsibilities. The nurse and other health care personnel must be especially supportive of the adolescent. In addition, the adolescent's own needs must be carefully assessed to determine the kind of postdischarge support she will need. The adolescent whose own family is supportive may be able to turn to her mother or other close older relative for help. However, adolescents often are rejected by their families and may be on their own with no family support system. Community resource referrals are necessary to fill the needs of the infant and young mother.

The adolescent who experiences the death of a fetus or newborn may be experiencing a close death for the first time. She also may be faced with great guilt about the death. She may feel that she did something that caused the condition that resulted in death. The nurse must be very sensitive, patient, and supportive in helping the adolescent deal with the loss and guilt. The adolescent usually has very few life experiences that will help her resolve her grief. The nurse may need to be innovative in providing support for the adolescent, using all the resources available to their greatest extent. The adolescent who is alone needs to have a contact person who will follow up and support her after discharge from the facility. Seeking support from a group such as SHARE or Compassionate Friends may be very important step for the adolescent.

Cultural Considerations

Chapter 17 discussed the belief in some cultures that their newborn is subject to the curses of an "evil eye." This belief may contribute to the way in which the family copes with the birth of a special-needs child. Great guilt can be the result of some of these cultural beliefs. Also, if the neonate died of a previously known hereditary condition, the family may have guilt for allowing the pregnancy to happen. The grandmother often has a strong influence on the family and their reaction to the neonate. Some cultural practices may not be permitted because of the condition of the neonate. For example, the Jewish male may not be able to be circumcised on the eighth day of life if his condition does not permit it. This may be upsetting to the family. The nurse must be sensitive to the family's feelings.

The response of the family to the death of a fetus or neonate is very dependent on cultural beliefs. Persons from some cultures may respond to death with wailing and noisy mourning, and others may seem quiet and detached, almost as though nothing has happened. The nurse must accept each of these ways of grieving and respect the family's needs. Funeral and burial arrangements may vary with cultural customs, also. The nurse must be supportive but let the family take the lead in these plans. If necessary, the nurse can tactfully inquire about the family's desires. Throughout the entire ex-

---

✓ NURSING DIAGNOSES CHECKLIST

Nursing Diagnoses Related to Care of the Newborn With Special Needs

Family anxiety, related to unfamiliarity with newborn's condition and potential outcome.

Interrupted Breastfeeding, related to newborn's physical condition

Ineffective Breathing Pattern, related to immaturity of central nervous system

Impaired Gas Exchange, related to insufficient surfactant stores, weak respiratory effort.

Anticipatory Grieving, related to instability of newborn's condition.

Ineffective Infant Feeding Pattern, related to muscular weakness and high caloric requirement

High risk for infection, related to lack of skin integrity and open spinal cord

Family Health Seeking Behaviors, related to the neonate's long term care requirements

Altered Parenting, related to lack of opportunity for bonding

High risk for ineffective family coping, related to the neonate's death

perience, the nurse must remain openly caring and supportive.

The Role of the Nurse

The role of the nurse who cares for the neonate with special needs is challenging and rewarding. The birth of a newborn with congenital anomalies or other special needs is distressing for the health care staff as well as for the family. The nurse must be aware of the need to avoid any negative reaction, either verbally or nonverbally. In addition to providing the skilled nursing care that the neonate needs, the nurse has the responsibility of teaching, supporting, listening to, and responding to the needs of the family. The family is undergoing a crisis situation, and the nurse must respond in a way that helps relieve some of their feelings of fear and anxiety. The role is a strenuous one.

A detailed assessment helps the nurse develop an individualized plan of care. Based on assessment data that the nurse gathers, nursing diagnoses are developed for the special-needs newborn. Although prenatal testing frequently is reliable in predicting the impending arrival of a special needs neonate, there are still unexpected births that bring unforeseen devastation. The nurse must be alert to any signs and symptoms that may indicate additional problems. The nurse provides care for the neonate and the family to achieve the highest level of care possible for them. Nursing diagnoses related to the care of the newborn with special needs are presented in the Nursing Diagnoses Checklist.

REVIEW

In this final chapter, the text has focused on the neonate with special needs. Nursing assessments and interventions in the initial period immediately after birth were discussed. The discussion also focused on the immense emotional factors that are involved for family and health care personnel. Transportation of the neonate to a specialized NICU was discussed.

Some of the conditions presented in this chapter were respiratory disorders, congenital anomalies, chromosomal disorders, inborn errors of metabolism, and incompatibilities of ABO and Rh. Much of the information was presented in table format to enable the reader to quickly find pertinent information about a specific condition. Infections that may affect the newborn were presented, including the infective agent, maternal and neonatal effects, and common treatment and methods of prevention. The grief process and the support and guidance the family needs during this time were discussed.

This text is an introduction to maternity-newborn nursing. It is hoped that the reader will use this as a base on which to build a strong foundation in caring for the family and the neonate in any setting. From here the reader is encouraged to continue to read, study, and research additional information to enhance nursing care.

◘ KEY POINTS

◆ Prenatal data such as maternal disease or results from diagnostic testing may indicate potential risks for the developing fetus. Intrapartum findings, including Apgar scores and the appearance of the amniotic fluid, may suggest problems in the newborn. Neonatal findings of variations from normal often predict the birth of a special-needs newborn.

◆ The family most often anticipate the birth of a healthy, perfect newborn. With the birth of a special-needs newborn, the family experiences grief over the loss of a perfect baby. The nurse provides support and guidance to help parents adapt to their special-needs newborn.

◆ Knowledge of resuscitation procedures are essential for nurses practicing in the birthing room or newborn nursery. Attention to maintaining an open airway and maintenance of the newborn's body temperature are top nursing priorities.

◆ The newborn may or may not be easily recognized during this early time. Some congenital problems are obviously apparent physically, such as cleft lip, omphalocele, gastroschisis, spina bifida, and club foot. Other indications of special needs are a poor Apgar score and respiratory difficulties.

◆ The nurse helps to set the tone of the birth area. The family watches for nonverbal clues when an air of possible emergency is evident. Arranging for another nurse to talk with the family and keep them informed is very helpful. The nurse helps maintain a calm, controlled atmosphere.

◆ The nurse prepares the family of the neonate who is to be transferred, telling the family about the physical aspects of the NICU. Rules, regulations, and protocol are explained. Their questions are answered, and they are encouraged to express their fears. The family is provided time with the neonate before the transfer if the neonate's condition permits.

◆ The most common fracture is the fracture of the clavicle.

◆ In utero or during birth, the fetus or neonate may suffer hypoxia. The rectal sphincter relaxes and meconium is expelled into the amniotic fluid. If the neonate inhales some of the meconium with the first breaths, it is aspirated and causes a blockage in the alveoli. It results in trapping air in the alveoli and causes overdistension of the alveoli. Pneumonia and pneumothorax result.

◆ Spina bifida occurs as spina bifida occulta, meningocele, or myelomeningocele. Occulta has only a bony defect, but no meninges or cord escape through the defect. It may only be

1. A history of hydramnios during the pregnancy should alert the nurse to pay specific attention to the infant's:

- ○ **A.** Vital signs
- ○ **B.** Feeding ability
- ○ **C.** Hemoglobin and hematocrit
- ○ **D.** Reflexes

2. How does RhoGAM prevent sensitization of an Rh negative woman?

- ○ **A.** RhoGAM prevents formation of antibodies
- ○ **B.** RhoGAM increases production of fetal red blood cells
- ○ **C.** RhoGAM increases the production of antibodies
- ○ **D.** RhoGAM neutralizes the fetus' Rh factor

3. Prompt management of phenylketonuria helps prevent:

- ○ **A.** Respiratory distress
- ○ **B.** Excessive weight gain
- ◉ **C.** Mental retardation
- ○ **D.** Congestive heart failure

4. Which of the following should be the nurse's *first* priority when caring for a newborn?

- ○ **A.** Thermoregulation
- ○ **B.** Maintaining an open airway
- ○ **C.** Prevention of infection
- ◉ **D.** Adequate nutrition

5. Signs of respiratory distress include all of the following EXCEPT:

- ○ **A.** Grunting
- ○ **B.** Nasal flaring
- ○ **C.** Decreased respiratory rate
- ○ **D.** Cyanosis

marked by a dimple and a hair tuft on the spinal column. Meningocele is the escape of meninges through the opening. Myelomeningocele is the involvement of the cord and its nerves as well as the meninges. Myelomeningocele is the most serious, leading to paralysis and incontinence.

◆ The family who experiences neonatal loss need support to begin grief resolution. Referral to family support groups allows continuation of grief resolution after discharge.

BIBLIOGRAPHY

Beachy, P., & Deacon, J. (1993). *Core curriculum: Neonatal intensive care nursing*. Philadelphia: W. B. Saunders.

Butler, K. M. & Pizzo, P. A. (1992). HIV infection in children. In Devita, V., Jr., Hellman, S., & Rosenberg, S.A. (Eds.), *AIDS: Etiology, diagnosis, treatment, and prevention* (pp. 285–305). Philadelphia: J. B. Lippincott.

Castiglia, P. T., & Harbin, R. E. (1992). *Child health care: Process and practice*. Philadelphia: J. B. Lippincott.

Clark, P. J., & Byrne, M. W. (1993). A step up from home: Enhanced care for medically complex HIV infected children. *The American Journal of Maternal-Child Nursing, 18*(2), 94–98.

Kelley, S. J., Walsh, J. H., & Thompson, K. (1991). Birth outcomes, health problems, and neglect with prenatal exposure to cocaine. *Pediatric Nursing, 17*(2), 130–135.

Kenner, C. A. (1992). *Nurse's clinical guide: Neonatal care*. Springhouse, PA: Springhouse Corporation.

Krause, K. D., & Younger, V. J. (1992). Nursing diagnoses as guidelines in the care of the neonatal ECMO patient. *Journal of Obstetric, Gynecologic, and Neonatal Nursing, 21*(3), 169–176.

Lewis, K. D., Schmeder, N. H., & Bennett, B. (1992). Maternal drug abuse and its effects on young children. *The American Journal of Maternal-Child Nursing, 17*(4), 198–203.

MacLaren, A. (1994). *Concepts and activities: Maternal-neonatal nursing*. Springhouse, PA: Springhouse Corporation.

Marks, M. G. (1994). *Broadribb's introductory pediatric nursing*. (4th ed). Philadelphia: J. B. Lippincott.

May, K. A., & Mahlmeister, L. R. (1994). *Maternal & neonatal care: Family-centered care* (3rd ed.). Philadelphia: J. B. Lippincott.

Merenstein, G. B., & Gardner, S. L. (1993). *Handbook of neonatal intensive care* (3rd ed.). St Louis: Mosby–Year Book.

Peterson, P. K. (1992). Spina bifida: Nursing challenge. *RN, 55*(1), 40–47.

Pillitterri, A. (1992). *Maternal and child health nursing*. Philadelphia: J. B. Lippincott.

Primeau, M. R., & Recht, C. K. (1994). Professional bereavement photographs: One aspect of a perinatal bereavement program. *Journal of Obstetric, Gynecologic and Neonatal Nursing, 23*(1), 22–25.

Ross, T., & Dickason, E. J. (1992). Nursing alert: Vertical transmission of HIV and HBV. *The American Journal of Maternal-Child Nursing, 17*(4), 192–195.

Speers, A. T., & Speers, M. (1992). Care of the infant in a Pavlik harness (congenital dislocated hip). *Pediatric Nursing, 18*(3), 229–232.

Sullivan, J., Boudreaux, M., & Keller, P. (1993). Can we help the substance abusing mother and infant? *The American Journal of Maternal-Child Nursing, 18*(3), 153–157.

APPENDIX A

Assessment Tool for Prenatal Visits

Date:

Name:

Address:

Phone Number:

Emergency Person and Number:

Social Security Number:

Means of Transportation:

Employment Status:

Significant Other/Support Person:

Insurance/Medicaid:

GTPALM:

Ages of Other Children:

Allergies:

Medical History (Systems analysis, including diseases such as diabetes, heart, lung, respiratory, and endocrine disorders, hypertension, medications):

Obstetric History (Include complications for antepartum, intrapartum [during childbirth], postpartum periods; fetal complications):

Family Health History (Include medical disorders treated with medications, age and health status of parents):

Family Obstetrical History: (Include significant problems for antepartum, intrapartum, postpartum periods; fetal complications)

Vital Signs:

    Temperature

    Pulse

    Respirations

    Blood Pressure

Height:

Prepregnancy Weight:

Present Weight:

Physical Examination:

HEENT (Head, Eyes, Ears, Nose, Throat)

Cardiovascular

Lungs and Thorax

Abdomen

Fundal Height

Musculoskeletal (Range of motion, pulses, reflexes)

Psychosocial Assessment:

History of Alcohol, Smoking, Drugs, Abuse (physical, sexual, substance)

Support Person

Housing

Heat/Running Water

Sanitary Conditions

Financial Status

Stress Adaptation

Problem-Solving Abilities

Attitude Toward Pregnancy

Transportation

Laboratory Tests:

Complete Blood Count

    Hgb

    Hct

    RBC

    WBC

    Platelets

Electrolytes

    Glucose

    Na

    K

    Cl

    Blood/Urea/Nitrogen

    Creatinine

    CO_2

    Urinalysis

    VDRL

    Blood Type

    RH Factor

Indirect Coombs'

HIV (informed consent)

Rubella Titer

Hepatitis B Titer

Pelvic Examination:

Date of Last Pap Smear and Result

Pap Smear Sent This Examination

Physical Findings:

Chadwick's Sign

Goodell's Sign

Hegar's Sign

Vagina

Cervix

Uterus

Fallopian Tubes

Ovaries

Rectum

Vaginal Discharge

Pelvic Measurements:

True Conjugate

Diagonal Conjugate

Fetal Heart Tones:

Rate

Location

Fetal Movements:

Gestational Age:

Weeks

Months

Disparity

Sonogram Recommended:

Other Diagnostic Tests Ordered:

Recommendations:

APPENDIX B

Normal Laboratory Test Values During Pregnancy

Laboratory Test	Normal Range	Abnormal Findings (woman and fetus)
Hgb	12–16 g/dL	Low levels may indicate anemia in the woman
Hct	37%–47%	Low levels may indicate anemia in the woman
WBC	5000–10,000	Low levels may indicate compromise in immune system
		High levels may indicate infection
RBC	3.6–5.0	Low level may indicate anemia
		High level may indicate polycythemia (excess of red blood cells) as in dehydration
Platelets	150,000–350,000	Low level may indicate prolonged bleeding
		High level may indicate malignancy
Glucose	60–80 mg/dL	Low level may indicate hypoglycemia (low blood sugar)
		High level may indicate diabetes
Na	135–148	Low level may indicate retention of excess body water
		High level may indicate dehydration
K	3.5–5 mEq/L	Low level may indicate food fast
		High level may indicate renal problems
Cl	98–106	Low level may indicate vomiting
		High level may indicate dehydration
Creatinine	0.6–1.2 mg/dL	Low level may indicate impaired renal function
BUN	7–18 mg/dL	High level may indicate impaired renal function
		Low level may indicate liver failure
CO_2	23–30	High level may indicate vomiting
VDRL	Nonreactive	Reactive indicates syphilis antibodies
Blood type	A+/–, B+/– O+/–, AB	Indicates presence of antigens
Indirect Coombs'	Negative	Positive test indicates anti-Rh antibodies
HIV	Negative	Positive test indicates presence of infection
Rubella	Immune	No immunity to rubella virus
Hepatitis B	Negative	Positive result indicates exposure

APPENDIX C

Blood Group Table

Antibodies Found in Crossmatching		
Blood Grouping System	*Antibody*	*Description*
Rh-hr	Anti-D	Rh1
		May cause severe hemolytic disease of newborn
	Anti-C	Rh2
		Often found with anti-D, -Ce(rh$_i$) or -C^w
	Anti-E	Rh3
		Often found with anti-c
	Anti-c	Rh4
		Often found with anti-E
	Anti-e	Rh5
		Often found with anti-C
	Anti-C^w	Rh8
	Anti-V	Rh10
		Alternate antigen names: ce^s, hr^v
Kell	Anti-K	K1
		Some non–red cell immune
		Occasional Kell system antibodies may not react
	Anti-k	K2
		Antigen may be depressed by the presence of Kp^a
	Anti-Kp^a	K3
		Few non–red cell immune
	Anti-Kp^b	K4
	Anti-Js^a	K6
		Few non–red cell immune
	Anti-Js^b	K7
Duffy	Anti-Fy^a	Some antibodies exhibit dosage.
	Anti-Fy^b	Some antibodies may bind complement.
Kidd	Anti-Jk^a	Antibodies may exhibit dosage.
		May cause severe delayed hemolytic transfusion reactions
Kidd	Anti-Jk^b	Antibody titers may drop rapidly below detectable levels.
		Antibodies may require anti-C3 for detection.
Lutheran	Anti-Lu^a	Antibody gives mixed-field–like agglutination
	Anti-Lu^b	

(continued)

(continued)

Blood Grouping System	Antibody	Description
	Antibodies Found in Crossmatching	
MN	Anti-M	Common antibody
		Seldom clinically significant or implicated in HDN
		May be pH-dependent or exhibit dosage
	Anti-N	Rare antibody
		Rarely causes HDN
		Formaldehyde-induced anti-N commonly found in dialysis patients
	Anti-S	Antibody may be enhanced if incubated below 37°C before AHG.
	Anti-s	
	Anti-U	Autoanti-U identified as rare cause of WAIHA
Lewis	Anti-Le^a	Frequently found in serum of pregnant women
	Anti-Le^b	Neutralized by soluble antigen
	-Le^{bh}	Anti-Le^b often found with anti-Le^a
	-Le^{bL}	Anti-Le^b usually made by Le(a-b-) individuals
P	Anti-P$_1$	Antigen strength variable; neutralized by soluble antigen
	Anti-P	Biphasic hemolytic IgG autoantibody in PCH
		Alloantibody is usually potent IgM hemolysin.
	Anti-PP$_1$P^k (Tj^a)	
Xg	Anti-Xg^a	X-linked
Colton	Anti-Co^a	Rare antibodies
	Anti-Co^b	
Dombrock	Anti-Do^a	Incidence of Do^a lower in African Americans, Native Americans, and Orientals
	Anti-Do^b	Infrequently reported antibodies
Diego	Anti-Di^a	Di^a antigen frequency higher in Orientals and native Americans
	Anti-Di^b	
Wright	Anti-Wr^a	IgM and IgG forms of antibody reported
		Frequently occurring antibody
Vel	Anti-Vel	Antibodies usually IgM
		Antigen strength variable
		Binds complement
Sid	Anti-Sd^a	Antigen weaker during pregnancy
		Wide variation of antigen expression
		Agglutinates have refractile, mixed-field appearance.
HLA associated	Anti-Bg$_a$	Antigen strength variable
	-Bg$_b$	Antibodies often found in multitransfused or
	-Bg$_c$	multiparous patients
	-Bg	Antibodies characteristically weakly reactive
		Bg/HLA Bg^a/HLA-B7
		associations: Bg^b/HLA-Ba17
		Bg^c/HLA-A28
Cartwright	Anti-Yt^a	Antibody not uncommon in Yt(a-) individuals
	Anti-Yt^b	Rare antibody usually found in combination with other antibodies

(continued)

(continued)

	Antibodies Found in Crossmatching	
Blood Grouping System	*Antibody*	*Description*
HTLA (high titer low avidity)	Anti-CHª -Rgª -Knª -McCª -Ykª -Csª -Gyª -Hy -JMH	Antigen strength variable Antibodies characteristically weakly reactive
I	Anti-I	Most frequent cold autoagglutinin Anti-I in CHD has wide thermal range, high titer; binds complement; seen as alloantibody in i adults
	Anti-i	Antibody seen in serum of patients with infectious mononucleosis Rare cause of CHD Antigen very weakly expressed on the cells of most adults

(From Fischbach, F. [1992]. *A manual of laboratory and diagnostic tests* (p. 550, Table 8-8). Philadelphia: J. B. Lippincott.)
(*Adapted from Baxter Healthcare Corporation, Dade Division, Miami, FL, Baxter Healthcare Corporation, 1987*)

APPENDIX D

Normal Laboratory Test Results

Test	Results Prepregnant	Results At Term	Purpose
CBC			
RBC	4,000,000/mm^3	25–30% increased	Detect physiologic anemia in increased plasma volume
Hematocrit	36–46%	32–39%	
Hemoglobin	12–16 g/100 mL	12.3 g/mL	Detect anemia—present if below 32%
WBC	4500–10,000/mm^3	18,000–25,000/mm^3	
Platelets	140,000/mm^3	140,000/mm^3	Detect anemia—present if below 10.5 g/mL
			Elevated in infection, hemorrhage, and eclampsia
			Assess coagulation factors
Indirect Coombs'	Negative	Negative	Positive in Rh incompatibility
VDRL	Negative	Negative	Positive indicates syphilis
Hepatitis Screen	Negative	Negative	Screen for hepatitis B
Sickle cell prep	Negative	Negative	Screens for sickle hemoglobin, but does not indicate if neonate will be a carrier or have the disease
Urinalysis			
Sugar	Negative	Negative or 1+	Screen for gestational diabetes
Albumin	Negative	Negative	Screen for pregnancy induced hypertension
Microscopic	Negative	Negative	Screen for urinary infection
Glucose Screen	75 mg/100 mL (fasting)	65 mg/100 mL (fasting)	Screen for gestational diabetes
Rh factor	Rh+ or Rh–	Same	Test to determine Rh factor, alert for possible Rh factor problems with neonate
Blood typing	O, A, B, AB	Same	Blood typing for possible transfusion; also to alert to possible ABO incompatibility in neonate

APPENDIX E

Blood Incompatibilities

Categories	Maternal Blood Type	Incompatibility Blood Types	Compatible Fetal Blood Types
Rh incompatibilities	Negative	Positive	Negative
	Positive	None	Negative/Positive
ABO incompatibilities	O	A or B	O
	A	B or AB	O or A
	B	A or AB	B or O
	AB	None	A, B, or O

Answers to Self-Assessment Questions

Chapter 1: Directions in Family-Centered Maternal-Newborn Care

1. D. A neonatologist should be present at a delivery of **a patient at 30 weeks' gestation.**
Rationale: A neonatologist should be present at the delivery of a high-risk infant such as one born at 30 weeks.

2. C. Goals of family-centered maternity care do <u>not</u> include **making decisions for the family during the intrapartum period.**
Rationale: Although nurses should assist and support families in decision making, they should not make decisions for them.

3. C. The following nurse's note is an example of the evaluation phase of the nursing process: **"The patient states incisional pain has decreased following the administration of Demerol."**
Rationale: This note evaluates the effectiveness of the care provided.

4. B. Economic status plays the greatest role in predicting infant mortality.
Rationale: Poverty has been identified as the single most reliable predictor of infant mortality.

5. D. Data regarding maternal/fetal morbidity/mortality indicates that **low birth weight is a major problem in the United States.**
Rationale: Approximately two thirds of infant deaths in the United States are associated with low birth weight.

Chapter 2: Reproduction and Human Sexuality

1. C. Decreased secretion of estrogen and progesterone results in **menstruation.**
Rationale: If fertilization does not occur, the corpus luteum begins to break down, resulting in decreased amounts of estrogen and progesterone. As a result, the endometrium begins to shed (menstruation).

2. B. The role of secretions from the prostate gland and bulbourethral glands is to **increase sperm motility.**

Rationale: Secretions from the prostate and bulbourethral glands are alakaline and help the sperms' motility in the acidic vaginal environment.

3. A. Prolactin is responsible for milk production.
Rationale: Prolactin, which is secreted from the anterior pituitary gland, helps produce milk by stimulating cells in the alveoli.

4. C. Women are more prone to urinary tract infections than men because of **the length of the urethra.**
Rationale: Bacteria can enter the woman's body more easily because of the shorter length of the urethra.

5. C. Ovarian functioning is influenced by secretion of the **follicle-stimulating hormone and luteinizing hormone.**
Rationale: The follicle-stimulating hormone (FSH) stimulates the follicles in the ovaries while the luteinizing hormone (LH) enhances its maturation.

Chapter 3: Family Planning and Infertility

1. B. Inadequate amounts of **progesterone** can prevent implantation of a fertilized ovum.
Rationale: Progesterone plays an important role in preparing the endometrium for implantation and in maintaining a resulting pregnancy.

2. C. You would advise a woman who forgot to take one birth control pill yesterday to **take 2 pills that day and continue the pack as prescribed.**
Rationale: A single missed pill should be taken as soon as possible.

3. C. A man's age is <u>least</u> likely to cause male infertility.
Rationale: Male infertility results primarily from ejaculatory, sperm, or testicular causes.

4. D. An intrauterine device (IUD) prevents pregnancy by **preventing implantation.**
Rationale: By irritating the uterine lining, a fertilized egg is unable to implant in the uterus.

5. A. The **female condom** is the safest contraceptive method for a woman with a history of toxic shock syndrome (TSS).
Rationale: *There is no evidence at this time linking TSS and the female condom (perhaps because of its short time on the market).*

Chapter 4: Women's Health Care

1. B. To decrease the incidence of incorrect Pap smear results, **the slide should be immediately sprayed with fixative.**
Rationale: *The fixative helps prevent deterioration of the specimen.*

2. C. A woman with fibrocystic breast disease should be instructed to **have a mammogram every year.**
Rationale: *Yearly mammograms will help monitor the disease's progress.*

3. A. A woman with PMS should be instructed to increase her intake of **oranges** before her menstrual period.
Rationale: *Fruits are natural diuretics, which can help alleviate water retention.*

4. C. Dysmenorrhea is primarily due to increased production of **prostaglandins.**
Rationale: *Prostaglandins cause uterine muscles to contract, thus causing cramps.*

5. C. Decreased estrogen production during menopause has <u>not</u> been associated with **weight loss.**
Rationale: *Decreased estrogen production is associated with weight gain.*

Chapter 5: Normal Prenatal Physical and Psychosocial Changes

1. D. A pregnant woman who has had one full-term infant, two preterm infants (one of whom died), and one miscarriage would be classified as **G5P1212.**
Rationale: *Counting the present pregnancy, the woman has been pregnant 5 times. She had one full-term infant, two premature infants, one miscarriage, and has two live children.*

2. B. A woman complains of urinary frequency when she is 10 weeks' pregnant. It would be appropriate for the nurse to **inform her this is common at this point of pregnancy.**
Rationale: *Pressure from the enlarging uterus on the bladder causes urinary frequency during the first trimester.*

3. D. Using Naegele's rule, a woman's due date would be **January 20th** if the first day of her last menstrual period was April 13th.
Rationale: *Using Naegle's rule, add 7 days to the first day of the last menstrual period and subtract 3 months. Thus:*
April 13 + 7 days = April 20, April 20 – 3 months = January 20

4. C. A pregnant patient should be encouraged to assume a **left lateral** position whenever possible.
Rationale: *Lying in a left lateral position decreases pressure on the inferior vena cava and promotes venous return from the lower extremities.*

5. B. Potential complications from pica do <u>not</u> include **excessive weight gain.**
Rationale: *Pica, the ingestion of nonfood items, is more likely to lead to a loss, not a gain, due to options A, C, and D.*

Chapter 6: Prenatal Visits and Assessments

1. B. Decreased hemoglobin and hematocrit levels during pregnancy are due to **hemodilution.**
Rationale: *During pregnancy, the total blood volume increases while the portion of red blood cells remain the same.*

2. C. During her first prenatal visit at 8 weeks, an overweight patient expresses concern over gaining more weight. She should be encouraged to **gain between 15 and 25 pounds.**
Rationale: *It is recommended that overweight women gain between 15 and 25 pounds during the entire pregnancy.*

3. C. You would expect a **glucose** lab test ordered for a woman at 27 weeks' gestation.
Rationale: *It is recommended that all pregnant women be screened for gestational diabetes between 26 and 28 weeks.*

4. A. A patient's fundal height measurement is greater than expected. The physician is likely to order an **ultrasound** for further evaluation.
Rationale: *An ultrasound is useful in identifying possible causes of increased fundal height such as hydramnios and multiple gestation.*

5. D. A woman's baseline B/P is 140/70. A blood pressure of **124/88** would be of the greatest concern at 25 weeks' gestation.

Rationale: An increase of ≥30 mm Hg systolic or ≥15 mm Hg diastolic over the baseline requires further evaluation.

Chapter 7: Prenatal Health Promotion

1. D. A patient complains of shortness of breath (SOB) at 35 weeks' gestation. The nurse's initial action should be to **explain that this is a common finding at this point in pregnancy.**
Rationale: The enlarging uterus limits lung expansion and presses against the diaphragm. Though a common finding, the extent of SOB should be investigated.

2. A. Adequate intake of vitamin K during pregnancy helps with **blood clotting.**
Rationale: Produced in the liver, vitamin K is necessary for the production of the blood-clotting factor, prothrombin.

3. C. To limit common discomforts of pregnancy, the woman should be instructed to **increase her fruit intake.**
Rationale: Constipation can be prevented by increasing intake of fruits, vegetables, and high-bulk items.

4. D. Management of lower leg cramping includes **frequent rest periods.**
Rationale: All women should be encouraged to rest with their legs elevated several times a day to prevent leg cramps.

5. B. Limiting sodium intake during pregnancy can help minimize **edema.**
Rationale: Sodium intake leads to water retention and edema.

Chapter 8: The Family at Risk During the Antepartum Period

1. D. An anemic pregnant woman must be watched for signs of **infection.**
Rationale: Women with hemoglobin levels less than 11g/dL and hematocrit levels less than 35% are considered anemic and susceptible to infection.

2. B. A pregnant woman **with restricted activity** is at highest risk for developing a deep vein thrombosis (DVT).
Rationale: Women at risk of developing a DVT include women on bedrest and those who are overweight or over 30 years old.

3. B. Methotrexate may be used in the management of **ectopic pregnancy.**
Rationale: Methotrexate is a chemotherapy drug that stops products of conception from growing.

4. A. Painless vaginal bleeding is the most common symptom of placenta previa.
Rationale: The most common sign of placenta previa, implantation of the placenta near or over the cervix, is painless varginal bleeding.

5. D. A pregnant woman with a history of cardiac disease is considered high-risk due to **increased blood volume.**
Rationale: The heart's workload is increased as the blood volume increases 40% to 50% higher than pre-pregnant levels.

Chapter 9: Normal Fetal Development

1. C. The term **embryo** describes the products of conception during the first 8 weeks of gestation.
Rationale: Embryo is the proper term to use at this time of gestation.

2. D. The placenta is able to sustain a pregnancy by **12** weeks' gestation.
Rationale: The placenta is able to transport oxygen and nourishment to waste products from the fetus by 12 weeks' gestation.

3. C. The statement **"testes in the inguinal canal; abundant vernix"** best describes an infant born at 28 weeks' gestation.
Rationale: These are normal findings from 28 to 31 weeks' gestation.

4. C. Monozygotic twins occur when **one ovum is fertilized by one sperm.**
Rationale: After one ovum is fertilized by one sperm, it splits into two identical monozygotes.

5. A. Fertilization most frequently occurs in the **fallopian tube.**
Rationale: The outermost portion of the fallopian tube is the most frequent site of fertilization.

Chapter 10: Assessment of Fetal Health

1. C. Variable decelerations are due to **cord compression.**
Rationale: Early decelerations result from head compression and late decelerations are due, in part, to maternal hypotension.

2. D. Nursing interventions for late decelerations do <u>not</u> include **increasing infusion rate of oxytocin.**
Rationale: Uterine hyperstimulation may cause late decelerations. Uterine stimulation can be decreased with the stopping of oxytocin.

3. A. Meconium in the amniotic fluid may indicate **hypoxia.**
Rationale: An inadequate amount of oxygen in utero may result in anal sphincter relaxation and the passage of meconium.

4. C. Vibroacoustic stimulation may be performed following a nonreactive NST.
Rationale: Vibroacoustic stimulation can stimulate a sleeping fetus, one possible cause of a nonreactive NST.

5. B. The following statement regarding the fetal heartbeat is <u>incorrect</u>: **It can be measured by counting the uterine souffle.**
Rationale: The uterine souffle reflects the maternal, not fetal, pulse rate. The funic souffle rate is the same as the fetal heart rate.

Chapter 11: Process of Labor and Delivery

1. A. A fetus is considered engaged when the presenting part is level with **the ischial spine.**
Rationale: A fetus is "engaged" when the presenting part is at "0" station, level with the ischial spine.

2. C. If a patient asks what it means that her baby is in a longitudinal line, you would answer **the baby's spine is parallel to the mother's spine.**
Rationale: The fetal lie refers to the relationship of the fetal spine to the maternal spine.

3. B. A contraction pattern of **every 4 minutes, lasting 110 seconds,** should be immediately reported to a physician.
Rationale: Contractions that last more then 90 seconds can dramatically decrease the fetal oxygen supply.

4. D. Common subjective symptoms following lightening do <u>not</u> include **dysuria.**
Rationale: Dysuria is a symptom of a urinary tract infection.

5. B. A woman at 38 weeks' gestation reports having a blood-tinged mucous discharge. The nurse should advise her to **watch for signs of labor.**
Rationale: The patient is describing "show," the mucous plug from the cervical canal. The appearance of

"show" generally appears several hours or days before the onset of labor.

Chapter 12: Nursing Care During Normal Labor and Childbirth

1. D. A woman in the transitional stage of labor is most likely to be **agitated and overwhelmed.**
Rationale: As contractions become harder and more frequent, it is not unusual for women to feel a sense of panic.

2. C. A woman who is 9 centimeters dilated expresses the urge to push. The nurse's initial response should be to **discourage her from pushing.**
Rationale: Though a woman may have an urge to push as she approaches full dilation, she should be discouraged from doing so since premature pushing can cause cervical edema.

3. B. Upon assessment at 1 minute of life, the nurse notes the following: blue extremities and pink body, heart rate 110, irregular breathing, no response to suction catheter, and slight flexion of the extremities. The infant's Apgar score is **5.**
Rationale: One point is given for color, two points for heart rate, and one point each for respiratory rate and muscle tone; no points for reflex irritability.

4. C. Nitrazine paper turns **blue** when it comes in contact with amniotic fluid.
Rationale: Nitrazine paper turns blue when it comes in contact with the alkaline pH of amniotic fluid.

5. A. Several hours after delivery, the nurse palpitates a patient's uterus one finger breath above the umbilicus and displaced to the left. This finding is most likely the result of **a distended bladder.**
Rationale: A distended bladder can displace the uterus and prevent it from clamping down.

Chapter 13: Nursing Care in the Complicated Intrapartum Period

1. B. A woman who delivers at 34 weeks' gestation is least likely to experience a uterine rupture.
Rationale: A preterm delivery is not associated with uterine rupture. Possible causes include large fetal size, malpresentation/malposition, traumatic delivery, improper use of oxytocin, prolonged labor, previous uterine scar, and maternal abdominal trauma.

2. C. The nurse must carefully assess the mother who delivered twins for **postpartum hemorrhage.**

Rationale: Uterine overdistension due to multiple gestation increases the risk of postpartum hemorrhage.

3. A. Hydramnios places the woman at higher risk for **a prolapsed cord.**
Rationale: The force created by the rupture of excessive amniotic fluid may cause the umbilical cord to slip down in front of the presenting part.

4. C. Following artificial rupture of membranes (AROM), the nurse's most important action should be **noting the color of the amniotic fluid.**
Rationale: The nurse must note the time of AROM as well as the color, odor, and amount of the amniotic fluid.

5. D. When the fetus is in a persistent occiput posterior (OP) position, the patient will most likely experience **severe back pain.**
Rationale: Women commonly experience severe back pain or "back labor" when the baby is in an OP position.

Chapter 14: Normal Postpartum Physical and Psychosocial Changes

1. D. Vaginal hematoma found during the first 24 hours postpartum should be immediately reported to the physician.
Rationale: A vaginal hematoma is a collection of blood that must be carefully assessed for size, location, and degree of discomfort.

2. B. A **pinkish** color best describes lochia 1 week after delivery.
Rationale: Lochia serosa, which generally occurs 4 to 10 days following delivery, is pinkish to pinkish brown.

3. A. Typical maternal behavior during the taking-in stage includes **recounting her L & D experience.**
Rationale: The taking-in stage may last from several hours to 2 days. During this time, the woman is generally tired and frequently repeats her birth experience.

4. C. The nurse should advise a patient who asks how long stretch marks last that **they may be permanent.**
Rationale: Stretch marks, which result from stretching and minute tearing of the skin, may not disappear completely, despite any maternal effort.

5. B. Fetal presentation is <u>least</u> likely to affect fundal height following delivery.
Rationale: Fetal position before delivery does not affect fundal location after delivery.

Chapter 15: Nursing Care Following Normal Childbirth

1. B. The statement **"I should apply breast cream to my nipples before each feeding"** indicates that a breast-feeding woman requires additional teaching.
Rationale: If used, breast creams should be rubbed thoroughly into nipples after breastfeeding.

2. C. Three days after delivery, a patient complains of severe breast tenderness and a feeling of fullness. The nurse's initial action should be to **encourage the woman to wear a supportive bra.**
Rationale: Breast engorgement generally occurs 3 to 4 days after delivery. Congestion from increased blood and lymph in the breast causes the breasts to become larger, firmer, and tender.

3. C. Perineal care does <u>not</u> include **removing the perineal pad from back to front.**
Rationale: To avoid contamination from the rectum, perineal pads should be applied and removed from front to back.

4. C. Healing of episiotomy may be slowed by **prolonged use of cold applications.**
Rationale: While cold application in the immediate postpartum period provides comfort and reduces swelling, use after the first 24 hours may interfere with healing because of vasoconstriction.

5. B. A breast-feeding woman should change her diet to include **more calories and calcium.**
Rationale: A breast-feeding woman should increase her calorie intake to 2700–2800 calories per day and consume at least 3 milk servings a day to ensure adequate calcium and phosphorus levels.

Chapter 16: Nursing Care in the Complicated Postpartum Period

1. A. Vital signs would be least helpful in the early diagnosis of shock due to postpartum hemorrhage.
Rationale: Because of the increased blood volume during pregnancy, a woman's vital signs may not reflect excessive blood loss until the total volume decreases 30% to 35%.

2. D. A woman with endometritis is <u>not</u> likely to exhibit **dysuria.**
Rationale: Dysuria is associated with a urinary tract infection, not endometritis.

3. B. Methergine may be ordered following delivery to prevent **postpartum hemorrhage.**

Rationale: By causing the uterus to contract, Methergine helps prevent postpartum hemorrhage.

4. D. Management of mastitis would <u>not</u> include the **application of a cold compress.**
Rationale: Application of a warm, not cold, compress helps relieve clogged milk ducts.

5. C. Fleet's enema is an inappropriate medication for a patient with a fourth-degree laceration.
Rationale: Because of fourth-degree lacerations to the rectal mucosa, neither enemas nor suppositories should be introduced into the rectum while it is healing.

Chapter 17: The Newborn's Transition to Extrauterine Life

1. B. Vitamin K is administered to newborns to prevent **excessive bleeding.**
Rationale: Vitamin K helps with the production of certain coagulation factors. It takes several days for intestinal bacteria to produce sufficient amounts of vitamin K.

2. C. The presence of IgM in the neonate may be indicative of **intrauterine infection.**
Rationale: The presence of IgM immunoglobulin at birth may indicate fetal production in response to intrauterine infections such as TORCH.

3. D. Oxygen administered to the neonate must be warmed to prevent heat loss via **convection.**
Rationale: Heat loss via convection occurs when the infant is exposed to cool air.

4. A. Acute cold stress in the neonate can lead to **hypoglycemia.**
Rationale: When cold stressed, the neonate uses glucose, which can lead to hypoglycemia.

5. C. After the umbilical cord is cut, respiratory centers in the brain are activated in response to **decreased arterial oxygen tension.**
Rationale: Cutting the umbilical cord results in decreased arterial oxygen tension, increased arterial carbon dioxide tension, and decreased arterial pH.

Chapter 18: Nursing Care of the Normal Newborn

1. C. During a newborn assessment, the nurse notes that the infant's hands and feet are cyanotic. The nurse's initial action should be to **document the finding.**
Rationale: Acrocyanosis, bluish discoloration of the newborn's hands and feet, is a normal finding in skin color.

2. B. When there is a significant difference between the blood pressure in an infant's upper and lower extremities, the nurse should anticipate further evaluation of the **cardiac** system.
Rationale: Blood pressure measurements are approximately equal in the four extremities. Significant differences may indicate a congenital heart disorder.

3. D. The **Moro** reflex may be abnormal when there has been an injury to the clavicle during delivery.
Rationale: Clavicle injury may interfere with the Moro reflex in which there is bilateral abduction and extension in the infant's arms.

4. A. The nurse recognizes a sunken fontanel to be a possible sign of **dehydration.**
Rationale: Fontanels are normally soft and flat. A sunken fontanel may indicate dehydration, while a bulging fontanel may indicate increased intracranial pressure.

5. C. Estrogen from the mother is responsible for **witch's milk.**
Rationale: Maternal estrogen may cause a milky white discharge, known as "witch's milk," from the breasts of either newborn sex.

Chapter 19: Nursing Care of the Preterm Neonate

1. B. Preterm infants have problems with thermoregulation primarily because of **lack of body flexion.**
Rationale: Preterm infants generally assume an extended instead of a flexed position because of muscle weakness. This position exposes a large amount of body surface through which heat can be lost.

2. B. Indomethacin may be given to a premature infant for the management of **patent ductus arteriosus.**
Rationale: Indomethacin is a prostaglandin inhibitor that helps constrict the ductus arteriosus.

3. C. Bilirubin levels must be carefully monitored to prevent **brain damage.**
Rationale: Brain damage may result from kernicterus, a condition in which serum bilirubin levels ≥20 mg/mL.

4. D. Nosocomial infections in the newborn can best be prevented by **good handwashing techniques.**
Rationale: A 2 to 3 minute scrub at the beginning of each shift, followed by frequent handwashing, helps prevent nosocomial infections.

5. A. Abundant lanugo and vernix would be expected in an infant born at 28 weeks' gestation.

Rationale: At this point in pregnancy, the body would be covered by both lanugo (fine downy hair) and vernix (a white creamy substance).

Chapter 20: Nursing Care of the Newborn with Special Needs

1. B. A history of hydramnios during the pregnancy should alert the nurse to pay specific attention to the infant's **feeding ability.**
Rationale: Excessive amniotic fluid could indicate difficulty with swallowing.

2. A. RhoGAM prevents the formation of antibodies, thereby preventing sensitization of an Rh negative woman.
Rationale: By neutralizing and destroying fetal blood cells in the mother, RhoGAM prevents maternal development of antibodies.

3. C. Prompt management of phenylketonuria helps prevent **mental retardation.**
Rationale: Absence of the liver enzyme phenylalanine hydroxylase prevents the conversion of phenylalanine to tyrosine. As the breakdown products of phenylalanine—phenylketones—accumulate in the brain, mental retardation occurs.

4. B. The nurse's <u>first</u> priority when caring for a newborn should be **maintaining an open airway.**
Rationale: Newborns have small airways that can become blocked easily, thus interfering with gaseous exchange.

5. C. Signs of respiratory distress do <u>not</u> include **decreased respiratory rate.**
Rationale: Infants in respiratory distress have tachypnea, with respirations as high as 140/min.

Glossary

abortion. Termination of a pregnancy before the fetus is old enough to survive outside of the uterus.

abruptio placentae. Premature partial or complete separation of the placenta from the uterine wall after 20 weeks' gestation.

abstinence. Refraining from having sexual intercourse.

acceleration. Increase in the fetal heart beats per minute.

acme. Point of greatest intensity of a uterine contraction.

acquired immunodeficiency syndrome (AIDS). Fatal disease that destroys the body's natural immune system and renders it ineffective in fighting opportunistic infections.

acrocyanosis. Normal cyanotic appearance, or bluish discoloration, of the hands and feet in the neonate.

active phase. Period of labor from 4 cm dilatation of the cervix to 7 cm dilatation.

adolescence. Period of development that begins in puberty and ends at full physiologic maturity.

afterbirth. The fetal and placental membranes expelled after the expulsion of the fetus.

afterpains. Mild uterine contractions experienced approximately 2 days after birth. Discomfort is typically more severe with breast-feeding.

albuminuria. Presence of protein (albumin) in the urine.

alpha-fetoprotein. Antigen carried by the fetus that is used in determining neural tube defects and diagnosing Down syndrome.

alternative birthing center. Specially designed centers for the no-risk family who have a desire to experience closeness in childbirth outside of the hospital setting.

amenorrhea. Absence of normal menstrual flow.

amniocentesis. Removal of amniotic fluid by puncturing the amniotic sac with a large-bore needle and syringe.

amniotic fluid. Fluid in the amniotic sac that surrounds the fetus and allows for movement and heat conservation.

amniotomy. Purposeful (artificial) rupture of the amniotic sac.

analgesia. Relief of pain without loss of consciousness by means of medication administration.

anemia. A condition in which the tissues receive inadequate oxygen due to a decrease in red blood cells, hemoglobin, or in total blood volume.

anesthesia. Complete or localized loss of sensation associated with the administration of an agent used for this purpose.

anoxia. Absence of oxygen to supply the tissues, often resulting in inadequate circulation.

antenatal. Before birth.

antepartum period. Period of time in pregnancy that begins at conception and ends with the first true uterine contraction.

antibodies. Immunoglobulins formed as a result of antigen formation that fight to protect the body from infection.

antigens. Stimulate the body's natural immune system in the production of antibodies.

Apgar score. Systematic measurement of the neonate's physical condition at 1 minute and 5 minutes after birth; based on heart rate, respiratory effort, muscle tone, reflex irritability, and color of the neonate.

apnea. Cessation of respirations.

appropriate for gestational age (AGA). Neonates that weigh less than the heaviest 10% and more than the lightest 10% of neonates of the same gestational age.

asphyxia neonatorum. Insufficient oxygenation in the neonate that results in respiratory failure.

ataractic. An agent that produces detached serenity with decreased mental alertness; tranquilizing agent.

atelectasis. Partial or complete failure of the lungs to inflate in the newborn.

atony. Without tone or strength.

attachment. Bonding with the newborn through touch, eye-to-eye contact, and talking to the infant.

Babinski's reflex. Reflex seen in the infant. There is dorsiflexion of the great toe and a spreading of the rest of the toes. A positive Babinski's after the first year of life indicates neurologic damage.

ballottement. Through the use of palpation, the floating fetus will rebound off the examiner's finger.

barbiturates. Central nervous system depressants used for pain relief in labor.

Bartholin's glands. Glands located on either side of the vaginal opening, believed to provide lubricating mucus during sexual arousal.

basal body temperature. Temperature of the body at rest.

bilirubin. Yellowish pigment in bile that is produced from the hemoglobin of red blood cells.

Billing's cervical mucus method. Charting of changes in cervical mucus that indicates increased or decreased fertility.

blastocyst. Formed from the division of the morula.

boggy. Soft and without tone; as in a boggy uterus where the risk of hemorrhage is great.

brachial palsy. Also called Erb's palsy. Paralysis of an arm, usually as a result of nerve damage during the birth process; usually temporary but may be permanent.

Bradley method. Named after Robert A. Bradley. Supports labor as a natural process using a calm environment, the use of diversionary activities during labor, a comfortable position for delivery, and slow deep breathing.

bradycardia. Decreased heart rate. In the fetus or newborn, a heart rate of less than 100 beats per minute.

Braxton Hicks contractions. Painless irregular uterine contractions that allow for expansion of the uterus but do no work of labor.

breech presentation. The fetus is turned so that the buttocks or feet lead into the birth canal. May be classified as frank, complete, or footling.

caput succedaneum. Collection of fluid (swelling) on the fetal head in response to pressure during labor.

cephalic. Pertaining to the head.

cephalhematoma. Collection of fluid and blood underneath the periosteum of the skull of the newborn resulting from blood vessels ruptured during labor.

cephalocaudal. Neurologic growth of the newborn in a head-to-toe and proximal-to-distal fashion.

cephalopelvic disproportion (CPD). Disproportion in the size of the fetal head and the maternal pelvis; the fetal head is too large to fit through the maternal pelvis and vaginal birth is not possible.

certified nurse midwife. Licensed registered nurse who provides normal gynecologic care to women, and supports, counsels, and monitors pregnant women through birth.

cervical cap. Pliable birth control device that fits over the cervix.

cervical os. Usually the outer opening of the neck of the uterus, called the cervix or cervical canal.

cesarean birth. Incision through the abdominal wall and uterus for removal of the fetus and placenta.

Chadwick's sign. Probable sign of pregnancy, where there is a purplish discoloration of the vulva and vagina.

chlamydia infection. Genital sexually transmitted infection of males and females with purulent vaginal discharge, frequent burning on urination, and lower abdominal discomfort.

chloasma gravidarum. Increase in facial pigmentation in pregnancy that fades after delivery. Often referred to as the "mask of pregnancy."

chorion. Extraembryonic membrane that is formed from the trophoblast.

chorionic villi. Root or fingerlike projections in the external fetal portion of the placenta that are filled with capillaries and through which the gases and nutrients are exchanged between the fetal and maternal circulatory systems.

chromosome. Carry the genetic code for each unique individual. There are 23 pairs in each soma cell; one chromosome in each pair is from each parent.

circumcision. Surgical removal of the foreskin of the penis.

cleft lip. Congenital incomplete closure of the lip. May be unilateral or bilateral.

cleft palate. Congenital fissure, or incomplete closure of the roof of the mouth.

clinical nurse specialist. Licensed registered nurse who manages the gynecologic and childbearing needs of women.

clitoris. A small amount of sensitive erectile tissue located at the anterior juncture of the labia majora; corresponds to the penis in the male.

club foot. Congenital deformity of the foot in which it is twisted out of its normal position. Also called talipes.

coitus interruptus. Removal of the penis from the vagina during intercourse before ejaculation occurs.

colostrum. Thin yellow fluid that contains antibodies, nutrients, and laxative properties. It is the initial nourishment for the breast-feeding neonate.

conception. Fertilization of the female ovum by the male sperm.

condom. Sheath worn over the penis during sexual intercourse to prevent sperm from entering the vagina.

congenital. Condition present from birth.

congenital anomaly. Any variation or deformity present at birth.

congenital hip dysplasia. Condition at birth in which the hip socket (acetabulum) is not well formed and the head of the femur slips out of place, resulting in a limp, if not treated.

conjugate. The anteroposterior diameter of the pelvic inlet.

contraceptive. Any device or method that prevents fertilization of the ovum.

contraction stress test/oxytocin challenge test. Used to determine the response of the fetal heart in relation to uterine contractions.

corpus luteum. Yellowed body formed within a ruptured ovarian follicle that secretes progesterone.

couplet care. Also known as mother–baby nursing, the mother and newborn are cared for by one nurse.

crepitation. Crackling sound or sensation of fractured bone ends rubbing against each other.

crowning. Visualization of the fetal head in the vulva.

cryptorchidism. When one or both testicles fail to descend into the scrotal sac at the time of birth.

culture. A person's perceptions and interpretations that direct one's socialization within a specific group and in relating to others outside the group.

extended family. A family consisting of relatives beyond the nuclear family to include aunts, uncles, and grandparents.

external os. The portion of the cervix that opens into the vagina.

decelerations. Decrease in the fetal heart rate.

decidua. The term used for the endometrium of the uterus during pregnancy.

decrement. Decrease in intensity of a uterine contraction.

dehiscence. Rupture of a surgical wound or scar; may cause uterine rupture.

deoxyribonucleic acid (DNA) Deoxyribonucleic acid; spiral-shaped double helix containing the chemical formation of genetic code present in genes and carrying specifications for all of the characteristics of a cell.

descent. Downward movement of the presenting part of the fetus into and through the birth canal.

diagonal conjugate. Distance between the sacral promontory and the lower border of the symphysis pubis.

diaphragm. Cup made from rubber or pliable plastic that fits over the cervix to prevent fertilization of the ovum.

diaphragmatic hernia. A weakness in the muscle of the diaphragm that allows the abdominal organs to protrude through into the chest cavity, resulting in crowding of the heart and lungs.

Dick-Read method. Named for Dr. Grantly Dick-Read. Promotes relaxation by eliminating fear of the unknown. The families are given ample information about labor and birth, taught relaxation techniques, and are given a sense of control during the birthing process.

dilatation. Opening of the external os of the cervical canal in labor to a maximum of 10 cm.

disseminated intravascular coagulation (DIC). Coagulation disorder in which the maternal blood does not clot. Anemia and hemorrhagic conditions may develop.

dizygotic twins. Twins that develop from two separate fertilized ova; fraternal twins.

Down syndrome. Also known as trisomy 21, a congenital abnormality with specific physical characteristics and varying levels of retardation.

dorsiflexion. Movement of a body part toward the posterior side of the body.

ductus arteriosus. Transports oxygenated blood from the fetal pulmonary artery and aorta for distribution to the body.

ductus venosus. Umbilical vein that transports fetal blood to the portal vein of the liver and the inferior vena cava.

dysmenorrhea. Painful menstruation.

dyspnea. Difficulty in breathing associated with pain.

dystocia. Painful or difficult labor; often slower than usual.

ecchymosis. Appearance of a blackish-blue area on the skin associated with bleeding into the area.

eclampsia. Occurrence of coma and/or convulsions in the woman diagnosed with preeclampsia.

ectopic pregnancy. Implantation of a fertilized ovum outside of the uterus. The fallopian tubes are the primary site for this occurrence.

effacement. Softening, shortening, and thinning of the cervical canal in labor; obliteration of the cervix.

effleurage. Rhythmic stroking of the abdomen during labor to intensify concentration during a uterine contraction.

embolectomy. Removal of an embolus from a blood vessel.

embryo. From 4 to 8 weeks after fertilization occurs, it is formed from the inner cell mass of the blastocyst.

endometritis. Inflammation of the endometrium.

en face. Mother turns her newborn toward her to look directly at the infant.

engorgement. Enlargement and increased tenderness of the breasts approximately the 3rd postpartum day, caused by congestion of blood and lymph as lactation occurs.

epididymis. Firm, coiled, oblong canal where the sperm mature and gain motility.

epidural. Anesthetic injected into the epidural space of the spinal column to provide continuous pain relief in labor or when a cesarean birth is necessary.

episiotomy. Surgical incision or cut of the perineum to prevent lacerations in the second stage of labor and to hasten birth.

erythema toxicum. Self-limiting rash of the newborn found on the trunk. It is characterized by areas of redness with yellow-white centers.

erythroblastosis fetalis. Hemolytic disease of the newborn associated with Rh and ABO incompatibilities.

estrogen. Female hormone that stimulates the development of sexual characteristics.

expected date of delivery (EDD). Anticipated date childbirth will occur.

expulsion. Refers to the term used in the second stage of labor; the birth of the neonate.

extension. During birth, the passage of the head under the symphysis pubis, resulting in the expulsion of the head from the birth canal.

extracorporeal membrane oxygenation (ECMO). Heart–lung machine that provides cardiopulmonary bypass for the neonate with meconium aspiration syndrome.

fallopian tube. Duct along which the ovum travels from the ovary to the uterus.

false labor. Uterine contractions that are irregular and do no work of labor. They are typically confined to the abdomen and disappear with rest.

family. Two or more interacting persons that share common beliefs and goals, and support each other physically and emotionally.

family-centered care. Nursing care designed to support and care for the special needs of the family.

ferning. Characteristic frondlike appearance of amniotic fluid when viewed microscopically.

fertility. Degree to which one can reproduce or be fertile.

fertilization. Joining of the female ovum and the male spermatozoa.

fetal alcohol syndrome (FAS). Condition resulting from maternal alcohol consumption during pregnancy. Characterized by mental retardation and physical defects.

fetal blood sampling. Sample of blood is drawn from the presenting part of the fetus in labor.

fetal death. Death of a fetus before birth.

fetal distress. A change in the condition of the fetus signifying that the fetus is in difficulty.

fetal heart rate (FHR). Rate of heart beats per minute of the fetus. Normal is 120 to 160 beats per minute.

fetal heart tones (FHT). The sounds of the fetal heart.

fetal presentation. Fetal part that is located in the lowest portion of the woman's pelvis.

fetal position. Relationship of the fetal presenting part to the woman's pelvis.

fetus. Infant in utero after the 8th week of pregnancy to birth; this follows the embryonic period.

fibrocystic breast disease. Benign irregularities in breast tissue.

fibrolytic therapy. Medication administered to dissolve an existing blood clot.

first stage of labor. The stage of effacement and dilatation, beginning with the first signs of labor such as bloody show and regular contractions until the cervix is dilated to 10 cm. Divided into three phases: latent, active, and transition.

flexion. Movement of a joint to decrease the angle.

follicle stimulating hormone (FSH). Hormone secreted by the anterior pituitary gland that influences ovarian activity.

fontanelle. Space formed between the skull bones of the fetus located anteriorly and posteriorly. The anterior fontanelle is commonly referred to as the soft spot.

foramen ovale. Opening in the fetal heart between the atria.

forceps delivery. Use of extractors placed on the fetal presenting part, usually the head, to assist in birth.

fourth stage of labor. The stage of recovery lasting up to 4 hours after birth.

functional residual capacity. Air that remains within the alveoli during expiration, preventing the alveoli from closing completely.

fundal height. Used as a measurement in determining fetal gestational age.

fundus. Large base of the uterus palpated in the upper abdomen of the pregnant woman.

funic souffle. Audible sound of blood pulsing through the blood vessels of the umbilical cord.

gamete. Sex cells located in reproductive glands.

gene. DNA components that determine heredity.

gestation. Length of time from conception to birth.

gestational diabetes. Diabetes occurring in pregnancy due to altered carbohydrate metabolism.

gestational trophoblastic neoplasm. Known as hydatidiform mole, is a rapid growth of benign trophoblastic cells.

gonorrhea. Sexually transmitted disease that infects the genital mucosa.

Goodell's sign. Softening of the cervix in pregnancy.

grasp reflex. The neonate's response of grasping tightly when pressure is placed on the palms of the hands.

gravida. Refers to a woman who is or has been pregnant.

GTPALM. Used for recording a woman's pregnancy history, its letters stand for: Gravida, Term pregnancies, Premature births, Abortions, number of Living children, and Multiple gestations and births.

heel stick. Gathering a blood specimen by puncturing a small vein in the neonate's heel with a sharp microlancet.

Hegar's sign. Softening of the lower segment of the uterus in pregnancy.

hemangioma. Cluster of blood vessels that form a lesion.

hemolysis. Release of hemoglobin through the destruction of red blood cells.

hepatitis B. Inflammation of the liver spread by blood and body fluid contact.

high risk. Increased chance in incurring disease or injury.

human chorionic gonadotropin (hCG). Hormone responsible for maintaining the corpus luteum in early pregnancy.

human immunodeficiency virus (HIV). Virus that causes the fatal disease AIDS.

human placental lactogen. Hormone in late pregnancy that prepares the breast to produce milk.

hydramnios. Excessive amount of amniotic fluid (more than 2000 mL).

hyperbilirubinemia. Excessive amount of bilirubin in the blood; over 12 mg/100 mL.

hyperemesis gravidarum. Excessive nausea and vomiting in pregnancy. This condition may lead to dehydration, electrolyte imbalances, and weight loss.

hypochondriasis. A condition in which normal sensations and minor complaints are exaggerated, suggesting serious illness.

hypoglycemia. Occurs when the serum blood glucose levels are abnormally low.

icterus neonatorum. Physiologic jaundice that occurs frequently in neonates after the first 24 hours of life.

immunoglobulin. Antibodies found in the immune system.

implantation. The process of the embedding and attachment of the fertilized ovum into the endometrium.

incomplete abortion. Occurs when part of the products of conception are retained in the uterus.

increment. Increase in intensity of a uterine contraction.

indirect Coombs' test. Serologic exam that identifies the presence of antibodies to the Rh factor in an Rh-negative woman.

induced abortion. Intentional termination of a pregnancy.

induction of labor. Intentional initiation of uterine contractions for birth.

infant mortality rate. Number of infant deaths under the age of 12 months per year.

infertility. Diminished or absent ability to be fertile or to reproduce.

inlet of the pelvis. The brim of the pelvic cavity.

internal rotation. Movement of the fetal head to an anterior position just before birth.

intrapartum period. Period of time that begins with the first true uterine contraction and ends with the birth of the newborn.

intrauterine catheter. After rupture of the membranes, a waterfilled catheter is introduced into the uterus to monitor uterine contractions.

intrauterine device. Appliance inserted into the uterus to prevent conception.

intrauterine growth retardation (IUGR). Fetuses who are small for their gestational age.

involution. Return of the uterus and other organs to a pre-pregnant state following pregnancy.

jaundice. Yellow discoloration of the skin in response to elevated bilirubin levels.

kernicterus. Extreme elevation of bilirubin levels in the neonate that can lead to brain damage if untreated.

labia. The plural of labium, often referring to the two pairs of skin folds protecting the entrance to the vagina.

labia majora. The outer fatty skin folds covered with hair forming each side of the vulva.

labia minora. The smaller inner skin folds between the labia majora and the vagina.

labor. The process of rhythmic contraction and relaxation of the uterine muscles in the effort to expel the products of conception. Divided into four stages.

labor–delivery–recovery room (LDR). Specially design rooms to accommodate the labor, delivery, and recovery of the pregnant woman and support person(s).

laceration. Tear in the perineum that occurs during birth.

lactation. Production of breast milk in the postpartum mother.

Lamaze method. Childbirth method that advocates mental conditioning and relaxation for limiting pain in labor and birth.

large for gestational age (LGA). Neonate weighing greater than 90% of other neonates of the same gestational age.

last menstrual period (LMP). First day of the last menstrual period.

latent phase. Early part of the first stage of labor during which the cervix dilates to 4 cm; the longest phase of first stage of labor.

lecithin/sphingomyelin ratio (L/S ratio). Test used to determine fetal lung maturity.

Leopold's maneuvers. External palpation of the uterus to assess fetal presentation and position.

let-down reflex. Release of milk into the breasts in response to stimulation.

letting-go. Postpartum woman uses independence in assuming the maternal role.

lightening. Descent of the presenting part into the pelvis before the start of labor.

linea nigra. The pigmented line running from the pubis to the umbilicus that appears on the abdomen during pregnancy .

local infiltration. Injection of anesthesia into the perineal tissue, typically for repair of an episiotomy.

lochia alba. Whitish-yellowish vaginal discharge typically seen from the 2nd to the 6th week postpartum.

lochia rubra. Bright red vaginal discharge typically seen from day 1 to day 3 postpartum.

lochia serosa. Pinkish vaginal discharge typically seen from day 4 and continues until day 10 to 14 postpartum.

luteinizing hormone (LH). Hormone secreted by the anterior pituitary gland that influences ovarian activity.

macrosomia. Large fetal size often occurring in response to elevated maternal blood glucose levels.

mastitis. Inflammation of the breast.

maternal mortality rate. Number of women who have died in childbirth.

maternal-newborn care. Nursing discipline concerned with the care of the woman and fetus in pregnancy and the neonate.

McDonald's rule. Method of determining gestational length in weeks and lunar months.

meconium aspiration syndrome (MAS). Aspiration of meconium by the fetus, usually during the birth process.

medial incision. Surgical opening made in the midline of the perineum when performing an episiotomy.

meiosis. Cellular divisions of the nucleus of sex cells.

menopause. Permanent cessation of the menstrual period.

menorrhagia. Excessive vaginal bleeding with the menstrual period.

menstruation. Cyclic discharge of bloody fluid from the uterus.

metrorrhagia. Uterine bleeding that occurs outside of the menstrual period.

micronate. Preterm neonate born before 26 weeks' gestation and weighing less than 500 grams.

milia. Tiny white papules found on the nose and chin of the newborn as a result of plugged sebaceous glands.

minerals. Inorganic compounds that occur in nature.

mitosis. Cellular division of somatic cells.

molding. Shaping of the fetal head caused by overlapping of the fetal skull bones during birth.

mongolian spots. Bluish-gray or darkened areas of the skin found on the newborn's lower back and shoulders; common in dark-skinned and Asian neonates.

monozygotic twins. Twins that develop from one fertilized ovum; identical twins.

Montgomery glands. Tubercles in the areola of the nipple that provide lubrication during nursing.

Moro's reflex. Reflex in neonate in response to noise or jarring resulting in abduction and extension of the arms and legs. Sometimes called the startle reflex.

morula. Solid mass that results from miotic division of the zygote.

mother–baby nursing. Care of the neonate and mother by one nurse. Also known as couplet care.

multi. More than one or more than once.

multigravida. Woman who is pregnant and has also been pregnant before.

myelomeningocele. Defect in the development of the fetal spinal column that includes the spinal cord and nerves.

Naegele's rule. Method of calculating the length of pregnancy; 3 months are subtracted from the first day of the last menstrual period and 7 days are added.

necrotizing enterocolitis (NEC). Acute inflammatory process of the bowel with necrosis, seen most frequently in preterm neonates.

neonatology. Study of the newborn.

neutral thermal environment. Balance of heat loss and heat production in the newborn.

nitrazine paper. A pH sensitive strip of paper used in assessing the presence of amniotic fluid.

nonstress test (NST). Noninvasive method of assessing fetal wellness in relation to its movement.

nuchal cord. Umbilical cord wrapped around the neck of the newborn at the time of birth.

nuclear family. A family constellation made up of mother, father, and their children.

nulli. None or never.

nulligravida. Woman who has never been pregnant.

nullipara. Woman who has not carried a fetus to the age of viability.

nurse practitioner. Registered nurse with advanced education and training in a particular area.

nursing process. Systematic and organized approach in planning and giving comprehensive family-centered nursing care.

nutrients. Essential elements mostly derived from food intake that are necessary for physiologic health and well-being.

nystagmus. Rapid, involuntary movement of the eyeballs.

occiput. Pertaining to the back of the head.

omphalocele. Congenital hernia of the umbilicus through which a part of the intestines protrude.

ophthalmia neonatorum. Severe purulent infection in the eyes of the newborn.

orgasm. Climax of sexual intercourse.

orthostatic hypotension. Drop in blood pressure when sitting or standing from a lying position.

Ortolani's maneuver. Test for congenital hip dysplasia. The legs are flexed and abducted laterally toward the surface of the bed or examining table.

ovary. The sex gland of the female in which the ova are developed. Each female has a pair of ovaries, one on either side of the uterus.

ovulation. The discharge of the ovum from the ovary, usually at the midpoint of the menstrual cycle.

ovum. Female germ cell that when fertilized develops into a new organism.

oxytocin. Hormone used to stimulate or augment labor.

oxytocin induction. Administration of oxytocin to initiate uterine contractions (labor).

Papanicolaou (Pap) smear. Sampling of cervical tissue for the detection of cancer cells.

para. Indicates the number of pregnancies that have reached the legal age of viability.

paracervical block. Anesthesia injected intravaginally into the rim of the cervix for pain control in labor and birth.

parametritis. Infection of the pelvic structures.

paravaginal hematoma. A collection of blood (hematoma) alongside the tissues of the vagina .

passage. The true pelvis through which the fetus travels during the birth process; consists of the inlet, the midpelvis, and the outlet.

pelvic inflammatory disease (PID). Inflammation and infection that has spread throughout the reproductive organs in a woman.

pelvic types. Method of classification of pelvic structure by shape and significant bony structures. Basic types include android, gynecoid, platypelloid, and anthropoid.

pelvimetry. The measurement of the pelvis to determine its adequacy for the passage of the fetus; may be performed internally or externally.

peritonitis. Inflammation of the membrane covering the walls of the abdominal and pelvic cavities or inflammation of the peritoneum.

phenylketonuria (PKU). Inherited disease where the newborn cannot oxidize phenylalanine, resulting in mental retardation if untreated.

phimosis. Narrowing or tightening of the foreskin on the penis.

phlebothrombosis. Venous clot without associated inflammation.

phototherapy. Exposure of the newborn's skin to artificial light for the treatment of elevated serum bilirubin levels.

pica. Cravings experienced by the pregnant woman for nonfood substances.

pigmented nevus. Birthmark classified as a mole.

placenta. The vascular, flat, oval structure that attaches to the uterus to provide nutrients to the developing fetus.

placenta accreta. Nonseparation of the placenta from the uterine wall due to abnormal implantation.

placenta previa. Implantation of the placenta near or covering the cervical os.

polydactyly. The presence of extra fingers or toes.

polyhydramnios. See hydramnios.

positive signs of pregnancy. Signs that confirm pregnancy: fetal heartbeat, palpation of fetal movements, and visualization of fetus by ultrasound.

postpartum depression. Transient negative emotional feelings felt by many women in the postpartum period.

postpartum hemorrhage. Loss of more than 500 mL of blood from the time after birth to the end of the postpartum period.

postpartum period. Period of time from birth of the newborn until involution is complete in the woman.

postterm. Neonate who has completed 42 weeks' gestation or more.

precipitous labor. Labor lasting less than 3 hours.

preeclampsia. Classification of PIH characterized by hypertension, edema, and albuminuria.

pregnancy. The state of having a developing embryo or fetus in the body as a result of conception.

pregnancy induced hypertension (PIH). Disorder in pregnancy classified as preeclampsia and eclampsia.

premenstrual syndrome (PMS). Reoccurrence of physiologic discomforts and emotional irregularities associated with the menstrual cycle.

prenatal. Before birth.

presentation. Position of the fetus as it enters the pelvic inlet.

presenting part. The part of the fetus that leads the way through the birth canal, such as the buttocks, feet, head, or shoulder.

presumptive signs of pregnancy. Physical signs that suggest pregnancy but do not provide definite diagnosis of pregnancy: amenorrhea, nausea and vomiting, breast changes, urinary frequency, fatigue, and Goodell's sign.

preterm. Neonate who has completed less than 37 weeks' gestation.

preterm labor. Onset of regular uterine contractions that result in cervical dilatation and effacement after 20 weeks' but before 37 weeks' gestation.

primi. Refers to first.

primigravida. Woman who is pregnant for the first time.

primipara. Woman who has delivered a potentially viable fetus, regardless of survival.

primordial follicles. Immature ovarian follicles that eventually mature and contain a single ovum.

probable signs of pregnancy. Objective signs that indicate pregnancy occurring between 12 and 16 weeks of pregnancy: pigmentation changes, enlarging abdomen, Chadwick's sign, Hegar's sign, ballottement, Braxton Hicks contractions, palpation of the fetal outline, quickening, and a positive pregnancy test.

progesterone. Hormone secreted by the corpus luteum that supports the lining of the uterus for implantation.

prolactin. Hormone that stimulates the acini cells of the breasts to produce milk.

prolapsed cord. Movement of the umbilical cord into the pelvic outlet and positioned in front of the presenting fetal part.

prostaglandin gel. Product made from prostaglandins which is inserted into the vagina to stimulate cervical changes and uterine activity.

prostaglandins. Naturally occurring substances in the body that produce forceful contractions of uterine muscle.

protein. Compounds abundant with essential amino acids.

pseudomenstruation. Slight whitish or bloody vaginal discharge in the newborn resulting from the influence of maternal hormones.

puberty. Time of growth when physical and sexual maturity is achieved.

pudendal block. Anesthesia injected around the pudendal nerve for the relief of pain in labor and birth.

puerperal. Refers to the period after childbirth.

puerperium. Synonymous with the postpartum period.

pulmonary vascular resistance. Opposition to blood flow in the blood vessels of the fetal lungs.

pyelonephritis. Inflammation of the kidney and renal pelvis.

quickening. Sensations felt by the pregnant woman with the first fetal movements.

radioimmunoassay. Test used in diagnosing pregnancy by determining the presence of hormones in the woman's blood.

REEDA. An acronym to help remember the points to cover when inspecting the episiotomy: **R**edness, **E**dema, **E**cchymosis, **D**ischarge, and **A**pproximation of wound edges.

respiratory distress syndrome (RDS). Serious inability of the premature newborn to maintain adequate respiratory effort as the result of the lack of surfactant in the lungs; also called hyaline membrane disease.

restitution. External rotation of the fetal head to align with the shoulders.

Rh factor. Antigen found in red blood cells.

RhoGAM. Immune globulin given intramuscularly to women who are Rh− and have delivered Rh+ newborns.

rooming-in. When the neonate and mother are together in the same room for the entire hospital stay.

rubella. German measles.

salpingitis. Inflammation of the fallopian tubes.

second stage of labor. The expulsion stage of labor. The stage of the birth of the neonate.

sexually transmitted diseases (STD). Group of conditions that have serious health concerns and are passed to another person through sexual activity.

sickle cell anemia. Inherited disorder caused by abnormal hemoglobin that causes a sickling of red blood cells.

sitz bath. Immersion of the perineal area in warm water to promote comfort; frequently administered after childbirth.

small for gestational age (SGA). Neonate weighing less than 90% of other neonates of the same gestational age.

smegma. Collection of cheesy-like secretions which may be found under the foreskin of the penis in an uncircumcised neonate.

soma cells. Body's cells; building blocks.

sperm. Fluid ejaculated from the male penis containing spermatozoa.

spermatozoa. Mature male germ cell.

spina bifida. A congenital anomaly of development in which there is defective closure of the spinal column. One or more vertebral arches may be missing. Also called neural tube defect.

spinal block. Anesthesia injected into spinal fluid in the spinal canal for the relief of pain in labor and birth.

spinnbarkeit. Refers to the elasticity of cervical mucus.

spontaneous abortion. Termination of pregnancy without outside intervention.

station (of presenting part). The position of the fetal presenting part in relation to the maternal ischial spine.

step (dance) reflex. Occurs when the neonate is held upright with the feet touching a surface. The neonate appears to take steps as in walking.

sterilization. Surgical intervention to render the body permanently incapable of reproducing.

strabismus. The appearance of crossed eyes resulting from weak or immature eye muscles.

striae gravidarum. Pinkish or reddish lines that occur as a result of stretched skin, appearing on the abdomen, breasts, and thighs during pregnancy.

subinvolution. Failure of the uterus to return to its prepregnant condition and place.

surfactant. Phospholipid, secreted in the alveoli, necessary for neonatal respiratory adaption.

symptothermal method. Technique that assists couples in determining the time of ovulation for increasing or decreasing the chances of conception occurring.

syndactyly. Webbing between two digits so that they are attached, more common in hands than feet.

syphilis. Sexually transmitted disease with chronic reoccurrences.

systemic vascular resistance. Opposition to blood flow in the vessels of one's body.

tachycardia. Fetal or newborn heart rate above 160 beats per minute.

tachypnea. Rapid respiration in the neonate.

taking-in. Dependent, self-centered behavior of the new mother soon after birth.

taking-hold. Behavior of the new mother that demonstrates concern for herself but also some responsibility for infant care.

teratogen. Any agent that interferes with the normal development of the fetus.

term infant. A newborn resulting from a 38- to 42-week gestation.

testosterone. Primary male hormone responsible for male characteristics.

thermogenesis. Production of heat.

thermoregulation. Control of heat production.

third stage of labor. The stage of labor during which the placenta is expelled.

thrombophlebitis. Inflammation of a vein related to the formation of a clot (thrombus).

tocolysis. Administration of beta mimetic drugs to stop uterine contractions.

tokodynamometer. Instrument for measuring the force of uterine activity.

tonic neck reflex. A reflex seen in the supine neonate in which the head is turned to one side, the arm and leg on that side extended, while the arm and leg on the opposite side are flexed.

TORCH. Infectious conditions known as Toxoplasmosis, Other infections, Rubella, Cytomegalovirus, and Herpes.

toxic shock syndrome (TSS). Appearance of multiple symptoms as the body responds to the toxins produced by the *Staphylococcus aureus* bacterium.

transient tachypnea of the newborn (TTN). Temporary increase in neonatal respirations in an effort to rid the lungs of amniotic fluid.

transition period. The 6- to 8-hour period during which the neonate adjusts from intrauterine to extrauterine life.

transition phase. End phase of the first stage of labor where the cervix fully dilates.

trimester. A 3-month period in pregnancy. A pregnancy is divided into 3 trimesters.

trophoblast. Outer wall of the blastocyst.

true conjugate. Area between the sacral promontory and the symphysis pubis.

true labor. Uterine contractions that cause effacement and dilatation of the cervix in preparation for childbirth.

ultrasound. Use of sound waves to outline internal structures, such as a fetus.

umbilical cord. Connection between the fetus and the placenta for transportation of blood.

uterine contraction. Rhythmic tightening of the muscles of the uterus to dilate and efface the cervix.

uterine inversion. Partial or complete turning inside-out of the uterus in the 3rd or 4th stage of labor.

uterine rupture. Tearing of uterine muscle that creates a life-threatening situation for the woman and fetus due to hemorrhage.

uterine souffle. Swishing sound produced by maternal blood as it enters the large uterine vessels.

vacuum extraction. Vacuum cup that is attached to the fetal head and the air is removed to cause a vacuum. Gentle traction is then applied to the device to deliver the fetus.

vaginal sponge. Device that is inserted into the vagina to cover the cervical os in preventing pregnancy.

variability. Refers to changes in the fetal baseline heart rate.

varicose veins. Veins that are swollen and distended as a result of sluggish circulation.

vas deferens. Duct that transports sperm from the testes to the urethra.

VBAC. Acronym for vaginal birth after cesarean.

vernix caseosa. Cheesy yellow-white substance found on the neonate's skin.

vertex. Refers to the top of the head; used in describing presentation of the neonate at birth when the crown of the head presents first.

viability. Fetus who has reached 24 weeks' gestation, weighs more than 500 grams, and is capable of surviving outside of the uterus.

vibroacoustic stimulation. Acoustic stimulator placed on the pregnant woman's abdomen which transmits sound to awaken the fetus during a nonstress test.

viscosity. Tendency of fluids to be thick and flow slowly, or thin and runny; resistance to flow.

vitamins. Organic substances that regulate the body's metabolism.

x chromosome. The female chromosome. Females have two x chromosomes.

y chromosome. The male chromosome. Males have one x and one y chromosome. Females do not carry y chromosomes.

zygote. Fertilized ovum until the first cleavage.

Spanish Phrases Helpful in Maternal and Neonatal Nursing

ENGLISH-TO-SPANISH PHRASES

Prepared by Judith Chavez, RN, BSN, Staff Nurse and Translator, San Francisco General Hospital

A woman and her family will be more at ease and feel relaxed if someone on the staff speaks their language. Some health care facilities provide interpreters. When an interpreter is not available, the nurse can use a few phrases that have been learned. The following table presents English phrases with the corresponding words in Spanish. The third column is a key to pronunciation, given in phonetics. The syllable to be accented is in *italic* type.

English	*Spanish*	*Pronunciation*
Please*	Por favor	Por fah-*vor*
Thank you	Grácias	*Grah*-see-ahs
Good morning	Buénos días	*Bway*-nos *dee*-ahs
Good afternoon	Buénas tárdes	*Bway*-nas *tar*-days
Good evening	Buénas nóches	*Bway*-nas *noh*-chays
My name is	Mi nómbre es	Me *nohm*-bray ays
Yes/No	Si/No	See/No
I am a student nurse	Estoy estudiénte enferméra	Es-toy ays-stoo-dee-*ayn*-tay ayn-fay-*may*-rah
Remove your clothing	Quítese su ropa	*Key*-tay-say soo *roh*-pah
Put on this gown	Pongáse la bata	Pohn-*gah*-say lah *bah*-tah
Need a urine specimen	Es necesário una muéstra de su orina	Ays nay-say-*sar*-ee-oh oo-nah moo-*ay*-strah day oh-*ree*-nah
Be seated	Siéntese	See-*ayn*-tay-say
Recline	Acuestése	Ah-cways-*tay*-say
Sit up	Siéntese	See-*ayn*-tay-say
Stand	Parése	Pah-*ray*-say
Bend your knees	Dóble las rodíllas	*Doh*-blay lahs roh-*dee*-yahs
Relax your muscles	Reláje los músculos	Ray-*lah*-hay lohs *moos*-koo-lohs
Try to	Aténte	Ah-*tayn*-tay
Try again	Aténte ótra vez	Ah-*tayn*-tay *oh*-tra vays
Do not move	No se muéva	Noh say moo-*ay*-vah
Turn on (or to) your left side	Voltése a su ládo izquiérdo	Vohl-*tay*-say ah soo *lah*-doh is-key-*ayr*-doh
Turn on (or to) your right side	Voltése a su ládo derécho	Vohl-*tay*-say ah soo *lah*-doh day-*ray*-choh
Take a deep breath	Respíra profúndo	Ray-*speer*-rah pro-*foon*-doh
Hold your breath	Deténga su respiración	Day-*tayn*-gah soo ray-speer-ah-see-*ohn*

*You should begin or end any request with the word "please" (por favor).

(continued)

English	*Spanish*	*Pronunciation*
Don't hold your breath	No deténga su respiración	Noh day-*tayn*-gah soo ray-speer-ah-see-*ohn*
How long?	¿Hace cuánto?	¿Ah-say kwahn-toh?
How much?	¿Cuánto?	¿*Kwahn*-toh?
How do you feel?	¿Como se siénte?	¿*Koh*-moh say see-*ayn*-tay?
Do you have allergies?	¿Tiéne alérgias?	¿Tee-*ay*-nay ah-layr-hee-ahs?
Are you warm?	¿Tiéne calór?	¿Tee-*ay*-nay kahl-*or*?
Are you warm enough?	¿Esta suficiénte caliénte?	¿*Ay*-stah soo-fee-see-*ayn*-tay kahl-ee-*ayn*-tay?
Are you cold?	¿Tiéne frío?	¿Tee-*ay*-nay free-oh?
Do you have pain?	¿Tiéne dolór?	¿Tee-*ay*-nay doh-*lorh*?
Where is the pain?	¿Adónde es el dolór?	¿Ah-*dohn*-day ays ayl doh-*lorh*?
Do you want medication for your pain?	¿Quiére medicación para su dolór?	¿Key-*ay*-ray may-dee-kah see-*ohn* pah-rah soo doh-*lorh*?
Are you comfortable?	¿Está comfortáble?	¿*Ay-stah* kohm-for-*tah*-blay?
Your membranes have ruptured?	¿Sus membránas se rupturarón?	¿Soos maym-*brah*-nahs say roop-too-*rah*-rohn?
Has your bag of water ruptured?	¿Se rómpio la bólsa de agua?	¿Say *rohm*-pee-oh lah *bohl*-sah day *ah*-gwah?
Are you feeling contractions?	¿Siénte contrácciones?	¿See-*ayn*-tay cohn-*trahc*-see-ohn-nays?
Is there vaginal bleeding?	¿Hay sangrádo vagínal?	¿I sahn-*grah*-doh vah-*hee*-nahl?
Breathe slowly—like this (in this manner)	Respíre despácio—asi	Ray-*speer*-ray day-*spah*-see-oh ah-*see*
This is oxygen	Este oxigéno	*Ah*-stay ohx-ee-*hay*-noh
Push like this (in this manner)	Púje asi	*Pooh*-hay ah-*see*
Push now	Púje ahora	*Pooh*-hay ah-or-ah
Don't push	No púje	Noh *pooh*-hay
Pant/Blow like this (in this manner)	Jadé/Sóple asi	Yah-*day*/*Soh*-play ah-*see*
Look	Míre	*Meer*-ray
An operation is necessary	Una operación es necesária	*Oo*-nah oh-payr-ah-see-*ohn* ays nay-say-*sayr*-ee-ah
You should (try to):	Tráte de:	*Trah*-tay day:
Call for help/assistance	Llamár para asisténcia	Yah-*marh* pah-rah ah-sees-*tayn*-see-ah
Empty your bladder	Orínar	Oh-*ree*-narh
Feed your baby	Dárle de comér a su bébe	*Dahr*-lay day Koh-*mayr* ah soo *bay*-bay
Change the diaper	Cambiár el pañal	Kahm-bee-*arh* ayl pahn-*yah*l
Ambulate	Caminár	Kah-mee-*narh*
It is important to:	Es importánte de:	Ays eem-por-*tahn*-tay day
Walk (ambulate)	Caminár	Kah-mee-*narh*
Drink fluids	Bebér líquidos	Bay-*bayr* lee-key-dohs
Feed your baby now	Dárle de comér a su bébe ahora	*Dar*-lay day koh-*mayr* ah soo bay-bay ah-or-*ah*
Place (position) the baby on its side	Posicionár el bébe en su ládo	Poh-zee-see-oh-*narh* ayl bay-bay ayn soo *lah*-doh
You will feel pressure	Vá a sentír presión	Vah ah sayn-*teer* pray-see-*oh*n
I am going to:	Voy a:	Voy ah
Count (take) your pulse	Tomár su púlso	Toh-*marh* soo *pool*-soh
Take your temperature	Tomár su temperatúra	Toh-*marh* soo taym-pay-rah-*too*-rah

(continued)

English	Spanish	Pronunciation
Take your blood pressure	Tomar su presión	Toh-*marh* soo pray-see-*ohn*
Examine your cervix	Examinár su cervíz	Ayx-ah-mee-*narh* soo sayr-*veez*
I am going to:	Va a:	Vah-ah
Start an IV line	Comensár una intravenósa	Koh-mayn-*sarh* oo-nah een-trah-vayn-*oh*-sah
Give you pain medicine	Dárle medicación para dolór	*Darh*-lay may-dee-kah-see-*ohn* pah-rah Doh-*lohr*
Empty your bladder with a small tube	Vaciár su vejíga con una túbo pequeño	Vah-see-*arh* soo vee-*hee*-gah Kohn *oo*-nah *too*-boh pay-*kay*-nyoh
Give you an enema	Dárle un lavádo	*Darh*-lay oon lah-*vah*-doh
Clean the umbilical cord like this (in this manner)	Limpiár el cordón umbílical así	Leem-pee-*arh* ayl korh-*dohn* oom-*bee*-lee-kahl ah-see
Clean the baby like this (in this manner)	Limpiár el bébe asi	*Leem*-pee-arh ayl bay-bay ah-see
Fold the diaper like this (in this manner)	Dóblar el pañal asi	*Doh*-blarh ayl pahn-*yahl* ah-see
Fasten the diaper like this (in this manner)	Segúre el pañal asi	Say-*gurh*-ah ayl pahn-*yahl* ah-see
Place the soiled diapers here	Pónga el pañal súcio aquí	*Pohn*-gah ayl pahn-*yahl* soo-see-ahoh-*key*
Are you hungry?	¿Tiéne hámbre?	¿Tee-*ay*-nay *ahm*-bray
Are you thirsty?	¿Tiéne sed?	¿Tee-*ay*-nay sayd
You may not eat/drink	No cóma/béba	Noh *koh*-mah/Bay-*bah*
You can only drink water	Solo puéde tomár água	Soh-loh *pway*-day toh-mar *ah*-gwah
You can only take ice chips	Solo puéde tomár pedazítos de hiélo	Soh-loh *pway*-day toh-*marh* pay-dah-*zee*-tohs day ee-*ay*-loh
It will be uncomfortable	Séra incomódo	Say-rah een-koh-*moh*-doh
It will sting	Va ardér	Vah ahr-*dayr*

(Used with permission from May, K.A. & Mahlmeister, L. R. (1994). *Maternal and neonatal nursing* (3rd ed.). (Philadelphia: J.B. Lippincott.)

NANDA Approved Nursing Diagnoses—1994

Activity Intolerance

Risk for Activity Intolerance

Adjustment, Impaired

Ineffective Airway Clearance

Altered Family Process: Alcoholism

Anxiety

Risk for Aspiration

Body Image Disturbance

Risk for Altered Body Temperature

Effective Breastfeeding

Ineffective Breastfeeding

Interrupted Breastfeeding

Ineffective Breathing Pattern

Caregiver Role Strain

Risk for Caregiver Role Strain

Impaired Verbal Communication

Potential for Enhanced Community Coping

Ineffective Community Coping

Acute Confusion

Chronic Confusion

Constipation

Colonic Constipation

Perceived Constipation

Decisional Conflict (Specify)

Decreased Cardiac Output

Defensive Coping

Ineffective Denial

Diarrhea

Risk for Disuse Syndrome

Diversional Activity Deficit

Dysreflexia

Energy Field Disturbance

Impaired Environmental Interpretation Syndrome

Ineffective Family Coping: Compromised

Ineffective Family Coping: Disabling

Family Coping: Potential for Growth

Altered Family Processes

Fatigue

Fear

Fluid Volume Deficit

Risk for Fluid Volume Deficit

Fluid Volume Excess

Impaired Gas Exchange

Anticipatory Grieving

Dysfunctional Grieving

Altered Growth and Development

Altered Health Maintenance

Health-Seeking Behaviors (Specify)

Impaired Home Maintenance Management

Hopelessness

Hyperthermia

Hypothermia

Bowel Incontinence

Functional Incontinence

Reflex Incontinence

Stress Incontinence

Total Incontinence

Urge Incontinence

Ineffective Individual Coping

Ineffective Infant Feeding Pattern

Risk for Disorganized Infant Behavior

Disorganized Infant Behavior

Potential for Enhanced Organized Infant Behavior

Risk for Infection

Risk for Injury

Decreased Adaptive Capacity, Intracranial

Knowledge Deficit (Specify)

Risk for Loneliness

Impaired Memory

Noncompliance (Specify)

Altered Nutrition: Less than body requirements

Altered Nutrition: More than body requirements

Altered Nutrition: Potential for more than body requirements

Altered Oral Mucous Membrane

Pain

Chronic Pain

Parental Role Conflict

Altered Parenting

Risk for Altered Parenting

Risk for Altered Parent/Infant/Child Attachment

Personal Identity Disturbance

Risk for Peripheral Neurovascular Dysfunction

Risk for Perioperative Positioning Injury

Impaired Physical Mobility

Risk for Poisoning

Post-Trauma Response

Powerlessness

Altered Protection

Rape-Trauma Syndrome

Rape-Trauma Syndrome: Compound Reaction

Rape-Trauma Syndrome: Silent Reaction

Relocation Stress Syndrome

Altered Role Performance

Bathing/Hygiene Self-Care Deficit

Feeding Self-Care Deficit

Dressing/Grooming Self-Care Deficit

Toileting Self-Care Deficit

Chronic Low Self-Esteem

Situational Low Self-Esteem

Self-Esteem Disturbance

Risk for Self-Mutilation

Sensory/Perceptual Alterations (Specify) (Visual, auditory, kinesthetic, gustatory, tactile, olfactory)

Sexual Dysfunction

Altered Sexuality Patterns

Impaired Skin Integrity

Risk for Impaired Skin Integrity

Sleep Pattern Disturbance

Impaired Social Interaction

Social Isolation

Spiritual Distress (distress of the human spirit)

Potential for Enhanced Spiritual Well Being

Risk for Suffocation

Impaired Swallowing

Ineffective Management of Therapeutic Regimen: Families

Ineffective Management of Therapeutic Regimen: Community

Ineffective Management of Therapeutic Regimen: Individual

Ineffective Thermoregulation

Altered Thought Processes

Impaired Tissue Integrity

Altered Tissue Perfusion (Specify Type) (Renal, cerebral, cardiopulmonary, gastrointestinal, peripheral)

Risk for Trauma

Unilateral Neglect

Altered Urinary Elimination

Urinary Retention

Inability to Sustain Spontaneous Ventilation

Dysfunctional Ventilatory Weaning Response

Risk for Violence: Self-directed or directed at others

(Nursing Diagnoses: Definitions & Classification 1995–1996, Philadelphia: North American Nursing Diagnoses Association, 1994)

Conversion Tables

Temperature Conversion Table (Centigrade to Fahrenheit)

Celsius (C°)	Fahrenheit (F°)	Celsius (C°)	Fahrenheit (F°)
34.0	93.2	38.6	101.4
34.2	93.6	38.8	101.8
34.4	93.9	39.0	102.2
34.6	94.3	39.2	102.5
34.8	94.6	39.4	102.9
35.0	95.0	39.6	103.2
35.2	95.4	39.8	103.6
35.4	95.7	40.0	104.0
35.6	96.1	40.2	104.3
35.8	96.4	40.4	104.7
36.0	96.8	40.6	105.1
36.2	97.1	40.8	105.4
36.4	97.5	41.0	105.8
36.6	97.8	41.2	106.1
36.8	98.2	41.4	106.5
37.0	98.6	41.6	106.8
37.2	98.9	41.8	107.2
37.4	99.3	42.0	107.6
37.6	99.6	42.2	108.0
37.8	100.0	42.4	108.3
38.0	100.4	42.6	108.7
38.2	100.7	42.8	109.0
38.4	101.0	43.0	109.4

Conversion of Celsius (Centigrade) to Fahrenheit: 9/5 × temperature) + 32
Conversion of Fahrenheit to Celsius (Centigrade): (Temperature − 32) × 5/9
(Used with permission from May, K.A. & Mahlmeister, L. R. (1994). *Maternal and neonatal nursing* (3rd ed.). (Philadelphia: J.B. Lippincott.)

Pounds and Ounces to Grams Conversion Table

Pounds	Ounces															
	0	1	2	3	4	5	6	7	8	9	10	11	12	13	14	15
0	—	28	57	85	113	142	170	198	227	255	283	312	340	369	397	425
1	454	482	510	539	567	595	624	652	680	709	737	765	794	822	850	879
2	907	936	964	992	1021	1049	1077	1106	1134	1162	1191	1219	1247	1276	1304	1332
3	1361	1389	1417	1446	1474	1503	1531	1559	1588	1616	1644	1673	1701	1729	1758	1786
4	1814	1843	1871	1899	1928	1956	1984	2013	2041	2070	2098	2126	2155	2183	2211	2240
5	2268	2296	2325	2353	2381	2410	2438	2466	2495	2523	2551	2580	2608	2637	2665	2693
6	2722	2750	2778	2807	2835	2863	2892	2920	2948	2977	3005	3033	3062	3090	3118	3147
7	3175	3203	3232	3260	3289	3317	3345	3374	3402	3430	3459	3487	3515	3544	3572	3600
8	3629	3657	3685	3714	3742	3770	3799	3827	3856	3884	3912	3941	3969	3997	4026	4054
9	4082	4111	4139	4167	4196	4224	4252	4281	4309	4337	4366	4394	4423	4451	4479	4508
10	4536	4564	4593	4621	4649	4678	4706	4734	4763	4791	4819	4848	4876	4904	4933	4961
11	4990	5018	5046	5075	5103	5131	5160	5188	5216	5245	5273	5301	5330	5358	5386	5415
12	5443	5471	5500	5528	5557	5585	5613	5642	5670	5698	5727	5755	5783	5812	5840	5868
13	5897	5925	5953	5982	6010	6038	6067	6095	6123	6152	6180	6209	6237	6265	6294	6322
14	6350	6379	6407	6435	6464	6492	6520	6549	6577	6605	6634	6662	6690	6719	6747	6776
15	6804	6832	6860	6889	6917	6945	6973	7002	7030	7059	7087	7115	7144	7172	7201	7228
16	7257	7286	7313	7342	7371	7399	7427	7456	7484	7512	7541	7569	7597	7626	7654	7682
17	7711	7739	7768	7796	7824	7853	7881	7909	7938	7966	7994	8023	8051	8079	8108	8136
18	8165	8192	8221	8249	8278	8306	8335	8363	8391	8420	8448	8476	8504	8533	8561	8590
19	8618	8646	8675	8703	8731	8760	8788	8816	8845	8873	8902	8930	8958	8987	9015	9043
20	9072	9100	9128	9157	9185	9213	9242	9270	9298	9327	9355	9383	9412	9440	9469	9497
21	9525	9554	9582	9610	9639	9667	9695	9724	9752	9780	9809	9837	9865	9894	9922	9950
22	9979	10007	10036	10064	10092	10120	10149	10177	10206	10234	10262	10291	10319	10347	10376	10404

(Used with permission from May, K.A. & Mahlmeister, L. R. (1994). *Maternal and neonatal nursing* (3rd ed.). (Philadelphia: J.B. Lippincott.)

Universal Precautions

Human immunodeficiency virus (HIV), the virus that causes acquired immunodeficiency syndrome (AIDS), is transmitted during sexual contact, through the sharing of intravenous drug needles and syringes while "shooting" drugs, through exposure to infected blood or blood components, and perinatally from mother to neonate. Currently there is neither a cure for nor an immunization to prevent AIDS. The increasing prevalence of HIV increases the risk that health care workers will be exposed to blood from patients infected with HIV.

The Centers for Disease Control in Atlanta has developed "Universal Precautions" (formerly called "Universal Blood and Body Fluid Precautions") as recommendations to all health care workers. Under universal precautions, blood and certain body fluids of **all** patients are considered potentially infectious for HIV, hepatitis B virus (HBV), and other bloodborne pathogens. Universal precautions are intended to prevent parenteral, mucous membrane, and nonintact skin exposures of health care workers to bloodborne pathogens. In addition, immunization with HBV vaccine is recommended as an important adjunct to universal precautions for health care workers who have been exposed to blood. (The implementation of control measures for HIV and HBV does not obviate the need for continued adherence to general infection-control principles and general hygiene measures.) The following is a summary of the CDC's recommendations.

Body Fluids to Which Universal Precautions Apply

Universal precautions apply to blood and other body fluids containing visible blood. **Blood is the single most important source of HIV, HBV, and other bloodborne pathogens in the health care facility.** Infection control efforts for HIV, HBV, and other bloodborne pathogens must focus on both preventing exposures to blood and delivering HBV immunization. Universal precautions also apply to semen and vaginal secretions, tissues, and the following fluids: cerebrospinal, synovial, pleural, peritoneal, pericardial, and amniotic.

Body Fluids to Which Universal Precautions Do Not Apply

Universal precautions do not apply to feces, nasal secretions, sputum, sweat, tears, urine, and vomitus unless they contain visible blood. The risk of transmission of HIV or HBV from these fluids is extremely low or nonexistent.

General Precautions

- Use universal precautions for all patients.
- Use appropriate barrier precautions routinely when contact with blood or other body fluids of any patient is anticipated.
  - Wear gloves when touching blood and body fluids, mucous membranes, or nonintact skin; when handling items or surfaces soiled with blood or body fluids; and when performing venipuncture and other vascular access procedures.
  - Change gloves after each contact with patients.
  - Wear masks and protective eyewear or face shields during procedures that are likely to generate drops of blood or other body fluids to prevent exposure to mucous membranes of mouth, nose, and eyes.
  - Wear gowns or aprons during procedures that are likely to generate splashes of blood or other body fluids.
- Wash hands and other skin surfaces immediately and thoroughly if contaminated with blood or other body fluids.
- Wash hands immediately after gloves are removed.
- Take precautions to prevent injuries caused by needles, scalpels, and other sharp instruments or devices during procedures; when cleaning used instruments; during disposal of used needles; and when handling sharp instruments after procedures.
  - Discard needle units uncapped and unbroken after use.
  - Place disposable syringes and needles, scalpel blades, and other sharp items in puncture-resistant containers.
  - Place puncture-resistant containers as near as practical to the area of use.

- Although saliva has not been implicated, to minimize the need for emergency mouth-to-mouth resuscitation, make mouthpieces, resuscitation bags, or other ventilation devices available for use in areas where the need for resuscitation is predictable.
- If you have exudative lesions or weeping dermatitis refrain from all direct patient care and from handling patient care equipment until the condition resolves.

Precautions for Invasive Procedures

- If you participate in invasive procedures, use appropriate barrier methods: gloves, surgical masks, protective eyewear, face shields, gowns, and aprons.
- If you perform or assist in vaginal or cesarean deliveries, wear gloves and gowns when handling the placenta or the infant until blood and amniotic fluid have been removed from the infant's skin and during postdelivery care of the umbilical cord.
- If a glove is torn or a needlestick or other injury occurs, remove the gloves and use a new glove as promptly as patient safety permits; remove the needle or instrument used in the incident from the sterile field.

Environmental Considerations

- Standard sterilization and disinfection procedures currently recommended for use in health care settings are adequate.
- Sterilize instruments or devices that enter sterile tissue or the vascular system before reuse.
- Clean and remove soiled surfaces on walls, floors, and other surfaces routinely; extraordinary attempts to disinfect or sterilize are not necessary.

- Use chemical germicides approved as hospital disinfectants (and tuberculocidals) to decontaminate spills of blood and other body fluids.

Precautions with Soiled Linen

- Observe hygienic and common-sense storage and processing of clean and soiled linens.
- Handle soiled linen as little as possible and with minimum agitation.
- Bag all soiled linen at the location where it is used.
- Place and transport linen soiled with blood or body fluids in bags that prevent leakage.

Infective Waste

- It is practical to identify those wastes with the potential for causing infection during handling and disposal and for which some special precautions seem prudent (e.g., microbiology laboratory waste, pathology waste, and blood specimens or blood products).
- Incinerate or autoclave infective waste before disposal in a sanitary landfill.
- Carefully pour bulk blood, suctioned fluids, excretions, and secretions down a drain connected to a sanitary sewer.

(From *Guidelines for prevention of transmission of human immunodeficiency virus and hepatitis B virus to health-care and public safety workers.* U.S. Department of Health and Human Services, Centers for Disease Control, Atlanta, GA, February 1989; Update: Universal precautions for prevention of transmission of human immunodeficiency virus, hepatitis B virus, and other bloodborne pathogens in health-care settings. *Morbidity and Mortality Weekly Report,* 1988; Recommendations for prevention of HIV transmission in health-care settings. *Morbidity and Mortality Weekly Report,* 1987.)

Drug Use During Breast-Feeding*

Drug or Agent	Contra-indicated	R_x With Caution	No Apparent Harm	Insufficient Information	Comment
Analgesics					
Acetaminophen			X		
Aspirin			X		
Propoxyphene (Darvon)			X		
Anticoagulants					
Ethyl biscoumacetate	X				Bleeding infant
Phenindione	X				Bleeding infant
Heparin			X		No passage into milk
Warfarin Na (Coumadin)			X		
Bishydroxycoumarin (Dicumarol)		X			
Anticonvulsants					
Phenobarbital			X		Low levels in infant
Primadone (Mysoline)			X		Drowsiness
Carbamazepine				X	Significant infant levels; no reported effects
Diphenylhydantoin (Phenytoin, Dilantin)			X		Low levels in infant, methemoglobin, 1 case
Antihistamines					
Diphenhydramine (Benadryl)			X		Small amounts excreted
Trimeprazine (Temaril)			X		Small amounts excreted
Tripelennamine (Pyribenzamine)			X		Small amounts excreted
Anti-infective Agents					
Aminoglycosides (Kanamycin, gentamcin)			X		Significant excretion in milk; not absorbed
Chloramphenicol	X				Bone marrow depression; gastrointestinal and behavioral effects
Penicillins			X		Possible sensitization
Sulfonamides		X			Hemolysis, G-6-PD deficiency, bilirubin displacement

(continued)

431

Drug or Agent	Contra-indicated	R_x With Caution	No Apparent Harm	Insufficient Information	Comment
Tetracyclines			X		Limited absorption by infant
Nalidixic acid		X			Hemolysis
Nitrofurantoin		X			Possible G-6-PD hemolysis
Metronidazole (Flagyl)		X			Low absorption but potentially toxic
Isoniazid		X			High levels in milk, possible toxicity
Pyramethamine	X				Vomiting, marrow suppression, convulsions
Chloraquine			X		Not excreted
Quinine		X			Thrombocytopenia
Anti-inflammatory					
Aspirin			X		
Indomethacin		X			Seizures, 1 case
Phenylbutazone		X			Low levels, ? blood dyscrasia
Gold	X				Found in baby; nephritis, hepatitis, hematologic changes
Steroids				X	Low levels with prednisone and prednisolone
Antineoplastic					
Cyclophosphamide	X				Neutropenia
Methotrexate	X				Very small excretion
Antithyroid					
Radioactive iodine	X				Thyroid suppression
Propylthiouracil	X				Thyroid suppression
Bronchodilators					
Aminophylline			X		Irritability, 1 case
Iodides	X				Thyroid suppression
Sympathomimetics				X	Inhalers probably safe
Cardiovascular Agents					
Digoxin			X		Insignificant levels
Propanolol			X		Insignificant levels
Reserpine	X				Nasal stuffiness, lethargy
Guanethidine (Ismelin)			X		Insignificant levels
Methyldopa (Aldomet)				X	

(continued)

Drug or Agent	Contra-indicated	R_x With Caution	No Apparent Harm	Insufficient Information	Comment
Cathartics					
Anthroquinones (Cascara, danthron)	X				Diarrhea, cramps
Aloe, senna		X			Safe in moderate dosage
Bulk agents, softeners			X		
Contraceptives, Oral†					
Diethylstilbestrol	X				Possible vaginal cancer
Depo-provera		X			May affect lactation
Norethisterone		X			May affect lactation
Ethinyl estradiol		X			May affect lactation
Diuretics					
Chlorthalidone				X	Low levels, but may accumulate
Thiazides		X			May affect lactation; low levels in milk
Spironolactone			X		Insignificant levels
Ergot Alkaloids					
Bromocriptine	X				Lactation suppressed
Ergot	X				Vomiting, diarrhea, seizures
Ergotamine				X	
Ergonovine	X				Brief postpartum course may be safe
Methylergonovine	X				Brief postpartum course may be safe
Hormones					
Corticosteroids				X	Low levels with short-term prednisone or prednisolone
Sex hormones (see above, Contraceptives, Oral)					
Thyroid (T_3 or T_4)			X		Excreted in milk; may mask hypothyroid infant
Insulin			X		Not absorbed
ACTH			X		Not absorbed
Epinephrine			X		Not absorbed
Narcotics					
Codeine			X		In usual doses
Meperidine (Demerol)				X	
Morphine			X		Low infant levels on usual dosage
Heroin	X				Addiction withdrawal in infants

(continued)

Drug or Agent	Contra-indicated	R_x With Caution	No Apparent Harm	Insufficient Information	Comment
Methadone		X			Minimal levels
Psychotherapeutic Drugs					
Lithium	X				High levels in milk
Phenothiazines		X			Drowsiness; chronic effects uncertain
Tricyclic antidepressants				X	Low levels; effects uncertain
Diazepam (Valium)	X				Lethargy, weight loss, EEG changes
Meprobamate (Equanil)	X				High levels in milk
Chlordiazepoxide (Librium)			X		Low levels in milk
Radiopharmaceuticals					
131I	X				72 hr, no breast-feeding
Technetium (99M Tc)					48 hr, no breast-feeding
131I albumin	X				10 days, no breast-feeding
Sedatives–Hypnotics					
Barbiturates		X			Short-acting, less depressant
Chloral hydrate		X			Drowsiness
Bromides	X				Depression, rash
Diazepam (Valium)	X				Depression, weight loss
Flurazepam				X	Chemically related to diazepam
Nitrazepam				X	
Social–Recreational Drugs					
Alcohol			X		Milk levels equal plasma, moderate consumption apparently safe, high levels inhibit lactation
Caffeine			X		Jitteriness with very high intakes
Nicotine			X		Low levels in milk
Marijuana			X		Minimal passage in milk
Miscellaneous					
Atropine		X			May cause constipation or inhibit lactation
Dihydrotachysterol		X			Renal calcification in animals

(From Avery, G. B. [ed.]. 1967, *Neonatology* [3rd ed.]. Philadelphia: J.B. Lippincott.)
*Drug use during breast-feeding remains controversial.
†Controversy in literature, long-term effects uncertain, one case of gynecomastia.

Cervical Dilatation

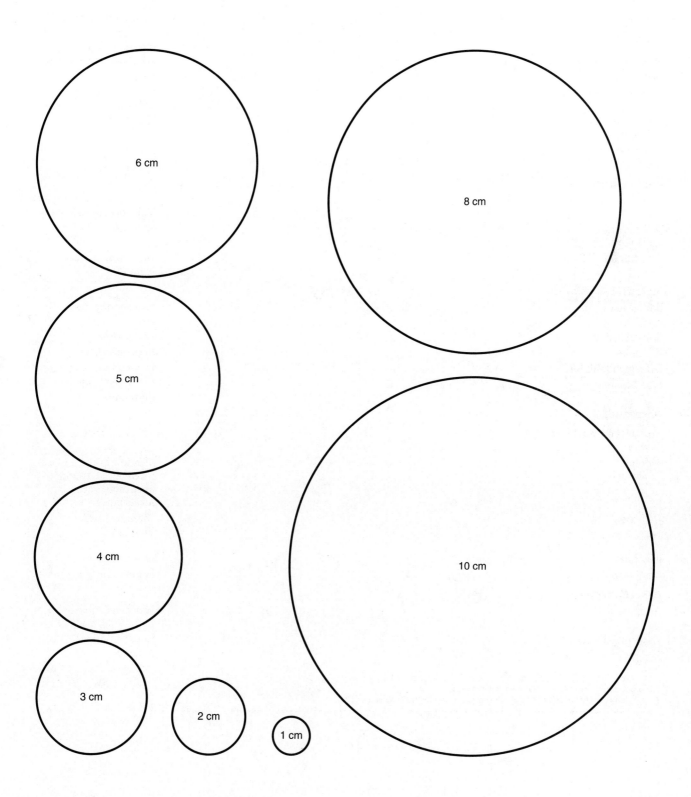

Index

NOTE: A *t* following a page number indicates tabular material, an *f* following a page number indicates a figure, a *c* following a page number indicates a checklist, and a *d* following a page number indicates a display.

A

Abdomen
    enlargement of, as probable sign of pregnancy, 77, 79*d*
    of newborn
        assessment of, 307*c*, 312
        measurement of circumference of in gastrointestinal anomalies, 366
ABO incompatibility, 96, 128
    hemolytic disease of newborn and, 377
Abortion, 12, 128–129
    incomplete, 129
    induced elective, 129
    inevitable, 129
    missed, 129
    spontaneous, 79, 128–129
Abruptio placentae, 132–133
Abstinence, for contraception, 38
    failure rate of, 42*t*
Abstinence syndrome, neonatal, 381–382
Abuse
    child, prevention of, 324
    physical, during pregnancy, 113
    substance. *See* Substance abuse
Accelerations, in nonstress test, 164
Accident prevention, teaching about, 324
Acidosis, neonatal respiration stimulated by, 292
Acquired immunodeficiency syndrome (AIDS), 68–69.
                    See also HIV infection
    in newborn, 377–381
    during pregnancy, 137
Acrocyanosis, 307*c*, 308
Active phase of labor, 182
Activity
    in newborn, teaching family about, 329
    during pregnancy, health teaching about, 108
Acyclovir, for herpes simplex infections, 68
Addicted mothers, 114
    newborn symptoms and, 381–382
    postpartum considerations and, 283
Admission care and procedures, 190–193
Adolescent pregnancy, 11–12
    fetal assessment and, 167
    fetal development and, 156
    health promotion and, 116, 117–118
    high-risk factors and, 138

labor and, 186, 209
newborn with special needs and, 385
newborn's transition to extrauterine life and, 300
nursing care of normal newborn and, 333
nursing care plan for, 116
physical and psychosocial changes and, 86
postpartum care and, 263
postpartum changes and, 246
postpartum complications and, 283–284
prenatal visits and assessment and, 97
preterm neonate and, 349
Adolescents. *See also* Puberty
    contraceptive use among, 52
    gynecologic care for, 70
    pregnant. *See* Adolescent pregnancy
    sexual activity among, 11–12
    sexuality and, 32
Adoptive family, 5*d*, 6*f*
β-Adrenergic agonists, for preterm labor, 215*t*, 216
AFP. *See* Alpha-fetoprotein
After-pains, 238, 258
AGA neonate. *See* Appropriate for gestational age neonate
AIDS. *See* Acquired immunodeficiency syndrome
Airway, in preterm neonate, 345
Alcohol consumption, during pregnancy, 113
    newborn symptoms of (fetal alcohol syndrome), 113, 154*t*, 382
    teratogenic effects of, 154*t*
Aldosterone, in pregnancy, 82
Alpha-fetoprotein, in amniotic fluid, 161
Alveolar surface tension, first respirations opposed by, 293
Alveoli, breast, 27
Ambiguous genitalia, 313, 369
Amenorrhea, 63–64
    as presumptive sign of pregnancy, 76, 79*d*
Amniocentesis, 161–162
    sex determined by, 142–144
Amnion, 145, 146
Amniotic fluid, 146
    analysis of. *See* Amniocentesis
    functions of, 147*d*
    meconium in, 162. *See also* Meconium
Amniotic sac, 146, 147*f*
Amniotomy, 192–193
    for induction of labor, 218
Analgesia, during labor, 196

Hospital-based childbirth, 9
hPL. *See* Human placental lactogen
HPV. *See* Human papillomavirus
Human chorionic gonadotropin (hCG), 82, 147
    pregnancy tests based on, 78
Human papillomavirus, 68
Human placental lactogen (hPL), 82, 147
Human sexuality. *See* Sexuality
Hyaline membrane disease, 345–346
Hydantoins, teratogenic effects of, 154*t*
Hydatidiform mole, 131
Hydramnios (polyhydramnios), 146, 223
Hydrocephalus, in newborn, 368*t*, 370*f*
Hydroxyzine, for analgesia in labor, 196*t*
Hygiene
    general, teaching family about, 330
    during pregnancy, health teaching about, 107
Hymen, 24
Hymenal tags, in newborn, 313
Hyperbilirubinemia
    in hemolytic disease of newborn, 375
    in preterm infant, 347
Hyperemesis gravidarum, 122
Hypertension, pregnancy-induced, 124–128
Hypertonic uterine dysfunction, 219–221
Hypoglycemia
    monitoring in newborn of diabetic mother, 381
    in preterm neonate, 344
Hypospadias, 367*f*, 367*t*
Hypotension
    orthostatic, during pregnancy, 83
        health teaching about, 112
    supine, during pregnancy, 82–83
Hypothyroidism, congenital, 374
    screening for, 320, 374
Hypotonic uterine dysfunction, 219–221
Hypoxia, in newborn, 362
Hysterosalpingogram, for infertility, 52*t*

I

Icterus neonatorum (physiologic jaundice), 295–296, 321
Identical twins (monozygotic twins), 152
Identification bracelets, on mother and newborn, 206, 319
IgA, in newborn, 297
IgG, in newborn, 297
IgM, in newborn, 297
Ileum, 26, 27*f*
Illness, in newborn, signs and symptoms of, 332*c*, 333
Imagery (guided), for pain management during labor, 194
Immune system
    newborn adaptations in, 297
    in preterm infant, 344
Immunity, passive, in preterm neonate, 344
Immunoglobulins. *See also specific type under Ig*
    in newborn, 297
Imperforate anus, 365*t*
Implantation, 145
Implementation. *See* Intervention
Inborn errors of metabolism, 373–374
Incompetent cervix, 129
Incomplete abortion, 129
Indigestion during pregnancy, 84
    relief of, 110

Indirect Coombs' test, in prenatal assessment, 96
Indomethacin, for patent ductus arteriosus, 347
Induced elective abortion, 129
Induction of labor. *See* Labor, induction of
Inevitable abortion, 129
    incompetent cervix causing, 129
Infant car seat, 323
Infant mortality rate, 11
Infections
    in newborn, 377, 378–379*t*
        nursing care plan for, 380
        in preterm neonate, 344, 348
        prevention of, 321–323, 377
    during pregnancy, 136–138
        teratogenic, 136–137
Infertility, 38, 50–52
    nursing diagnoses related to, 51*c*
Innominate bones, 26
Integumentary system
    maternal
        postpartum changes in, 242
        pregnancy affecting, 84–85
    in newborn
        adaptations in, 296
        in preterm neonate, 343–344
Intensity, of uterine contraction, 178
Intensive care unit, neonatal, 346*f*, 357
Intercourse (sexual), 31
Internal electronic fetal monitoring, 165–166, 166*c*
Internal os, 25*f*, 26
Internal rotation, fetal, 183, 184*f*
Intervention (implementation), in nursing process, 14*d*, 15
Intracranial hemorrhage, in newborn, 359*t*
Intrapartum period, 173–188. *See also* Birth; Labor
    admission care and procedures and, 190–193
    adolescent considerations and, 186, 209
    complicated, 213–234
    cultural considerations and, 186, 209
    definition of, 4
    role of nurse and, 186–187, 209
Intrauterine device, 45–46
    failure rate of, 42*t*
    warning signs for users of, 46*c*
Intrauterine growth retardation, amniocentesis in identification of, 161
Intrauterine pressure catheter, for monitoring contractions, 219–220
Intraventricular hemorrhage, in preterm neonate, 347
In vitro fertilization, 52
Involution, 238
Iodine, recommended intake of, 105*t*
Iron
    recommended intake of, 105*t*
    requirements for during pregnancy, 103
    supplemental
        for newborn, 324
        during pregnancy, 123
Iron deficiency anemia, in pregnancy, 123
Ischemic phase of uterine cycle, 29*f*, 30, 30*d*
Ischium, 26, 27*f*
Isolette, for temperature maintenance in newborn, 354
Isoniazid, for tuberculosis, 137
Isthmus, of uterus, 26
IUD. *See* Intrauterine device
IUGR. *See* Intrauterine growth retardation

8/14/94

Caput

present @ birth
crosses suture lines
↓ after birth
Pit on pressure
disappers about 3 days

Cephalahematoma

About 24hrs 48hrs
on one side
↑ before it decreases
No pitty
Several wks to disappear.
Does not cross suture line

12 danger signs for the baby

Cynosis
Rapid or difficult respiration
Delayed or inadquate Voiding
Vomitting
Excessive Salvation
No Meconium Stool first 24hrs
Abdomnal Mass or distention
Jaundice within 1st 24 hrs pathological
If there Muscle twitchy or Convulsions
If theres Lethargy (Listlessness)
Shrill or Weak Cry
History of low Apgar Score

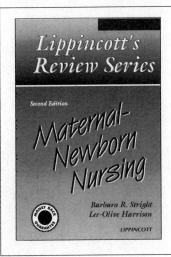
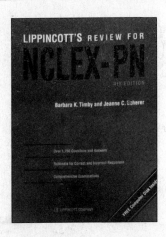
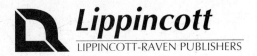